FOUNDATIONS OF PSYCHOLOGY

WILEY PUBLICATIONS IN PSYCHOLOGY

FOUNDATIONS OF PSYCHOLOGY
By Edwin G. Boring, Herbert S. Langfeld, and Harry P. Weld
INTRODUCTION TO PSYCHOLOGY
By Edwin G. Boring, Herbert S. Langfeld, and Harry P. Weld
SOCIAL PSYCHOLOGY
By Daniel Katz and Richard L. Schanck
HEARING—ITS PSYCHOLOGY AND PHYSIOLOGY
By S. Smith Stevens and Hallowell Davis
MANUAL OF PSYCHIATRY AND MENTAL HYGIENE, Seventh Edition
By Aaron J. Rosanoff
STATISTICAL METHODS IN BIOLOGY, MEDICINE, AND PSYCHOLOGY, Fourth Edition
By C. B. Davenport and Merle P. Ekas
MOTIVATION OF BEHAVIOR
By P. T. Young
PSYCHOLOGY—A FACTUAL TEXTBOOK
By Edwin G. Boring, Herbert S. Langfeld, and Harry P. Weld
PSYCHOLOGY IN BUSINESS AND INDUSTRY
By John G. Jenkins

HERBERT S. LANGFELD
Advisory Editor

METHODS OF PSYCHOLOGY
T. G. Andrews, Editor
THE PSYCHOLOGY OF EGO-INVOLVEMENTS
By Muzafer Sherif and Hadley Cantril
MANUAL OF CHILD PSYCHOLOGY
Leonard Carmichael, Editor
EMOTION IN MAN AND ANIMAL
By P. T. Young
UNCONSCIOUSNESS
By James Grier Miller
THE PSYCHOLOGY OF PERSONAL ADJUSTMENT
By Fred McKinney
THE PSYCHOLOGY OF SOCIAL MOVEMENTS
By Hadley Cantril

FOUNDATIONS OF PSYCHOLOGY

EDITED BY

Edwin Garrigues Boring
HARVARD UNIVERSITY

Herbert Sidney Langfeld
PRINCETON UNIVERSITY

Harry Porter Weld
CORNELL UNIVERSITY

1948

JOHN WILEY AND SONS, INC., NEW YORK
CHAPMAN AND HALL, LIMITED, LONDON

SECOND PRINTING, NOVEMBER, 1948

PRINTED IN THE UNITED STATES OF AMERICA

CONTRIBUTORS

ANNE ANASTASI
Fordham University

M. E. BITTERMAN
Cornell University

EDWIN G. BORING
Harvard University

HADLEY CANTRIL
Princeton University

LEONARD CARMICHAEL
Tufts College

LEO P. CRESPI
Princeton University

FORREST L. DIMMICK
U. S. Naval Medical Research Laboratory at New London

FRANK A. GELDARD
University of Virginia

DONALD R. GRIFFIN
Cornell University

CARL I. HOVLAND
Yale University

WILLIAM A. HUNT
Northwestern University

DONALD W. MacKINNON
University of California

CLIFFORD T. MORGAN
The Johns Hopkins University

EDWIN B. NEWMAN
Harvard University

CARL PFAFFMANN
Brown University

T. A. RYAN
Cornell University

LAURANCE F. SHAFFER
Teachers College, Columbia University

CARROLL L. SHARTLE
Ohio State University

S. SMITH STEVENS
Harvard University

PREFACE

THE strongest evidence of the rapid advance of psychology is the need of frequent revisions of textbooks. It is nine years since our last book, *Introduction to Psychology,* was published. In the meantime we have had a long war and a victory which psychological research helped attain. In this wartime research much new and valuable knowledge came into being. In addition there has been the more normal acquisition of facts as well as a clearly distinguishable change in point of view. This advance in our science had to be covered in a revision, but we soon found that instead of a revision we were going to have a book so nearly new that it needed a new title. And so we present here the third book that has appeared under our combined editorship.

To describe in detail the changes in this book over the last would be to describe a large part of its contents. We must confine ourselves to indicating a few of the more significant differences. It is about twice as large as the *Introduction* of 1939. Approximately 80 per cent of the material is either new or freshly described. What has been taken from the previous book has been re-edited. There are eighteen contributors, of whom fifteen are new. A number of new chapters have been added, two of which introduce the student to problems of personal adjustment. Some of the material of the old chapters has been differently distributed among the chapters of this book. Some of the topics have been given more detailed treatment; no material of importance has been omitted. There are also a large number of new illustrations, and many of the old ones have been redrawn. In selecting the illustrations we have intended to include only those which we feel would help the student to understand the text.

The order of the chapters is completely changed. In our first book we held to the conventional arrangement of sensation at the beginning and thought and personality at the end. In the second book we reversed this order. We had a principle in mind with each book: synthesis in the first order, analysis in the second; but we must confess to a certain dependence on trial and error. Now, with the trials and, we hope, the errors past, and giving attention to the opinions expressed by some teachers of introductory courses, we present what is partly a compromise between the two orders and partly a reflection of psychology's changed orientation. In 1948 the important thing about the organism is not that it is conscious, but that it reacts to stimulation. So we are having the book start with response—its nature, its mechanics, its maturation, its dependence on motive. After that the student is prepared to study learning as change in the organism's response repertoire, and then perception as a form of the organism's adjustment to its physical environment. Such an approach leads on naturally to the study of the facts of individual difference, to the problems of human efficiency and personal adjustment, and finally to the understanding of attitudes and social relations.

The amount of necessary editing has varied considerably. Some chapters remain very much as they were presented by the collaborator. Some had to be rewritten. In several instances we transferred material from one chapter to another. Some material was deleted, some new material added. For the sake of unity and style all chapters had to undergo at least some changes by the editorial pen.

From this explanation the reader will see the reason for the wording of our acknowledgment of the authorship of each of the chapters. We as editors must assume responsibility for any errors that may have occurred in the text. We wish, on the other hand, to give full credit to the collaborators for their contributions to this book and to thank them for their generous cooperation, which we realize was motivated by their loyalty to their science.

We are also grateful to our former collaborators, all of whom helped to make this book possible. They are C. W. Bray, J. G. Beebe-Center, Warner Brown, D. W. Chapman, K. M. Dallenbach, H. B. DeSilva, S. Feldman, Norman Frederiksen, George Humphrey, Daniel Katz, Carney Landis, R. B. MacLeod, J. A. McGeoch, C. C. Miles, D. McL. Purdy, M. A. Tinker, E. G. Wever and M. J. Zigler. We note a special debt to Dr. Wever for his continued advice.

We acknowledge an especial debt of gratitude to the secretarial staff of the Harvard Psychological Laboratories, who retyped entirely the much-edited manuscript; to Elizabeth MacLeod, who administered the retyping and its proofing; to Robert S. Harper of Harvard University, who, with some assistance from Mabel Mills, prepared the figures for our publisher's artist; and to Helen Orr of Princeton University, who lent us her very considerable editorial experience in reading both manuscript and proofs.

E. G. B.
H. S. L.
H. P. W.

January 11, 1948

C O N T E N T S

CHAPTER 1

The Nature of Psychology

PSYCHOLOGY is the study of *human nature.* It is the study of man, man as a living being, acting in an ever-changing world, responding to things and events and other people. If you know what man is, if you know the full answer to the question about the nature of man, then you know what human nature is and what psychology comprises.

The single person is the psychological unit. He acts more or less consistently with himself, although often differently from other persons. There is, moreover, a great deal of interaction among persons. They act together in groups: families, societies, parties, nations. They communicate with one another by language. They talk as man to man, and also as author to his readers or statesman to his radio audience. With language they incite each other to action. The mother incites her son to be good. The propagandist incites a nation to accept or reject a government. There is always a good deal of conflict between persons and between groups, for the same people get incited in different directions simultaneously. Sometimes they actually get pushed around or made to go where they do not want to go, but mostly the forces of social interaction are expressed by words. The first thing we note about a man is that he is a unit in a complex field of *social relations.* It is the psychology of these social functions that supplies the details as to just how man fits into the social structure and how he adjusts to it or resists it.

The fundamental nature of man does not appear, however, merely in his relation to his fellows. We have also to consider him as a single individual. While chemically he seems to be only an active mass of protoplasm, he turns out to have many consistencies of behavior which make up what is called his *personality.* His particular pattern of behavior may, however, vary greatly from the patterns of other men. He may be introverted or extraverted in his relation to his world, ascendant or submissive in his relation to his fellows, persistent or volatile in his activities, a radical or a conservative in his thought. He may have a high or low level of aspiration in his motivation. The number of traits and attitudes which would describe these consistencies of mind and conduct is enormous. If we ask why men differ in these various respects, we learn that it is because of their differences in inheritance, in education, in physiological constitution, in past emotional experience, in the secretions of their endocrine glands and in a myriad of other properties of this active

This chapter was prepared by Edwin G. Boring of Harvard University.

mass of protoplasm, which is a man, and which psychologists call *the organism*.

To understand why man acts as he does in different circumstances, psychology has to study all the properties of this organism. Just what, we may ask, is an organism? An organism is a mass of protoplasm that responds to excitation. It has certain necessities for response, and they are called its *needs*. Man has a need for food, and, if we keep a man from food, he will be driven to seek it until he gets it. In this way a need unsupplied creates a *drive*. Every need leads to a drive which is terminated by the satisfaction of the need. Man has a great capacity for needs. His primary needs become differentiated, and in that way he acquires many new needs. A child may need not only food, but candy; a youth not only love, but good clothes. Around man's needs and drives centers the psychology of his *motivation*.

Man's *emotions* are closely related to his needs. In his need for self-preservation may arise his emotion of fear. In his sexual need may arise his emotion of love. Like his needs, his emotions become differentiated and specific. The fear of insult and the love of music are important, useful, acquired emotions, whereas the fear of mice and the love of liquor are acquired but less useful.

Since man is a doer, he satisfies his needs by doing something about them. He *acts*. His action is, however, never fortuitous or spontaneous, for it occurs always as a response to excitation. Why? Because of the *nervous system*. To understand man, the doer, we must understand his nervous system, which activates his muscles and his glands.

The nervous system connects *stimulus* with *response*, making excitation effective. It has simple levels for *reflex action*, levels that may not even involve the brain. It has complex levels, where action depends on elaborate connections in the brain. Because no animal that does not respond to stimulation can be said to have a mind, the nervous system is often said to be the organ of man's mind.

Responses develop as the individual *grows up*. The embryo can squirm as a whole. The infant can clench his fist. The adult can trill a note or say a tongue-twister. Some responses are primitive and automatic, like winking, whereas others are complex and voluntary in the sense that they are excited by ideas, like going shopping. Still others are complex and learned, like walking. The essential cause of a response may be social pressure, emotion, need, thought, learning, idea or simple stimulation. To understand thoroughly the causes of the organism's responses would be to understand man himself.

Next in importance to the fact that man can respond with movement to excitation is his characteristic of being able to alter his modes of response. He can *learn*. Learning is the establishment of new relations between stimulus and response. Food in a man's mouth makes his saliva flow; that is an inherited relationship. Man can, however, learn what food looks like so that his saliva flows at the mere sight of food. His mouth may even learn to water at the sound of a dinner bell.

It often happens that a complex response seems entirely new because it is a brand new combination of old response elements, as in the learning of a poem or of a stroke at tennis. Man makes these new *integrations* of responses under the pressure of some need, primitive or sophisticated. He learns to recognize food, because he needs to eat to live; and he learns to recognize musical intervals because he needs to play the violin in order to enjoy the life in which he lives. Sometimes he perceives a new relationship suddenly, and ever afterward acts differently about what he has perceived. That is *insight.* More often he learns slowly, with many repetitions, a little at a time. Learning accounts for most of the differences between the adult and the infant. It is so important that some animal psychologists have said that without learning there can be no mind, although it is probably more accurate to say that mind exists wherever response exists.

It turns out that learning is not permanent in man. He forgets. In general his *forgetting* goes on continually. His recent memories are more numerous than his old ones. One cause of his forgetting is his limited capacity for the acquisition of response relationships. He cannot learn more than so much at a time and thus generally for complete learning he requires many repetitions. What he succeeds in learning, however, interferes with what he has already learned, so that the new acquisitions cancel out some of the old. Perhaps if a man could sleep without thinking or learning at all for a hundred years, he would, like the sleeping beauty, wake up with no forgetfulness and go on just where he had left off.

Next in importance to learning is man's capacity for *representation.* He can respond to an absent object because he can learn to let a present object represent it, or because he creates within himself a representative. These internal representatives have been called *images.* Out of sight is not out of mind for man. In terms of his imagery he can recollect and he can think; he can imagine and dream the bizarre dreams of sleep or the wise dreams of creative genius. By images he can solve problems in *thought.* Similarly he can use *words,* either imaged or spoken, to represent absent objects or abstract generalizations. With them he can think, and create, and solve problems. This great capacity to utilize the symbolic power of words and images is the chief distinction between man and the animals.

There is also the question as to how man learns about the world in which he lives, how he finds out what is there. That is the problem of *perception.* Man does not perceive his environment exactly as it is, but alters what he perceives in accordance with his needs, for the outside world is too complicated and variable for him to be able to perceive it in all its chaotic changefulness. Needing to simplify his environment for his own purposes, the first thing man does is to divide it up into *objects.* Objects are thus man-made. Perception pulls many items of experience together into an object and puts other items off on the outside, so that man, when he sees the world as a collection of objects, has done something to the world in perceiving it. An object must have a certain amount of stability in order that it may always seem to be itself and not to be forever becoming something else. Thus we find man equipped with a set of laws of perceptual constancy: seen objects tend to stay the same size, even when they vary in distance; they tend to stay the same shape, even when viewed at different angles; they tend to stay the same color, even when the intensity and hue of the illumination change.

Since man needs to know where he is and where other things are, we find that he can perceive the locations and distances of many objects, as well as their shapes and sizes. From various clues that come to him he correctly reconstructs some of the data of his environment—or rather his nervous system is such that it makes these 'inferences' about the outer world for him and presents them to him as his perceptions. Man is so built that he gets in this way the picture of the world that he needs.

It is via the five *senses* that the nervous system gets the data which it works over into perceptions of objects. Psychology had a great deal to say about the senses because they constitute its oldest field of research, and much is now known about it. It is an historical accident that we know more about tones than about needs, more about colors than about prejudices, but there will not always be this discrepancy. Eventually, as research continues, the laws of thinking and wishing will become fully as explicit as the laws of seeing and hearing are now.

So this is what psychology is about—man, the organism: man's capacity (1) for perceiving, (2) for response, (3) for learning and (4) for symbolization. The organism has these various properties, man has these various capacities, and man uses them all in a world filled with things, which have been created by his own perceiving, and with other people, who themselves have comparable capacities and whose relations and responses to one another are of the utmost importance to all.

BEHAVIOR AND CONSCIOUSNESS

Psychology deals with both the *behavior* of man as it appears in his responses and with *consciousness* as he finds it in his immediate experience. We need now to consider a few matters about each of these two kinds of data.

Behavior

If behavior is just movement of the organism, why does it come into psychology? Is not physiology the field where bodily movement is studied? People are always asking that question, asking where the line between physiology and psychology comes, where one science leaves off and the other begins; but there is no line. Sciences never have sharp boundaries.

Think, for instance, about the behavior of the stomach. You put food into it and then study how it contracts while the gastric juice flows in rapidly. In doing that you are being a physiologist, studying digestion. But suppose you keep food out of the stomach and then see how, after several hours, it starts its long slow contractions that make men restless and make them say, "Oh, how hungry I am!" Then you are being a psychologist, studying hunger as motivation. Or you start finding out how continued worry makes the stomach keep contracting too much and the gastric juice flow too much, forming presently a stomach ulcer, and then you are—what? A psychologist. A physiologist. A physiological psychologist. A scientist interested in what is now called *psychosomatic medicine.* The terms do not really matter.

Actually a psychologist ought to know, besides psychology, a great deal of physiology, physics and sociology, and have some acquaintance with the history of science and enough knowledge of philosophy to prevent him from trying to make too rigorous a definition of psychology for students to learn. Actually he has to be content with less.

Consciousness

Psychology studies consciousness as well as behavior. Only a hundred years ago you would have been told that psychology *is* the study of consciousness, that men have minds and bodies, and that psychology studies the minds and physiology the bodies. That is really how this distinction between physiology and psychology developed, the one group of men studying the workings of the body and the other consciousness—sensations, perceptions, feelings, emotions, imaginations, memories, thoughts and volitions. The two sciences would never have overlapped had it not been for the fact that consciousness *depends on* the body and its nervous system. No scientist has ever been able to observe a disembodied consciousness. There is always a body around, and the body is behaving—talking or acting in some way. So, although it is true that psychology studies both consciousness and behavior, you never find consciousness in anyone but yourself except by observing his behavior. The basic rule is: no behavior, no consciousness. It is for this reason that the psychologists, who began with the study of consciousness, got to studying behavior, so that after a time the sharp line between physiology and psychology disappeared.

The fact that consciousness can be known only through behavior reduces to the simple statement that there are three kinds of behavior which psychologists study. (1) First, there is the behavior which gives information about *consciousness,* like laughing or crying or saying the words, "It's pink," or telling about a dream. (2) Then there is the behavior which gives information about *unconsciousness*—for psychologists believe in the paradox of an unconscious kind of consciousness. This is the behavior that implies that you are acting on wishes which you do not know about and would, perhaps, deny having, like wishful forgetting when you remain happily unconscious of something you ought to remember and do not want to remember. Rebuking a person you know well and do not like by forgetting his name is a good instance. (3) And then there is just plain *behavior,* like putting the 5644th candy neatly in a box in a candy factory because you have learned to do it and it is now a habit which you carry on, hour after hour, while you occupy your consciousness with memories of last night's date. It all gets back to behavior in this way, even if you start with consciousness.

On the other hand, even though you have to study the behavior of other people to know about their consciousnesses, your own consciousness always seems to be known to you yourself immediately. You do not need a mirror to find out that you are angry. A science of psychology cannot, of course, be built up on any one man's experience, so most of consciousness for every psychologist is the experience of others. Nevertheless it is interesting to pause to consider just what sort of stuff your own experience is and how it differs from what you know exists in the world about you.

Begin with an experiment. Look at Fig. 1. See the spirals. Find the letter *A* at the top of the figure on one of the spirals. Follow that spiral with your eyes or your pencil around the figure until you come back to the top again. There you are, back at the letter *A*. What you were following was not a spiral after all, but a circle—in fact a perfect circle, as you could discover if you had a compass. Nevertheless what you see is a spiral, even though what you follow is a circle. Therein lies the distinction which we are considering. The spiral is your consciousness. The circle, which is there and which you cannot see, is the physical stimulus for your perception of

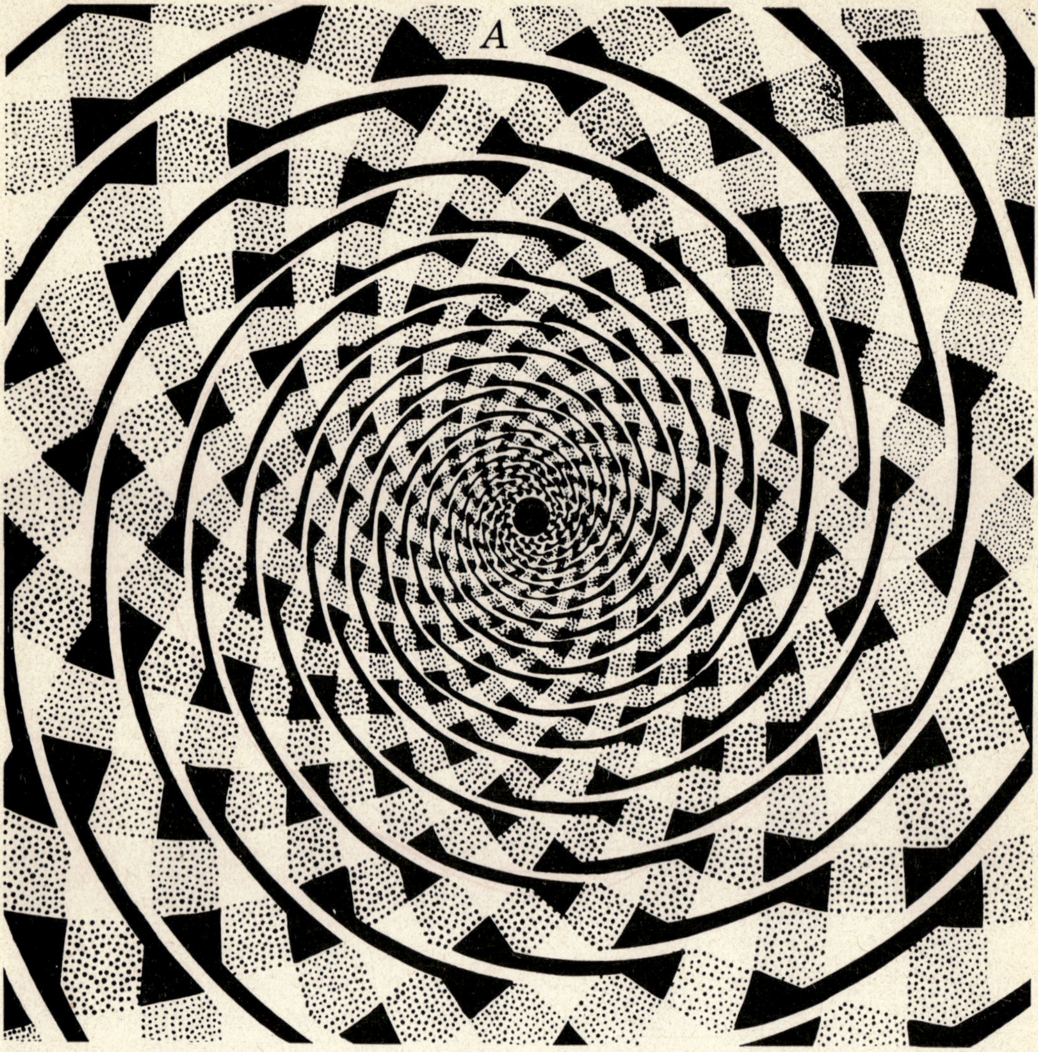

FIGURE 1. STIMULUS VS. CONSCIOUSNESS: THE TWISTED CORD ILLUSION

The conscious data are the spirals, which are seen immediately and persist in spite of sophistication. The stimuli for the spirals are perfect circles. Start at *A* at the top and follow all the way around; you come back to *A* again. [Adapted from J. Fraser, *Brit. J. Psychol.*, 1908, 2, 307, Fig. 3.]

the spiral. This is an illusion, a perception in which consciousness and its stimulus coexist in a lawful, scientifically understood disagreement.

In others words, consciousness is what you experience *immediately*. Physical objects, unless you have already learned about them, have to be figured out. It takes a compass to discover the circularity of the spiral's stimulus. One of the commonest illusions is seeing a single object as single with two eyes. You can find out that that sort of stimulation is double only by first shutting one eye, then opening it and shutting the other. Consciousness, on the other hand, is the sort of experience which you can describe immediately without hesitation or reasoning.

Unconsciousness has to be figured out—by yourself, your friends, your psychiatrist or someone else. Maybe *I* am wise enough to know more about your motives than you yourself when you address the letter meant for Boston to Baltimore where lives the girl you met last night. Motives are very likely not to be directly conscious.

ORIGINS OF SCIENTIFIC PSYCHOLOGY

Psychology has had a long history, and we had better have some words about how it came to be the way it is.

The first name to mention is that of the philosopher-physiologist Descartes (1596–1650), whose effect upon psychological thinking is still felt. Descartes made these two important contributions. (1) He argued that animals are automata, that they act like machines, and that men do too in their irrational conduct. Based on this view is the modern notion that, if you knew enough about the nervous system, you could make a mechanical or electronic robot who could act and think like a man. (2) Descartes also argued that soul and body, consciousness and nervous system are quite separate, forming different worlds, which nevertheless interact, each affecting the other, at a specific point in the brain. Consciousness is in the body but it occupies no space within it—is, as Descartes put it, "unextended substance." This view of quite different body substance and mind stuff is called *dualism.* It is responsible for the modern common-sense notion that the mind is something within the head, taking up no separate space of its own, yet working there to perceive the outside world, to do its own thinking and to control the actions of the body—a little extra person immured in the skull, perpetually busy, as news comes in along one set of nerves, sending out orders along another set.

Next we must put in our record the long tradition of British psychology that began in 1690 with the philosopher John Locke (1632–1704) and continued up into modern psychology two centuries later. This school is sometimes called British *empiricism* and sometimes British *associationism.* It was empiricism first when Locke argued —he was trying to refute Descartes in this matter—that all content of the mind comes from experience. The infant's mind, he said, is just a piece of white paper on which experience writes. Actually he had hold of half the truth, for there is nothing in a man's consciousness or behavior that is not partly learned, although heredity also plays its role. Having made learning so important, Locke then had to say how learning works. He suggested that *association* is the principle. Ideas that belong together tend to stay together in the mind; that is what association is. Locke's view led eventually to a kind of mental chemistry, in which perceptions and ideas were thought of as complex molecules made up of atoms of sensations and images held together by association.

Dualism remained the rule in psychology pretty much up to the end of the nineteenth century. You had mind and you had body. There were many guesses as to how the two were related, but, in the middle of the nineteenth century, the general acceptance of the notion of the conservation of energy led psychologists to accept, for the most part, the conception of *parallelism.* That view is that man is a machine in which all conduct is to be explained by the action of the sensory nerves, the spinal cord, the brain and the motor nerves, and that certain of these events—some of those that occur in the brain—are paralleled by the occurrences in consciousness.

Against this parallelistic-dualistic view of the relation of the mind to the body were put forward various kinds of *monism,* the view that mind and body are the same kind of stuff or at most different aspects of the same basic events. These views of the relation of mind to body matter to us only in respect of what they led to. Parallelistic dualism led to introspectionism. Monism has realized itself in modern times in behaviorism. These two schools of psychology we shall consider presently, but first we must get back to the nineteenth century.

When physiology was growing into a science, some of the physiologists became interested in what are really psychological problems. There was, for instance, Johannes Müller (1801–1858), called the father of experimental physiology, who in 1826 laid down the theory that the nature of sensory quality depends on which particular nerve is excited. Press on your eyeball, and you see colors; get your ears boxed, and they will ring. Müller was a dualist. He was supposing that the mind, within the brain, would be noting: "This is something that can be seen, a sight not a sound, because it is the optic nerve that is being stimulated." There was also E. H. Weber (1795–1878), who gave us Weber's law in 1834, the law which asserts that the just perceivable difference between two stimuli gets larger as the stimuli get larger. Two men shouting make more noise than one man, but, if you add only one extra shouter to fifty shouters, you will never hear the difference. In such ways it was getting quite clear toward the middle of the nineteenth century that you could experiment with the mind—at least with sensations—as well as with the brain.

At that point experimental psychology began. Three men contributed to its founding. There was Hermann von Helmholtz (1821–1894), perhaps the ablest scientist who has as yet touched psychology, the man who set the physiologists by the ears in 1850 by measuring the velocity of the nerve impulse and who wrote and published what are still the great classical volumes on visual and auditory sensation in the decade following 1856. There was also G. T. Fechner (1801–1887), who worked out the methods for measuring sensation and published them in 1860. And then there was Wilhelm Wundt (1832–1920), who coined the phrase *physiological psychology* to stand for the kind of work Müller and Weber and Helmholtz and Fechner had been doing. He wrote in 1874 the first systematic handbook of physiological or experimental psychology (the classic up to its sixth edition in 1911), he founded the first important laboratory of experimental psychology at Leipzig in 1879 (William James had a little laboratory at Harvard a few years earlier) and he really got the new experimental psychology under way as a separate social institution. Wundt was a dualist and parallelist in his theory of mind and body. He took over the notion of association from British empiricism. He was a mental chemist, and he believed that we can, by *introspection,* analyze consciousness into the mental elements of which it is composed. Introspection is the having of experience and describing it. When we note that the curves in Fig. 1 are spirals, we are introspecting. Introspection is the way to get at consciousness.

As late as 1910 most psychologists regarded introspection as the basic method of psychology, that is to say, most psychologists were dualists: they believed that physiology studied the body, that psychology studied consciousness and that introspection was the direct way of getting at consciousness.

Meanwhile, in 1859, Darwin had contributed the theory of evolution to science. It created a revolution in scientific thinking and cast some doubt upon dualism. Before that time consciousness had been thought of as practically the same stuff as the soul. Now Darwin suggested that mental characteristics—especially emotional behavior—might be inherited by man from his animal ancestors. Consciousness was thus being biologized. Darwin's famous cousin, Francis Galton (1822–1911), published in 1869 a study of British genius, in which he sought to show that genius is inherited. Several investigators in England and America became interested in mental evolution and so in animal psychology, and in 1898 Thorndike in America published what were almost the first systematic psychological experiments on animal intelligence. He studied how cats can learn to get out of puzzle boxes.

From this point it will be easy for us to follow the main developments in the history of scientific psychology by noting how the four most important schools of modern psychology waxed and waned from the end of the nineteenth century until the present. We turn to them now.

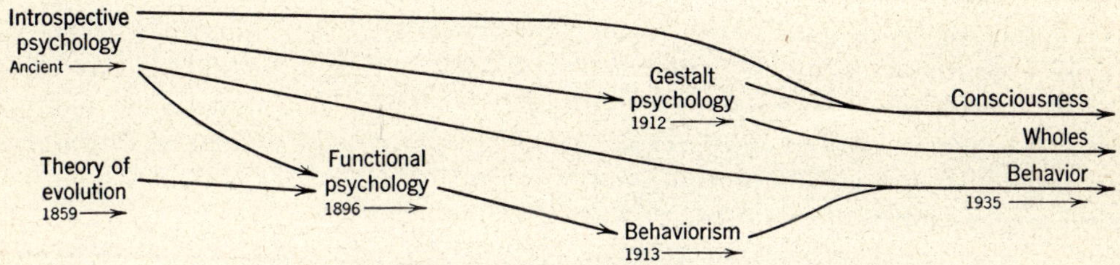

FIGURE 2. SCHOOLS OF PSYCHOLOGY

Diagram shows the relationship of four schools of psychology to each other and to the theory of evolution. Modern psychology tends to ignore schools but to deal with both consciousness and behavior in integrated wholes.

SCHOOLS OF PSYCHOLOGY

There have, then, been these four schools of psychology. They are of different ages, but the last two were contemporaneous. See Fig. 2 for a diagram of their relationships.

(1) Introspective Psychology

That is the school which regards consciousness as the important object of study. It was the school of Wundt and for the most part it used some kind of introspective analysis of consciousness, a kind of mental chemistry. In America it was most strongly defended by Titchener (1867–1927) at Cornell. The school was at its greatest power about 1910. No one nowadays calls himself an introspectionist, but everyone has to know about this oldest of the schools in order to understand the others.

(2) Functional Psychology

The theory of evolution was marvelously well fitted to thrive in the American atmosphere, where competition and the struggle for success resembled Darwin's principle of the survival of the fittest. It was natural for American psychology to be functional, to consider mind in terms of its uses to the organism in its effort to succeed. William James (1842–1910) at Harvard was the first American to react against introspectionism, and most of the other American psychologists in the period 1890–1910 believed that psychology should deal primarily with human abilities and capacities. The school that was called the functional school was established by John Dewey (1859–) at the University of Chicago about 1896 and was carried on there later by James R. Angell (1869). This school was dualistic, interpreting consciousness in terms of its use, and, because it was concerned primarily with human abilities, it provided a friendly background for both the mental tests and animal psychology, neither of which is primarily concerned about consciousness. The school of functional psychology may be said to have evaporated when behaviorism became well established, but the spirit of the school is still the dominating force in American psychology. Mental testing and applied psychology have thrived in America because they are useful psychologies and accord well with the spirit of competition that marks the American culture.

(3) Behaviorism

The next step in functionalistic progress in America was the founding of behaviorism about 1913 by John B. Watson (1878–). Watson had been working with rats at Chicago under Angell. His early interests were in animal psychology, and the conventions of his day held that animals, in learning to solve puzzles, to find food in mazes and to discriminate the correct food box, were displaying consciousness and that the psychologist ought, therefore, to assess their consciousnesses. Watson argued that you never know much about the consciousness of a rat, although you can study his abilities and capacities, and that such study is properly to be regarded as psychology. He laid down the law that psychology should deal only with behavior. Introspection he ruled out, and consciousness he ignored. His behaviorism proved practicable for the very reason that you never learn about the consciousness of any organism, human or animal, unless the organism behaves somehow in its introspection. Thus Watson could really keep introspection in behaviorism by calling introspection "verbal behavior." Nevertheless, interest in consciousness was diminishing and interest in behavior increasing. Behaviorism was consistent with mental testing and animal psychology. The study of consciousness was still further depreciated about the turn of the century when the psychoanalytic doctrine of Sigmund Freud (1856–1939) began to direct the thinking of the psychologists toward unconsciousness. Partly on this account and partly because of the outcome of experiments on thought and action, they came to realize that a great deal of motivation is unconscious and quite unavailable to introspection. By 1930 introspection had become only a secondary method of psychology, except as it was used in simple sensory discriminations or employed loosely in social psychology and psychotherapy.

(4) Gestalt Psychology

The success of behaviorism was somewhat diminished by the appearance of Gestalt psychology in Germany about 1912. The new movement had caught American interest by the 1920's, and then in the 1930's its leaders migrated to America when the Nazi power destroyed German freedom. *Gestalt* means *form,* and the name was derived from certain studies of visual perception of spatial form. It is better translated, however, as *structure,* for the thesis of the school, which was founded by Max Wertheimer (1880–1943), is that psychologists must deal with total structures and the system of their internal forces, eschewing the mental chemistry and the analysis that both introspectionism and behaviorism favored. The Gestalt psychologists say that, in looking at a square, it is the total figure that makes the square look square, not the parts. A square is more than four black lines. It is four black lines in a particular relation to one another, and squareness really depends on the relation and not the lines. Four dots will also make a square, as will four red lines. The mental chemists were always talking about the sensations, the parts that made up the square, as if the squareness of a red square were different from the squareness of a blue square. By the late 1930's this school had accomplished its main purpose of getting the attention of psychologists directed to larger systems of interrelated facts. The movement did not revive American interest in consciousness, though for a while it delayed the general shift of the Americans toward behaviorism. Meanwhile the Nazi power had destroyed German psychology, and America took the lead in the new science.

(5) Modern Psychology

During the 1930's the *isms* pretty well dropped out of psychology. The functionalists first gave place to the behavior-ists, but nowadays you ne call himself a *behavioris* may still hear about *beh* been even longer since label himself an *introspectio* are, perhaps, still a few *Gestaltists,* but that is only because Germans like *isms* better than Americans do.

What has actually happened is that consciousness, inherited from introspectionism, is used in psychophysics (for example, in discrimination of colors, tones, visual distances and all the other sensory capacities for which perceptual accuracy must be determined) and, at the other extreme, in psychotherapy where experiences from waking life or dreams need to be recorded and studied. The spirit of functional psychology pervades the modern American scene which studies *mind in use for the organism* as a matter of course. Behaviorism has contributed behavior and the modern stimulus-response psychology. This kind of psychology also claims to be studying consciousness, because consciousness is revealed to scientific observation only through behavior of some kind. Gestalt psychology disappeared as an *ism* because, after a battle, nearly everyone had accepted its basic tenet that too much analysis gives false results, that wholes are safer objects of study than their parts, that you must always take into consideration enough of the interrelated forces to make you fairly safe about not having omitted any essential.

From here we can go on to the fields of modern psychology. The only reason for mentioning these four schools in this book is that the student hears about *behaviorism* and *Gestalt psychology* and has a right to be told what they are and that they are no longer important as schools. What was good in all the schools is now simply part of psychology.

FIELDS OF PSYCHOLOGY

The way in which modern psychology has become further complicated appears if we pick out and define eleven of its more important fields. Let us do it.

(1) *General psychology* includes the fundamental principles of all psychology. It also deals particularly with the normal human adult, leaving other matters to special fields. It is sometimes divided into the smaller fields of (*a*) sensation and perception, (*b*) feeling and emotion, (*c*) learning and motivation and (*d*) the higher processes, including thought.

(2) *Physiological psychology* studies the functions of the nervous system which control behavior and consciousness and of other similar mechanisms like the endocrine glands. It often uses operative techniques, investigating the functions of animal brains, for instance, by removing portions of the brain tissue and noting the effect upon behavior. This kind of experiment is older than experimental psychology, going back to the early nineteenth century.

(3) *Comparative psychology* is the name given to the study of the comparison of the behaviors of different animal species. It is the natural history of animal conduct. Most of the psychological work with animals is now in the hands of physiological psychologists, but there are still some comparative psychologists left.

(4) *Psychology of individual differences* is the name given to the measurement and assessment of human abilities, largely by the employment of mental tests. The use of mental tests for this purpose goes back to Francis Galton in England in 1883, but the development of the tests has been greatest in America in the last forty years. Both the World Wars greatly stimulated research in these modes of the appraisal of human abilities.

(5) *Industrial psychology* includes all the means of personnel selection by the use of tests, interviews and other devices, and all the means of training on the job and of measuring efficiency of work. It is not new, but it has been accelerated by the success of these procedures in the Second World War.

(6) *Child psychology* studies the development of the child, assesses his abilities by the use of tests, seeks evidence on the problem of the relative effects of heredity and environment upon ability, and also considers the adjustment of the child, a form of clinical psychology (vide infra).

(7) *Educational psychology* examines the educational process in terms of child psychology, clinical psychology and the dynamic psychology of learning and motivation (vide infra).

(8) *Abnormal psychology* has to do with the deviation of the human adult from the normal. It is allied to *psychiatry,* the medical field for the treatment of psychological disorders and maladjustments. Since about 1930 this field has been greatly influenced by *psychoanalysis,* and the psychoanalytic conceptions of unconscious motivation are now used by all.

(9) *Dynamic psychology* is the result of this interpenetration of abnormal psychology by psychoanalysis and of other researches that have indicated how often motivation is unconscious. Dynamic psychology can be defined, therefore, as the psychology of normal motivation. While its origins can be traced far back into the French abnormal psychology of the nineteenth century, its important development lies entirely in the present century.

(10) *Clinical psychology* is the practical application of dynamic and abnormal psy-

chology to the problems of human adjustment. It has been stimulated by the demand for psychological assistance for the many veterans of the Second World War who suffer from psychoneurosis.

(11) *Social psychology* is the study of the individual in the group and the relations of groups to one another. Thus social psychology considers the psychological interrelations of people forming families, crowds, societies and mobs, and of the leader with his followers. It includes the study of the formation of group attitudes and opinions and of the assessment of social attitudes and public opinions. It is thus forced into a consideration of social and national conflict, of race prejudice and similar manifestations of the interrelations of the conflicting needs of many individuals. Social psychology is as old as sociology and cultural anthropology, but its specific development along psychological lines is usually traced from the writing of William McDougall in 1908.

The present book has something to say about these kinds of psychology: general, physiological, individual differences, industrial, dynamic and social. The other five fields enter only incidentally, often by way of illustration. In general this book limits itself to the scientific core of psychology. The other fields are more specialized or are fields of application.

SCIENTIFIC METHOD

We ought now to say something about how the scientist works. He does not follow rigid rules. Usually he has a hunch that something might be true and tries it out in an experiment. If his hunch proves wrong, he does not, as a rule, publish that fact; so perhaps someone else will make the same guess and try it out again, and find again that the guess is wrong. The scientist is sometimes motivated by intellectual curiosity, sometimes by that esthetic feeling which makes a man want to make concrete a good idea and sometimes by the desire to advance civilization or to solve a particularly pressing practical problem; but all the other human competitive motives work too—the need for money, the need for prestige, the need to prove yourself right and the other man wrong. The rules for research have been worked out, not to constrict scientific imagination and constrain drive, but to stimulate men into what are usually the more profitable avenues of work.

Experiment

The basic scientific method is experiment. Experiment is the observation of *concomitant variation* and the interpretation of the concomitances as causes and effects. You change x, and y happens. So y is observed as a function of x. You prick a man's finger with a pin, and he quickly withdraws his finger. The prick is x, the *independent variable,* which the experimenter controls. The withdrawal, y, is the *dependent variable,* which the experimenter observes as a result of x, the prick.

Sometimes you have to wait for nature to do the independent varying for you. The astronomer does. His independent observation is often a date and a moment at which he makes the observations which his hypothesis (or hunch) requires. It is also impossible for the psychologist to create individual differences in intelligence, but he can choose persons who have different scores on an intelligence test (independent variable) and then see whether they do differently as clerks or salesmen (dependent variable).

It is fair to define the scientist as the

man who is always after *generalizations,* and the engineer or applied scientist as the man who is solving *particular* problems. A generalization would be the statement: All dreams are partially concealed expressions of unconscious wishes. A particular problem of psychiatric 'human engineering' would be the use of John's dreams to show why *he* had had a nervous breakdown. John is an immediate problem for 'human engineering,' but he is interesting to science only if he serves to represent some larger class of objects—like all men, or all the dreamers with psychoneuroses. Usually 'pure' and applied science go ahead together. Work in the one contributes to the advance of the other, but it is important to remember about generalization. The whole value of science is that it reduces the complexities of the world to general rules, which, once established, enable you to explain or predict many, many individual cases.

You cannot generalize without *repetition.* If y changes when x is changed, that may be chance. Try it again. If it happens ten times, perhaps it is 'right,' that is to say, perhaps the general rule can be accepted. More cases make you more sure. Yet you are never entirely certain; the future may still reveal some discrepancy.

Control

You also need control if you are to generalize. That means ordinarily that you must keep all the conditions constant when you repeat or you may not get the same result. If conditions are going to be allowed to change, you had better change them at will and then you may learn something extra. If you withdraw your finger when it is pricked and you are awake, what will you do when you are asleep? But the experimenter must not let you sleep and wake at random. He must control your sleeping, keeping it constant or varying it at his will.

On the other hand, hunch comes into this business too. No one can keep all the conditions constant, and the experimenter has to guess which conditions are the most important. Suppose you discovered on a Tuesday that a certain percentage of automobile drivers cannot tell a red traffic light from a green, except by knowing that the red is on top. (You could do it by interchanging the red and green in one signal, provided you prevented accidents in some other way.) Well, that was Tuesday. Would you have to repeat the experiment on Wednesday and all the other days? No, you assume that the day of the week makes no difference, that eyes see the same on Tuesdays and on Wednesdays. Nor does the phase of the moon matter, nor the last name of the driver. It is by hunch that you leave these matters out of control. You hope they make no difference. Sometimes, when a long-accepted generalization turns out later to be wrong, it is because some such essential condition was not controlled when the original generalization was formed. For instance, most people would expect sex to make no difference in observing traffic lights, but it does. Very few women are color-blind.

In reading about experiments you often see the phrase *control series* or *control group* or you meet the criticism that an experiment was *uncontrolled.* What do those statements mean? This. The experiment consists of seeing whether y varies when x varies. The *control* consists in seeing whether y does *not* vary when x does *not* vary. You want to see whether men can do better on an intelligence test when you give them some of the drug benzedrine sulphate. So you divide the men into two groups. To the *experimental group* you give the benzedrine in capsules without telling them what it is. To the *control group* you give sugar in capsules without telling them what it is. If the experimental group does better or worse than the control group, maybe benzedrine has some effect. If both groups do as much better with the capsules as without, perhaps the improvement is due merely to the confidence of the men that a psychologist's capsule will make them more efficient. If you do not have two groups, but only one, you must have *control series* with the sugar, and *experimental series* with the benzedrine, both for the same people.

There is a great deal of pseudoscience which fails to get reliable results just because it has no controls. Colleges, for instance, keep changing their course requirements in order to manufacture better A.B.'s. How do they know when the A.B.'s are better unless they keep half the students as a control on the old plan and put the other half on the new plan and also know how to compare the two finished products after Commencement?

Hypothesis

Now one word about the use of hypotheses in science. If a psychologist gets a hunch that blond women are more placid than brunettes, he is privileged to try to prove his hypothesis by experiment if he has the time and facilities for such research. The safe rule for research, however, is to use it to test plausible hypotheses which grow out of other research. That is, by and large, the way science has progressed. Here, then, is the best way, which has been burdened with the name *hypothetico-deductive* method.

(1) On the basis of general knowledge, previous research and insight into the relationships of the available facts, you form an *hypothesis*. It had better be a sensible one, but you are the judge of its plausibility. If you are trying to serve science, you choose an hypothesis the proof or disproof of which would advance scientific knowledge.

(2) The hypothesis is a generality, the sort of proposition that makes a law when it is proved. So you *deduce* from it some particular consequence that ought to follow, one that can be subjected to experimental test.

(3) Then you set up the *test experiment* and see whether the deductive prediction is verified or not.

(4) If the prediction is verified, you may assume tentatively that the hypothesis is strengthened. You may even decide to accept it, always subject, of course, to the possibility that it may be overthrown later.

(5) If the experiment gives negative results, does not justify the hypothesis, then, if you are very anxious to understand the phenomena being investigated, you will have to use your wits to find another plausible hypothesis to test out.

(6) When an hypothesis is verified, you are very likely to find that it sets you new problems. So now you think up new finer hypotheses to direct you toward finding out *why* the hypothesis just verified is true, and that process of refinement can go on practically forever.

The study of the moon illusion shows this process operating. It was early observed that the full moon looks larger on the horizon than up in the heavens. Many hypotheses were advanced—that the difference is due to refraction at the horizon, or due to the atmospheric haze at the horizon, or due to the fact that the moon looks farther away at the horizon and thus would have to be big in order to give the normal-sized image on the retina. The first two hypotheses fail when tested by the camera. A photograph of the horizon moon is as small as the photograph of the moon in elevation. The third hypothesis fails because the horizon moon no longer looks large when you bend over and view it between your legs. The next hypothesis is that the illusion depends on looking up, and that hypothesis has been proved. It holds even for experimental moons only thirty meters away. So now you know; the phenomenon is an illusion and not an astronomical change, and it depends on looking up. But *why,* you ask at once. That needs another hypothesis. Perhaps what shrinks the moon is raising the eyes, or perhaps it is bending the neck. That question has been answered. The raised-eyes hypothesis is right, the bent-neck hypothesis is wrong. So, by forming and testing new hypotheses, you have refined your knowledge. *Now* you want to know *why* raising the eyes shrinks the moon, but no one has yet been clever enough to formulate for test the crucial hypothesis that will answer that question. Sometime it will be done.

DEFINITIONS

Nearly all the definitions of terms come up in their proper places in this book. We may, however, examine here a very few special words that we need to use at the outset.

Stimulus. A stimulus is any change in external energy that gives rise to such an excitation of the nervous system as arouses a response. (See pp. 20, 217, 251.) A stimulus cannot exist without a response because it is defined as producing a response, but in this sense a conscious event must be regarded as a response.

Stimulus object. An object, like a colored paper that is seen or a sweet substance that is tasted, is often called a *stimulus,* but it is more correct to call it a *stimulus object,* since it determines a change of energy but is not the change.

Situation. When a stimulus object is extremely complex or has special meaning to the observer, it is often loosely called a *situation.* A red light may be a stimulus, but an enemy is a situation.

Proximal stimulus. Since energy changes progress serially from a stimulus object to the organism, it is plain that stimuli can be more or less proximal (near the nervous system). When the pistol shot makes you jump, the pistol is the stimulus object, the sound in the air is a stimulus, the motion of your eardrum is a more proximal stimulus, and motion of the hair cells where the sensory nerve fibers are in your inner ear is a still more proximal stimulus. *The* stimulus does not exist, for there is always a series of more and more proximal energy changes when stimulation occurs.

Response. A response is the second and later event in a stimulus-response pair. In man it is usually a muscular movement or the secretion of a gland. When a psychologist is dealing with consciousness, he thinks of a sensation as a response. Response exists only in relation to a stimulus, and in man it is always an end result of the action of the nervous system. Responses, like stimuli, can be more or less proximal. The contraction of a muscle is more proximal than the finger movement which the muscle's contraction causes.

Behavior. When the responses are very complicated, it is better to call them *behavior.* Behavior has the same relation to a situation that a response has to a stimulus.

Subject and observer. The psychologist does his research with the stimulated responses of men and lower animals. These organisms on which he works are his *subjects*—the subjects of his experiment. The psychologist performing an experiment is the *experimenter.* Sometimes, when a human subject is asked to observe his own consciousness, he is called an *observer.* That means that the human subject has been able to take over a part of the experimenter's responsibility for the accuracy of observation. In an experiment with animal subjects, it is always the experimenter who is the observer, for animals cannot be trusted with responsibility for scientific results.

With all these matters out of the way, we can now turn to the real business of this book, and we shall begin with the mechanism of response, which is, in man, the nervous system.

REFERENCES

1. Boring, E. G. *A history of experimental psychology.* New York: Appleton-Century, 1929.

A thorough-going history, from 1690 to about 1920, of psychologists and their schools within the scientific tradition in psychology.

2. Boring, E. G. *Sensation and perception in the history of experimental psychology.* New York: Appleton-Century, 1942.

The history of research and ideas in the field of sensation and perception from the seventeenth century down to about 1930.

3. Cohen, M. R., and Nagel, E. *An introduction to logic and scientific method.* New York: Harcourt, Brace, 1936. Chaps. 10–16. Or abridged ed. London: Rutledge, 1939. Chaps. 5–10.

Discussion of experimental method, classification, use of hypotheses, probability, induction, measurement and statistical method by two logicians.

4. Dennis, W., *et al. Current trends in psychology.* Pittsburgh, Pa.: University of Pittsburgh Press, 1947.

Eight lectures by eight distinguished psychologists showing how the Second World War altered the scientific picture in eight of the most important fields of scientific and applied psychology.

5. Ellis, W. D. *A source book of Gestalt psychology.* London: K. Paul, Trench, Trubner, 1938.

Thirty-four selections from the writings of seventeen Gestalt psychologists translated into English.

6. Fearing, F. *Reflex action: a study in the history of physiological psychology.* Baltimore: Williams and Wilkins, 1930.

A good and quite detailed survey of the history of physiological psychology from Descartes to about 1930.

7. Flugel, J. C. *A hundred years of psychology.* New York: Macmillan, 1933.

A picture of modern psychology from 1833 to 1933 with especial emphasis upon the psychology of Great Britain and psychoanalysis.

8. Guilford, J. P. (Ed.) *Fields of psychology.* New York: Van Nostrand, 1940.

Twenty-two chapters by thirteen authors on the content of physiological, animal, differential, child, educational, industrial, abnormal, clinical and social psychology.

9. Hartmann, G. W. *Gestalt psychology.* New York: Ronald Press, 1935.

A good interpretation and summary of the theories and researches that belong to the school of Gestalt psychology and other closely allied schools.

10. Heidbreder, E. *Seven psychologies.* New York: Appleton-Century, 1933.

A clear summary of the psychology of the schools of introspective, functional, behavioristic, dynamic and Gestalt psychology.

11. Keller, F. S. *The definition of psychology.* New York: Appleton-Century, 1937.

Brief discussions of the principles involved in introspective, functional, behavioristic and Gestalt psychologies.

12. Köhler, W. *Gestalt psychology.* (2nd ed.) New York: Liveright, 1947.

A clear, readable exposition of Gestalt psychology by one of its leading exponents, somewhat revised since the 1929 edition.

13. Moore, J. S., and Gurnee, H. *The foundations of psychology.* (2nd ed.) Princeton: Princeton University Press, 1933.

A good, although not recent, discussion of the fundamental concepts and principles of psychology.

14. Murphy, G. *An historical introduction to modern psychology.* New York: Harcourt, Brace, 1929.

An excellent detailed and accurate history of modern psychology, not limited to the experimental tradition.

15. Petermann, B. *The Gestalt theory and the problem of configuration.* New York: Harcourt, Brace, 1932.

A straightforward exposition and evaluation of the Gestalt psychology of the three leading exponents of the school.

16. Watson, J. B. *Behaviorism.* (2nd ed.) New York: Norton, 1930.

A readable and elementary presentation of this school of psychological thought, by the founder of the school long after the founding.

17. Woodworth, R. S. *Contemporary schools of psychology.* New York: Ronald Press, 1931.

Clear chapters on introspective, behavioristic, Gestalt, dynamic and purposive psychologies.

18. Zilboorg, G., and Henry, G. W. *A history of medical psychology.* New York: Norton, 1941.

A vividly written history of psychopathology from the Greeks to the present with especial emphasis on the psychoneuroses and their antecedents.

CHAPTER 2

The Response Mechanism

NOW that we have seen what psychology in its essentials is, and how it came to be what it is, we are prepared to go ahead with the study of psychology's actual facts. We start with the topic of the nervous system. Psychology is not physiology, but it has constantly to consider that part of physiology which explains the mechanisms of human action. Psychology studies man, the doer. Man's doings are responses—responses to stimulations, to situations, to his own needs and ideas. The nervous system, considered together with the system of endocrine glands, is the principal response mechanism. These two systems are basic to all human behavior.

This chapter sketches the machinery of the body which enables man to perceive and to respond to his environment in intelligent fashion.

As a matter of fact, nearly every part of the human body is involved either directly or indirectly in behavior, for each part plays some role in the smooth functioning of the whole body. The digestive tract is the portal of entry for food and water without which other tissues of the body cannot survive or carry on their functions normally. The liver stores food materials which the brain uses. The heart pumps blood which carries these materials to the sense organs, the brain and the muscles. The lungs provide oxygen for the use of the food materials in tissues of the body, and they carry away carbon dioxide resulting from such use. The kidneys, similarly, rid the body of the poisonous products which are generated in the activities of the body's tissues. These are but a few of the interrelations of organs of the body; the list could be greatly enlarged.

The response mechanism in man and in the higher animals includes (1) the sense organs or *receptors,* which react to stimulation and set in operation the processes of excitation in the living individual, (2) the *nervous* system, which transmits and conducts excitation, and (3) the muscles and glands, or *effectors,* which make actual response possible. Combined in a highly complex mechanism, these three principal parts give the living organism means of responding in an organized fashion to the physical energies of the environment which stimulate him. The immediate analogy is a system of push-buttons and buzzers. Each button (receptor) is connected (nervous system) to its own buzzer (effector). A particular buzz is a response. Actually this analogy is much too simple. Different patterns of pushes should produce different patterns of buzzes, and the system of connections should change from time to time

This chapter was prepared by Clifford T. Morgan of The Johns Hopkins University.

as situations change. We must, however, understand the simplest things first.

DIFFERENTIATION OF THE RESPONSE MECHANISM

All around us, all the time, energy changes are going on. Light is emitted by the sun, stars, fires and man-made light bulbs; it is reflected by the moon, the walls of our rooms, the plants, our clothes and the earth. Heat is given off in the absorption of light, in chemical process in our bodies, from machinery and from hot objects; it is absorbed by the cold objects in our environment. Electromagnetic waves are sent out by our radio and radar transmitters and picked up by sensitive receivers. Sounds are made by the whirling of the wind, the boiling of the water or, generally, whenever one object strikes or rubs against another. Changes in chemical energy occur in food as it is being cooked, in the barnyard, in the brewery, in the plants around us and in the tissues of our bodies.

The Stimulus

Many, but not all, of these energy changes affect living tissues. Radio and magnetic waves do not, some frequencies of light and sound do not and some chemical substances are relatively inactive. On the other hand, X-rays can destroy living tissue, infrared rays heat it up, ultraviolet rays assist in the synthesis of vitamin B in the body. Heat causes changes in chemical reactions in our tissues and, if extreme enough, can destroy them. Sounds set tissues into vibration, causing mechanical changes in them and, at certain frequencies and intensities, destroying them. Chemical reactions are necessary for the growth and maintenance of living cells but, if of the wrong kind, can kill them.

Of those energy changes which affect living tissues, some produce responses in the organism, others simply affect the tissues directly. Those energy changes which produce responses are defined, for the purposes of scientific psychology, as *stimuli*. Thus, in man, who is equipped with receptors and effectors for responding, the word *stimulus* is used to describe any change in the energies outside a receptor which is responsible for altering the physical-chemical state of the receptor in such a way that excitation is initiated. The essential characteristics of a stimulus, we may note, are described in the same quantitative units as are employed in the sciences of physics and chemistry.

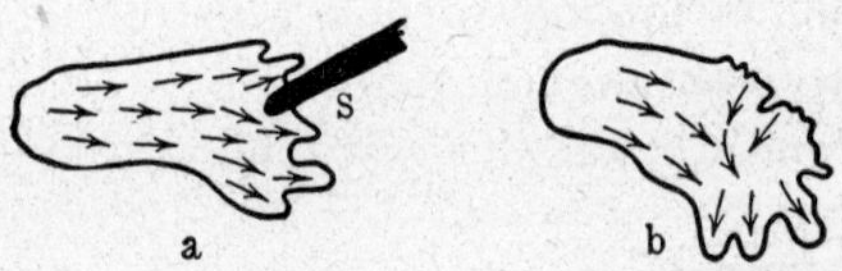

FIGURE 3. RESPONSE OF AMOEBA TO STIMULATION

(*a*) Just stimulated by glass rod, *S;* (*b*) change of flow of protoplasm and response of amoeba to such stimulation.

Man's response mechanism is very complex. We may, however, more easily understand it by seeing how it got to be the way it is, how the response mechanism evolved from the simple to the complex.

Look at a simple unicellular animal, the amoeba. It has no specialized receptors, no organs for the reception of stimuli, for the transmission of excitation or for the effecting of response. Yet the amoeba is a self-contained, living system, which may be acted upon and changed by many of the same physical stimuli which are significant in complex animal behavior and, indeed, in the whole psychological life of man. Radiant energy, vibrations in its surrounding medium, chemical and other energies act upon the amoeba and initiate processes in the single cell. If strong light or heat, for example, is projected upon one side of an amoeba, the creature contracts its body on the stimulated side in such a way as to effect its withdrawal from the stimulus. As the result of processes so initiated the orientation of the organism in relation to its environment may be changed. The amoeba, like man, responds to the stimuli in its environment.

Evolution of the Response Mechanism

Between the amoeba and man, there is obviously a vast difference, not only in the complexity of the organism as a whole, but also in the response mechanism. It is a difference in the number of cells involved and in the specialization of their functions.

Above the amoeba in the evolutionary scale are the simple multicellular organisms like the sponge and the jellyfish. In them we see the first steps in the differentiation which finally results in the complex response mechanism of man. The very first step, the most primitive differentiation, consists in the appearance of the independent muscle-effector cell, as seen in the sponge. These independent effectors of the sponge are more sensitive to external physical stimuli than primitive undifferentiated cells like amoebae. They contract more readily and vigorously than primitive cells, thus featuring response to external stimulation.

After the specialization of cells for response had begun in the evolutionary development, there came the differentiation of special cells for excitation by stimuli, the receptor cells. In such primitive animals as the sea anemone, these receptor cells took the form of diffuse nerve nets which are excited by external stimuli and distribute the excitation to effector cells. It was in this way that the *receptor-effector* mechanism first appeared (Fig. 4, *A*).

Finally, in somewhat higher animal forms, specialized nerve or ganglion cells (adjustors) came to be interposed between the receptors and effectors to make up a true nervous system for conducting excitation from receptors to effectors (Fig. 4, *B*). Such a ganglionic nervous system, or *receptor-adjustor-effector* mechanism, is seen in worms. Thereafter, this mechanism increases in complexity and also in effectiveness in the series of vertebrate and mammalian animals to reach its highest development in man.

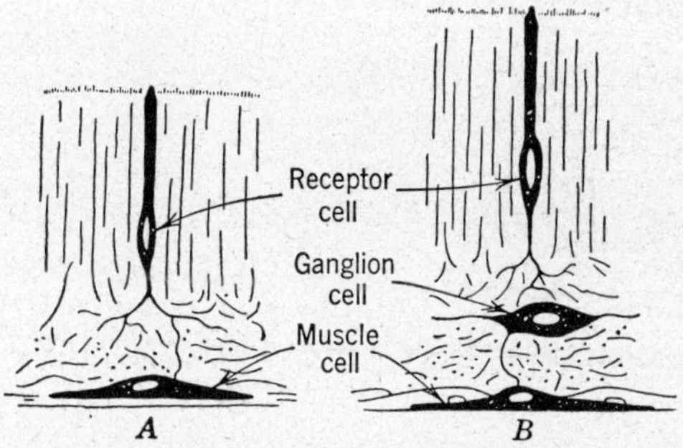

FIGURE 4. PRIMITIVE RESPONSE MECHANISMS

(*A*) A simple receptor-effector mechanism; (*B*) a receptor-adjustor-effector mechanism. [From G. H. Parker, *The elementary nervous system*, Lippincott, 1919, pp. 201 f.]

The Effectors

To the muscle cells, which were the first effectors to appear in evolution, was later added another class of effectors, the glands, so that, in man, we must distinguish two main classes of effectors, the *muscles* and *glands*. The glands secrete chemical substances, needed in the body's functions, and deliver them into the blood stream for general circulation or into special cavities of the body like the mouth or stomach.

The muscles are of three kinds, varying according to the amount and kind of differentiation which they have undergone (Fig. 5). (1) Most primitive, or least differentiated, of the muscle effectors is the unstriped, or *smooth,* muscle cell (*D*). It is found, for example, in the walls of the intestine. Typically a spindle-shaped cell, it contains within it a special substance, the fibrillae, upon which its contractual properties depend. (2) More elaborate in form, however, is a second class of muscle cells, the *striped* muscle cells (*A, B*), which are typical of arm and leg muscles. They are much more elongated than smooth muscle cells and are enclosed in a special elastic membrane, the sarcolemma. In them the contractile fibrillae are differentiated into two substances, one darker than the other, the regular alternation of which throughout the length of the fiber gives the muscle cell its striped appearance. (3) A third type of muscle, the *cardiac* muscle of the heart (*C*), is actually a special kind of striped muscle. Its chief distinction is that its fibers are not arranged parallel or enclosed in a membrane as are the striped muscle cells, but branch and unite with each other in a network.

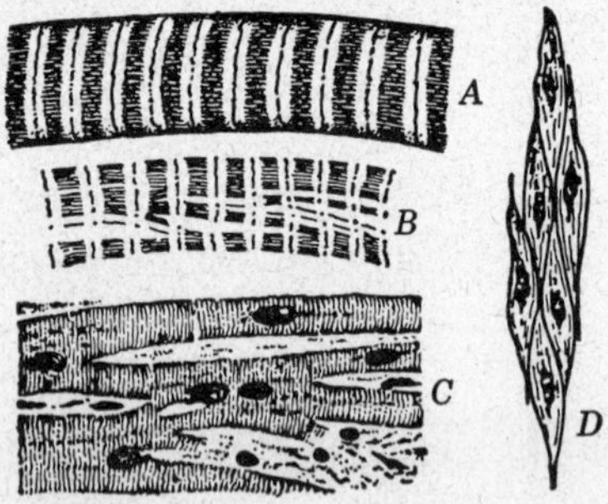

FIGURE 5. TYPES OF MUSCLE FIBERS

(*A, B*) Striped muscle fibers; (*C*) heart muscle fibers; and (*D*) smooth muscle fibers. [From M. F. Guyer, *Animal biology* (3rd ed.), Harper, 1941, p. 405.]

All muscle—be it smooth, striped or cardiac—is specialized for but one function, *contraction.* The excitation transmitted through the adjustors of the nervous system initiates the essential physical and chemical events in the muscle, events which lead to the release of the muscle's stored energy in the form of a contraction. Contraction is the final step which determines the behavior of the stimulated organism.

Because glandular cells, in most instances at least, are connected with the cells of the nervous system and respond, like muscle cells, to excitation transmitted by the adjustors, they too are called effector cells. The differentiation by which glands have developed their secretory function is not particularly prominent in their structure, for they look very much like simple cells of the skin. They differ, however, in their chemical function and in the way in which they deliver their secretions into the body. In fact, glands may be classified into two

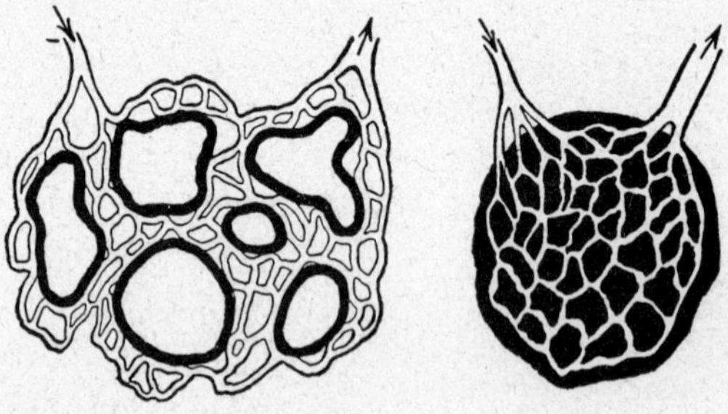

FIGURE 6. DIAGRAMS OF ENDOCRINE GLANDS

(*a*) Gland composed of irregular sacs (heavy black lines) surrounded by tissue and blood vessels (e.g., thyroid and ovary); (*b*) gland simply consisting of epithelium (black) penetrated by networks of blood vessels (white). Most endocrine glands belong to this type (adrenals, pancreas, parathyroids, hypophysis). [From A. A. Maximow and W. Bloom, *A textbook of histology* (4th ed.), Saunders, 1941, p. 291.]

principal groups: (1) *duct* or exocrine glands, like the salivary and the tear glands, which pour the product of secretion through a tube into a cavity of the body or out upon the body surface, and (2) *endocrine* glands, as shown in Fig. 6, of which the thyroid and the adrenal glands are typical, and which have no ducts but pour their secretions directly into the blood stream. Such endocrine secretions, called *hormones,* must be taken into consideration for a complete understanding of the response mechanism. We, therefore, must consider them in more detail.

Endocrine Effectors

The *adrenal glands,* for example, are known to be directly involved in the physiological expression of emotion. Two forms of secretion, both of which are circulated in the blood stream, are produced by these glands: the hormone from the *medulla* of the gland, which is called *adrenalin* (sometimes epinephrine), and the hormone of the *cortex* of the gland, which is called *cortin.* Cortin is made up of several chemically distinct hormones, active in several bodily functions. Thus cortin has a slight effect on the sugar content of the blood and tissues, but more significant is its role in controlling sodium and water content. If cortin is withdrawn by removal of the adrenal cortex, sodium is excreted through the kidneys, and the sodium level falls in the blood stream and tissues of the body. Sodium, in turn, is necessary for the retention of water in the body, and lack of cortin therefore causes dehydration. Sodium is also necessary for nervous excitability, and without it animal organisms become inactive and may eventually go into a coma and die. This condition occurs with a severe deficiency of cortin, but it may be partially remedied by feeding large amounts of sodium chloride (common salt) to make up for the large amounts lost from the body.

Besides cortin, the adrenal cortex secretes in small amounts some of the so-called androgenic hormones, hormones having the same physiological effects as the hormones secreted by the glands of sex (see below).

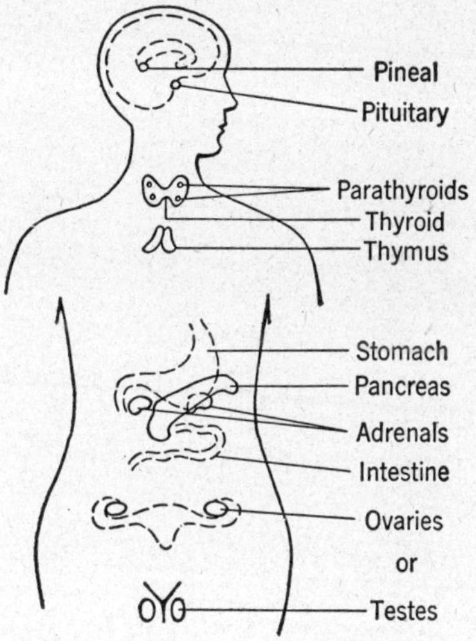

FIGURE 7. SILHOUETTE OF THE HUMAN FIGURE SHOWING LOCATION OF ENDOCRINE GLANDS

[From R. G. Hoskins, *Tides of life,* Norton, 1933, p. 19.]

Cortin is itself closely related chemically to these hormones and is derived from the same tissues in embryological development.

In many of the commonly observed features of emotion we can see the physiological effects of the hormone adrenalin which is poured into the blood stream in times of emotional reaction. An increase in the amount of adrenalin in the blood has the following effects upon physiological activity: (1) it increases the tremor in striped (voluntary) muscles; (2) it causes relaxation of smooth (involuntary) muscle; (3) it counteracts fatigue in striped muscle, by facilitating the transmission between the adjustor and the muscle effector; (4) it alters distribution of the blood in the body, sending more blood to the voluntary muscles, less to the digestive tract; (5) it increases blood pressure; (6) it hastens clotting of blood; (7) it relaxes the bronchioles in the lungs; (8) it causes the liver to release sugar into the blood stream; and (9) it causes the spleen to secrete or release red corpuscles into the blood stream. All these physiological changes brought about by adrenalin may be considered emergency reactions which prepare an organism to meet situations calling for quick and probably prolonged discharge of energy. (See pp. 95 f.)

The *thyroid gland* is directly related to the metabolism of the body, that is to say, to the destructive and constructive changes in the body tissues. Its hormone, *thyroxin,* acts as an agent which facilitates the breaking down of waste products so that they can be readily eliminated from the body. If the thyroid gland is underactive, partially decomposed proteins are retained in the tissues, oxidation is lessened, blood pressure falls and metabolic processes are generally slowed up. If the thyroid gland is overactive, on the other hand, metabolism is increased and body tissues are overstimulated.

Situated just behind the stomach, the *pancreatic gland* is attached to the intestinal tract by a duct. Through this duct, the pancreas delivers secretion to the digestive tract, thereby aiding digestion; in addition, it manufactures a hormone, *insulin,* which it pours directly into the blood. This hormone is concerned primarily in the utilization of sugar by the tissues of the body. When insulin concentration is low, as in diabetes, blood sugar does not get into the tissues to be used but remains in the blood at abnormally high levels. When insulin concentration is excessively high, the opposite process occurs, and sugar leaves the blood to be deposited in the liver, the muscles and the brain. Sugar in the blood is utilized as fuel by the brain and muscles. It is especially important for the brain, which uses sugar almost exclusively.

The *gonadal glands* are important in the development of secondary sex characteristics and also, to a considerable extent, in sexual motivation. (See pp. 116–118.) The adult's secondary sex characteristics, which are determined in great part by the gonadal hormones, include height, weight, the distribution of hair over the body, subcutaneous fat and the development of the mammary glands, all of which are features distinguishing the two sexes. In animals, moreover, these hormones are important as determiners of sexual behavior, and they are undoubtedly of significance too in the sexual behavior of man, although it has been shown that man's sexual conduct is also influenced greatly by his customs and moral codes.

The *pituitary gland,* sometimes called the master gland and located deep within the skull at the base of the brain, manufactures many different hormones. Among them are many whose principal function is to stimulate or regulate other glands of the body. There is also the growth hormone which comes from the pituitary gland and is important in regulating body growth. Deficiency of the growth hormone in childhood creates a dwarf; excess may produce a giant, a very tall person with a long spindly frame. In general, impairment of pituitary function in childhood results in a deficient body structure, weakened striped muscles and underdeveloped sex organs.

The Receptors

Receptor cells are cells upon which the physical stimuli of the environment act and which start in motion the processes by which the organism makes adjustment to stimulation. It is instructive to observe how receptors have been differentiated in evolution, changing their structures, their positions in the body and their chemical make-up so as to respond to different types of physical energy. The first primitive step (noted above) in the differentiation of receptors is the relative increase in excitability of receptor cells as compared with other tissues. Further evolution has carried this trend forward by specializing certain receptors to respond to one kind of stimulation and other receptors to be excited by other kinds. (See Fig. 8.)

As a result of this differentiation, in man, receptors may be divided into four classes: thermal (warmth and cold), mechanical, chemical and light receptors. The fourth class, the light receptors, differs from the others, in that it has arisen through the differentiation of special chemical materials in the cell which are responsive to light. In none of these specializations, however, does a receptor completely lose sensitivity to other kinds of energy change; its development results only in a special increase in one type of sensitivity. Thus the thermal receptors are more sensitive to changes in temperature than other receptors, but they can be chemically stimulated. For the mechanical receptors a mechanical stimulus is more effective than other kinds of stimuli, yet thermal stimulation may affect them.

The kind of stimulus to which a receptor is most sensitive because of its specialization is known as the *adequate stimulus;* other kinds of energy changes which will excite the receptor if presented in unusual amounts are sometimes called *inadequate stimuli,* being inappropriate and therefore less adequate. As a result of this differentiation with respect to stimuli, we have the following specific types of receptors in man: photic receptors—the eyes; mechanical receptors—the ears and the pressure receptors in the skin; chemical receptors—taste, smell, and the common chemical receptors in the mouth and nose; and thermal receptors—the receptors in the skin responsive to changes in temperature and giving rise to the sensations of warmth and of cold.

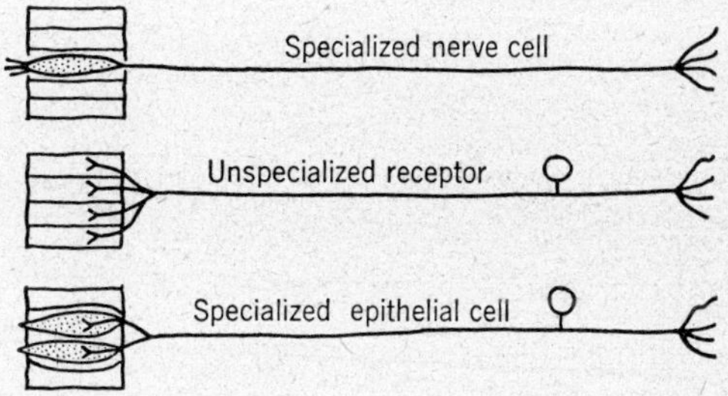

FIGURE 8. TYPES OF SPECIALIZATION OF RECEPTORS AND EPITHELIAL CELLS

[After G. H. Parker; from C. T. Morgan, *Physiological psychology,* McGraw-Hill, 1943, p. 25.]

Along with this functional differentiation of the receptors have gone changes in their structure—from simple to complex. Those chemical receptors, which are activated only by high concentrations of chemical substances, are very simple in structure and not highly differentiated in function. The receptors for taste are chemical organs which have become much more complex in structure and precise in discrimination. The receptors for smell are the most highly developed of the chemical receptors. They are nerve cells with different chemical compositions. The same differences occur for mechanical stimulation. The receptors for touch are relatively simple, for hearing (a mechanical sense) extremely complex.

We may note also how receptors have taken different positions in the body in order to be available for the different kinds

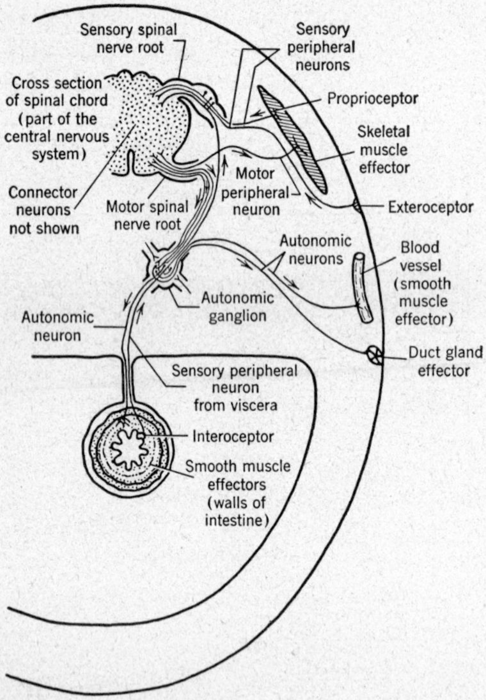

FIGURE 9. RELATIONSHIP BETWEEN THE VARIOUS CLASSES OF RECEPTORS, THE NERVOUS SYSTEM AND THE EFFECTORS

A diagram to show the relationship of exteroceptors, proprioceptors and interoceptors to the peripheral, central and autonomic nervous systems, and to the muscular and glandular effectors of the body. [Adapted from various sources.]

of stimulation which come to act at the different positions. Some of the receptors are at the surface of the body, so located that they may easily be affected by external environmental forces. These, called *exteroceptors,* are exemplified by the receptor cells of the eye. Some receptors, on the other hand, are embedded in the bodily substance itself. Typical of such receptor cells are the sensory cells of the muscles, which are stimulated by the movement of the muscle substance. Such receptors are called *proprioceptors. Proprio* means *self,* and these receptors inform the organism about itself. There are also receptors associated with the lining of the digestive tract, sometimes called *interoceptors.* (See Fig. 9.)

The Adjustors

The central nervous system—the adjustor mechanism—makes possible the different connections between receptors and effectors and consequently between the impulses coming in from receptors and going out to effectors. The possibility of this switchboard-like action is due in part to the fact that the continuity of the nervous system, as it was seen in the old nerve-net stage, has given place in the receptor-adjustor-effector system to relatively independent nerve cells or *neurons.* In understanding the function of the human nervous system, a clear knowledge of the structure, function and interdependence of neurons is important. (See Fig. 10.)

STRUCTURE AND FUNCTION OF NEURONS

First we need to establish the meanings of a few terms. The *central nervous system* consists of the brain and the spinal cord. In it lie all the adjustor mechanisms. The *peripheral nervous system* is the totality of the nerves which connect the central nervous system with the receptors and effectors. The *afferent* nervous system is the totality of nerve fibers which connect receptors with the spinal cord and the brain. It is the input or *sensory* half of the peripheral nervous system. The *efferent* nervous system

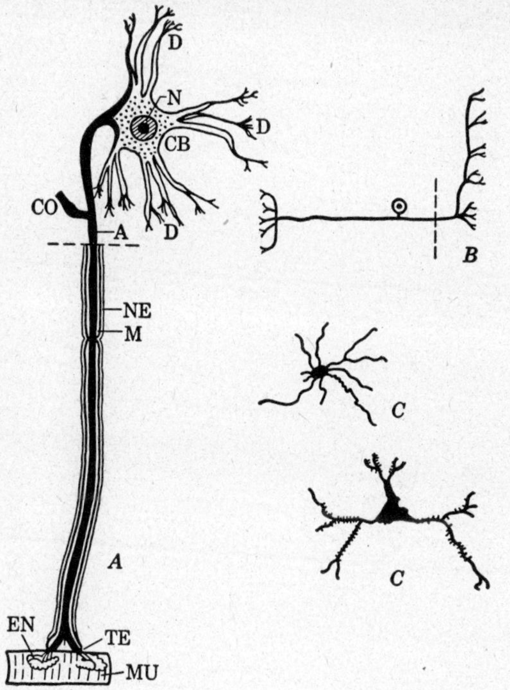

FIGURE 10. STRUCTURE OF SOME TYPICAL NEURONS

(*A*) A typical efferent (motor) neuron. (*B*) A typical afferent (sensory) neuron (in less detail than *A*). (*C*) Typical central (connector) neurons (in less detail than *A*). Abbreviations: D = dendrites, N = nucleus, CB = cell body, CO = collateral, A = axon, NE = neurilemma sheath, M = myelin (medullary sheath), MU = muscle, EN = motor end plate, TE = terminal arborization or end brush.

is the totality of nerve fibers which lead from the spinal cord and brain to the effectors. It is the output or *motor* half of the peripheral nervous system.

The basic unit of the nervous system is the *neuron,* which is a nerve cell having a cell body and nerve fibers leading to it and away from it. Impulses are ordinarily admitted to a neuron by fibers called *dendrites* and are passed on to the next neurons by the fibers called *axons.* Within the single neuron, therefore, impulses are normally transmitted from dendrite to axon.

In the simplest cases in the human body, a receptor is merely a free ending of an afferent neuron of the peripheral nervous system. More often, however, as we have just seen, a receptor is a specialized cell associated with such a neuron. The afferent peripheral neuron itself is typically a continuous thread of protoplasm connecting a receptor with the neurons of the central nervous system. The peripheral fiber of a single neuron may thus be several feet long, for it is unbroken from receptor to central nervous system, although it is microscopic in diameter. In most cases each neuron fiber is insulated by special sheaths. A great many insulated fibers are ordinarily held together by other tissue to form a cable called a *peripheral nerve.* Such nerves usually contain, at least for certain distances, many independent fibers of which some may be efferent and others afferent.

Stimulation

The energy changes which make up the world's stimuli act upon receptors or afferent neurons to cause physical and chemical changes in the fibers of the neurons. These disturbances travel—propagate themselves—along the fibers and cause similar disturbances, in turn, in neurons of the central nervous system, and eventually in the effectors. Stimulation in an animal thus initiates processes which usually lead in the course of time to effector response and a change of the individual in relation to its environment.

Stimulation is in some respects analogous to the finger pressure on the trigger which initiates the release of energy in the gunpowder of a cartridge, and thus leads to the expulsion of a bullet from a gun. Obviously, in the cartridge, the explosion of the stored energy, not the movement of the finger, is what drives the bullet. In the same way, the release by stimulation of energy stored in the receptor or neuron is what starts the nervous impulse off. Unlike the bullet, however, the impulse is not a thing which moves along a fiber. It is merely a *progressive release of energy;* that is to say, the physical energy of the stimulus does not itself go through the receptor but releases certain energies of the organism

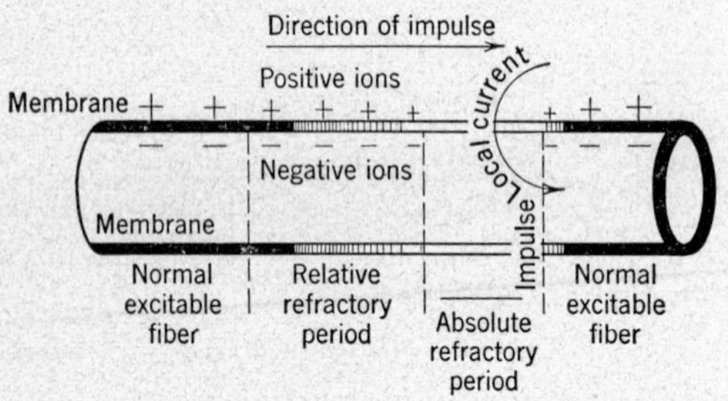

FIGURE 11. SCHEMATIC DIAGRAM OF EXCITATION AND CONDUCTION IN THE NERVE MEMBRANE

The semipermeable membrane is shown in black with the positive ions on the outside and the negative ions on the inside. A local current flows when the polarization of the membrane breaks down. That part of the membrane which is being restored after the passage of the impulse is shaded. Thus the diagram also shows the refractory periods. [Adapted from E. G. Boring.]

located in the receptor, whereupon other progressive releases of energy follow all the way along the excited fiber. Movement is analogous to the movement of fire along a train of gunpowder in which each bit of powder is ignited by a preceding bit and in turn ignites still another bit.

Recent research has shown that there are complex chemical and electrical events occurring in a receptor, neuron or effector when it is excited by a stimulus. The place of these events, it is now known, is in the membranes, not in the interior, of the microscopic neuron fiber. Across this membrane, in the normal resting neuron, there is always a difference of electrical potential, represented in Fig. 11, created between the positive ions accumulated on the outside and the negative ions accumulated on the inside of the membrane. This electrical difference, because of the arrangement of chemical ions on the two sides of the membrane, is known as *polarization* of the membrane.

The effect of the trigger-like action of a stimulus applied to the membrane is to set off a series of chemical reactions in the membrane. The most important result of these reactions is a release of energy consequent upon a sudden depolarization of the membrane and a rapid change in the resting potential across the membrane. This sudden and progressive electrical change *is* the *nervous impulse.*

If a single neuron is excited by a stimulus which sets up a nervous impulse, the neuron is always excited to its maximum extent. This principle is known as the *all-or-none law.* The law may be stated formally as follows: The magnitude of the activity in any single neural functional unit is as great as it can be in that unit at that time and is independent of the magnitude of the energy exciting it, provided only that the stimulating energy is sufficiently strong to excite the neuron at all. This law follows from the more general principle that the characteristics of the impulse at any point depend upon the state and properties of the fiber at that point and not upon the nature of preceding events.

The nervous impulse arises at any point on the neuron at which the stimulus is applied. Once initiated, it in turn becomes a stimulus to adjacent points on the membrane and thus the impulse propagates itself along the neuron fiber, like a burning train of gunpowder or a burning string, except for the fact that burning is chemical, whereas the neural impulse is an electrical depolarization which is set off by an immediately preceding depolarization. It is important to remember that the energy of the nervous impulse depends upon the energy released in the neuron, not upon the energy of the original stimulus.

The progress of a nervous impulse along a fiber may be recorded on a galvanometer (as represented in Fig. 12). On this instrument, the active region of the neuron fiber is seen to be electrically negative in relation to the unexcited portion of the same fiber, because, in nervous excitation, the normal polarization of the membrane with positive ions on the outside is destroyed and the region of depolarization (the region of the impulse) is therefore less positive and thus more negative than it was before the impulse arrived. This region of negativity, which is the measure of the impulse, travels on down the neuron. Though the impulse travels in mammalian neurons at varying speeds, a speed of approximately one hundred meters a second, or two hundred miles an hour, may be taken as typical. Such a speed, though relatively fast, is, of course, in no way comparable to the speed of light or the speed of an electrical impulse in a wire. It is only about a quarter as fast as the speed of sound.

Returning for a moment to the analogue of the burning trail of gunpowder, we may note that, once a gunpowder trail has been burned, it cannot be ignited again until new energy in the form of a new trail of powder has once more been laid down. In the nerve, there is a similar effect. Immediately following the peak of the nervous impulse, there is a period during which the nerve fiber cannot be activated again, no matter how strong the stimulus. The potential difference has been used up. This time interval is known technically as the *absolute refractory period.* Then, following this period, there is an interval of continuous recovery during which the neuron may be stimulated again, provided the stimulus is stronger than the minimal stimulus which ordinarily is effective. This

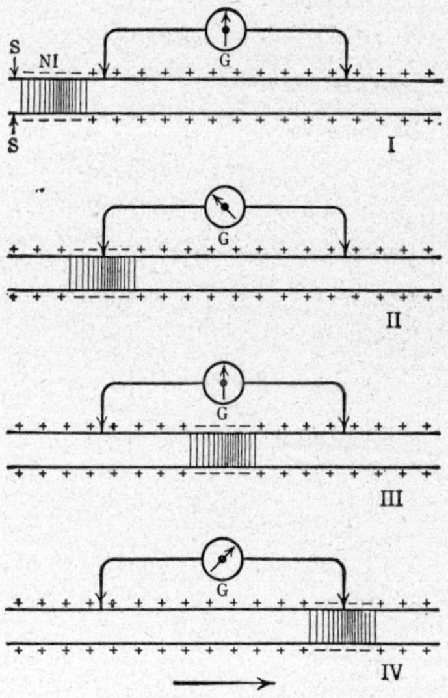

FIGURE 12. PROPAGATION OF AN ELECTRICAL DISTURBANCE ALONG A NEURON FIBER

I, II, III, IV show successive time intervals as the impulse passes from left to right. The galvanometer deflection is indicated in each case. It will be noticed that the impulse is marked by a negative deflection. Abbreviations: S = stimulus, NI = nerve impulse, G = galvanometer.

second interval is called the *relative refractory period.* At the end of the relative refractory period, the excitability of the neuron has completely recovered and the neuron is again ready for activation by a stimulus of normal degree. In certain neurons, especially in the larger sensory neurons and when the neurons are not greatly fatigued, it has been demonstrated that there may be a brief period, immediately following the relative refractory period, during which a stimulus of an intensity less than that normally required to excite the resting nerve may be effective. The time during which this phenomenon is possible has been called the *supernormal* period. A diagram of the relation of these various periods is given in Fig. 13.

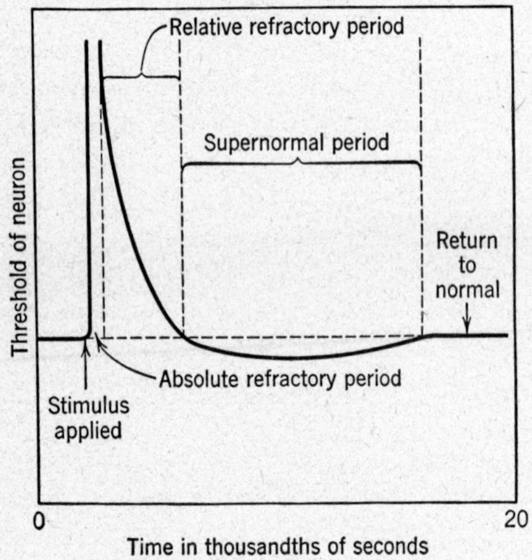

FIGURE 13. NERVE EXCITATION

Graph shows schematically the absolute and relative refractory periods and the supernormal period.

Mechanisms of Intensity

Because animals and human beings are quite capable of appreciating differences in the intensity of various stimuli, it is interesting to see how nervous impulses may represent these differences in the intensity of stimulation. Increasing the intensity of stimulation may affect nervous impulses in two ways: (1) it may increase the frequency of successive nerve impulses in a particular neuron fiber and (2) it may increase the number of fibers in which there are nervous impulses.

Laboratory experiments show how increasing the intensity of the stimulus may increase the number of nerve impulses in a single neuron fiber. If a stimulus is applied continuously to a fiber, a strong stimulus will reexcite the fiber at an earlier stage of the refractory period than a weak one. Consequently, an intense continued stimulus produces a relatively rapid series of successive impulses, whereas a weak stimulus may produce a less rapid series. The rate of discharge in a peripheral nerve fiber thus tends to become greater the more intense the physical energy of the stimulus applied to it. The total limits of this frequency are, as can be seen (Fig. 13), always determined by the time limits of the relative and absolute refractory periods of the neurons in question.

The second neural mechanism of intensity is an increase in the number of neurons being excited. To understand this mechanism, it should not be forgotten that, in many of the sense organs, as well as in centers of the nervous system, there are many receptors or neurons exposed at the same time to every strong stimulus. The neurons and receptors differ among themselves with respect to their excitabilities, so that a stimulus of a particular physical intensity may call into action some, but not all, of the neurons being stimulated.

From this description it can be seen that, when the intensity of the stimulus applied to a group of neurons increases, an increasing number of individual neurons is activated as each neuron reacts in an all-or-none manner. It thus appears that an increase in the intensity of a stimulus may be associated in the peripheral nervous system with an *increase in number of units* affected as well as with an increase in the *number of impulses per second* in each fiber involved. These two factors jointly determine the intensity of sensation.

Synaptic Connections

In order to come to an understanding of the response mechanism, we have dealt with the structure and properties of individual neurons. Not single neurons, however, but myriads of them, connected with each other in many diverse ways, make up the central nervous system. Someone has calculated that there are approximately twelve billion neurons in the central nervous system. At first, this inconceivable complexity might seem to balk any hope of understanding the mechanisms of the nervous system. It is well to remember, however, that, no matter what the complications of this system may be, it is possible to look at it as basically organized for the purpose of making connections between incoming and outgoing nerve impulses.

Neurons, according to most observers, are not actually connected one with another, for each is an individual cell with its own membrane. Nevertheless, the fibers of the neurons interlace to form functionally effective junctures, which are known as *synapses*. Nowadays a general understanding of the nervous system requires a knowledge not only of the properties of the individual neurons but also of the special anatomical and functional characteristics of synapses.

Three of these synaptic characteristics are worthy of special attention. (1) In the synapse, fibers tend to divide many times into small terminals which come in contact with the terminals of other neurons or, in some cases, with the body of another neuron. (2) By virtue of the fact that each neuron has, usually, several collaterals or branches of its fibers, one neuron usually makes connections with many other neurons, both afferent and efferent. Thus, synapses may be regarded as 'choice points' from which nervous activity may be transmitted along different neurons. (3) The synapse acts as a valve, permitting passage of the impulse only from axon to dendrite. It is the synapses that limit the nerve fibers to one-way traffic.

For many years psychologists have thought of the synapses as having resistance, just as water in a large main meets resistance when it comes to a small outlet, or as an electrical current is resisted when it is conducted through a very small wire. The notion of synaptic resistance should be regarded only as an analogy, but there are conditions at the synapse which give it resistive characteristics. For one thing, we know from the all-or-none law that the size of the nervous impulse is reduced when it comes to the very small terminals which are common at the synapses. For another thing 'conduction across a synapse' means, of course, that the nerve impulse at the terminals of the fibers of one neuron must initiate an impulse in a second neuron, in spite of the discontinuity of the membranes. For this reason one would expect transmission of the nerve impulse to be more easily blocked at a synapse than along a neuron fiber.

Out of these anatomical and functional characteristics of the synapses arise some properties of the central nervous system which are not ordinarily seen in peripheral nerves. One of these properties is *spatial summation*. In many cases an impulse coming along a fiber to a synapse is not sufficiently strong to excite, by itself, the nerve fiber on the other side of the synapse. Instead, it is necessary that two, three or even more impulses arrive along different fibers and stimulate the same region across the synapse simultaneously. In this way the effect of impulses arriving at the central nervous system over afferent neurons is summative. Such spatial summation is encountered in sensory phenomena and reflex behavior. For instance, a tiny spot of light, too faint to be perceived, may become visible if its size is doubled, simply because more adjacent fibers are activated simultaneously and their impulses are summated at some synaptic point.

Another important characteristic of activity in the central nervous system is *reverberation.*

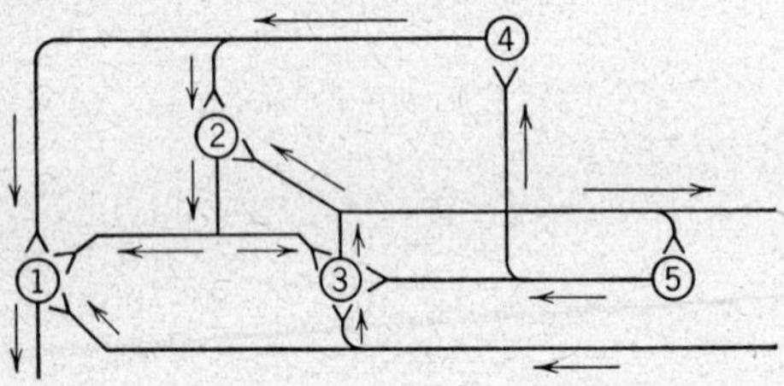

FIGURE 14. RECURRENT (REVERBERATORY) NERVE CIRCUITS

The circles represent cell bodies; the lines represent the axons and dendrites. Direction of the nerve impulse is indicated by the arrows. [From C. T. Morgan, *Physiological psychology,* McGraw-Hill, 1943, p. 64.]

By tracing, with electrical recording, the impulses in groups of neurons in certain centers of the nervous system, it has been possible to demonstrate that neurons are frequently arranged in circuits in which the fiber of one neuron comes back and ends on the neuron whose fiber stimulated the first neuron. A typical arrangement of neurons in such a *recurrent nervous circuit* is shown diagrammatically in Fig. 14. Such an arrangement of neurons means that in the central nervous system activity may be set up by a stimulus and, unlike the situation in peripheral neurons, may continue for some time after the stimulus has disappeared. This principle of reverberation has many important applications in understanding the response mechanism and human psychological capacities. It accounts in some instances for the persistence of sensory motivation. A pang of hunger or surge of fear, for example, may start activity. Often the activity persists, even though the hunger or fear subsides. The nervous system seems often to hang on to such motives, and reverberation may well be the mechanism.

A third characteristic of central nervous function is *recruitment.* This term refers to a progressive increase in the number of nerve fibers giving nervous impulses as the exciting impulse is repeated. The phenomenon of recruitment is based on the fact that the excitability of a neuron varies from time to time and that, on repeated stimulation, the fiber that fails to respond on the first or second try may be activated on the third or fourth because by that time it has, in the random variation of its sensitivity, become more excitable. Once excited, there is a tendency for a nerve fiber to continue giving nervous impulses because of the chance of stimulation during the supernormal phase.

Recruitment has also been demonstrated in peripheral nerves, but it is a more important phenomenon in the central nervous system. Recruitment, especially when taken in connection with reverberation, explains many cases in which persistent activity becomes more vigorous as it persists. Reverberation and recruitment are stabilizing factors in the lives of the higher vertebrates. They keep the organism from mirroring in its behavior every casual change in its stimulating environment.

STRUCTURE OF THE NERVOUS SYSTEM

It is now time, after being introduced to neurons and synaptic functions, to take up the nervous system as a whole and to consider its general structure and functions. This system, in man, is made up of the brain, the spinal cord, the autonomic nervous system, the afferent peripheral nervous system, the receptors, the efferent peripheral nervous system and the effectors (Fig. 15).

The *spinal cord* is the part of the nervous system that is enclosed in the jointed bony case of the vertebral column. It is connected with receptors and effectors by more than thirty pairs of spinal peripheral nerves. The spinal cord is primarily to be thought of as a cable of insulated fibers, by means of which impulses initiated at the receptors may be transmitted to and from the higher centers of the brain. Yet the cord is also in its own right a center for the connection of afferent and efferent neurons taking part in the action of relatively simple reflexes.

Continuous with the spinal cord and protected by the bony case of the skull is a very complex system of nerve centers and communication tracks known as the *brain.* Immediately above the cord and in continuity with it is located the *medulla oblongata.* Like the cord, the medulla is an important adjustment center in its own right, but it is primarily—again like the cord—to be regarded as a great cable of fibers connecting the spinal system below with the higher brain centers above. In addition, however, it plays a vital role in the control of certain bodily functions, such as breathing, heart rate and circulation of the blood.

Situated above the medulla, and, as it were, off the main track of the central nervous system, are the two hemispheres of the *cerebellum,* which functions in the coordination of bodily movements. In front of the cerebellum, there is a large structure, the *pons,* made up of fiber tracks and specialized adjustment centers. Above the cerebellum and pons is an elaborate series of special connecting centers, all of which play an important part in the adjustment

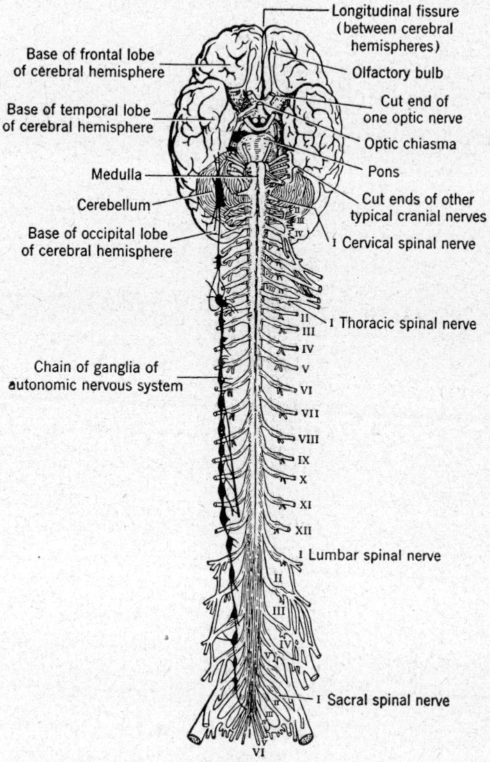

FIGURE 15. BASE OF BRAIN AND SPINAL CORD

Heavy black structure at left of cord indicates part of autonomic nervous system. [Adapted from C. J. Herrick, *An introduction to neurology,* 1931; by permission of the W. B. Saunders Co.]

of impulses and in the adaptation of the organism to its environment. Much is known concerning these centers, and much is still to be discovered. It is impossible to review here their anatomical relationships. It is important to note, nevertheless, that, before we reach the cerebral cortex, the upper level of the central nervous system, we pass through a complex group of amplifying and contributing centers known as the *thalamus,* or thalamic region. The thalamus proper is concerned mainly with relaying afferent impulses on their way from the sense organs to the cerebral cortex, but the parts known as the subthalamus and *hypothalamus* are concerned with the control and coordination of bodily functions involved in metabolism, and the hypothalamus has also a special role in the expression of emotion. More will be said elsewhere (see p. 100) concerning this function of the hypothalamic region.

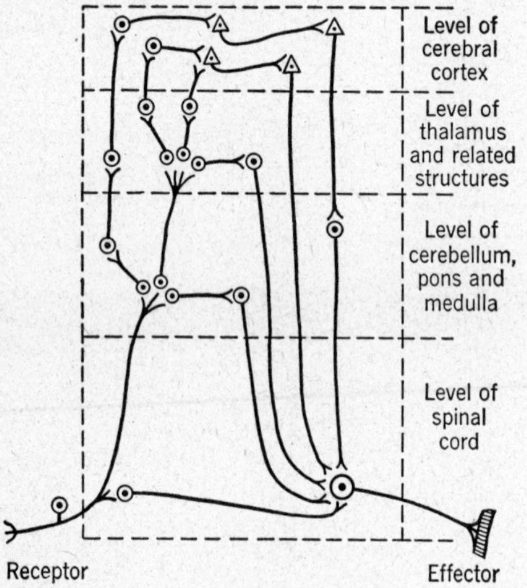

FIGURE 16. LEVELS OF THE CENTRAL NERVOUS SYSTEM

Schematic diagram showing alternative loops at various levels of the central nervous system. Many other schemes of levels in the nervous system have been proposed. The diagram given here does not represent an accepted view of the hierarchy of governing centers but is given to emphasize the fact that there are levels in the brain and that they influence each other. [Adapted from W. M. Bayliss, *Principles of general physiology,* 1927; by permission of Longmans, Green.]

In man, by far the largest part of the brain is the great *cerebrum,* which is divided into two *cerebral hemispheres.* Large, closely organized masses of neurons, these structures almost fit the skull. The surface of the hemispheres is the cerebral *cortex.* It is convoluted and deeply fissured, and in it lie the cell bodies of the cerebral neurons, the gray matter of the brain. The cerebrum is constructed both to receive impulses from and to send impulses back to the lower levels of the central nervous system. It thus forms an adjustment center for recircuiting and patterning impulses, a center superimposed, as it were, upon the lower, more immediate, connecting centers of the central nervous system. Sometimes the activities of the cerebral hemispheres facilitate processes already in progress in lower centers; sometimes, on the contrary, they inhibit such processes.

The Efferent Peripheral Nervous System

We have seen how sensory activity tends to spread out over many paths, ultimately involving many regions of the central nervous system. Often it is this total complex of excitation that determines just which effectors shall be activated and how. Distributed excitation must be brought together to act along particular efferent paths upon specific effectors if response is to be adequate to the needs of the organism. We may think then of the efferent system as the place where excitation converges upon final common neural paths to produce response.

The *final common path* is the name applied to the avenue along which all impulses, no matter whence they come, must travel, if they are to act on particular muscle fibers or glands and bring about the corresponding response. Thus activities in various parts of the brain and spinal cord, which have resulted, it may be, from exteroceptive stimulation, can be brought into relation with impulses from other parts of the central nervous system which have themselves originated, for example, in the proprioceptors of certain muscles. Some of these impulses may mutually strengthen or *facilitate* one another; some may act in such a way as to lead to mutual extinction or *inhibition.* In the normal individual the outcome of such complex adjustment is the finely graded and precisely timed effector response. In this way activities occur which make up adaptive, intelligent behavior.

The Autonomic Nervous System

In a complete consideration of the motor aspects of the response mechanism, it is necessary to deal with the so-called autonomic nervous system, a motor nervous system which enjoys a measure of independence from the great peripheral and central systems already considered. This system, together with the secretions of the endocrine glands, constitutes a *neurohumoral* system which, to a large degree, controls the organic functions of the body—the digestive functions, the circulatory functions and others that are connected with efficient action.

The autonomic nervous system is essentially a nerve net of interconnections. Anatomically, it is divided into the *sympathetic* and *parasympathetic* divisions. The parasympathetic division is composed of the *cranial* and *sacral* sections. Figure 17 is a schematic diagram of the interrelations of these divisions and their relationship to the various bodily organs.

Generally speaking, the activity of the sympathetic division is antagonistic to that of the parasympathetic; for example, the heart rate is inhibited by nervous excitation reaching it over the parasympathetic, while it is accelerated by excitation from the sympathetic. On the whole, the action of the autonomic nervous system, which serves involuntary muscles and glands, is diffuse and relatively slow in effect compared with that of the central nervous sys-

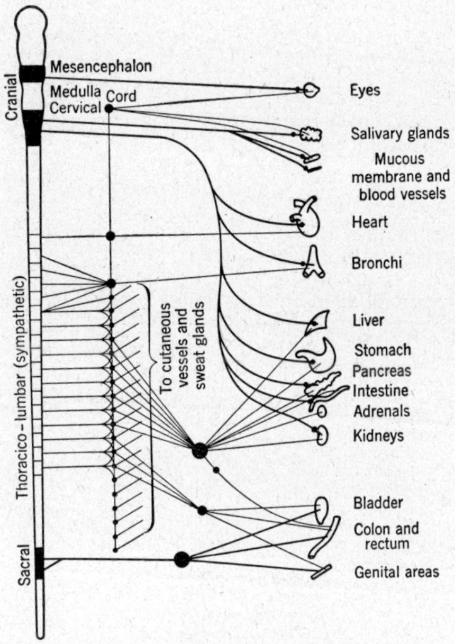

FIGURE 17. AUTONOMIC NERVOUS SYSTEM—SCHEMATIC DIAGRAM

[Reprinted from *Bodily Changes in Pain, Hunger, Fear and Rage* by Walter B. Cannon, by permission of W. W. Norton & Company, Inc. Copyright 1915, 1920 by D. Appleton-Century Co., copyright 1929 by Walter B. Cannon.]

tem. (See the further discussion of the uses of this system in emotion, pp. 94 f.)

FUNCTIONS OF THE BRAIN

There are certain general problems of the central nervous system in which the student of mental phenomena is keenly interested.

One of these, about which there has been much speculation, is the relationship between brain weight and intellectual ability. When a formula is used which makes possible the comparison between the ratios of brain weight to body weight, it is found that there is some positive relationship between the relative brain weight and adaptability, as far as the various species of animals in the evolutionary series are concerned. Animals with brains that are large in proportion to the size of their bodies tend to be more adaptable, more clever. It has not been demonstrated, however, that this relationship also holds true statistically in comparing human beings of different intellectual abilities.

Localization in the Brain

Another problem of interest in the functioning of the central nervous system is the localization of various psychological functions in the brain. This problem has been extensively investigated in recent years by a variety of techniques: by observing the effects of accidental destruction of brain tissue in human individuals, by experimental removal of parts of the brain in animals preceded and followed by tests of behavior of various sorts, by directly stimulating with electrical stimuli centers of the brain in animals and in human beings to get observations or verbal reports of the effects and by using various methods of the electrical recording of activity in the nervous system.

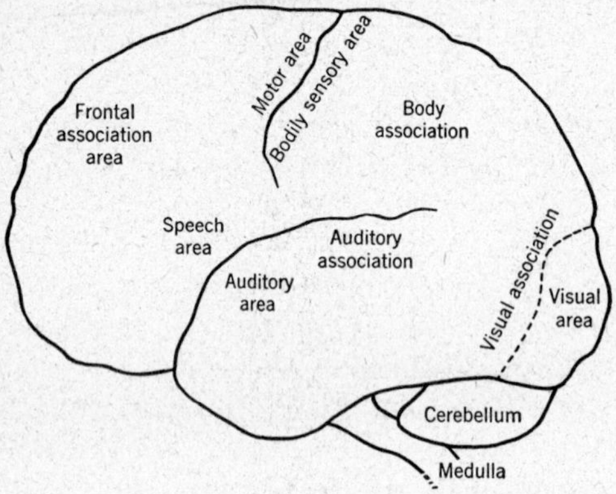

FIGURE 18. HUMAN CEREBRAL CORTEX SHOWING LOCALIZATION OF MENTAL FUNCTIONS

Diagram of side-view of cortex. [From C. T. Morgan, *Physiological psychology,* McGraw-Hill, 1943, p. 16.]

We know now that there is a considerable amount of localization of psychological functions in the brain; on the other hand, there is also a considerable independence of the various parts of the brain, such that many mental functions depend on several different areas of the brain or even, in some cases, it would seem, on the brain as a whole.

The simplest aspects of perceiving and acting are well localized. In rats and other animals below man these functions are localized in part at subcortical levels; but in man, though the subcortical centers still exist, they are concerned mainly with simple reflex reactions to stimuli, and the primary centers for perceiving and acting are cortical.

In the occipital region at the extreme back of the head is the area for seeing. Destruction of this area causes almost complete blindness in man, leaving him with only the crudest appreciation of light and dark but depriving him of ability to see objects and to perceive color. In the temporal lobes at the side of the head are the primary cortical areas for hearing. We know less about them than the visual areas, but their loss, by destruction or operation, causes 'cortical deafness' which is considerable, if not complete. Along and behind the central fissure in the cerebrum, a fissure which lies under the skull on a line running roughly from the center and top of the head toward the ear, is the area representing the sensations of the body—pressure, pain and temperature as well as proprioceptive sensations from the muscles. It is interesting to note that when this area is exposed under local anesthesia and stimulated by electricity, it is possible to obtain reports from the patient of the occurrence of the proper sensory experiences.

Just in front of, but also running along, the central fissure is the *motor area* of the brain. It is not so well defined in lower animals, but in monkeys and in man it is the area through which 'voluntary' acts of behavior are controlled. By direct electrical stimulation of different parts of the motor area one may produce movement of the fingers, the legs or the mouth, depending upon just which spot is stimulated. By exciting the right spot it is possible to get 'forced' vocalization, voiced sounds from the larynx. Extirpation or destruction of this area causes paralysis of muscles in voluntary acts. This is what we see in a person who has suffered a 'stroke' or apoplectic attack.

Both the motor area and the bodily sensation area lying near it are laid out like a map of the body, with those spots near the top of the head representing the feet and legs, those along the sides the hands and arms, and those farther to the sides the face and mouth.

Although simple perceiving and acting depend on specific areas, more complex perception, learning and memory are not so well localized. There is, however, good reason to believe that there are sensory association areas, situated immediately adjacent to the primary areas for sensation and concerned in the more complex perceptions of the respective senses. Thus the *visual association area* seems to be necessary for coordinated responses to seen objects and may well play a role in visual remembering. The *auditory association area* is needed in auditory space perception, the orienting of the body in relation to the direction of the source of sound. It is thought also to be essential to auditory recall. These functions, however, are not fully established, and much more research is needed before this chapter of brain psychology can be written.

For the majority of complex memories and intellectual activities in man there is only a rough localization of functions. It is possible to distinguish between *receptive* memory functions, involving the recognition and naming of objects and the meaning of experiences, and *expressive* functions, consisting of memories for skills and ways of doing things. In general, receptive types of memories, as in simple perception, reside in the back portion of the cerebral cortex, particularly in the areas not directly concerned with sensation, whereas expressive types of memory are dependent on the frontal areas of the cortex lying ahead of the motor area.

Worthy of particular mention is recent research concerning the function of the extreme *frontal association areas.* Although the whole cerebral cortex seems to be concerned in reasoning and thinking, a man's ability to order his behavior and direct it toward a goal depends especially on these areas. In certain standard tests with monkeys, for example, in which it is necessary to use tools or rakes in a certain order—first a short rake is used to obtain a longer rake, and then that rake in turn is used to obtain a longer rake, in order eventually to obtain food—in these tests monkeys deprived of their frontal association areas are unable to solve the problem. In man, similarly, destruction of the frontal areas interferes with ability to synthesize acts into a complete pattern and, in particular, to plan and administer daily activities.

This function of the frontal areas of the

cortex has been recognized in the surgical treatment of mental disorders. Certain types of patients, who suffer from such an excess of anxiety and planning of their lives that they are depressed or are obsessed with complex, compulsive rituals of behavior, have been treated by partial removal of the frontal areas (prefrontal lobectomy) or by interrupting the fibers which go to and from these areas (prefrontal lobotomy). This treatment has had some success in relieving patients. Along with the good results there has been some loss in their ability to plan their behavior; yet, all in all, the results have been good.

REFERENCES

1. Adrian, E. D. *The mechanism of nervous action: electrical studies of the neuron.* Philadelphia: University of Pennsylvania Press, 1932.

   A short series of lectures outlining the methods of electro-physiology and the nature of action potentials in various types of nerves.

2. Boring, E. G. *Sensation and perception in the history of experimental psychology.* New York: D. Appleton-Century, 1942. Chap. 2.

   Chapter 2 gives a brief history of experiments in nerve conduction.

3. Cannon, W. B., and Rosenblueth, A. *Autonomic neuro-effector systems.* New York: Macmillan, 1937.

   A monograph summarizing a great deal of research on the functions of the autonomic nervous system and particularly on the role of chemical messengers in synaptic conduction.

4. Creed, R. S., Denny-Brown, D., Eccles, J. C., Liddell, E. G. T., and Sherrington, C. S. *Reflex activity of the spinal cord.* Oxford: Clarendon Press, 1932.

   A summary of experiments on reflex action and synaptic functions in the nervous system.

5. Erlanger, J., and Gasser, H. S. *Electrical signs of nervous activity.* Philadelphia: University of Pennsylvania Press, 1937.

   A monograph covering experiments on action-potentials. It illustrates especially well the methods by which one can determine the functions of different groups of fibers in different nerves.

6. Forbes, A. The mechanism of reaction. In C. Murchison (Ed.), *A handbook of general experimental psychology.* Worcester, Mass.: Clark University Press, 1934. Chap. 3.

   A comprehensive review of the functions of the nervous system forming the background of behavior. It is now a little out of date.

7. Freeman, W. J., and Watts, J. W. *Psychosurgery.* Springfield, Ill.: C. C. Thomas, 1942.

   An account of use of brain operations in human patients performed to alleviate or cure certain types of mental disorder.

8. Fulton, J. F. *Selected readings in the history of physiology.* Springfield, Ill.: C. C. Thomas, 1930. Chaps. 6 and 7.

   Excerpts from the classical writings on the action of the nervous system and of muscles by thirty-two physiologists from the second century down to 1926. A third of the excerpts belong to the twentieth century.

9. Fulton, J. F. *Physiology of the nervous system.* (Rev. ed.) New York: Oxford University Press, 1943.

   A comprehensive, up-to-date textbook on the functions of the nervous system.

10. Gardner, E. *Fundamentals of neurology.* Philadelphia: Saunders, 1947.

    Contains excellent illustrations of the nervous system.

11. Herrick, C. J. *Brains of rats and men.* Chicago: University of Chicago Press, 1926.

    An elementary description of brain anatomy and functions.

12. Hill, A. V. *Muscular activity.* Baltimore: Williams and Wilkins, 1926.

    A summary of classical researches on muscle contraction, the nervous excitation of muscles and muscular work.

13. Lillie, R. S. *Protoplasmic action and nervous action.* (2nd ed.) Chicago: University of Chicago Press, 1932.

    A discussion and summary of biochemical problems of propagation and integration of nervous impulses.

14. Marquis, D. G. The neurology of learning. In F. A. Moss (Ed.), *Comparative psychology*. New York: Prentice-Hall, 1942. Chap. 7.

An excellent summary, not too technical, of what is known of brain functions in learning and memory.

15. Papez, J. W. *Comparative neurology*. New York: Thomas Y. Crowell, 1929.

An old but useful introduction to neurology in animals and man.

16. Parker, G. H. *The elementary nervous system*. Philadelphia: J. B. Lippincott, 1919.

A classical description of the evolution of the nervous system in simple invertebrate animals.

17. Weisenburg, T., and McBride, K. *Aphasia*. New York: The Commonwealth Fund, 1935.

An advanced but readable treatment of the localization of psychological functions, particularly language functions, in the human brain.

CHAPTER 3

Response

MAN is seldom, if ever, quiet in his waking moments, nor is he very tranquil in sleep. In response to stimulation he is constantly making movements, though often they are hardly noticeable. There are the incipient movements of his vocal organs and other muscles while he is thinking, the ever-recurring eyewink, the shifting of his limbs, the restless movement of his body, the frequent turning of his head, as well as the more coordinated activities like walking, talking, piano playing and tennis. All such behavior is directed primarily toward a manipulation and understanding of things of the external world. It is this behavior with which the psychologist is chiefly concerned. Such movements are dependent, for the most part, on the striped muscles. There are, in addition, the actions of the smooth muscles, like those connected with the functions of nutrition and of reproduction, but these movements are mainly of interest to the physiologist.

The importance of the behavior which the psychologist studies need hardly be emphasized. If we may judge from the lower forms of life, such as the sponge whose muscles are stimulated by direct contact only, behavior was present in the evolution of life even before the development of a nervous system. It is the means by which the organism, in order to survive, becomes adapted to the ever-changing external situation. We have seen in the previous chapter what are the physiological mechanisms which affect the behavior of the organism. Our present task is to survey the kinds and characteristics of the various responses which make up this behavior.

VARIETIES OF BEHAVIOR

There are many ways to classify human and animal behavior. We may inquire whether an act has been learned through experience or whether it is an innate characteristic of the organism, whether it is evoked by external stimuli or whether it arises from a need within the organism, whether it is automatic or conscious and voluntary, and whether it is a movement of the body as a whole or of a part or limb in particular. All these distinctions have their place in helping us to understand man's behavior, and we shall employ them in a description of the varieties of behavior.

Locomotion and Manipulation

Since the maintenance of life is dependent upon the physical environment—the supply of food, water, oxygen and sunshine, and protection from extremes of tempera-

This chapter was prepared by Clifford T. Morgan of The Johns Hopkins University.

ture—living things either must use what is available as plants do, or they must try to change their environment as animals do. Most behavior may be classified in terms of whether the individual changes its environment by moving about, or by manipulating or altering it to suit his needs. For example, in the autumn many of the birds migrate from north to south to obtain a warmer climate and a more abundant food supply. Man, on the other hand, can build and heat a shelter, and can grow, preserve and store food for the winter months. The former action we call locomotor behavior, the latter manipulatory behavior.

Locomotor behavior is the more primitive. It is interesting to note that in lower invertebrate forms, such as the worm, and also in the lower vertebrates, such as fishes, organisms must adjust to their environment merely by swallowing some of it or by moving to and fro within it. The higher invertebrate and vertebrate forms, however—insects, most of the mammals, monkeys and man—have evolved appendages with which they can manipulate objects in their environment, and in this way they adjust themselves to it or adjust it to themselves. Thus the worm or the fish can avoid light only by moving away from it, but man can turn the light out. The fish procures its food by swimming to it and grabbing it in its mouth, but the monkey can use its hands to pick bananas from the tree, and man can eat by manipulating a fork and a spoon. A worm gets a home by burrowing in the ground, but man, by handling a hammer and saw, builds himself a house.

As we look at evolutionary history, we see that the development of appendages, an important aid to locomotion, accompanied change of the animal's habitat from the water to the land. An earlier step was taken, however, when animals began to use their mouths to manipulate the environment. This is the only way in which many animals can alter their environments. The insects, for example, carry food to their nests by clasping it in their mandibles. Birds construct nests with their beaks. The dog retrieves a stick by carrying it in his mouth.

It was late in evolution that animals began to use their limbs for manipulation. A rat can, under appropriate circumstances, learn to pull a string with its forefeet in order to obtain food. Monkeys are skillful with their hands, and chimpanzees can handle tools to solve many problems. Man, however, represents a tremendous refinement in manipulative ability: in the precise movements of his hands and fingers and in the extremely delicate coordination of his vocal apparatus and of his eyes. It is his use of a very small part of himself to alter his environment that has made man capable of his mechanical and engineering achievements.

Tropisms and Reflexes

The distinction between the use of the whole body or some part of it in an act of behavior is also useful in understanding two other varieties of behavior, the tropism and the reflex. Both types of behavior, unlike any others, are relatively stereotyped immediate reactions to stimuli. The tropism, however, is an orientation or movement of the whole body with respect to a stimulus, whereas the reflex is the movement of a specific part, such as a leg or an eyelid, in response to a stimulus.

We get the concept of the tropism from observation of the behavior of plants, such as the sunflower's turning its face toward the sun in the daytime and drooping it toward the ground in the night. Orientation toward the sun is a *heliotropism,* and orientation toward light in general is a *phototropism.* Many of the lower animals, especially the insects, also show phototropic behavior. Some, like the night bugs which seek the light on a summer evening, are positively phototropic; others, like the cockroach which scurries out of the light into the dark corner, are negatively phototropic.

There are many other kinds of tropism. The larval salamander, for example, displays a *galvanotropism* to electrical stimulation. It lowers its head and tail, arching the body concavely, when the positive electrode is near the head and the negative one near the tail; it raises its head and tail, arching its body convexly, when the direction of electrical stimulation is reversed. Many animals which live in the water show a *rheotropism,* an orientation and a swimming movement opposite to the current. We may see such a rheotropism in fish swimming upstream or attempting to jump a falls. There is also *geotropism,* a response elicited by the force of gravity (the cat lands on its feet), and *stereotropism,* elicited by the surfaces with which the body makes contact (the mouse hugs the wall as it runs). These are but a few of the tropistic responses. All of them have the characteristics that (1) they are not learned, (2) they are controlled by external stimuli rather than by volition, (3) they are orienting responses involving approach to stimulation or withdrawal from it, and (4) they involve the entire organism rather than some part of it.

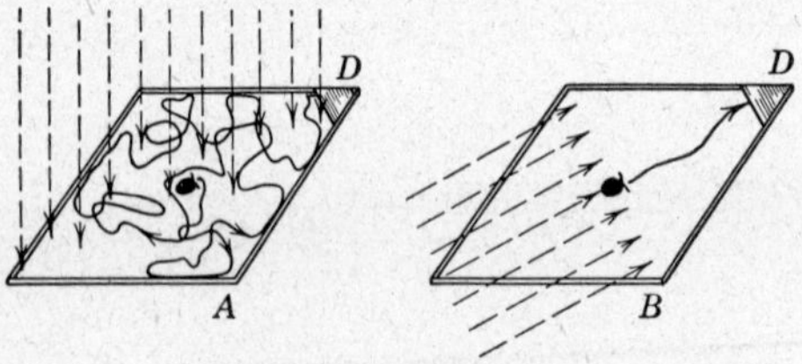

FIGURE 19. NEGATIVE PHOTOTROPIC BEHAVIOR IN THE 'SOWBUG'

(*A*) When light from above illuminates diffusely the surface, the bug wanders around randomly until it accidentally finds the dark corner (*D*). (*B*) When light is directed from one side, the bug moves directly away from it to the dark corner. [From N. R. F. Maier and T. C. Schneirla, *Principles of animal psychology,* McGraw-Hill, 1935, p. 131.]

We see little that can be called tropistic behavior in man and the higher animals. Just as specific manipulative responses have in large part displaced locomotion as a means of adjusting to the environment, so reflex responses of parts of the organism have, in man and the higher animals, taken the place of the gross orienting movements in the tropistic behavior of the lower animals.

The *reflexes* may be defined as involuntary and prompt responses of the striped or the smooth muscles of the body. In the human repertoire of behavior there is a great variety of such reflex acts. If liquid gets into the throat of an infant, its muscles immediately respond and the liquid is swallowed; if there is too much liquid, the infant chokes. It begins breathing at birth as a reflex response to lack of oxygen and accumulation of carbon dioxide in its blood. Its eyelids close automatically at a loud noise or when something moves rapidly toward its eyes. These are a few early examples of man's many reflexes.

It will aid our understanding of the reflex to consider briefly its physiological mechanism. The simplest form of reflex would require a receptor, a sensory neuron, a motor neuron and an effector. Such a simple *reflex arc,* however, is not found isolated functionally from all other parts of the nervous system in a mature human organism. Take, for example, the following illustration of a spinal reflex. If we pinch the paw of a dog whose spinal cord has been cut just below the brain, we can still obtain a withdrawal or flexion of the one paw accompanied by a forward thrust of the other paw. A relatively simple neural arc is involved in the flexion of the paw, but even here more than one motor neuron is necessary to bend the leg; and, besides, there must be a connection in the spinal cord between the sensory neuron and the motor neuron going to the opposite leg to produce the thrust of that leg. There are also connections between these arcs and many more remote reflexes, which, if stimulated at the same time, may exert either an inhibitory or facilitating effect upon the first reflex. Furthermore, when the central nervous system is intact, the legs may be moved voluntarily—a fact which means that there are connections between the spinal reflex arc and the cerebrum. This brief sketch of the physiology of the reflex arc is given to emphasize once more the fact that even the simplest form of response involves a complicated neural and muscular pattern.

By observing reflex acts in young infants, or even in human and animal fetuses before birth, one can see that the maturing of certain parts of the response mechanism is necessary for the appearance of reflexes. There may be, in addition, some stimulation necessary for their appearance (see below), but in the broad sense of the term reflexes are unlearned acts. Once firmly established, they remain stable and predictable, many of them being common to all organisms of the same species.

Conditioned Response

Pavlov, a famous Russian physiologist, was the first to demonstrate experimentally that there are learned reflexes, and that they appear through the *conditioning* of unlearned reflexes. Pavlov stimulated a dog with the sound of a bell for a brief period, then gave it food and measured the resulting flow of saliva. After a considerable number of such pairings of bell with food, the sound of the bell alone would call forth the saliva in somewhat the same manner as had the food, that is to say, the bell had taken the place of the food as a stimulus to salivation. Pavlov called this fact a *conditioned reflex.*

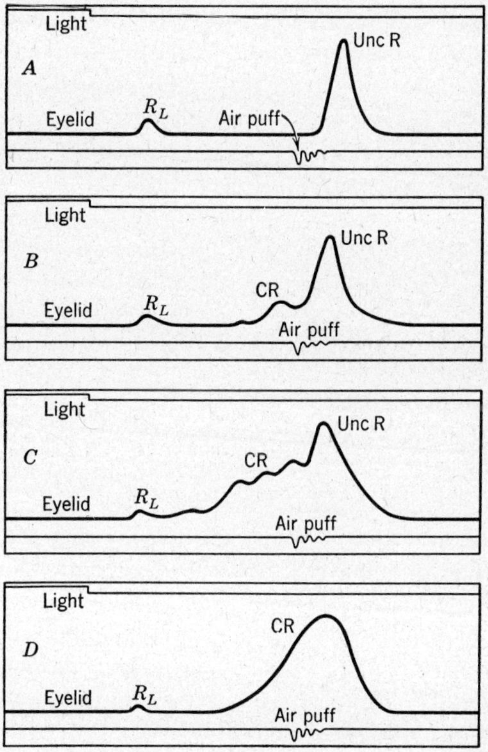

FIGURE 20. RECORDS OF CONDITIONING OF THE RIGHT EYELID TO LIGHT

(*A*) Reaction of the eyelid (Unc R) to a puff of air before conditioning. (*B, C*) The beginnings of conditioning (CR), in which the closure of the eyelid anticipates somewhat the puff of air. (*D*) Full conditioned response to light. R_L is the light reflex. [From E. R. Hilgard and D. G. Marquis, *Conditioning and learning,* Appleton-Century, 1940, p. 38.]

Later work, however, has shown that many responses other than simple reflexes can be conditioned. For instance, a man places his hand on a grid of electric wires, a bell is rung, and then, a second later, the man receives a shock in his hand. Quickly he withdraws his hand. After this sequence of events has happened often enough, the man begins to withdraw his hand at the sound of the bell, thus escaping the shock. Since the conditioned withdrawal was a learned response and not a simple reflex, it seems better in general for us not to speak at all of a conditioned reflex, but to call it a *conditioned response*. (For a further description of conditioned responses, see pp. 139–144.)

The Reflex Circle

There are several situations in human behavior, particularly at the early stages of infancy and childhood, when a reflex pattern of behavior may be strengthened or perpetuated through conditioning. Consider, for example, the grasping reflex. If a stick is placed on the palm of an infant's hand, its fingers will curl about the stick and hold on with considerable strength. Indeed, shortly after birth an infant can be raised from the ground by its hold on the stick. Although this reflex is present at birth, it is probable that the grasping response is not due entirely to inherited factors, but involves the formation of a reflex circle through conditioning. It is easy to see that, in this case of grasping, when a movement occurs, the resulting stimulation of the proprioceptors—the receptors in muscles, tendons and joints—produces a sensory impulse which goes into the central nervous system and that this impulse may then become connected by conditioning to the motor response of the original movement, so that it acts to continue the original movement. The grasping is strengthened because it becomes conditioned upon itself by way of proprioception. This type of reflex circle which involves proprioceptors is called a *circular response*.

It is through the mechanism of a reflex circle that various other responses are sustained and perpetuated, often by means of exteroceptors. For example, if an infant utters the sound *ah,* this sound stimulus affects its ear, and impulses travel along the auditory nerve to the brain. Since the muscles of the vocal organs are the ones that have just moved, this motor path tends to be reactivated by the impulses from the auditory nerve, and the infant says *ah* again. It is clear that until there is a break in this circle, the infant would continue to say *ah,* but the reiteration always gets terminated presently by some other stronger stimulation from outside the circle.

Even in older children this circular phenomenon is frequently observed. They delight in repeating sounds—to the annoyance of their parents, who may think the children do it purposely to irritate them. One boy of eight would bleat like a sheep and keep on until, only with difficulty, he was made to stop. There was a mental defective who sat in a corner, day in and day out, hitting his two index fingers together and murmuring "Beelzebub." The normal adult also has many such continuous circular responses—like chewing gum, twisting a lock of hair, turning a coat button while thinking.

Conditioned Voluntary Responses

Other complex aspects of human behavior may be understood, at least in part, in terms of the method and phenomenon of conditioning. It is even possible to obtain voluntary control of what is for most persons an involuntary reflex.

In one experiment of this nature, the pupil of a man's eye was trained to contract at command. In the first stage of training, a bell was rung immediately before a light was shone in his eyes. After some trials, the sound of the bell alone would cause his pupil to contract. Then the man was instructed to close and open the circuit for both bell and light by closing and opening his hand at the verbal command of the experimenter. In this way verbal command became connected through the hand movement and the sound of the bell to the pupilary reflex. The next step in the experiment was to eliminate both the hand movement and the bell. This left only the vocal instruction of the experimenter as the conditioned stimulus, and the man's pupil now contracted to it alone. The last stage of the experiment consisted in having the subject himself repeat the verbal instructions, first aloud, then in a whisper and finally subvocally. Each of these forms of stimulation, it was found, could become the condition for the contraction of the pupil. So the man could, at the end of the experiment, effectively command his own pupilary reflex, and this ability was still present fifteen days later, without practice in the meantime.

MOTIVATED BEHAVIOR

Thus far we have been dealing with the kinds of behavior which are directly and immediately controlled by stimulation. Tropisms are orientations of the whole organism with respect to external stimuli. Reflexes are responses of specific parts of the organism to stimuli. Conditioned responses are reflexes, which, through learning, have come under the control of new stimuli. In addition to these stimulus-controlled responses, however, there are many varieties of behavior which arise from needs located within the organism. Such behavior, although it may use various stimuli as cues or signals, depends in its character and manifestation primarily on the motive of the organism. Now we shall consider such behavior.

Instinct

It is common among laymen to call reflex action instinctive, because both reflexive and instinctive behavior are, in the first instance, unlearned responses which depend upon innate connections in the nervous system. In the vocabulary of the psychologist, however, the instinct differs from the reflex because it is in part activated by internal needs of the organism. Responses are called instinctive when they involve not only innate reflexes in their response patterns, but also organic needs or drives as their immediate causes. Complicated responses, however, often owe their development to experience as well as to innate connections, and it is to the interest of the psychologist to determine by observation and experimentation how much may rightly be classed as instinctive or innate and how much is acquired.

An interesting form of behavior, which is in part instinctive, is the pecking response of chicks. Shortly before the chick is hatched, its whole body moves violently in the shell. The movements of its head take on the form essential to pecking, and its legs thrust upward against the shell. It is during one of these agitated movements that the shell cracks open and the chick emerges. The chick's action in breaking out of the shell is instinctive in the sense that it is caused by the internal development of the organism. It is not instinctive in the popular but incorrect sense that the *idea* of getting out of the shell at the right time was inherited by the chick.

After the chick is thus released, it uses its pecking response for eating, but it has to learn to peck effectively. At first the chick often misses the grain of corn that it strikes at. It may strike the corn but not seize it, or it may seize the grain but not swallow it. Only after some days does the chick peck accurately and eat with the proficiency of the adult hen. If some of the chicks are fed artificially for several days and not allowed to peck during that time, they will nevertheless very soon learn to peck as accurately as the chicks who had been 'practicing' earlier. Thus we see, even in this relatively simple response of pecking, that both instinctive response and learning play a part.

Many animals build nests according to a pattern which varies little within the species. In some instances, the offspring have had no opportunity to learn from their progenitors. There must, therefore, be at least some innate tendency controlling the activity. That such behavior, however, cannot possibly be an instinct in the sense in which an instinct is sometimes defined (that is to say, a series of chain reflexes whose connections are innate and fixed) is evident from the fact that the animal must change the nature and sequence of its responses in order to fit its behavior to the particular surroundings in which it finds itself and to the kind of material immediately available for the purpose.

In other cases, so-called instincts, both in animals and in man, are learned behavior. Naturalists frequently have reported, for example, that some wild animals they have encountered were not 'instinctively' either afraid of man or inclined to attack him until they had had unpleasant experiences with him. Hunters in Africa have frequently been able to approach by automobile within a few yards of a lion without the lion's paying particular attention to them. There are many other confusions of instincts with learned behavior, and it is a wise and prudent principle, when explaining a particular response, to endeavor first to determine all the factors of experience that could possibly have been operative in the development of the behavior in question before concluding that it is instinctive.

It may safely be stated, however, that there are many aspects of behavior which are primarily instinctive. Many fishes carry out long and complex cycles of migration and spawning. The salmon, for example, spawns in fresh water streams, and the young swim downstream to the sea. Later and at the proper time in their maturity, they swim back up the rivers and tributaries from which they came, there to spawn again. Some species of birds migrate back and forth between particular areas in the north in the summertime and in the south in the wintertime. (See Fig. 195.) Birds too not only build complex nests characteristic of their species but also display well-patterned activity in procuring food and feeding their young. The maternal behavior of many animals is largely instinctive; they deliver their young, clean them, construct nesting places, retrieve the young when they venture from the nest and suckle them. The complex sequences of sexual behavior—courting and strutting, billing and cooing, the male's pursuit of the female and finally the complex responses in copulation—are all largely innate and instinctive. Vestiges of these instinctive activities may often be seen in man's behavior, but learning, habit, intelligence and culture have so overridden them that it is seldom proper to speak of instinctive behavior in man.

Needs and Activity

Tropisms, reflexes and instinctive acts are all relatively definite, invariable and stereotyped kinds of behavior. If we know the stimulus conditions in the environment and, in the case of instinctive acts, the needs of the organism, we can predict with relative accuracy the kinds of acts which will occur. There is, however, much behavior in man and animals that is not so predictable; it is simply a pacing to and fro, or running through the wilds or exploring hither and yon. Such behavior may appear to be random, because we cannot see a stimulus or any other immediate cause for it, nor can we see any definite, repeated pattern in it.

We therefore often call such behavior *general activity* or *general exploratory behavior.* This kind of activity is important to the psychologist, for it is from general, exploratory and apparently aimless movement that patterns of learned behavior, and eventually of thinking, arise. Upon close observation, it is possible to conclude that most general exploratory behavior is the result of primitive needs or tensions within the organism. (See p. 114.) The organism is cold or hot, it is hungry, it is in need of water, or it is suffering sexual deprivation. Many experiments in which general activity has been measured in various animals show that large increases in activity and exploration occur when one or another of these needs is present.

Problem-Solving Behavior

It is no accident that general exploratory behavior accompanies the presence of needs in the organism. In the evolution of the response mechanism and in the adjustment of the organism to its environment, general activity becomes the first step in insuring that the organism has an opportunity to obtain the satisfaction of its needs. By foraging around the wild animal has a good chance to come upon food; by exploring a maze a rat finally, if somewhat randomly, finds the food at the end of it; and, similarly, the thirsty deer by roaming about comes to a stream and finds water. Thus general activity has use. It is instrumental in satisfying needs.

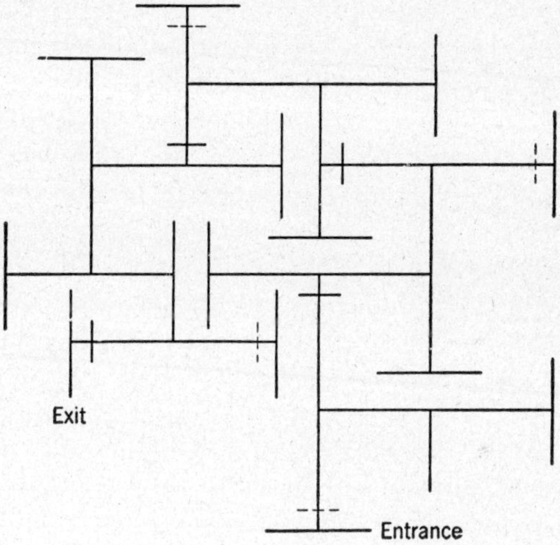

FIGURE 21. MULTIPLE-T MAZE FOR STUDYING PROBLEM-SOLVING BEHAVIOR IN RATS

[After C. P. Stone; from F. A. Moss (Ed.), *Comparative psychology* (2nd ed.), Prentice-Hall, 1942, p. 221.]

Although, in a new and unfamiliar situation, general exploration is the only available means for finding the satisfaction of a need, when the need arises again and again in the same situation, learning has an opportunity to take place. Activity then becomes less random and more stereotyped, and specific learned patterns of behavior emerge. Thus, the first time a hungry rat is placed in a maze, it wanders randomly in and out of many of the blind alleys, but after it has been placed in the maze many times, each time finding food at the end, it gradually eliminates its random behavior and, instead, runs rapidly through the maze along the shortest true path. Such learning behavior is called *problem-solving behavior.*

Problem-solving behavior as thus described involves a need which at first gives rise to general activity. It also may involve conditioning. Just as, in conditioning, the bell comes to elicit the salivary response originally evoked only by the sight of food, so, in establishing habits for problem-solving, stimuli like odors, shadows, cracks and sounds come to serve as signals for the correct responses which were originally only a part of general random activity. In this way conditioning establishes behavior patterns for solving problems. (Figure 21 shows a maze used in problem-solving studies.)

Covert Behavior

In animals and in children we can usually see many random movements in the course of their solving of a problem, but adult human individuals do not display so many random movements. In solving a puzzle, for example, an adult is likely to study the parts, not making any trial solutions, but putting two pieces together only when he has 'decided' that they will fit. He seems to think the solution out rather than to attain it by trial-and-error. Many experiments indicate, however, that the problem-solving behavior is there, even though it is not seen, that it is simply reduced in magnitude to very small muscular contractions. Even in the problem solving of animals, it may be shown that, when random responses seem to drop out, actually they are simply reduced in magnitude to the point where the eye cannot see them.

Such *covert behavior,* sometimes called *implicit behavior,* has been measured by mechanical and electrical methods of recording activity in muscles. In some experiments, for example, an apparatus was constructed for showing slight movements of the tongue. Subjects were then instructed to think of certain words, and, while they were thinking, the movements of their tongues were recorded. The thinking was found to be accompanied by definite movements of the tongue. In other cases, electrical voltages arising in various muscles were recorded while subjects were engaged in 'mental' problem solving, for example, the solution of arithmetical problems. In such subjects, muscle contractions almost always appeared in the course of problem solving, even though they could not be seen by the eye, and the electrical records showed that these contractions were similar in pattern to the responses obtained when the subjects were solving the problem 'out loud' or with observable movements. Thus it is important to realize that covert movements may be going on, and, in fact, that a person may be behaving all the time, even when no behavior is observable by the casual observer.

In the following experiment covert behavior is clearly demonstrated. If a recording instrument is placed on a person's head so that a graphic record of his head movements can be obtained, it is found that when, with his eyes closed, he merely thinks of his head's moving to the right, the records show that his head actually makes a slight movement to the right. When he thinks of moving his head to the left, the record indicates that such a movement to the left is made. Yet the person himself is unlikely at any time during the experiment to realize that he has made an actual movement.

The feat of muscle reading, a form of 'mind reading,' is based on this fact of covert behavior. If the individual, whose hand is held by the performer, thinks of going toward the window, his hand will make a slight movement in that direction, which the performer, who is especially sensitive to such weak muscular responses, will immediately feel and use as a clue. Animals are particularly acute in noticing such involuntary movement. A trained dog may be able to pick out the correct one of a series of playing cards spread on the floor if persons who know the correct card are near by. In thinking of the card, these onlookers are likely to turn their heads involuntarily for a fraction of a second toward the card in question, a hint which is not lost on the dog.

Set and Readiness

There is another aspect to the behavior of problem solving and conditioning, which is known as *set* or readiness to respond. An odor at a particular point in the pathway of a maze may be a signal to a rat to turn right, but it may be more than that. It may not only tell him to turn right but may also prepare him for making a second right turn after that. A pianist in learning to play the piano must learn not only to play one note at a time from the score but also to read ahead and to be ready to strike other notes at the appropriate time. He must let himself be 'set' for the particular key in which the piece is written and must not have to be constantly reminding himself about the sharps or the flats.

A more detailed example of *set* may be taken from laboratory experiments in which a subject is asked to push a key with his right hand when a red light appears and to push another key with his left hand when a green light appears. In this situation the subject of the experiment may at first repeat the instructions to himself. He may also consciously associate his right hand with the red light and his left hand with the green light. He will probably, in addition, feel some tension in his arms. In such terms as these the task or problem is represented in the subject's mind before a reaction takes place. This attitude of the subject is called the *set* toward the task. The set will, however, become increasingly less conscious, so that eventually the movement will occur immediately and automatically upon the appearance of the stimulus without any intervening mental state at all. Such a set may be either positive or negative. In the experiment with the red and green lights, the set for the right hand is positive for the red light and negative or inhibitory for the green light. The subject is set *not* to move his right hand for the green light. It would be much harder to reverse the meanings for red and green now for the two hands than to set up new sets for yellow and blue.

An experiment can be arranged to investigate a motor set by placing a rubber ball on the reaction key in order to measure the amount of pressure of the finger. By such means it has been found that the finger frequently makes an actual anticipatory movement of downward pressure on the key before the real movement is carried out. Another good example of motor set is that of the football player who has in mind just what to do in answer to the play of his opponent. As soon as he sees the play, his intended response follows immediately without further thought. Off-side play is frequently due to an overintensified set. The player is so ready to act, that he responds to the wrong stimulus or even to an imaginary stimulus. (For the relation of *set* to *need* and *attitude*, see p. 126.)

VOLUNTARY AND AUTOMATIC BEHAVIOR

We are now ready to consider briefly more complex forms of behavior, including voluntary behavior. A person decides to go to town. He walks down the stairs, puts on his coat and hat, opens the door, gets into his car and starts the engine. Common sense says that he has willed to do these various acts. Or again someone is trying to read a difficult passage in a textbook. His mind continues to wander from the book to irrelevant matters, until finally with great effort he succeeds in concentrating on the work at hand. It is usual to say that he has had to use his will power. No fault can be found with such an expression in ordinary speech, but the psychologist desires to know what is the general process that one calls 'will.'

The Will

In a voluntary act there is no special force that can be called the 'will.' Most important is the preliminary set or attitude already described. In addition, what is felt in an experience of 'will power' is the muscular tension involved—tension in the arms, for instance, in acts where arm movement is involved, or tension in the muscles of the forehead when the brow is wrinkled in an effort to concentrate on a mental task. It has been argued that, since a person paralyzed in one leg experiences an effort of will when he tries to move the inert limb and yet does not move it, the will experienced obviously cannot come from these muscles. What actually happens is that, unknowingly, he moves some other member. It is these other muscular sensations, imagined by their owner as coming from the missing member, that give him the impression of will power.

The will, then, so far as experience is concerned, turns out to be the preliminary set *plus* the experience of movement *plus* the knowledge that the movement follows directly on the set and has not been caused by any external force. We *know* that we have made the movement. It is unfortunate that *will* is a noun, as if it were an agent, a faculty or a special kind of energy. There is 'willing' but not a 'will.' *Willing is a process which one calls a voluntary act.*

Voluntary Control of Movement

What do we have to do in order to gain voluntary control of a response? It was at one time supposed that, if we could call to mind how the muscles would feel when moved in a certain way—in other words, if we had a clear memory of the proprioceptive sensations produced by the movement—we could then move those muscles appropriately. It was even sometimes supposed that such a memory of a movement must necessarily precede the movement which we desire to make. That this assumption is not true was demonstrated in the experiment already described, the one showing that voluntary control of a reflex can be obtained by the method of conditioning (pp. 44 f.).

Not only, however, is this anticipatory proprioception not necessary, but research has also shown that proprioception alone—or even when combined with a visual image of what the movement should be—is not a sufficient preliminary process to produce 'at will' a movement never before voluntarily initiated.

In certain experiments, persons who could not move their ears voluntarily had their ear muscles stimulated electrically so as to produce the movement. These persons felt the movement and saw it in a mirror. Still they could not move their ears voluntarily. In attempting to move them, they had the same sense of helplessness which they had experienced before the electrical stimulation. In their attempts, however, they moved the voluntarily controlled muscles of the brow, jaw and cheek, in such a way that the muscles of the ear were accidentally moved with them. Thus the ear muscles were brought into the reaction pattern, with the result that there occurred both afferent impulses to the muscles and proprioception from their contraction. It was only then that the proprioception, by becoming a link in a reflex circle, helped to develop full voluntary control of the ears.

These facts give us a picture of the origin and development of voluntary movement. It is clear from them that the *first movement* of our muscle groups are unconscious and *involuntary,* and that they come under conscious voluntary control only later, after the muscles have been 'accidentally' innervated.

Reflexes, Conditioned Responses and Voluntary Acts

In many instances of human behavior there is no difficulty in distinguishing a simple reflex from the more complicated conditioned response or from a voluntary response. Simply by observing the antecedents to the movement, we can tell, for example, whether an eyewink has occurred voluntarily or has been caused by some stimulus. In the case of the conditioned knee jerk, however, an investigator may not always be able to tell whether the movement of the leg in response to a bell as a conditioning stimulus is an involuntary conditioned response or whether the subject is 'faking' results by voluntarily moving his leg when he hears the bell.

Numerous experiments have been devised to obtain some objective criterion for the differentiation of these three forms of response. It has been found that the reflex is, on the average, more rapid than either the conditioned response or the voluntary response. Experiments in which the pupilary light reflex was conditioned showed that the average *latency* (the time between the presentation of the stimulus and the onset of the response) of the conditioned dilation of the pupil was 1.56 seconds and of the conditioned contraction 2.29 seconds, whereas the simple reflex to light is generally 0.2 to 0.5 second. The average *duration* of the conditioned dilation response was 8.24 seconds and of the conditioned contraction response 10.93 seconds, whereas the duration of the simple reflex to light is usually 1 to 4 seconds.

There may be overlapping, however, in the speed of these different forms of response. In the case of the eyelid response, it was found that, through practice in opening the eyes as quickly as possible immediately after the eyes had closed, the speed of such voluntary opening increased above the speed of the reflex. Yet this result does not mean that the voluntary response has developed into a reflex.

The conditioned response, moreover, usually differs qualitatively from the unconditioned. The conditioned knee jerk is not quite the same as the reflex knee jerk, nor is the conditioned wink response identical with the reflex eyewink. Under most experimental conditions the conditioned response is seldom as great in magnitude as the unconditioned.

Another objective difference between the reflex and the voluntary response appears in an analysis of the total time of the wink. If this time is analyzed into the time of opening and the time of closing the eye, it is found for the reflex that, as the time of closing decreases, the time of opening also decreases. In voluntary response this relationship is changed.

A further difference is that voluntary response is more readily modified by instruction than the reflex. At times the change of the reflex is found to be opposite in direction from the change in voluntary response. For example, subjects were told to relax as much as possible during both voluntary and reflex action. When the records of the eyelid movements were analyzed, it was found that the latency of response was generally slightly decreased for the reflex, whereas the latency of the voluntary response increased under relaxation. These last results are readily understood. The football player has to be 'keyed up' to start immediately upon the snapping of the ball. If he relaxes for a moment, he may be caught off his guard. The reflex, on the other hand, seems to work best when we are caught off guard. If our attention is concentrated on the appearance of the stimulus for, let us say, the knee jerk, there is likely to be a slight inhibitory effect on the reflex.

Experiments have also been made to determine whether any differences between reflex and voluntary activity can be discovered in the electrical potentials as the impulses pass along the nerves involved. The results indicate that the pattern of these potentials is more stereotyped in the reflex, a discovery which is in accord with the conception of a reflex as a *fixed* form of response as compared with the *variability* of voluntary response.

Voluntary Acts and Learning

The fact that voluntary acts have been so highly developed in man gives him a considerable advantage in learning various sorts of behavior, for he employs voluntary acts in his initial solutions. When, for example, a man starts to learn some difficult movement, like a new kind of dive, he has an idea of the form of movements that he wishes to make and then voluntarily attempts to carry out the movements. During the dive he will be aware to a certain extent of the position of his limbs, and after the completion of the dive he will have a memory of what he has done. On the next occasion, he may make use of this experience by voluntarily attempting to alter the form of his dive. By successively and voluntarily altering his behavior on subsequent occasions, he is able to learn much more rapidly and to achieve a higher degree of proficiency than if learning had to take place through random trials or conditioning.

After a great deal of practice, acts which were originally voluntary become more and more involuntary and finally result in automatic acts or habits. Thus, in learning to operate a typewriter, each pressing of a key is at first a voluntary act, but, after a reasonable degree of proficiency has been attained, the typist thinks no more of individual finger movements and may type automatically, while thinking about something else. By practice, the component voluntary acts become integrated into a smooth sequence of movements which do not, for the most part, enter consciousness. In fact, if the person becomes aware of the acts and attempts voluntarily to carry them out, his performance is usually impaired. Let a person suddenly become fully conscious of what he is doing, while he is performing some well-coordinated response, and there is likely to be an interference in the smoothness of the response. When he is very eager not to make a mistake in the letter he is typing, he is almost sure to do something wrong. If he thinks of voluntarily moving his legs when going rapidly upstairs, he is likely to trip. This change from an automatic response to a voluntary act throws the individual back to the initial stages in the development of his habit.

There are many examples in everyday life of the way in which acts which were originally voluntary become automatic. A pitcher, when he throws a ball, does not have to think of the movement he is going to make. The act is voluntary in the sense that he intends to pitch the ball, but, as he starts the swing of his arm, he is likely to be looking at the plate, his mind occupied with little else than the corner of the plate he wishes to 'cut.' Seldom are you conscious of the movements of your vocal organs while you are talking, nor are you often conscious of how you are going to move them before you start. For the most part, you are occupied with the direction of your thought and the effect you are achieving. You hear your own voice vaguely. If you want to know what words you are actually using to express your ideas, you have got to listen to yourself talking. In rapid conversation there is no feasible way of being aware of your own words before they are uttered. Conversation is only one example of habituated automatic action. A day is replete with such semivoluntary acts, acts that hardly touch the conscious level at all.

There are examples of voluntary acts which have become even more automatic. We curl a strand of hair, bite our pencil tip, tap on the floor, rattle our keys, entirely unaware that we are doing anything. While walking with a friend, we engage in animated conversation, completely unconscious of the action of our legs. Such automatic acts can be as complex and can involve as highly an integrated set of reactions as any fully voluntary response. This fact is well demonstrated by instances of automatic writing, where a person writes the answers to questions put to him without the least ability to say what it is he has written. Since it seems evident in such cases that the hand has been guided by 'unconscious' processes, the method is often used to discover what lies below the level of conciously controlled behavior.

The examples which we have examined in these last paragraphs illustrate the various forms of action, from wholly voluntary to unconscious automatic acts. Such a classification, however, is by no means clear-cut. We can have acts that are entirely automatic and unconscious, and acts that are entirely voluntary, but almost all voluntary acts contain some automatic process. In fact, such acts as piano playing, when performed by a proficient player, contain so much automatic response that it is customary to use the word *automatic* rather than *voluntary* in regard to them. Here action has become so well established a habit that correct response follows immediately upon stimulus, whether the musician is using the score or playing from memory, that is to say, whether the stimuli are the printed musical notations and the preceding finger movements or the latter alone. It is, indeed, frequently difficult to say whether an action is entirely automatic or not, as when the musician plays softly over the keys while conversing with a friend, or when a telegraph operator taps SOS on the desk with his finger while he is reading an engrossing detective story. The important point is that most of our responses are a mixture of the two types, being both automatic and voluntary.

ACTS AND IDEAS

Closely related to the complex voluntary and automatic acts which we considered in the last section are the forms of behavior which are controlled by ideas rather than by external stimuli, needs or volition. Although some animals can solve elementary problems involving reasoning and ideas, only man's behavior can be controlled in any considerable way by ideas. The fact that ideas may cause acts of behavior is called *suggestion.* Sometimes such suggestion comes from within the individual, sometimes from external events which he is observing and sometimes from the actions or words of other individuals. We shall now consider these forms in turn.

Ideomotor Action

If the idea of an act impels a person to carry out the act, we speak of ideomotor action. This form of action may be illustrated by the dislike of some persons for high places. The idea of jumping comes so strongly to them that they fear it will break over into action. Nearly everyone has had at some time so vivid an idea of the act of jumping out of the window at which he was standing that he has wished to withdraw from the spot in order to avoid the danger. Another example is the desire to knock off the top hat of a fellow traveler, an idea which, once brought to mind, may prove almost irresistible. Advertising has made good use of the principle of ideomotor action. The tired tennis player is portrayed in the act of smoking a certain brand of cigarette, so that the reader may be induced by the idea to do likewise. Innumerable examples of a similar nature could be taken from daily life, for ideomotor action is a very common experience.

Empathy

Still more frequent, however, are the incipient movements, sometimes too slight to be readily detected, at other times quite noticeable, which are aroused in us by movements in our environment. An obvious example may be observed at a football game where the home team, let us say, is holding on the one-yard line. An enthusiastic and partisan spectator may push actively and urgently with the players, until suddenly he realizes that he is actually pushing his neighbor. Or again, when spectators watch an acrobat climb to the top of a pole balanced on the head of a colleague and swing back and forth with the tottering pole, the whole crowd sways in unison.

In looking at statues and buildings and pictures, or in listening to music, this sort of movement likewise occurs. We may feel the thrust of the foot or the tension of the outstretched hand of a statue, the weight of the arch on its columns or the rise of the columns themselves, and the direction of the lines and weight of the represented mass in the picture. Listening to music, we often find ourselves following the rhythm with some part of our bodies. Even the rhythmical click of the car wheel over the rail may arouse a motor response. Since we are occupied with the perception of the object, we are for the most part not conscious of these movements in ourselves. Nevertheless our responses, though unconscious as such, give dynamic quality to these perceptions. The lines of the picture become lines of force, the represented mass has weight, the rhythm of the music seems to flow smoothly, the curves of the architecture appear to have the grace of a moving object. It is as if we had projected our own unconscious movements into the object of our perception. Because of this 'projection' the experience has been termed *empathy,* a feeling of oneself into the object of regard.

An example of empathy is presented in Fig. 22. It is assumed that the trainer is unconscious of the movement of his leg; he is only aware, through projection of his own movements, of the effort being made by the jumper, that is to say, of the dynamic quality of the perception. Without this assumption of projection the illustration would be merely an example of imitation and not of empathy.

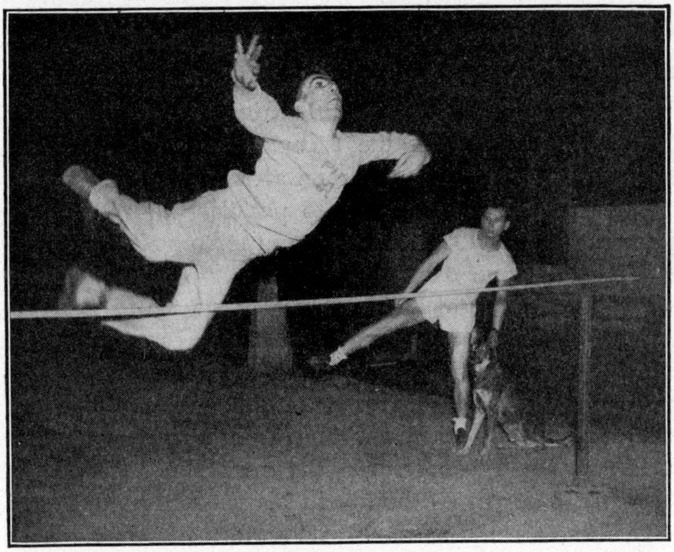

FIGURE 22. EMPATHY

Blind Bill Kelley clearing the pole, with his trainer, Peter Bennett, watching. Notice the empathic response of the trainer. [By permission of Pictures, Inc.]

Suggestion

In the broad sense of the term, suggestion plays a large role in our lives of action. The immediate perception of an object most frequently leads to some response which depends upon previous experience with the object. The flame suggests withdrawal of the hand. The sight of a half-read book suggests continuing the story; without any intervening thought the student picks it up, when he had fully intended to settle down to study. The sleight-of-hand performer, by a movement of the other hand, suggests a shift of the attention of the audience away from the hand that is doing the trick. In the empathic perception of lines and mass there is the direct suggestion of some motor response. The individuals of a mob are extremely suggestible to the action of one or more of their companions. Although the term suggestion is used legitimately in all these instances, it is usually restricted to that action which is brought about by a verbal instruction. We act through suggestion when we respond to the written or spoken word *uncritically.* In most instances such a response is immediate, but it may on occasions be delayed.

Children, being obviously less critical than adults, are more suggestible. As a consequence their testimony is particularly untrustworthy. This trait may be easily demonstrated. The child is asked to place his hand on an electric heater and told to say when he feels the warmth. After the experimenter has made the motion of turning on the current (without actually throwing the switch), the child will soon report that he feels the heat.

On occasion, however, adults can be just as suggestible as children. Given the proper emotional setting, they will imagine the impossible. An excellent example is what occurred in the autumn of 1938 when the story of the Martians came over the radio. Many persons 'actually' smelt the poisoned fumes which the men from Mars were supposed to have spread on Earth.

A person is said to be highly suggestible when he lacks firm convictions of his own. Though most of us can act through suggestion a thousand times a day without losing individuality, there are the extreme cases where a person has so few firm convictions of his own that no counter argument enters his mind when he is presented with an important course of action. Conversely, there is the negatively suggestible person. He almost invariably has some reason for not doing what is desired of him. The first type cuts out the coupon of the advertisement at once and mails it. The second type immediately throws the advertisement in the wastebasket. It is thus that attitudes toward suggestion determine action in the large as well as the small affairs of life. Degree of suggestibility is an essential feature of personality.

Hypnotism

The hypnotic trance and its manifestations are the result of an extreme state of suggestibility. It is a state which may be induced in varying degrees in most normal persons who are willing to cooperate with the hypnotist. Except that he can respond adequately to external stimulation when the hypnotist suggests it, the person who has been hypnotized is in a condition resembling sleep. If the subject's mind is free from the ordinary inhibitions and resistance, he readily carries out the instructions given him by the hypnotist, provided that the task does not conflict with his most fundamental convictions. He will commit an artificially arranged crime but, contrary to popular belief, he cannot easily be induced to commit an offense if it really contravenes strong tendencies of ethical conduct, as we shall see presently.

It has been supposed that under hypnosis a person's senses are keener and his strength greater than normal. Experiments, however, have shown that this is not the case. There is little if any difference in his sensitivity, and the feats of strength he performs under hypnosis he can also do in his normal state if he is willing to make great effort. It has also been found experimentally that persons who acted through hypnotic suggestion as if they could not see, actually had normal vision.

The state of hypnosis is characterized by its *contradictory phenomena.* The hypnotized person behaves as if he were enthusiastically acting out a big lie in order to please the hypnotist, acting it out and believing it as he acts. Sometimes he has to perceive something in order to know that it is something he is supposed not to perceive. For instance, the subject may be told that he is now blind in his left eye, can see only with his right. Immediately he begins to act consistently as if he were blind in his left eye. The hypnotist then shows him a little box into which he can look with both eyes. First the hypnotist lets the subject see that a red disk is inserted at the back of the box at the left and a green disk at the back at the right. Then he tells the subject to look into the box with both eyes and asks him what he sees. The subject reports that he sees a green disk, because the red disk is at the left and he is simulating blindness with his left eye. Actually the box, by the use of prisms, reverses the images of the disks left for right, so that the reported green disk is really seen with the left eye. Thus it appears that the subject really can see with his left eye when it helps him to play the game of being blind in his left eye.

Experiments of this sort make hypnosis resemble faking, but it is a very insistent and enthusiastic kind of faking. For instance, it is easy to suggest successfully to a subject that he is insensitive to pain in some part of his body and then to burn or cut him in that region while he carries on a gay conversation with the hypnotist. In fact, hypnosis was used successfully in many cases for surgical anesthesia just before the discovery of ether in 1846. It certainly takes a good deal of enthusiastic cooperation to fail to notice the pain when your leg is being amputated, with no anesthesia but with the hypnotic suggestion that you are not to feel anything in the leg.

This desire to please the hypnotist has to take its chances along with all the other desires that fight for dominance. Will a subject under hypnosis stab a man with a dagger? He will stab a friend with a cardboard dagger if he knows the dagger is cardboard. An habitual stabber might be persuaded to stab an enemy with a real dagger. A college student was once induced under hypnosis to throw what he knew certainly to be strong nitric acid at the face of a very good friend. The acid never reached its goal because invisible glass was interposed, but the student did not know about the glass. Still he did know that he was in a psychological laboratory where strange things may happen without permanent harm to any one, and he may have been trusting the hypnotist to protect him from the apparent consequences of his act. Hypnotic suggestion is only one among many motives that act upon the hypnotized subject.

Suggestion may also operate after a subject has been awakened from the hypnotic state. That phenomenon is called *posthypnotic suggestion.* For instance, the subject may be told: "After you awaken and before you leave the room, you will take that chair and stand it on the table." Then the subject awakens, looks at the chair, and puts it on the table. He gives all sorts of excuses. It is in the way on the floor. It looks better on the table. He was thinking he would like to sit way up there on the top of the table. One such subject looked at the chair and exclaimed: "I want to put that chair on the table. I bet it is because you told me to in hypnosis. I am *not* going to do it!" He left the room, banging the door. In five hours he was back, a little sheepish. He looked at the chair and the table. "Well," he said, "I may as well get it over with!" And he lifted the chair and put it on the table. Then he heaved a sigh of relief for a duty at last accomplished.

REACTION

The preceding sections have dealt principally with the qualitative aspects of volitional acts.

Reaction Time

We turn now to the speed of response and the conditions which determine the speed.

The problem of the reaction time arose in 1796, when a certain astronomer at the Greenwich Observatory in England dismissed his assistant because the latter's observations of the time at which stars cross a cross-hair in the field of the telescope were almost a second later than his own. Twenty years later it was discovered by checking the observations of different astronomers that the discrepancies were due to more fundamental differences in the manner of reaction than would be produced by mere carelessness. The conclusion was reached that these measurements, which depend upon the speed of reaction of the observer, were affected by what was then called the *personal equation,* that is to say, constant individual differences in reaction time. When the first psychological laboratory was established in Leipzig in 1879, experiments on reaction times were undertaken. Ever since, the determination of reaction times has represented an important technique in experimental psychology.

One of the most accurate arrangements for the measurement of human response is illustrated in Fig. 23. Its main feature is a chronoscope or timing device, consisting of a synchronous motor and a dial whose hand is attached to a magnetic clutch. Two telegraph keys are wired to the instrument in such a way that when one key is pressed the clutch engages with the motor and when the other key is pressed the motor is released. In the simplest experiment the subject is seated at one key and the experimenter at the other, and the motor is started. The experimenter presses his key, which gives the desired stimulus to the subject and engages the clutch so that the hand on the dial revolves. As quickly as possible upon perceiving the appropriate signal, the subject presses his key, thereby releasing the clutch, so that the hand on the dial stops. The revolutions of the hand are recorded on the dial. As the speed of revolution is already known, the time that elapsed between the pressing of the two keys—in

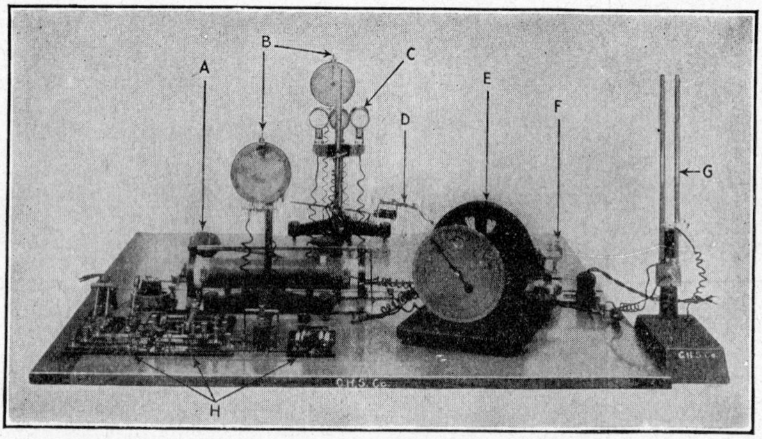

FIGURE 23. INSTRUMENT FOR TIMING REACTIONS

(*A*) Bulb for response key; (*B*) voice keys; (*C*) light stimulus; (*D*) relay for touch stimulus; (*E*) chronoscope; (*F*) relay for sound stimulus; (*G*) tuning fork for time control; (*H*) stimulus keys. [Courtesy of the C. H. Stoelting Company of Chicago.]

short, between stimulus and response—may be read from the dial in milliseconds.

Various stimuli and types of response may be used. For example, the experimenter may signal by means of a clicking sound produced by a relay, or he may give a tactual stimulus by means of a magnetic contrivance that presses on the subject's hand. He may flash an electric lamp as a visual stimulus; or, if a discrimination reaction is desired, he may illuminate in haphazard order a green and a red lamp, requiring the subject to react to one color and avoid reaction to the other. For word reactions he uses a voice key containing a thin diaphragm which vibrates when spoken against, thus temporarily breaking the electric circuit. The experimenter may speak into one voice key, starting the clock, and the subject may speak into the other key, stopping it. There are other possible arrangements and other forms of electric clocks, but in each of them the clock is started and stopped automatically and reaction times are obtained which are accurate within a few milliseconds.

Simple Reactions

In the *simple* reaction experiment, the subject is generally instructed to respond by pressing a telegraph key as quickly as possible after the signal is given by the experimenter. Not only do individuals vary among themselves in speed of reaction, but also the reaction time of the same individual varies according to the *sense organ stimulated.* The following table will give an idea of the approximate range of the reaction times in seconds for the different senses.

The reaction times to painful stimuli are especially long, owing in part to the fact that there is a considerable lag between the application of a stimulus and the consciousness of pain. The reaction times for warmth and cold vary according to the manner of application of the stimuli. The reaction to taste varies with the part of the tongue stimulated and the kind of stimulus; the time is shortest for salt and longest for bitter. The time for touch varies according to the part of body stimulated and to the limb making the response. The reaction time for a stimulus applied to the forehead is longer than for one applied to the hand, although the forehead is nearer the brain. The reaction of one hand to a tactual stimulus applied to the same hand is quicker than to a stimulus applied to the opposite hand. The reaction to light is faster when the light falls on the fovea (the area of clearest vision near the center of the retina of the eye) than when it falls on an eccentric part of the retina, the time increasing continuously with the distance of stimulation from the fovea. Reaction is more rapid to binocular than to monocular stimulation.

Kind of Stimulation	*Reaction Times (Seconds)*
Visual	0.150 to 0.225
Auditory	0.120 to 0.185
Tactual	0.115 to 0.190
Olfactory	0.200 to 0.800
Gustatory	0.305 to 1.080
Pain	0.400 to 1.000
Cold	0.150
Warm	0.180

In most experiments upon reaction time, a preparatory signal is given before the presentation of the stimulus. It is found that the reaction time varies with the *length of the interval* between the preparatory signal and reaction signal. Constant intervals between 2 and 4 seconds give the shortest times. If the preparatory signal is varied within a series, so that the subject never knows exactly how long he will have to wait for the reaction signal, the optimal interval ranges between 12 and 16 seconds. The act of preparation seems to be the chief factor involved in these results. If the interval is too short, the subject has not sufficient time to 'get set' and the stimulus may come before he is quite ready. If he has to wait more than 4 seconds, the interval becomes too monotonous for him to hold his attention entirely on the task. If the interval is varied, he is unable to assume a constant attitude of expectation and therefore requires a longer interval for his quickest reaction than when the interval is constant.

Distraction usually lengthens reaction time, but sometimes the supposedly distracting stimulus acts as a spur and decreases the time. This paradoxical effect, which has been found in other experiments where concentration is necessary, is explained by the fact that some persons use more effort to concentrate when there is an obstacle to overcome. City dwellers become so accustomed to concentration 'in spite of' the noise of the street that they often have difficulty at first in working efficiently when they go into the country. Students, studying with the radio turned on, may be more alert to their work because they are fighting the radio as a potential distractor—more alert than they would have been in the quiet without the radio's challenge. (For further description of the effects of distraction, see pp. 477 f.)

Reaction times to all kinds of stimuli decrease with an increase in the *intensity* of the stimulus. This decrease in time is most marked in the range of weak intensities.

Although an individual's reaction time varies according to the nature of the stimulus, the question arises whether, if he is quicker than his fellows in his response to visual stimuli, he will also respond more quickly to auditory and tactual stimuli. In other words, is there a speed characteristic of response that runs through all a person's motor reactions? In a series of experiments it was found that the correlation of simple visual, auditory and tactual reaction times is really quite high. Thus if a person excels in speed of reaction to one kind of stimulus, there is a good chance that he will also be quick in his reactions to other kinds.

Sensory and Motor Reactions

If a runner starts sooner than his rival at the crack of the pistol, it is owing in part to the difference in set of the contestants. It has been shown in the laboratory that there are two types of reaction, *sensory* and *motor*. In the sensory type, the subject's attention is directed by the initial set to the stimulus, and in the motor type to the response which he is to make. In the extreme form of sensory reaction, the expectation of the subject is directed almost exclusively to the coming stimulus, often with a steady fixation in the direction of its appearance. In the extreme motor reaction the idea of the movement to be performed in terms of proprioception is dominant. If the subject is allowed to react 'naturally,' there is usually an attitude midway between these two forms, or an alternation of the two.

These differences in set cause differences in reaction time. When the reaction tends toward the sensory type, the time is longer than when it tends toward the motor type. In the table on reaction times (p. 59) visual reactions range from 0.150 second to 0.225 second. It is probable that the time 0.150 second was obtained under a motor set and the 0.225 second under a sensory set. With practice one tends to become increasingly motor until the reaction becomes practically automatic; then the finger movements occur with little conscious intention as soon as a signal is given. With this ex treme motor set, however, premature reactions are not infrequent, as we find not only in the laboratory but also in such situations as racing. A runner who is of the extreme motor type often makes a false start. Some runners, however, prefer to be sure of the signal, even though they are a little late. These different types are found among people in general; there are those who are slow, safe and sure, and those who go off 'half-cocked.'

Discrimination and Choice Reactions

Most of our reactions in life are not like the simple reaction experiments. It is seldom in everyday life that we can be so sure of what is going to happen as to set ourselves to react automatically at maximum speed. The runner who is not alert may, for example, start at the sound of an automobile backfiring instead of at the pistol shot. Consequently some *discrimination* is generally necessary for a correct response.

In the laboratory this more complicated situation is produced by varying the stimuli. The subject may be instructed to react only to a red light, when both red and green signals are used in haphazard order. This is a *discrimination reaction.* It is obvious that this problem is similar to that confronting the locomotive engineer and the automobile driver. The necessity of recognizing the correct signal increases the average reaction time above the time of the simple reaction; and, the more motor the set of the subject is, the more likely he is to react to the wrong light. The discrimination situation may be further complicated by requiring a *choice* between two or more reactions as well as a discrimination between stimuli. The subject may, for example, be instructed to respond with the right hand if the light is red and with the left hand if the light is green, or with the right hand if the red light appears on the right of the green and with the left hand if the stimuli are reversed. The greater the complications in such *choice reactions,* the longer the reaction time.

In the discrimination reaction it is found that the more the stimuli resemble each other, the longer are the reaction times. If black and white are used as stimuli, the reactions are quickest. Red and green come next, then red and blue, followed by red and yellow, and finally red and orange. If tones are used, the reaction to tones differing by 16 cycles per second is quicker than to tones differing by 12 cycles, and much quicker than to tones only 4 cycles apart. When lines differing in length are the stimuli, the less the difference between the lines, the longer are the reactions. The reaction time is, for example, shorter for discrimination between lines of 10 and 13 millimeters than for 10 and 12 millimeters.

Word Reactions

The commonest reactions in life are *verbal.* To determine the nature and speed of such responses numerous experiments have been devised. The usual method is to present a word visually or vocally, the subject being told to respond as quickly as possible with the word that is suggested by the stimulus word. The time, which may be taken by a stop watch or by means of voice keys and a chronoscope, indicates the speed of the association of ideas for the person tested.

If the subject is told to respond with the first word that occurs to him, the association is termed 'free.' Frequently, however, the instructions are more limited. For example, a general term indicating a class, such as *animal,* is given and the subject is required to reply with the name of a member of this class, such as *bear;* or he is instructed to respond with a word opposite in meaning to the stimulus word. Many other variations in instruction may be given. These associations, being partially determined from the start, are called controlled associations. Experiments of this nature have been extensively employed in investigations of the nature of the thought process.

Practical Use of Reaction Experiments

An individual's ability in practical affairs depends in part upon his speed of reaction. It is, therefore, frequently of value to know both his speed of reaction in a given situation and how he compares with other individuals under similar circumstances. It is also of interest to know how much he may improve his speed and accuracy by practice as well as under the incentive of increased interest in the task.

Reaction time is an important factor both in vocational selection and in determining the individual's aptitudes as a basis for vocational advice. For example, in the selection of telephone switchboard operators, speed of response and relative freedom from errors are essential requirements. A consideration of the same characteristics is necessary in the selection of chauffeurs and machine operators. According to the results of tests of taxicab drivers, those men with the greatest number of accidents have the slowest reaction times. Those who have the fastest reaction times have also many accidents, perhaps because they are overconfident and take chances. It is therefore desirable to select drivers whose reaction times are neither very fast nor very slow.

The association-reaction experiments have been used with some success to determine guilt. Words which are related to the crime are interspersed with 'neutral' words. The words of this combined list are read to the subject, who must answer as rapidly as possible to each one with any word he can think of. Anyone knows from his own experience that when he is faced with an embarrassing situation—one that is emotionally toned—he is likely to hesitate and often to reply foolishly or irrelevantly. In the 'crime' experiment there is exactly such an embarrassing situation for the guilty person. Therefore the tendency is for the reaction time to the relevant words to be unusually long, or at least to vary more than the reaction times to the neutral words. In addition, the meaningful reference of the words is often different in the cases of guilt and of innocence.

This same method is used to discover suppressed complexes—the memory of painful experiences which, held in an unconscious state, often give rise to abnormal mental conditions. Because such complexes are, like the concealed knowledge of the guilty subject, highly emotional in nature, the two test situations are very similar.

REFERENCES

1. Crafts, L. W., Schneirla, T. C., Robinson, E. E., and Gilbert, R. S. *Recent experiments in psychology.* New York: McGraw-Hill, 1938. Chaps. 1 to 3.

   These chapters deal with 'instincts' (cats and mice, migration of birds and salmon) and with the behavior of newborn babies.

2. Estabrooks, G. H. *Hypnotism.* New York: Dutton, 1943.

   An up-to-date survey of hypnosis and suggestion in man.

3. Hilgard, E. R., and Marquis, D. G. *Conditioning and learning.* New York: Appleton-Century, 1940. Chaps. 2 and 13.

   A text and reference book which surveys conditioning and learning in both animals and man. Chapter 13 deals with physiological mechanisms in conditioning.

4. Hull, C. L. *Hypnosis and suggestibility.* New York: Appleton-Century, 1933.

   An old but useful summary of experiments and unsolved problems in the understanding of hypnosis and suggestion.

5. Morgan, C. T. *Physiological psychology.* New York: McGraw-Hill, 1943. Chaps. 15, 18, 19, 20, 21.

   An up-to-date textbook in physiological psychology. These chapters deal with reflexes, sleep and activity, instinctive behavior, mating behavior and bodily needs.

6. Shaffer, L. F. *The psychology of adjustment.* Boston: Houghton Mifflin, 1936. Chaps. 2, 3, 4.

   An elementary text on mechanisms of human adjustment approached from a biological point of view. These chapters consider the origin and modification of behavior and the role of motivation.

7. Tomkins, S. S. (Ed.) *Contemporary psychopathology.* Cambridge: Harvard University Press, 1943. Chaps. 34, 36.

   Selected readings from experiments and discussions dealing with abnormal behavior. Chapter 34, by H. S. Liddell, treats of the modification of instinct by conditioning. Chapter 35, by R. W. White, considers the nature of hypnosis.

8. Woodworth, R. S. *Experimental psychology.* New York: Holt, 1938. Chaps. 5, 13, 14.

   A comprehensive textbook of experimental psychology. These chapters deal with the conditioned response, the galvanic skin response and reaction time.

9. Young, P. T. *Motivation of behavior.* New York: Wiley, 1936. Chap. 5.

   The only text and reference book dealing entirely with motivation in relation to response. Chapter 5 deals specifically with set.

CHAPTER 4

Growth and Development

MAN is an organism, as the preceding chapters have shown, a mass of protoplasm moving about on the face of the earth. His movements are lawful. They depend on his properties as an organism, on his bodily structure and on his capacities for response to stimulation which in turn depend upon inherited and acquired characteristics of his nervous system.

This organism that is man has a life to live. It begins at the moment of conception when two parent cells unite to form a new individual. Then at once the new organism begins to grow and develop, at first as an embryo, then into a fetus, and then, being born, into an infant, a child, a youth, an adult and finally, if he lives, into an old person. Since growth and development are such important characteristics of man, it is proper that we should begin our detailed study of man's properties by seeing what happens to an individual organism as it grows and develops from conception to extreme old age.

GROWTH, DEVELOPMENT AND MATURATION

It will simplify our account of the processes of growth and development if, at the outset, we carefully distinguish between them. We shall use the term *growth,* as the biologists do, to mean merely increase in size, and it will apply not only to the overall dimensions of the body in terms of height (or length) and weight, but also to the parts of the body as, for example, the head, arms and trunk—the heart, brain, skeleton, muscles, etc. By the term *development* we shall mean the changes in the shape of the parts of the body and the integration of the various parts into functional units as growth goes on. Growth can be measured. Development can be observed by noting changes in shape as they occur and in modes of behavior as their maturation is completed.

We shall use the term *maturation* to mean the growth and development that is necessary either before any unlearned behavior can occur, or before the learning of any particular behavior can take place. For example, one of the first coordinated movements that any baby makes, is to raise its head, and to hold its head upright without support while sitting. The child could not perform this act earlier because its maturation was not complete, that is to say, the muscles at the back of its head and neck had not grown sufficiently, and the connections of nerve fibers and synapses leading from the muscles to the cerebral cortex and back again had not developed enough to activate the muscles. The maturation

This chapter was prepared by Leonard Carmichael of Tufts College.

of this bit of behavior is, therefore, complete as soon as the growth and integration of the parts have progressed sufficiently. The child does not learn to raise its head; maturation is all that is needed. But, later in life, it does learn to raise its head *in order to* see something, for that behavior means attaching the newly available movement to some stimulus. Similarly the child cannot *learn* to write until the growth of the small muscles in the fingers and their neural connections have developed sufficiently. It can learn to write only after it has developed the brain capacity for learning and the muscular capacity for fine movement.

Conditions of Growth

The first essential condition for growth is *food*. For a few days the newly fertilized cell finds its food in the cell itself. Then, as embryo and fetus, it derives its food from the mother and will continue to get it in this way throughout the prenatal period. If growing is to be normal, the mother must supply her child with a well-balanced diet, for the growing cells require proteins, carbohydrates, fats, vitamins and a variety of mineral salts. After birth the neonate, as the newborn infant is called, gets its food by mouth and must digest it himself. If he cannot digest his food properly, or if his mother's milk lacks needed elements for his diet, his growth will suffer.

A second important condition for human growth is the supply of the secretions called *hormones* from some of the endocrine glands. (See pp. 23 f.) Chief of these are hormones from various lobes of the *pituitary* body, a small gland situated at the base of the brain. One hormone affects the growth of the body as a whole—particularly the skeleton. If the amount of the secretion is too great, growth is abnormal and results in gigantism; if not enough, it results in dwarfism. Another hormone, called thyroxin and produced by the *thyroid* gland, influences the consumption of oxygen in the tissues and thereby influences metabolism and growth. An absence of this hormone in early childhood stops the growth of the brain, inhibits growth in stature—particularly of the arms and legs—and results in producing the kind of dwarf known as a cretin. The interstitial cells of the *sex glands* furnish a hormone that stimulates the growth of the secondary sex characters—the rapid growth and changes in figure, hair and voice that occur in early adolescence. A less dramatic but equally important part is played by hormones from still other glands in the assimilation of food and the removal of waste products which are necessary for growth.

A third condition of growth is *heredity*, which, of course, also determines the two previous conditions—food assimilation and the hormones. However, heredity also determines whether the fertilized cell, when grown and developed, will be a human being or some other animal and, if human, to what race it will belong; whether it will be a boy or a girl; whether, other things being equal, it will eventually be large, medium or small in size; whether the shape and size of many of its features (for example, eyes, nose, mouth, lower jaw, hands and fingers) will be like those of its father or mother or one of its grandparents or a more remote ancestor.

A detailed account of the laws of heredity would take us too far afield. We may say, however, that the basic factors for the transmission of characters from one generation to others are called *genes*. No two germinal cells have the same genes. Before fertilization there is usually only one ovum (female cell) but there are millions of sperms (male cells), only one of which joins the ovum. The newly fertilized cell has, therefore, an almost certainly unique combination of genes. If some other sperm had fertilized the ovum, the combination would have been different. If conception should take place a month later, the ovum would have a different set of genes and the fertilized cell would have quite another combination. These facts help us to understand why, for example, in a family consisting of a large number of children of the same parents, no two children (identical twins excepted) are of the same size and bodily contour. You can always tell one child from another (except, of course, with the identical twins).

Finally, a fourth condition of growth is *use* or *exercise*. General exercise, such as walking, gymnastics and sports, increases heart rate and blood pressure and the rate and depth of respiration. As a result, the blood, carrying an increased supply of oxygen and food, passes with new force into the smallest of the capillaries and thus reaches all the cells of the body. During the growing years the development of all parts of the body is thus quickened. In continuous and violent exercise the muscles particularly involved grow larger. The sprinter develops his leg muscles, the oarsman his arm, trunk and leg muscles, and, since the heart has an additional burden laid upon it, it is frequently permanently enlarged.

Integration and Maturation

Thus far we have regarded growth as if it were an end in itself, as if, for example, all that the brain does is to grow until it stops at maturity. Growth, however, is only one aspect—though a very important one—of a larger process of development. The end of development is the production of a living organism prepared to do all the things that man does. Development, therefore, requires not only the growth and formation of the structural parts but also, as we have seen, their integration into a functioning whole.

We may illustrate this process by a crude analogy. The structural parts of a gas engine—the cylinders and pistons, the battery, wires and timer, the carbureter and spark plugs—must be assembled, fastened into place, carefully adjusted and provided with fuel before the engine as an integrated whole is ready to run. The integration both of the engine and of the developing organism consists in uniting and coordinating the parts.

There are, however, two important differences between man and a gas engine. First, in man, under the guidance of the genes inherited from his ancestors, development takes place automatically. Second, when the gas engine leaves the assembly line its development ends. It can then do all the things it can ever do; it can start and stop, run at various speeds, and produce various amounts of horsepower. Except for limbering up and the effects of subsequent wear, its basic behaviors are all matured at once. In man, on the other hand, maturation of various forms of behavior goes on for a long time. Although at birth maturation of the functions necessary for the maintenance of life has been reached, it will be many months before the child has complete control of its muscles and years before it can reproduce its kind.

The Nervous System as Integrator

The great integrator and coordinator of the organism is the functioning nervous system. Its fibers pass into almost every structure of the body, few of which can function without nerve direction.

The rate of development of the nervous system is not, however, uniform throughout. The spinal cord is formed and developing throughout its entire length by the middle of the second month of the prenatal period. The lower parts of the brain —the medulla, midbrain and other parts necessary for automatic control—also develop early. Last of all the cortex develops.

We may illustrate the course of development in the lower centers by experiments that have been made with the larva of the salamander, *Amblystoma.* This salamander develops quickly under water from a fertilized egg which has its own rich supply of yolk. It becomes a free-swimming animal before it must seek for food. Thus it is an ideal animal in which to study the maturation of nerve and muscle coordination at the automatic level. The development which leads up to swimming behavior in this embryo (see Fig. 24) may be described in five typical stages, as follows: (1) a *nonmotile stage,* in which the direct muscle stimulation by electrical or mechanical means leads to muscular contractions which occur without bodily movement; (2) an early *C-flexure stage,* in which a light touch on the skin of any portion of the body leads to a bending of the head to one side; (3) a *tight-coil stage,* in which the contractions noted in stage (2) extend toward the tail to make a coil; (4) the *S-reaction,* which is characterized by a reversal of flexure before the previous C-flexure has been completely executed, thus leading to the sinuous behavior of the organism; and (5) the *speeding up of this S-reaction* so as to produce the typical swimming movement of the amphibian larva.

Studies were also made of the neural organization of the central nervous system at every one of these stages. It was found that development in specific chains of neurons in the central nervous system are necessary before the alterations of behavior from stage to stage can take place. These studies showed clearly that a particular set of connections must be produced by growth before particular responses occur. In general, it is found that the earliest movement is the bending of the head to one side. A little later the bending progresses downward toward the tail. The development of the swimming behavior is, therefore, in a head to tail, or *cephalocaudal* direction. This is a pattern of an orderly development of neuromuscular function which is also found in the maturation of bodily movements in the child.

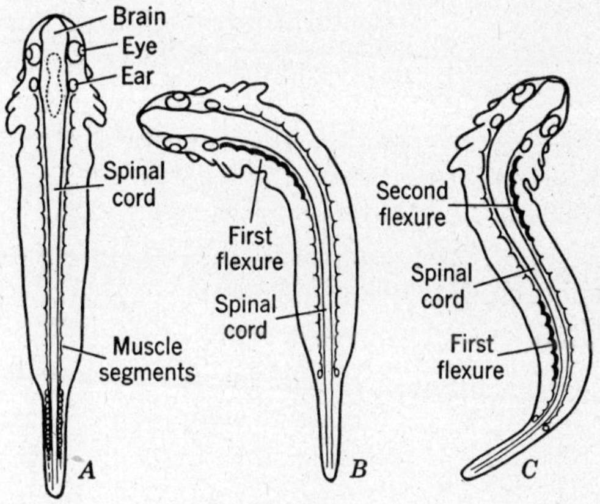

FIGURE 24. DEVELOPMENT OF SWIMMING IN THE YOUNG SALAMANDER

(*A*) Stage before neuromuscular activity has begun. In this stage muscles may be directly stimulated. (*B*) Beginning of C or reverse-C movement. (*C*) S-shaped swimming movement. The first reverse-C-flexure progresses toward the tail while another C-flexure begins at the head. Muscle contractions shown black at flexures. [After G. E. Coghill, *Anatomy and the problem of behavior,* Cambridge University Press, 1929, pp. 7 f.]

The development in the central nervous

system begins with the spinal cord and continues to higher and higher centers of the brain. As higher centers become effective, the lower centers, without ceasing to act, begin to be influenced by the higher in new ways. This development from lower to higher centers is spoken of as the *encephalization of function.* The word *encephalon* means brain, and encephalization occurs when the control of functions migrates in the developing child or in the evolution of animal species from the spinal cord to the brain. After encephalization has taken place, the same process of development is continued as *corticalization of function,* the migration in individual or evolutionary development of functional control from the lower centers of the brain to the cerebral cortex, where the highest centers lie. Thus, as development of the individual continues, the higher centers come to play a more and more important role in what the organism does. In man all voluntary movement and all learning are largely dependent upon the development of these higher centers.

GROWTH AND DEVELOPMENT BEFORE BIRTH

We turn now to follow the course of growth and development of a human being from a fertilized cell to his birth.

The Beginning of Human Growth

The growth of a human being starts first with the enlargement of the fertilized cell. Then, when the cell has reached a certain size, it divides into two smaller cells, each with a nucleus and surrounding protoplasm. These cells grow and again divide. The process continues, the number of cells increasing in geometrical proportion. Meanwhile the tiny individual is migrating from the oviduct, where fertilization took place, to the wall of the uterus, where it soon becomes attached. Here growth continues more rapidly until, two weeks after fertilization, the first period, called the *germinal period,* comes to an end. (See Fig. 25.)

The next five weeks of the life of the *prenate* (as the organism is called before birth) constitute the *embryonic period.* Growth goes on as before by cell enlargement and division, but differentiation also begins. These changes are the start of a long process, and some of the new structures do not become recognizable for several weeks. Others develop rapidly. By the end of the first week of the period (three weeks after fertilization) there occurs the first independent activity of the growing human embryo, namely, the beating of the cells which later develop into the adult human heart.

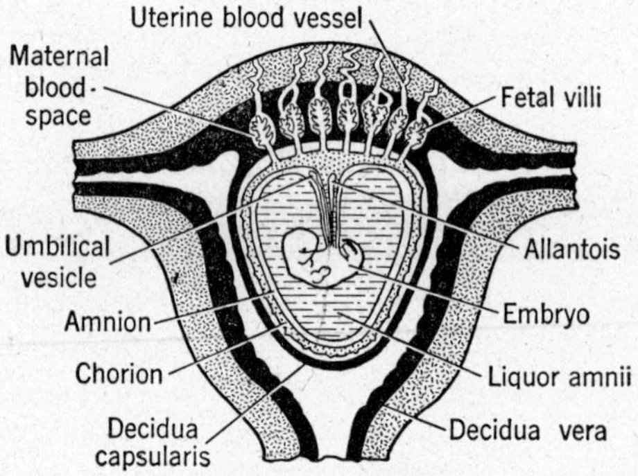

FIGURE 25. UTERUS, MEMBRANES AND EMBRYO IN EARLY PREGNANCY

[After L. Carmichael, *A handbook of child psychology* (2nd ed.), Clark University Press, 1933, p. 50.]

It may be remarked that at all times in the uterine life of the prenate, the circulatory system is completely separated from the maternal blood system by cell walls. A highly complex structure called the *placenta* develops to provide a means whereby the independent blood systems of the mother and child can communicate. (See Fig. 26.) Through the walls of this structure oxygen and food substances pass from the mother's blood to the independent blood stream of the embryo and fetus. Carbon dioxide and the other waste products from cell activity pass back into the maternal blood through the placenta. Furthermore, there is no neural connection at any time between the mother and the growing fetus. Contrary to superstitious belief, no transfer of ideas can take place between the mother and the fetus. Some drugs taken by the mother may, it is true, affect the fetus. It may be also that some strong emotions of the mother, which are related to changes in the chemical make-up of her blood, have some effect on the unborn child. If, however, the future mother wants a certain big strawberry and does not get it, this act does not produce a 'strawberry mark' on the unborn child which she is carrying, no matter what superstition may say.

By the end of the second month, the embryo begins to look like a human being, and thereafter until birth seven months later it is called a fetus. The *fetal period,* regarded as a whole, is first merely a continuation of the growth and development already begun. The external parts of the body—the features of the face, the arms and fingers, the legs and toes—become more clearly defined. There is also at this time a rapid increase in size. Beginning with the fourth month the cerebral cortex develops rapidly. Development of functional connections in the nervous system thus far has been restricted for the most part to the spinal cord and the lower parts of the brain —those parts which have the involuntary controls of the organs and muscles of the body. Now the cortex, man's most distinguishing feature, starts its rapid functional development. Presently, the fetus begins a wide variety of movements which, as its development proceeds, become more and more individualized. The first recorded movement, as the result of experimental

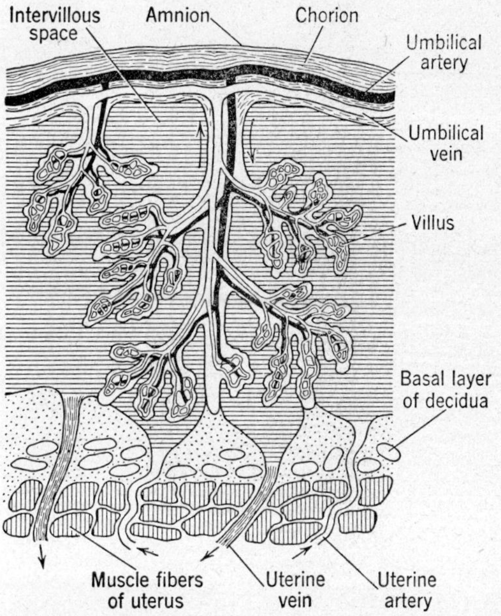

FIGURE 26. FETAL AND MATERNAL BLOOD STREAMS

In the placenta the fetal blood stream (umbilical artery and vein) and the maternal blood stream (uterine artery and vein) do not join. [From *Human Physiology* by Winton and Bayliss, by permission of J. & A. Churchill, Ltd., London.]

stimulation of fetuses that were born prematurely or removed from the mother by surgical means, occurred when the fetus was about eight and one-half weeks old. (See Fig. 27.) The stimulus was a light touch on the cheek near the mouth and it induced a contraction of the long muscles of the body and neck which resulted in a flexion of the body and accompanying movements of the arms. A week later a

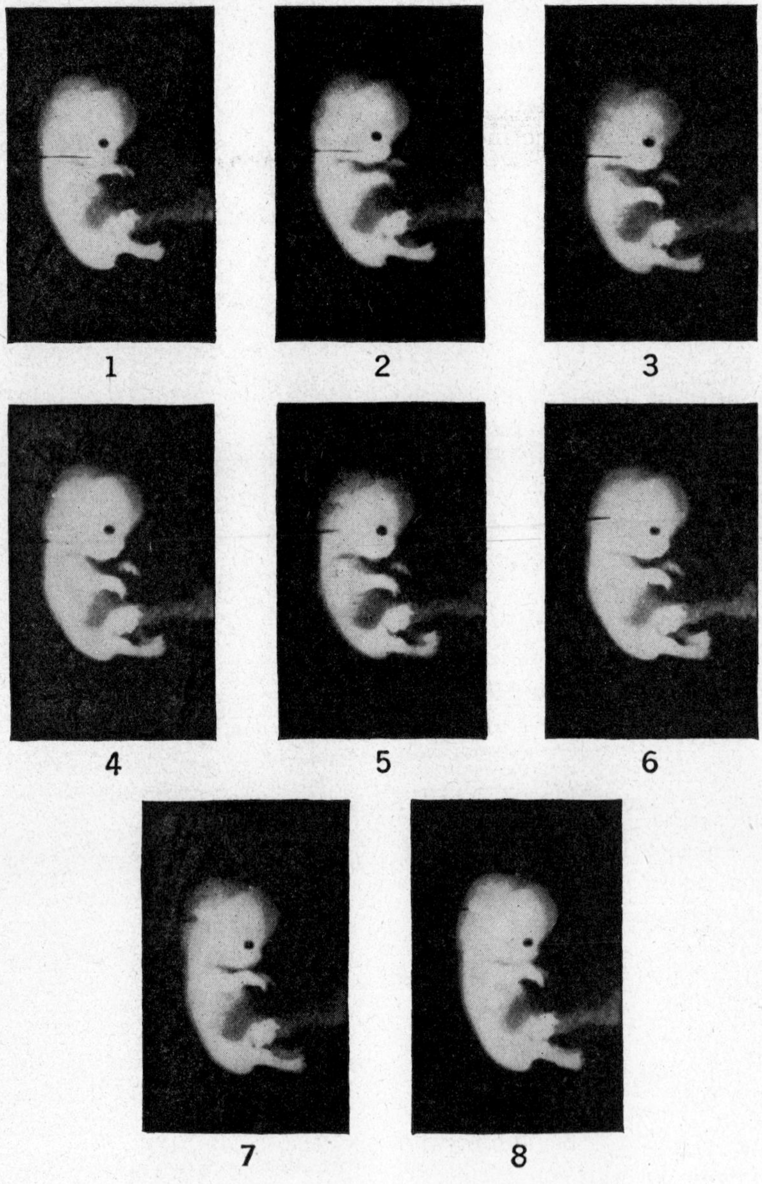

FIGURE 27. HUMAN FETUS WHEN ACTIVITY BEGINS

Photographs of response of fetus to touch stimulation at about eight weeks of age. [After D. Hooker, *A preliminary Atlas of early human fetal activity,* 1939, p. 15.]

similar stimulation produced a rotation of the pelvis in addition to a flexion of the body. By the twelfth week local movements resulted from stimulation of the arms and legs of the fetus. About the same time stimulation of the palm resulted in a partial closure of the fingers; this is the response which will later develop into the grasping reflex. These instances are perhaps enough to indicate the course of development of motor responses.

The responses of the prenate become more and more versatile and more and more effective as growth continues. In some mammals, such as the guinea pig, in which the development of behavior before birth has been studied in great detail, this sequence can be seen clearly. It is possible in the few weeks of prenatal development to observe how a first slight twitch of the forelimb develops into behavior which involves the effective use of almost every group of body muscles. Some of these late fetal sequences of response are marvelously well adjusted. In experimental work on still unborn guinea pigs it has been shown, for example, that the animals can localize and brush away with an appropriate paw a stimulus applied to almost any area of the skin. (See Fig. 28.) If this brushing response does not succeed in removing the stimulus, the guinea pig rotates its whole trunk in such a way as to favor removal of the touched spot from the noxious stimulus. If the stimulus still continues to be effective, it may be that the guinea pig's limbs begin to beat out a rhythmic swimming pattern which effectively moves the whole organism away from the stimulus save in so far as it is held fast by the umbilical cord. No one can watch such behavior in a fetus that has been prepared for experimental observation without recognizing the subtle perfection of the development for future activity that is begun before birth.

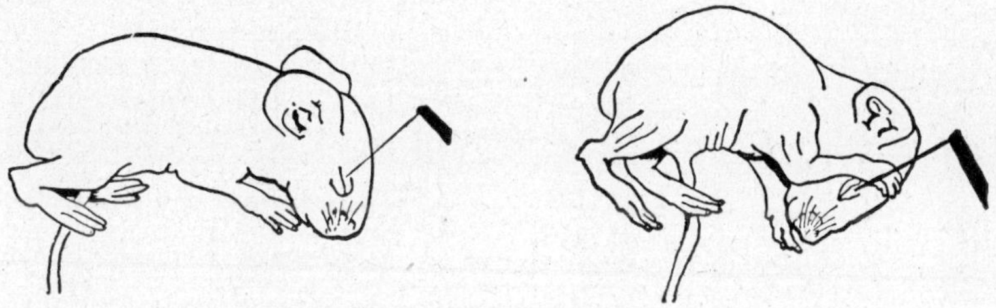

FIGURE 28. ADAPTIVE FETAL BEHAVIOR

Tracings of outline posture of the localizing paw movement of a guinea pig fetus a few days before the period of natural birth. Note the accuracy of this unlearned behavior. [After L. Carmichael and M. F. Smith, *J. genet. Psychol.*, 1939, **54**, 432.]

Rates of Prenatal Growth

Growth before birth is exceedingly rapid. The fertilized cell has a diameter of 0.013 millimeter or 1/2000 inch. By the end of the two weeks of the germinal period the prenate has a length of 6.0 millimeters or 1/4 inch, an increase 5 hundredfold in length (more than 100 millionfold in volume). During the eighth week the fetus is about an inch long and has increased its length 2 thousandfold since the beginning. At birth an average neonate has a length of 20 inches. That makes it about 40,000 times longer than the ovum from which it sprang, several thousand million times its original volume. The average rate per week for the 40 weeks of the uterine period is one-half inch. The growth per week at first increases rapidly and then after birth slows down. If the rate at birth were maintained until maturity, a grown man would be 45 feet tall.

the prenatal period, however, the brain reaches about two thirds of its adult size.

Before birth growth of the brain by the cell division of its neurons comes to an end. There are approximately twelve thousand million neurons in a normal brain at birth and there is no increase in this number during any part of postnatal life.

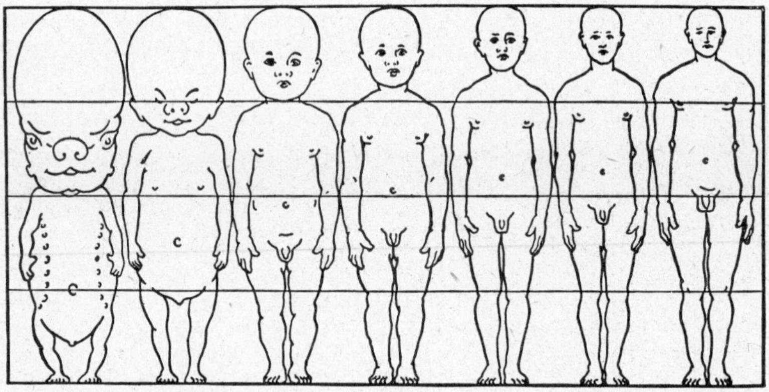

FIGURE 29. BODY PROPORTIONS DURING GROWTH

Changes in relative form and proportion of human body in fetal life, childhood, youth and adult life. [After C. M. Jackson; in W. J. Robbins, S. Brody, A. G. Hogan, C. M. Jackson and C. W. Green, *Growth*, Yale University Press, 1928, p. 118.]

The structures within the body also grow rapidly during the entire prenatal period. From about the third month until birth the weight of most of these structures increases at about the same rate; the small structures grow, in a given period, as much as the larger ones.

In the early days of the embryonic period, however, the heart and brain grow much more rapidly than other parts of the body. At about the fourth week, because of the large brain, the head constitutes nearly half the length of the embryo. Even at birth the size of the head is much larger in proportion to its body length than it will be at maturity. (See Fig. 29.) During

GROWTH AFTER BIRTH

Although, as we have seen, during most of the fetal period the structures of the body grow at about the same relative rate, after birth their rates and increments vary widely. Despite this variability, it has been found that the rates of many structures fall into groups for each of which the increments of growth through a number of years are so similar as to suggest types of growth.

Types of Growth

Four of these types with their typical growth curves are shown in Fig. 30. They represent only the growth that occurs between birth and the twentieth year. The increments shown in the figure are percentages of the total growth during that period.

The topmost curve is of the *Lymphoid Type.* It represents the growth of the thymus gland and a few lymphoid tissues. The curve rises sharply for eleven years and then falls until the end of the period of twenty years is reached.

The next curve is of the *Neural Type.* It includes the brain, the spinal cord and the eye. The curve of the pineal gland is similar but does not rise quite so rapidly. In this type, growth is rapid for the first six years, then slower for the next two years, and finally it nearly stops for the remainder of the period.

Below this in the figure is the curve of the *General Type.* It represents the growth of the body as a whole (excepting the head, neck and chest) in its external dimensions, the respiratory and digestive organs, the kidneys, the spleen, the muscles, the skeleton and blood volume. The curve rises rapidly until about the fourth year, much more slowly until about the twelfth year, rapidly again until the eighteenth year and slowly again until the end of the period.

The last curve is of the *Genital Type.* It shows the trend of growth for the testes,

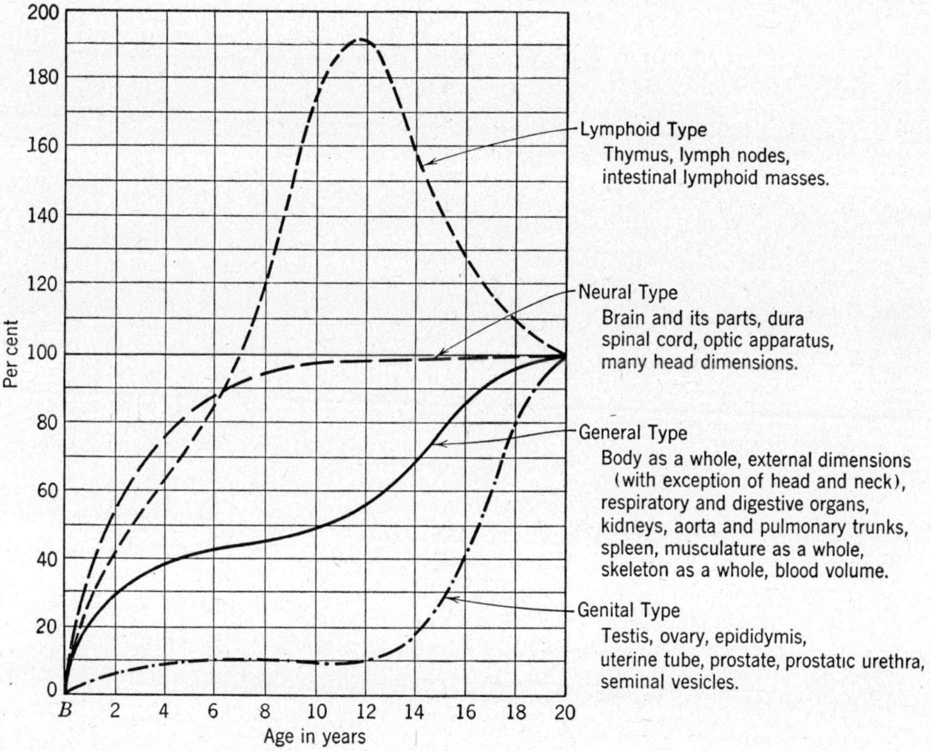

FIGURE 30. MAJOR TYPES OF POSTNATAL GROWTH OF THE VARIOUS PARTS AND ORGANS OF THE BODY

The several curves are drawn to a common scale by computing their values at successive ages in terms of their total postnatal increments (to twenty years). [From J. A. Harris, C. M. Jackson, D. G. Paterson and R. E. Scammon, *The measurement of man,* University of Minnesota Press, 1930, p. 193.]

ovaries, uterine tube, prostate gland and the seminal vesicles. There is first a slight growth for four years, then no growth at all until the twelfth year, after which there is a rapid growth until the end of adolescence.

Two things should be said about these typical curves. One is that they do not include all curves of growth. There are a few —those, for instance, of head, neck and chest circumference, of the weight of the suprarenal glands, the human uterus and the thyroid gland—that do not fit into any type. Second, it should be emphasized that the typical curves are merely graphic representations of trends of growth. As such they are exceedingly useful in aiding the understanding of the growth and development of the individual.

Maturity

Maturity means cessation of growth. A time is ultimately reached beyond which, normally, there is no further increase in size. Structures belonging to the neural type reach that stage, as we have seen, at about ten years after birth; those of the lymphoid type at twelve years; those of the general and genital types may continue to grow until at least the twenty-fifth year.

Increase in weight of the body may, of course, occur as a result of deposits of fat. When growth ceases, its curve either becomes a straight horizontal line and may so continue for thirty-five or forty years or even until death in extreme old age, or the curve turns downward representing a decrease in size, the regression of senescence.

MATURATION AT BIRTH

The newborn infant is called a *neonate*. We turn now to the appraisal of its maturation.

The Neonate in a New Environment

Development after birth is a continuation of prenatal development. At the moment of birth the neonate comes into a different world. For months he has been living as a prenate in a fluid medium of a constant temperature; he has been shielded by his liquid environment from all external stimuli and has derived his oxygen and food from his mother without breathing and without digestion. In a short interval he becomes an air-dwelling animal living in a variable temperature. He is now subject to a wide variety of external stimulation and must obtain his oxygen by his own breathing and his food by his own digestion. These new needs require that the great physiological functions—circulation, respiration and digestion—be maturated if the infant is to survive. Premature births show that the maturation of these functions is fairly well established as early as 220 days after fertilization, 60 days before normal birth. A baby born 180 days after fertilization rarely survives, principally because its digestive system is not at that time sufficiently developed.

We shall subsequently see that a number of other forms of behavior reach maturation at birth. The muscles of the trunk, legs and arms, however, have not yet reached sufficient development for their proper effective functioning in air. The liquid prenatal environment, because it is so nearly of the same specific gravity as the fetus, allows a complexity and precision of prenatal muscular response that the neonate cannot again achieve until some time after its birth. At birth the cortex of the brain, despite the fact that it has been developing since the latter half of the fetal period, is still immature.

Reflexes in the Neonate

During the first few days the complex feeding reactions, involving head orientation, lip reflexes, sucking and swallowing, mature. Soon after birth many infants can also grasp a rod and support their own weight if the rod is lifted. This *involuntary grasping reflex* ordinarily disappears during the first half year of life. Another reflex which soon disappears is the *Babinski reflex* in which the infant extends its toes when the bottom of the foot is tickled. (See Fig. 31.) This reflex is later replaced by the *plantar reflex* which consists of a curling up of the toes when the sole of the foot is stimulated. The plantar reflex depends upon certain motor tracts that lead from the brain to the spinal cord and appears when these fibers mature after birth.

An infant a few hours old, when held vertically in such a way as to support his head and trunk, and with the soles of his feet touching the floor, often makes prancing movements. These movements consist in alternately raising the legs and flexing them at the knee—behavior which is

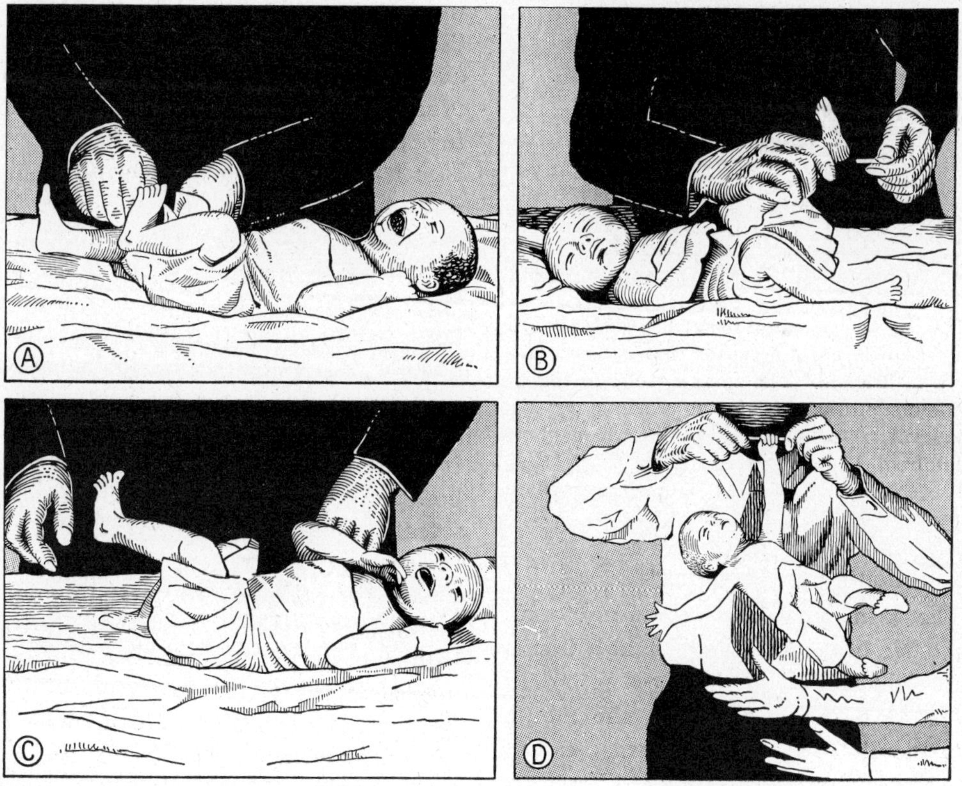

FIGURE 31. INFANTILE REFLEXES

(*A*) Defensive reflex with left foot to slight pinch on inner surface of right knee. (*B*) Stimulation for Babinski reflex. The blunt end of a match is rubbed across the sole of the foot. The result is shown in (*C*). The great toe shows extension, whereas the small toes shown 'fanning' or flexion. This is a variable reflex as far as the pattern is concerned. (*D*) The grasping reflex (infant 12 days old). [After J. B. Watson, *Psychology from the standpoint of a behaviorist,* Lippincott, 1919, p. 239.]

part of the leg movement in walking. (See Fig. 32.)

There are many other specific reflexes which develop in normal human individuals at various periods.

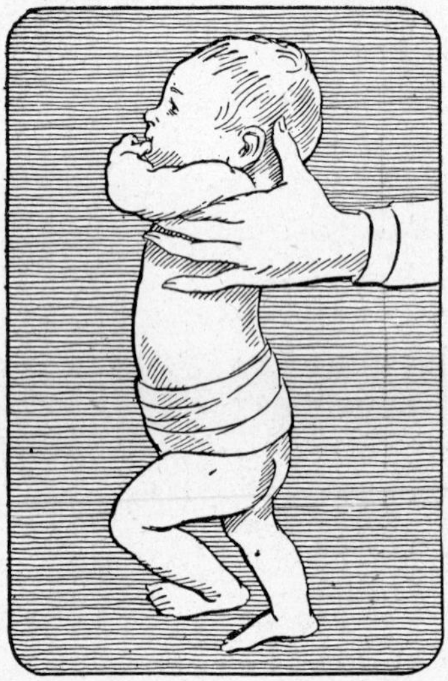

FIGURE 32. EARLY STEPPING MOVEMENTS

Infants a few hours old sometimes show prancing steps when they are supported under the arms, as shown in diagram. The patterns basic to this behavior are probably related to walking responses which will appear much later. [Sketch of photograph from M. B. McGraw, *Child development*, 1932, 3, 295; by permission of Williams and Wilkins Company.]

Maturation of the Receptors

The skin sense for pressure develops first. We have already seen that a human fetus eight and a half weeks old responded to pressure stimulation near the mouth. The mouth is the first area that can be activated by pressure stimuli. Later, effective areas for pressure stimulation spread over the entire skin surface. Such sensory development, like the development of movement, proceeds in a general cephalocaudal direction.

Responses to the stimulation of temperature and pain receptors can also be elicited during fetal life. The pain sense is, however, not well developed in the prenate. A needle prick or even a laceration of deep tissues in a fetus may not cause any more vigorous response than would a light touch with a soft hair. This late development of pain may have important value, for it may minimize the shock of the mechanical pulling and squeezing that are incident to birth.

It has long been known that at birth the receptors for smell, taste, vision and hearing (as soon as the liquid has drained from the middle ear) respond to their appropriate stimuli. The responses are movements usually of some part of the face like blinking, frowning or opening the eyes wide. The neonate does not distinguish objects until the higher levels of the brain have developed. Recently systematic observations have been made of a number of infants, some of whom were prematurely born babies that are called fetal infants because, except for the accident of birth, they would still be fetuses. They ranged in age from twenty-eight to forty weeks. It was found that they not only respond to both auditory and visual stimuli during the seventh month, but also that their responses may change in kind at a later time. For example, the first response of fetal infants to a bell may be a slight frown with a blink of the eyes, but during the ninth month its response changes to an opening of the eyes. Furthermore, the earliest movements are feeble and spasmodic, and, as a general rule, they cease entirely if the stimulus is frequently repeated. Later, they become stronger and more continuous. These facts mean that, with the earliest responses, development is not quite complete; a little more time or, it may be, some practice is necessary before it is complete.

Eye movements, which are later so important for visual perception, may also be observed in course of development in the fetal infant. During the seventh month the two eyes may move together in both horizontal and vertical directions, even before there is any definite response to a visual stimulus. During the eighth month the eyes may follow, with brief movements but without fixation, any object that moves slowly across the visual field. During the next month the eyes may definitely follow a moving object through an arc of forty-five degrees. All these eye movements mature quickly shortly after the time of normal birth.

There are located in each inner ear of a mammal, not only the complex sense organs which make hearing possible, but also stabilizing mechanisms, the static or vestibular receptors, which assist the organism in maintaining body balance. (See pp. 374–378.) There is good reason to believe that these inner-ear receptors are effective in fetal life. Before the eyes of the fetus have moved in response to stimulation by light, they can be made to move by changing the position of the fetus with respect to gravity in such a way as to stimulate the receptors in the inner ear. The maturation of such adjustments makes it possible for an infant, as he later develops, not only to maintain his posture but also to keep his eyes focused upon objects even when his own head and body move.

Maturation of Emotion

It is doubtful that the prenate and the neonate show clearly differentiated emotional responses, such as fear, joy and rage. Rather it appears that very young infants experience only a state of general excitation which results from certain so-called emotion-arousing situations such as undue restraint, sudden noises or being dropped onto a pillow. It is almost certain that the component movements of the behavior patterns of emotions are a result of maturation in the part of the brain called the *hypothalamus.*

The hypothalamus thus tends to induce certain emotional patterns, and the cerebral cortex tends to inhibit or limit this action of the hypothalamus. (See p. 100.) For instance, rage is natural to cats and dogs —the snarling, hissing attack of the cat, the growling, snapping attack of the dog. These behavior patterns are activated by the hypothalamus, but inhibited by the action of the cortex. The surgical removal of the cortex releases the thalamic action, and these animals, when disturbed, snarl and snap quickly and automatically in a manner so closely resembling a reflex that their behavior is called *sham rage.*

Thus it comes about that the development of the cortex makes possible the development of emotional restraint in man, as well as in the cat and dog. A child, using his cortex, gradually learns what emotional expressions are approved by the social groups to which he belongs, modifying his inborn behavior patterns accordingly. It follows that emotional maturity, the control of emotion, depends on the maturation of the cortex and learning—when the individual has a cortex with which to learn.

MATURATION AFTER BIRTH

Between the neonatal and adolescent levels of development comes childhood. In it adaptive behavior appears, the ability to learn develops and language is acquired.

The Maturation of Adaptive Behavior

As the child develops he progressively makes a large number of movements common to all human beings, which are unlearned and have only awaited maturation to be performed. These movements require the action of the higher brain centers and so are instances of the encephalization or corticalization of function. They are, in a sense, controlled movements and may be classified as voluntary. Examples of these forms of behavior are grasping, creeping, standing erect, walking, running. We may take the maturation of the act of walking as an illustration of their development.

The alternate innervation of the two legs in the prancing movement already described shows that a highly complex neuromuscular organization is well along at birth. Before the child can walk, however, he must first be able to hold up his head, then to hold his trunk erect without support while sitting. The maturation of erect sitting must await the stiffening of the spine. Next he must be able to stand erect, an act which he cannot do until the bones and muscles of his legs are strong enough to bear his weight. The order of these maturations, it will be noticed, follow the cephalocaudal rule. The child still cannot maintain his equilibrium until maturation effects the coordination of the sensory nerves from his muscles, the sensory nerves from his semicircular canals (see p. 378) and the motor tracts leading to his muscles. Only then can he transform the prancing into a walking movement by thrusting his flexed leg forward until it rests on the floor, at the same time letting his center of gravity also go forward. He must then maintain his balance on the one foot until the other is brought up and thrust forward. The repetition of this sequence is walking. Walking is the end product of a series of maturations which it takes the prancing infant about twelve to fourteen months to complete.

Norms of Early Development

There are tables and charts showing the general sequences of behavior which may be expected to take place during the first

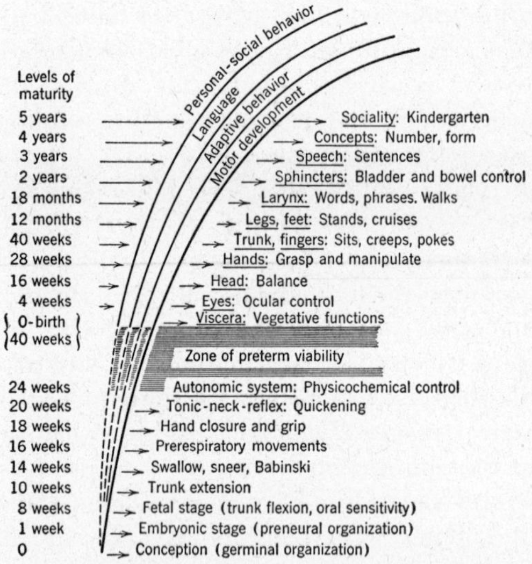

FIGURE 33. HUMAN BEHAVIOR GROWTH

Diagram to show gradual development of behavior in early life. [After A. Gesell and C. S. Amatruda, *Developmental diagnosis: normal and abnormal child development,* Hoeber, 1941, p. 9.]

five years. (See Fig. 33.) In the first year, the child gains control of his basic muscles so as to be able to grasp objects and stand erect and to do many other acts in his new nonaquatic environment. In his second year, typically, he walks and runs and articulates words and phrases. At this time he may acquire bladder and bowel control. In his third year, he speaks sentences and begins to comply with the demands of his home. In his fourth year, he asks many questions and becomes self-dependent in the routines of the house. At five he hops and skips, can tell a long story and is "a self-assured conforming citizen of his small world."

There are, nevertheless, great differences in the sequence of development in different children. No doubt some of these differences are due to differences in inherited rates of maturation. Some differences are also due to differences in environmental opportunity, as the studies of twins suggest. (See pp. 448 f.) It is also likely that there is a basis in maturation for the appearance of certain aptitudes, like musical ability.

Maturation of Ability to Learn

Thus far our discussion has been limited almost entirely to development in general and the maturation of unlearned behavior in particular. We can now turn to some of the relations between maturation and learning. It is, of course, impossible to say just when maturation ceases and learning begins. It may be that the fetal infant, by exercise or practice, 'learns' something from the feeble, spasmodic and discontinuous movements that he makes before the maturation of his eye movements is complete. It may be that the child can be said to learn from his successes and failures when he—as some of them do while taking their first steps—totters, staggers, falls down, gets up and tries again. The question of the effectiveness of such learning—assuming that it takes place—has been the subject of a number of investigations.

Experiments have been carried out on animals, birds and mammals to determine the effect of withholding exercise from certain young of a brood or litter, while allowing the others to exercise as they developed. Chicks, for instance, have been hooded or otherwise kept from visual experience after they hatch, to keep them from using the seeing-pecking behavior for food. Birds have also been prevented from flying until other birds of the same age were flying well. Figure 34 shows the result of some experiments in this field.

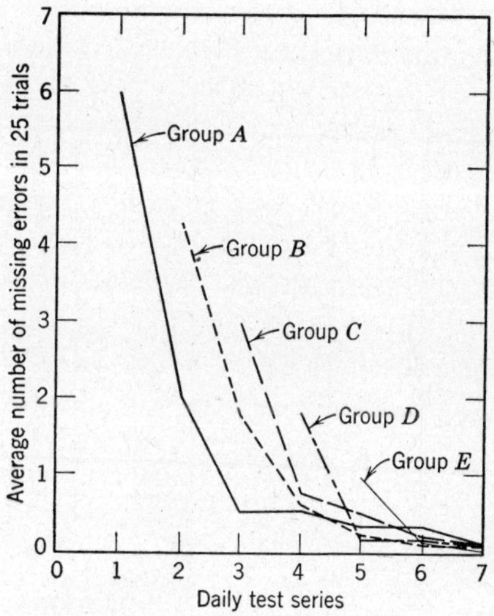

FIGURE 34. CHICK'S PECKING SKILL AND MATURATION

Errors of chicks given opportunity to peck for first time when 1 day old (Group *A*) up to when 5 days old (Group *E*). Curves show greater initial accuracy in older chicks, but learning is always needed to supplement maturation. Note speed of learning in 4-day groups. [From W. W. Cruze, *J. comp. Psychol.*, 1935, **19**, 391, Williams and Wilkins Co.]

In experiments with amphibians it has proved possible to raise experimental groups of larval *Amblystoma* (salamanders) in water containing a drug which kept the larvae from making any movements. At a later time, when a control group developed from eggs of the same age and raised in undrugged water were freely swimming, the experimental animals were placed in fresh water. In a few minutes the previously anesthetized animals swam in a way hardly to be distinguished from that of the animals that had been freely 'practicing' for some days.

All these experiments seem to show that the animal who was backward for want of exercise may overtake the animal who has had exercise all along after they have been given equal opportunity. Does this result hold also for the human organism? This question too has been put to experiment.

A detailed study has been made of a pair of twin boys from the age of twenty-one days to the age of twenty-two months.

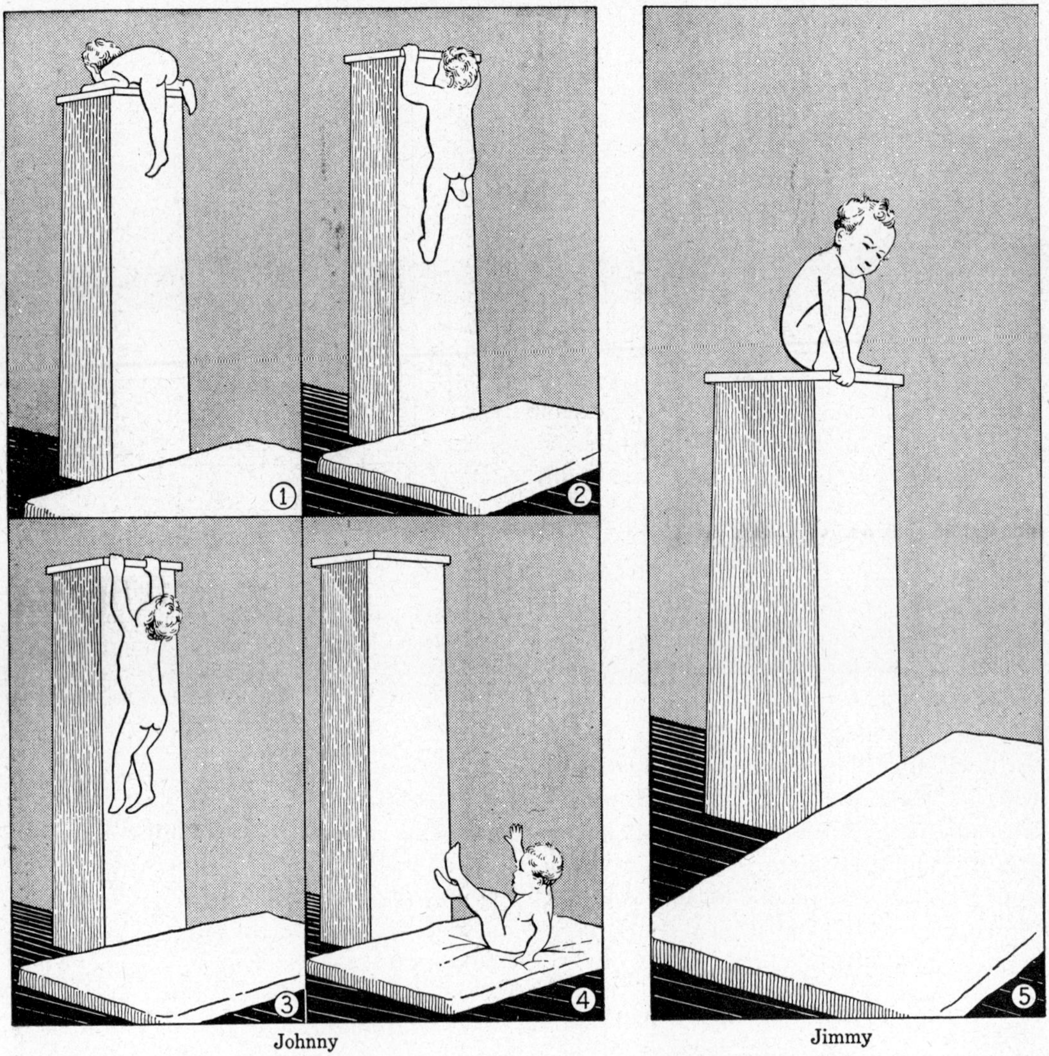

FIGURE 35. DEVELOPMENT OF TWINS' BEHAVIOR WITH PRACTICE

Johnny (*left*), who had been given a great deal of active exercise, tackles the problem of getting himself down from the pedestal with ease, whereas Jimmy (*right*), who had been given a minimum of active play, sits perched on top, unable to solve his problem. [After M. B. McGraw, *Growth: a study of Johnny and Jimmy,* Appleton-Century, 1935, pp. 156–157.]

Johnny, one of the twins, was regularly exercised in motor abilities, while his twin, Jimmy, was kept in a crib in the laboratory during the day. The two were compared with each other and with sixty-eight other children. This study showed that the behavior which every child must acquire in order to act as a biologically normal human being is not markedly modified by opportunity for practice. Maturation alone seems to take care of such responses. Specialized skills, on the other hand, are dependent on practice. Actually, Johnny, the exercised twin, continued all the way up to ten years of age to show greater muscular skill than his brother who received relatively little practice during the first two years of life. (See Fig. 35.) Human skills, unlike swimming of salamander larvae, depend on much more than inheritance. A good coach is an important factor in the success of a team.

This experiment, taken with the others, seems to show that the exercise of a behavior before its maturation is finished does no more than hasten the maturation. It can act in one or both of two ways. Exercise increases the growth and thus the strength of the muscles involved. That is one way in which exercise could hurry maturation. It is also conceivable that exercise hastens the integration of a neuromuscular pattern. In either case exercise would be doing little more than time alone would accomplish in completing the maturation. Furthermore it seems clear that, if there is any learning as a result of exercise, it affords little profit in so far as man's basic and fundamental acts of behavior are concerned. In the acquisition of specialized skills, on the other hand, learning is necessary, and what Johnny, the exercised twin, had learned, together with his greater strength, explains his superiority over his brother.

Since learning itself depends upon maturation, individual differences in the rate of maturation create individual differences in the capacity to learn. Children who mature earlier can learn specific skills earlier. Some infrahuman animals of a given age can learn more quickly than human children of the same age those forms of behavior that are common to both, simply because the child matures more slowly.

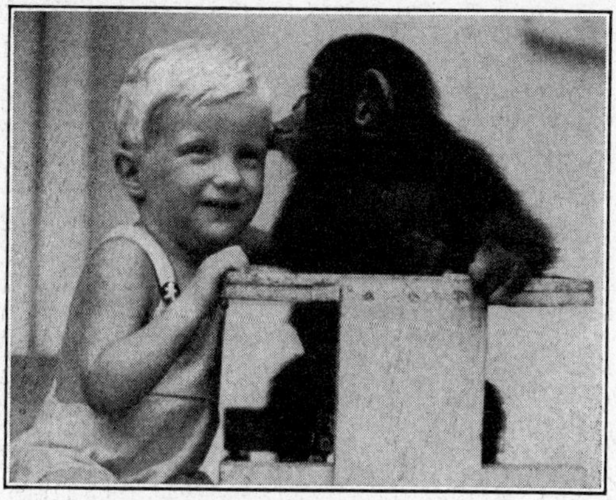

FIGURE 36. CHIMPANZEE AND HUMAN INFANT OF ABOUT THE SAME AGE

For two and a half years this chimpanzee lived in a human family with two children, one of them about its own age. (See also Fig. 216, p. 451.) [From R. M. Yerkes, *Chimpanzees: a laboratory colony,* Yale University Press, 1943, p. 191.]

There is an interesting example of this difference. A human infant and a chimpanzee infant of about the same age were brought together in the human child's home. (See Fig. 36.) Both were treated exactly alike. Each was fondled, kissed as he went to sleep and punished in the same way. Because the chimpanzee matured more rapidly, he outdistanced his human companion in many ways. At twelve months the chimpanzee could respond to twenty verbal commands such as "Open the door" and "Shake hands," but the human child could respond to only three. In control of bowels and bladder and in other skills the chimpanzee was superior to the child. The chimpanzee learned better to use a spoon and to drink from a glass. In general, at one year of age the chimpanzee could do better with a problem of learning than the child. This finding means simply that the physiological basis for learning had matured earlier in the ape than in the child. No ape, however, reared in human or other environment, has ever acquired the advanced use of language or of the other symbols that are basic to man's mental life. When the centers of the human brain, which are essential in the use of language and other symbolic processes, finally mature, a new kind of learning, not possessed by any organism other than man, becomes available. At this stage of maturation the human child soon outdistances all his animal competitors. (For details of a similar experiment, see p. 451.)

Maturation of Speech and Language

Speech implies both vocalization and symbolization—the production of sounds and their use as symbols. Both functions depend on learning, and both require the development of the higher brain centers before progress with respect to them can be made.

Vocalization consists in the coordination of the nerves and muscles which control movements of the throat, palate, tongue, lips and the lower jaw. Separately, as reflexes, all these movements are present at birth, and all are at least partially coordinated in the infant's first cry. The birth cry of the human infant has superstitiously been regarded from early times as having symbolic significance. It is, however, only a reflex which results from a stimulation of receptors and a coordination of groups of motor nerves in the medulla of the brain. For example, when the contraction of the walls of the empty stomach stimulates the receptors there, the baby cries. The cry has no symbolic significance whatever to the baby although to its nurse it means "the baby is hungry." Crying is not necessarily speech.

The coordination of the motor nerves necessary for speech occurs in the cortex of the brain in an area that is called the speech center. This coordination, the integration of the nerves to the various muscles of the throat and mouth, is sufficiently matured by the sixth or seventh month after birth to make possible the beginning of learning to talk. At this time the child begins to babble. Babbling consists in the automatic production of meaningless syllables; they are variable in sound, but generally the same syllable is repeated a number of times. The child hears, of course, the sounds of its own voice and apparently finds the experience pleasurable. Babbling is a period of practice in enunciation, particularly in the use of the tongue and lips. It has been said that before the period ends all the sounds are produced which occur in any language. This statement does not mean that the child can at will enunciate any speech sound that he hears and wishes to imitate. He needs much practice before he can command the sounds of his mother tongue.

When vocalization has become possible, then *symbolization* can follow. The sounds can acquire meanings. Symbolization is created by learning and the building up of conditioned responses. Since this process is discussed in a later chapter (pp. 594 f.), we need not consider it here.

When a vocalized sound has acquired a meaning, it has become a *word.* A repertoire of words is a *vocabulary.* At first the child acquires a vocabulary but slowly. When twelve months old he can usually respond to his own name and to two or three other words. At fifteen months he may know half a dozen more words; at eighteen months, twenty to fifty words. When he discovers that all objects have names, an event which occurs during his second year, his progress becomes much more rapid. By the beginning of his third year he will have learned some three hundred words. There can be no doubt that every one of these advances in his learning is preceded by a new stage of maturation, some new coordination or integration that occurs in the cerebral cortex.

ADOLESCENCE, ADULTHOOD AND OLD AGE

The period from adolescence to old age may be four times as long as the period from conception to adolescence, but it does not include nearly so much change. The adult reaches the height of his powers but slowly, and thereafter declines but slowly.

Puberty and Adolescence

Adolescence is the period of some eight or ten years during which the human individual develops from childhood to adulthood. The period is characterized by *pubescence,* the beginning of the procreative functions. It is the maturation of a complex mechanism which includes the sex glands, the external sexual organs and parts of the nervous system. The chronological age at which puberty begins is variable; it may, however, be expected during the thirteenth year in girls, and the following year in boys, and is generally regarded as established at the first menstruation in girls and at the appearance of pubic hair in boys. The common belief that puberty is reached early in tropical countries is not borne out by careful study. Girls in the United States reach sexual maturity on the average as early as any group that has been scientifically studied.

A second characteristic of adolescence is the rapid increase in the growth and development of the individual. As we have seen in the curve of the general type of growth in Fig. 30 (p. 73), the period begins during the eleventh year and the curve begins to flatten out about the sixteenth year, although it will continue to rise by smaller increments beyond the twentieth year. The change thus begins before puberty, and it commences earlier in girls than in boys, with the result that, although throughout childhood the boy has on the average been taller and heavier than the girl of the same age, from the eleventh to the fourteenth year this relation is reversed. Thereafter the boy will resume his superiority in this respect. We have also seen that the sex glands and all the internal and external sexual organs begin a period of rapid growth at about the twelfth year, starting at least a year earlier in girls than in boys.

This growth results not only in an increase in height, weight and the maturation of the sexual organs, but also in changes in the relative proportions of the head, the legs and arms, the trunk and the features of the face. Other changes are the secondary sexual characters noted previously. In a boy these changes are the starting of the beard and hair on other parts of the body and a lowering of the pitch of the voice, which sometimes amounts to as much as an octave. In a girl, the voice drops only slightly in pitch and she develops pubic hair and the soft downy hair on her face. There is also a widening of the pelvis and a consequent broadening of the hips and the development of the breasts.

A third characteristic of adolescence is the appearance of an increased emphasis upon certain previously existing interests and attitudes. The adolescent begins to be concerned about the other sex, and in romance and sexual matters. He feels a heightened self-consciousness, realizes more fully his position in the social group in which he moves. He gains a greater desire for independence and a tendency to resist parental direction. The girl, in particular, may become critical of her mother's dress and the way she does her hair. Both boys and girls acquire new attitudes toward social, economic and religious ideas which they formerly accepted without thought, but which now they question, at times with intolerance. Because he is still inexperienced the adolescent often says and does many things that he will later regard as radical or ill advised.

For many individuals this period is difficult. The adolescent has so many new adjustments to make. He yearns for action, but his goals are not yet clear. Nor does he yet know that his problems are characteristic of the period through which he is passing and that time alone will bring their solution.

Adulthood

There are wide individual differences in the chronological age at which the adolescent period ends. It ends earlier in women than in men, and within a sex it happens earlier in some persons than in others. It may be said to be all over by the age of twenty-five. By that time, as we have seen, the organism has practically completed its growth—only the skin, the nails and the hair continue to grow. Repair, however, will still go on.

When all maturation has come to an end, the normal individual does everything that all normal members of the human race do. His neuromuscular growth and development, however, are now such that he may learn to do many other things. His rate of metabolism is high; he has great stores of energy; he fatigues slowly and recuperates quickly. For this reason he is able to do more and harder work with fewer ill effects than at any other time in his life. He has presumably decided on his life's work—his trade, business or profession. His formal education is finished, and his apprenticeship or professional training is nearly completed. The end of maturation is, therefore, the beginning of another period, the period of adulthood, which may last for thirty-five or forty years, while the individual rears a family, masters a trade or profession and otherwise plays the part of a mature person in the culture to which he belongs.

The first twenty years of adulthood are, however, the most productive. A study of the recorded achievements of one thousand historically eminent persons showed that about a third of their best work was done between the ages of thirty and forty, and seventy per cent of it before the forty-fifth year. The causes for this difference must be very complex. The younger adult has more endurance; he can work harder and longer. He has higher motivation to work, not only because of his need to make a living for himself and his family, but also because he feels competition with his fellows more keenly when he is at the threshold of his career. It is not clear whether besides endurance and motivation there is something else that makes young animals and young people and younger adults more active, more aggressive, more enthusiastic, more 'energetic' than they will be later in life. It is certainly true that younger animals and persons expend effort more readily than older ones. What happens seems to be that this 'energy' diminishes with age while wisdom and skill increase, with the result that maximal effectiveness occurs

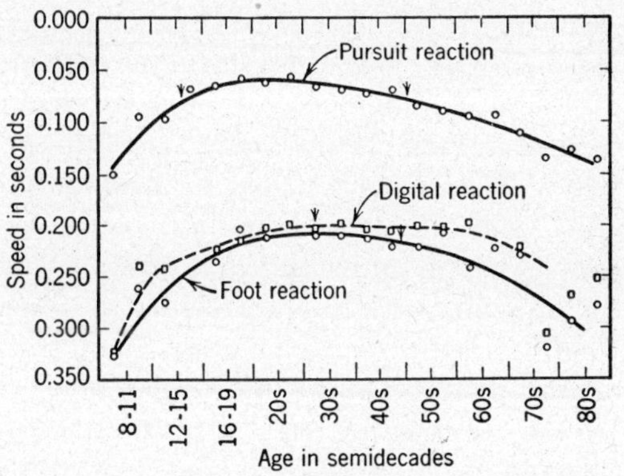

FIGURE 37. SPEED OF RESPONSE TO STIMULI AT VARIOUS AGES

Many other human functions follow similar curves. See also Fig. 30. [After W. R. Miles, *Proc. Nat. Acad. Sci.*, 1931, **17**, 631.]

for human beings in an intermediate decade around forty. There is possibly also a third effective factor: creative work in older adults becomes more difficult because society makes more demands upon older responsible people and seeks oftener to determine their activities. For instance, greatness, once achieved, may bring about its own limitation, for it takes time and is fatiguing to play the role of a famous person.

The high tide of muscular strength, endurance and speed of action at first recedes slowly and then, as the years go on, more rapidly. The professional baseball player, particularly the in-fielder, is frequently said to be an old man at thirty to thirty-seven years of age. He no longer has the blinding speed necessary to play his position with his former skill. Experiments also show that the speed of various movements of the hand, fingers and foot reaches its peak just before or soon after the twentieth year, and within the next decade begins a decline which continues for the remainder of life. The curves of some of these results are shown in Figs. 37 and 38.

After the forty-fifth year other decrements which at first were so small as to be unnoticed begin to be bothersome. The individual finds that his hearing is not so good as it was; he can no longer hear very high tones like the chirp of the cricket, and he frequently misses a word in a conversation. He discovers also that, although he

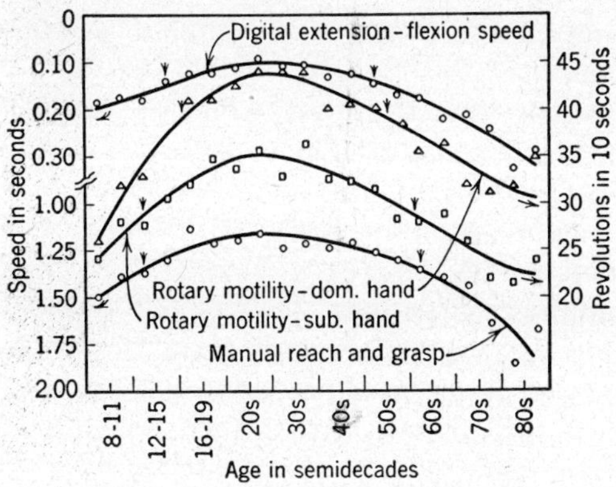

FIGURE 38. MOTILITY AT VARIOUS AGES

See also Fig. 37. [After W. R. Miles, *Proc. Nat. Acad. Sci.*, 1931, **17**, 629.]

can still see distant objects, he cannot focus his eyes to near objects as well as formerly. His memory too is often bothersome. At times he cannot recall proper and place names that are perfectly familiar. His immediate memory is bad. For example, he may look up a telephone number and then forget it before he puts in his call. He has trouble also in remembering facts that belong to a field which is unfamiliar. On the other hand, he may recall with fidelity the details of events that happened many years earlier, as well as new facts in a familiar field.

As a man grows older there is a decided shift in his interests and attitudes. He cares less for physical activity, and he gradually gives up those forms of sport that require strength, speed and endurance. If he continues to play tennis, he no longer tries to cover the court; instead he tries to win by strategy and greater accuracy. If he plays golf, he is satisfied with nine or perhaps six holes; and, if he defeats his younger opponent, it is through accuracy rather than distance. As observer, however, his interest in sports increases. He does not care so much for dancing or the cinema as younger persons do. The statistical studies show also that he has an increased interest in his home, in art galleries, in his church and in his clubs.

The least diminution with advancing years occurs in those human activities that depend less upon muscle and more upon brain. For example, tests of the kind of imagination which sees objects in the clouds or in ink blots show that there is little decline with age. Moreover, tests of comparison and judgment in which speed, immediate memory or recall of unfamiliar material are not involved, reveal that the older person does just about as well as the younger. On the whole, skill in verbal association, interpretation of meaning, generalization and the finding of relations resists the influence of age. Thus it comes about that the older man, provided he has escaped the hardening effect of habit, becomes a valued counselor; his long and varied experience renders his judgments more objective and impartial and gives his opinions greater breadth and perspective. Thus he finds compensation for the physical disabilities that overtake him.

Old Age

The period of old age is called senescence. There is no particular time at which senescence can be said to begin. The process of aging, like the process of maturing, is continuous and the two kinds of change are often just the obverse and reverse of the same process. Actually aging begins as soon as the ovum is fertilized. When the prenate, two weeks after development has started, passes from the germinal period to the embryonic period, its cells undergo a change. At first they are what is called *totipotent:* any cell could develop into a whole individual or into any of the kinds of tissue of which the individual is composed. Then the cells change, acquiring special functions, and it is no longer possible, for example, to get a nerve cell from a cell destined to be muscle. This specialization is a stage of maturation, but it is also a stage of prenatal aging. For the gain in special potency there had to be a loss in general potency. Senescence can be regarded simply as the ultimate maturity when the losses have become more noticeable than the gains.

Man does not grow old at the same rate all over. His vital organs, his glands, his bones and muscles, his senses and his psychological abilities age at different rates. It is only after a long time, somewhere between the ages of fifty and seventy-five, that all these symptoms combine to make up the picture of true old age. It may be even later before we find the extreme picture of age—the tottering step, the trembling hands, the filmed and watery eyes, the fluttering heart, the wrinkled skin, the extreme forgetfulness. Even then the old man has not lost his usefulness to society if his mind remains clear. He needs to resist the tendency to withdraw into himself, to nurse his growing infirmities, and thus to become solitary.

Postmortem studies show that all the structures of the body have degenerated in old age. Nearly all the internal organs and glands are atrophied and decreased in size. The muscles are shot through with fibrous tissue losing their elasticity and contractility. The cartilages are stiffened with deposits of lime. The arteries are hard and inelastic, a condition (*arteriosclerosis*) which results from a cellular change in the walls of the arteries, making it more difficult for the heart to force blood into the small capillaries of the brain, and thus depriving the brain of the needed food and oxygen. (See Fig. 39.) Sometimes, under high blood pressure, the blood vessels in some region of the brain burst, resulting in a 'stroke' (*apoplexy*), a partial paralysis. There is another kind of *sclerosis* which is a degeneration within the brain itself, and which, if it progresses far enough, may result in senile dementia, a form of mental disorder which sometimes occurs in the very old. Personality changes at various ages of the individual are discussed in a later chapter (pp. 505–509).

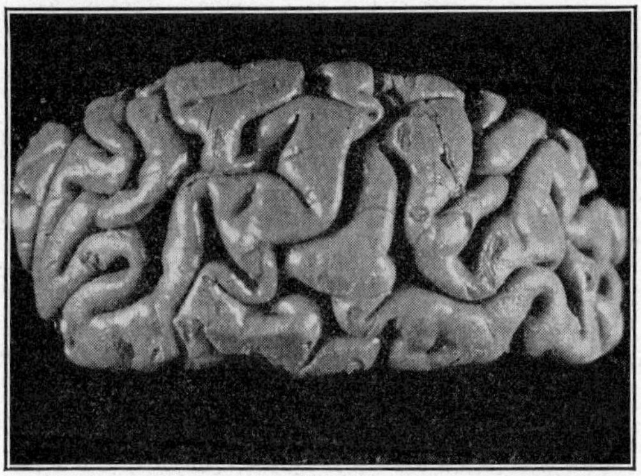

(*a*)

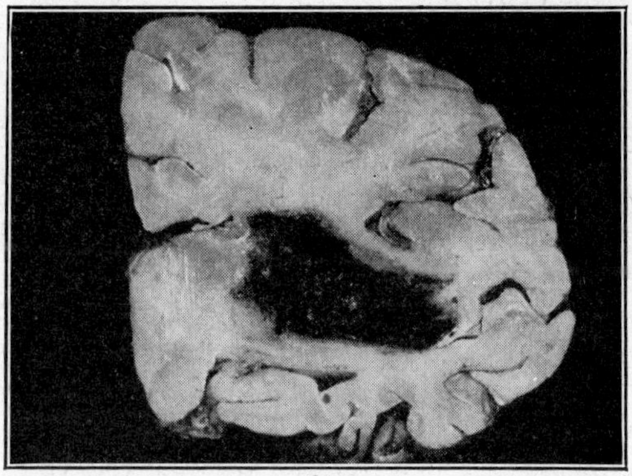

(*b*)

FIGURE 39. BRAINS OF OLD PEOPLE

(*a*) Small segment of the cerebral cortex with covering membranes removed. The deep wide fissures result from atrophy of the brain, common in senility. This brain weighed only 1000 grams, whereas the average normal brain weighs about 1300 grams. (*b*) Cross-section of one hemisphere of brain, showing in the center a large hemorrhage, such as often occurs in older people as a result of arteriosclerosis.

The Trajectory of Life

The course of human life throughout its ages has been likened to the trajectory of a bullet fired from a gun. The bullet first shoots upward and forward after leaving the gun, then levels off and eventually drops again to the earth. It is easy to see the analogy. From the moment of the fertilization of the egg until the end of adolescence there is an increase in size, in physical strength and endurance, in motor responses, in sensory capacity, in 'intelligence.' Ultimately a peak is reached at which the individual is at his best average in these respects. Then decline begins, at first very slowly and then more rapidly until death is reached in extreme old age.

This picture of the course of human

life is useful because it brings into bold relief an important truth. Notwithstanding the complexity of the course of growth and development which has been recounted in this chapter—the fact that every structure of the body has its own rate of growth and development, the fact that the maturation of the various structures and forms of behavior occurs at different times and yet all are about at their best when life is at its peak, the fact that the decline of the various psychological abilities is not uniform—notwithstanding these complexities, the course of life, regarded as a whole, is first an evolution, then a continuation and then an involution This is the basic life pattern of other living things, and, since man also conforms to it, the plan of his life course must surely have been laid down in heredity and directed by his genes. The wide individual variation in the chronological ages at which the several life periods are reached is not surprising. The marvelous timing of the genes is not done with respect to any astronomical calendar. The calendar of the genes is physiological, and some racial strains are longer lived than others.

Finally, it may be said that the task of heredity is finished only when it brings the organism to the peak of its powers and has enabled it to reproduce and rear its kind. What, in addition, man makes of his life, he does on his own initiative in relation to the social and other environmental forces which bear in upon him. What his resources are and what means he employs are set forth in subsequent chapters of this book.

REFERENCES

1. Brooks, F. D., and Shaffer, L. F. *Child psychology*. Boston: Houghton Mifflin, 1937. Chap. 7.

   A student textbook which reviews and interprets the scientific literature in its field.

2. Carmichael, L. (Ed.) *Manual of child psychology*. New York: Wiley, 1946.

   An advanced-level book on developmental psychology by nineteen experts. Excellent bibliographies.

3. Cowdry, E. V. (Ed.) *Problems of ageing.* (2nd ed.) Baltimore: Williams and Wilkins, 1942. Especially Chap. 28.

   A general book in a new field, including an excellent chapter on psychological aspects by Walter R. Miles.

4. Dewey, E. *Behavior development in infants: a survey of the literature on prenatal and postnatal activity, 1920–1934.* New York: Columbia University Press, 1935.

   A source book which gives a summary of scientific literature, some of which was previously available only in obscure journals.

5. Gerard, R. W. *The body functions: physiology*. New York: Wiley, 1941. Chap. 11.

   An excellent general summary which includes consideration of the physiology of development.

6. Gesell, A., and Amatruda, C. S. *Developmental diagnosis: normal and abnormal child development.* New York: Hoeber, 1941.

   A basic description, trait by trait, of typical and atypical early human development.

7. Gesell, A., and Amatruda, C. S. *The embryology of behavior.* New York: Harper, 1945.

   A general consideration of the growth of behavior discussed as the anatomist considers the growth of structure.

8. Gilbert, M. S. *Biography of the unborn.* Baltimore: Williams and Wilkins, 1939.

   A somewhat popular description of some aspects of prenatal life.

9. Hollingworth, L. S. *The psychology of the adolescent.* New York: Appleton-Century, 1928.

   A wise treatment of a difficult period of human development by a scientifically minded woman psychologist.

10. Kellogg, W. N., and Kellogg, L. A. *The ape and the child: a study of environmental influence upon early behavior.* New York: McGraw-Hill, 1933.

A detailed study of a chimpanzee and a human infant reared together in a human home.

11. McGraw, M. B. *Growth: a study of Johnny and Jimmy.* New York: Appleton-Century, 1935.

An elaborate experiment on twins, one of whom was given much exercise while the other was kept relatively quiet.

12. Miles, W. R. Age and human society. In C. Murchison (Ed.), *A handbook of social psychology.* Worcester, Mass.: Clark University Press, 1935. Chap. 15.

An excellent summary of the psychological factors that are important in human aging.

13. Munn, N. L. *Psychological development: an introduction to genetic psychology.* Boston: Houghton Mifflin, 1938.

A summary of the psychology of development with due reference to relevant biological facts.

14. Scammon, R. E. The measurement of the body in childhood. *The measurement of man.* Minneapolis: University of Minnesota Press, 1930. Chap. 4.

Facts and generalizations concerning the measurement of human growth in childhood.

15. Warthin, A. S. *Old age: the major involution.* New York: Paul B. Hocher, 1929.

A general book with special reference to medical problems.

16. Windle, W. F. *Physiology of the fetus: origin and extent of function in prenatal life.* Philadelphia: Saunders, 1940.

An excellent summary of the physiological functions of the mammalian and human fetuses before birth.

CHAPTER 5

Feeling and Emotion

FEW areas of human experience and behavior are as vital and interesting to the individual as his feelings and emotions. They occur in situations of special importance to him, when his interest is aroused, his attention held, and his energy increased and directed toward a definite goal. They range from the milder feelings which we call pleasantness and unpleasantness to stronger emotions like fear and anger. We do not know what the exact relationship may be between the *affective states,* as pleasantness and unpleasantness are called, and the stronger emotions, but this we do know: they both involve general reaction attitudes of the organism toward something in its environment.

PLEASANTNESS AND UNPLEASANTNESS

Pleasantness and unpleasantness, referred to either as *affective states* or as *hedonic tone,* correspond to broad attitudes of acceptance or rejection that the organism assumes toward various aspects of its environment. Pleasant things are the things that we like, that we desire and seek to obtain. Pleasant situations are ones that we attempt to maintain and prolong. Unpleasant things are not liked. We strive to avoid them. Unpleasantness is a condition which we try to terminate.

In one sense, pleasantness and unpleasantness may be said to be indicators of the organism's normal reaction tendencies toward stimulus objects. This interpretation is supported by laboratory experiments which show that under conditions where movement by the subject is not possible, pleasant stimuli lead to muscular relaxation, and unpleasant ones to muscular tension. Where movement by the subject is possible, where he sits unrestrained and the stimulus moves past him, pleasant stimuli produce movements of his approach to the stimulus, and unpleasant ones movements of his withdrawal. The actual behaviors involved in such acceptance or rejection vary from situation to situation, and from individual to individual, and resemble one another only in this one common characteristic, that they are designed to continue or to remove the source of stimulation.

Affective Value of Stimuli

Because pleasantness and unpleasantness serve as indicators of the direction an individual's behavior will take, it is important to know which stimuli are normally pleasant and which unpleasant. This knowledge should help us in predicting and controlling human behavior.

This chapter was prepared by William A. Hunt of Northwestern University.

There is some indication that pleasant stimuli tend to be those which are of positive biological value to the individual, and that unpleasant stimuli are in general biologically harmful. Thus the alkalies, which are often poisonous, are bitter and usually unpleasant; whereas the sugars, which have food value, are sweet and nearly always pleasant. Pain, which accompanies tissue damage or physiological disorganization, is notoriously unpleasant. The relationship is not exact, for many harmful stimuli are pleasant and many beneficial ones unpleasant. Few people relish the flavor of cod liver oil although its biological effect may be desirable; and diabetics continue to crave the sugar which has become bad for them.

This biological interpretation is supported by the relationship which exists between affectivity and the intensity of the stimulus. In general, pleasantness and unpleasantness vary in direct relation to the intensity of the stimulus, both the pleasantness and unpleasantness becoming greater as the intensity of the appropriate stimulus increases. In most cases, however, there comes a point beyond which an increase in intensity causes the pleasant stimulus to become unpleasant. Thus, as the concentration of salt in a solution is increased, the solution is at first indifferent, then it becomes pleasant as more salt is added, and finally, when the concentration is increased beyond a certain point, the solution becomes definitely distasteful and unpleasant. (See p. 356.) The biological importance of this general rule of intensity seems obvious—intense stimuli tend to be dangerous, and unpleasantness acts as a warning.

Whatever the biological significance of the affective states, it is possible to plot certain general relationships between pleasantness and unpleasantness, on the one hand, and their specific stimulus conditions, on the other. Human beings show broad resemblances in their preferences. For instance, they tend to prefer saturated colors to unsaturated. Primitive peoples and young children seem to prefer the 'warmer' colors like red, whereas our adult culture prefers the 'cooler' colors like blue. Certain combinations of tones have different hedonic value. The musical interval of the major third is usually considered most pleasant and the minor second least pleasant by musically sophisticated persons. Sweet is usually pleasant, and bitter unpleasant.

Although there is no doubt that these general tendencies exist, we must remember that they are only tendencies, broad generalizations concealing a great amount of individual variation among the members of the groups studied. Not only do pleasantness and unpleasantness change with learning, but they also depend on many other conditions. The breakfast food that is so pleasant today, through monotony may become unpleasant a few months from now. The favorite dress of ten years ago, discovered and put on today, may now look ridiculous.

The Relativity of Hedonic Tone

Not only are pleasantness and unpleasantness dependent on individual stimuli, but they also are affected by the relationships within a group of stimuli. If a less pleasant stimulus is presented as one of a group of more pleasant stimuli, its affective value may be enhanced by its inclusion, as belonging, within the group of more pleasant stimuli. This change is called *assimilation*. When you really like a person, you may find yourself liking even his (or her) faults. On the other hand, if the less pleasant stimulus is not assimilated into the group, it may seem even less pleasant or definitely unpleasant by contrast with the more pleasant stimuli present. This is called *affective contrast.* How much worse it is to spend an hour with the chap you do not like right after you have spent an hour with the chap you do like very much.

The affective value of a stimulus also is conditioned by the range of stimulus values presented to an individual. If we give a subject a series of odors which covers a wide range of hedonic tones, we can establish which odors are pleasant, indifferent or unpleasant to him. If we now remove the unpleasant odors, and continue to present to him over and over again the indifferent and the pleasant ones, some of the indifferent ones gradually become unpleasant and some of those previously less pleasant are presently judged to be indifferent. In other words, the subject rearranges his responses, spreading them over the present range of his olfactory experience. This phenomenon, known as *affective equilibrium,* is an example of the general principle of relativity of judgment with which we are all familiar.

Suppose, for example, a man found the food at a given restaurant so extremely unpleasant that he declared it the worst food he had ever eaten. Subsequently, if he has changed to a cheap boarding house where the food is even worse, it now seems to him that his present fare is really the worst food he has ever eaten. Should he then return to the original restaurant, the food there would seem much better, just as long as he keeps remembering about the food at the boarding house. If, however, he forgets all about the boarding house, the food at the restaurant is going to become worse again. To the Children of Israel in the wilderness the taste of the flesh pots of Egypt would have been very pleasant.

The same relationships work out at the other end of the scale. Our present pleasures fade before still greater ones; nor do the still greater ones long remain 'still greater.' This rule provides one of the reasons why wealth does not assure happiness. There seem, nevertheless, to be limits to such relativity. Some stimuli show great constancy in pleasantness or unpleasantness. Within a wide range, however, human beings do adjust their affective values to fit the experiences available to them, and this relativity has important consequences for man's contentment under varied environmental circumstances.

Dependence of Learning upon Hedonic Tone

Hedonic tone depends upon learning and, conversely, learning in part upon hedonic tone. This relationship between the two has received much attention in educational psychology. A child who likes candy learns to like the aunt who gives him candy; hedonic tone depends upon learning. Similarly, the child learns the multiplication table because the aunt, whom he now likes, teaches it to him and gives him the pleasure of her approval as a reward; learning depends upon hedonic tone. By such transfers of hedonic value, it might be possible to make a lover of candy into a mathematician, provided certain other capacities were available.

Pleasantness reinforces learning, and unpleasantness hinders it. For this reason either *reward* or *punishment* may be used to establish a learned response. Experiments with animals show that the task which is followed by the greater reward or by lesser punishment is the task that is learned most rapidly and effectively. Furthermore, reward or punishment is more effective the more immediate it is.

Hedonism

Because of the apparent importance of affectivity, or hedonic tone, in human motivation and behavior, it has frequently occupied a prominent part in some philosophical systems. These theories have assumed that hedonic tone *determines* action, a doctrine which is called *hedonism*. In its various forms hedonism reduces human motivation to a desire to seek pleasure and to avoid unpleasantness. Some of the theories base all present action on the part played by hedonic tone in the *past* when the action was learned; others hold that action is in direct accordance with *present* hedonic tone; still others maintain that action is determined by the *anticipated* pleasantness of the *future*.

These theories are too naive to explain adequately the complicated facts of human behavior. Hedonic tone is really not so much a determiner of human behavior as it is an accompaniment and indicator. Pleasantness indicates the existence of an attitude of acceptance and unpleasantness of an attitude of rejection.

Objection is often made to this statement because it implies that all positive action is pleasant, whereas it is obvious that man often 'chooses' unpleasant action or action with unpleasant consequences. Morality seems to depend on his capacity so to choose. Does the martyr like his martyrdom? Is it pleasant? That is the hedonic paradox.

This paradox arises because we tend to think of conflict situations in simple terms as if they were completely pleasant or completely unpleasant. If the martyr experiences no conflict, perhaps he can march to the lions with joy at this opportunity to glorify his faith, and soldiers similarly have been known to go into almost certain death with enthusiasm and without hesitation. Such instances are, however, rare. Expectation of death or pain normally leads to unpleasantness and the attitude of rejection, or, if opposed by some other motive, to a conflict and vacillation of acceptance and rejection. The stronger motive—courage or fear—is what wins out, but meanwhile there has almost always been a fluctuation of pleasantness and unpleasantness.

This matter, however, requires two further qualifications. (1) Often the only choice lies between two unequally unpleasant alternatives, courage with danger *versus* cowardice with shame. The hero may then choose unpleasant courage because it is less unpleasant than very unpleasant shame, may choose it without affective equilibrium's getting a chance to turn the less unpleasant courage into positive pleasantness. (2) Habit, moreover, enters into these equations. For instance, the purpose of military discipline is, in part, to substitute habit for choice when simple hedonistic preference would lead to the wrong action. Undoubtedly habituated action patterns have also lent support to martyrs.

EMOTION

Classed with pleasantness and unpleasantness under the general heading of *feelings* are such emotions as fear, anger, sorrow, love, joy, laughter. The emotions resemble the affective responses in that both represent general reaction attitudes of the organism and seem to have special biological significance for the organism. It is, moreover, an affective state that usually ushers in an emotion. As a rule you feel unpleasantness as a prelude to fear or anger, pleasantness as a prelude to joy or elation. In fact, all the emotions themselves may be roughly classified as either pleasant or unpleasant experiences. Affectivity is thus intimately connected with emotion.

The differences between the emotions and the affective responses are also marked, in some respects more marked than the resemblances. The reaction attitudes are more specific in the emotions than in the affective states. The general rejection that belongs to unpleasantness may be differentiated into actual flight in fear or actual attack in anger. The emotional behaviors themselves are more forceful, more extreme; they involve more of the body and involve it in a greater intensity of response. Attended by great feelings of excitement, they disorganize and disrupt other behavior patterns of the moment. We speak of being 'engulfed,' 'overwhelmed' or 'swept away' by emotion. We have only to remember the difference between disliking a person and being angry at him for the distinction between feeling and emotion to be clear.

The biological significance of emotional stimuli lies back of this intensitive difference. Emotions arise in situations which the individual feels are emergencies. We dislike things that are bad for us, but it is not until they become actually threatening, until an *emergency* arises, that we become emotional and respond with fear or with the aggressive attack that is typical of anger. We like pleasant things, strive to attain them and to keep them, but it is only the particularly desirable object or goal, the much-wanted or much-desired, whose attainment produces the excited response of elation or joy. Emotion accompanies an emergency, be it real or fancied. Emotion is typical of *crisis.*

Visceral Reactions and the Autonomic Nervous System

Emotions involve *generalized* reaction attitudes of the organism. Thus anger is always marked by some aggressive response, some kind of attack on the object that makes us angry; yet the specific behavior of attack varies from person to person and from situation to situation. We may attempt to dispose of an enemy by blackening his eye with a blow, by wounding his self-esteem with an epithet or by undermining his social reputation through derogatory remarks about his character. All strong emotion, however, does involve one common behavioral element: it is accompanied by increased visceral action, heightened response in the vital organs.

The importance of visceral response in emotion has been recognized since the earliest times. We speak of love as an affair of the heart, compassion as residing in the bowels and fear as striking in the pit of the stomach. Modern physiology has confirmed the general correctness of this literary usage. We know that the viscera are controlled by a special section of the nervous system, the *autonomic nervous system,* which is intimately involved in emotion.

The autonomic nervous system is a group of nerve centers or ganglia lying just outside the spinal cord. It controls those internal vital processes which have to do with metabolism and the vasomotor and glandular responses. Heart rate, blood pressure, salivation, digestion, elimination are a few of these involuntary functions that operate under the control of the autonomic nervous system.

This nervous system is divided into two parts (see Fig. 17, p. 35): the *parasympathetic* (craniosacral) and the *sympathetic* (thoracico-lumbar). The actions of these two branches are opposed; sympathetic stimulation, for example, increases the pulse rate, parasympathetic stimulation decreases it. These functions may be seen in Table I.

TABLE I

FUNCTIONS OF THE AUTONOMIC NERVOUS SYSTEM

Organ	*Sympathetic Function*	*Parasympathetic Function*
Heart	speeded up	slowed down
Surface arteries	dilated; more blood	constricted; less blood
Visceral arteries	constricted; less blood	dilated; more blood
Pupil of eye	dilated; more light	contracted; less light
Sweat glands	sweat secreted	
Hair on skin	hairs erected	
Adrenal glands	adrenalin secreted	
Liver	sugar liberated into blood	insulin liberated; blood sugar reduced
Salivary glands	salivation stopped	salivation increased
Stomach	contraction and secretion stopped	contraction and secretion increased
Intestines	contraction and secretion stopped	contraction and secretion increased
Rectum	defecation inhibited	feces expelled
Bladder	urination inhibited	urine expelled
Genital organs	seminal vesicles contracted	erection induced

The parasympathetic system governs those vegetative functions which are concerned with the normal metabolic activities of the organism, the functions which maintain the organism in everyday living; whereas the sympathetic system has an emergency function. It comes into action at times of crisis when normal metabolic function must be suspended and energy must be marshaled to counteract some threat.

In contrast to the parasympathetic system, the parts of which may act separately in activating specific individual organs, the sympathetic system tends to discharge itself as a whole, furnishing a general diffused excitation to all the organs under its control. It is this diffuse sympathetic action which provides the visceral response typical of all strong emotion. When you are angry or afraid and you feel as though the bottom of your stomach had 'dropped out,' feel yourself shaking and trembling, feel your heart racing and your blood pounding in your throat, it is a sign that your sympathetic nervous system has gone into action.

The parasympathetic system is also active in emotion, and its differential activation of various organs may account for some of the difference between such unpleasant emotional states as anger and fear; but this parasympathetic action usually is masked by the violent, generalized response of the sympathetic system. It is the sympathetic system that is primarily responsible for the bodily state of excitement common to all strong emotion.

Walter B. Cannon, in his *emergency* theory of emotion, has made the point that sympathetic action not only occurs commonly in all the emergencies which call forth emotion, but that the bodily results of such action place the individual in a state of physiological preparedness or efficiency to meet the threat of such emergencies. Sympathetic action occurs because it is useful in an emergency. Digestive functions are stopped, and the blood supply of the body is directed to the voluntary muscles—the attack muscles, the flight muscles. The heart beats more rapidly supplying more blood to these muscles. At the same time, blood sugar is liberated from the liver to furnish extra fuel for heavy muscular activity. The bronchioles to the lungs dilate, making it easier to breathe and insuring a greater supply of oxygen. The sympathetic innervation of the adrenal glands results in the secretion into the blood stream of a hormone, *adrenalin,* which acts directly upon the viscera in the same manner as direct sympathetic stimulation. Adrenalin thus becomes a sustaining or reinforcing agent, building up the sympathetic response. Because of this action it is called a sympathomimetic chemical agent, for it duplicates the effects of the sympathetic system.

Adrenalin also has some particular properties of its own which it contributes to the general bodily picture of efficiency for action during an emergency. It hastens the coagulation time of the blood, helping to counteract hemorrhage in a surface wound; and it is thought also to have some direct action in counteracting the effects of fatigue.

The actual efficiency of such an emergency response in the complicated conditions of present-day civilized living is dubious. We no longer fight wild beasts in hand-to-hand combat, but there are many social relations, ranging from an argument between two persons to war between nations, where perceived aggression begets aggression in the perceiver by way of these automatic reaction mechanisms of the sympathetic nervous system. Usually civilized man avoids fight with his muscles, using words or the police as his agents. Yet the visceral response of emotion is still present, and the effort to suppress emotion in civilization is often costly to him who is moved. Later we shall return to a consideration of this matter, when we come to the discussion of the measurement of emotion, and also when we deal with some of the harmful effects of emotion upon the body, a subject of great importance today in the medical specialty called *psychosomatic medicine*.

Direct Action of the Nervous System

The pattern of sympathetic excitation just described results in energizing the organism. The person experiencing emotion is ready for action; he is 'rarin' to go.' This fact has been shown in experiments where the visceral pattern of emotion has been artificially produced by the injection of adrenalin, whose action, as we have just learned, duplicates that of sympathetic stimulation. Few subjects report feeling a genuine emotion under these circumstances, but most of them report feeling tense, excited and moved to action. This state has sometimes been called a 'cold emotion.' Subjects say: "I want to have an emotion and get it over with" and "I feel all wrought up and want to get it off my chest."

When the emotional stimulation is particularly strong or when the usual channels of emotional expression are blocked, the excitation initiated may overflow into other nervous pathways to result in confusing, extraneous responses which are not part of the usual pattern. Thus an impatient man may relieve his tension by tapping his foot; an angry man attempting to control his rage may grind his teeth. In one experiment of infants' reactions to a sudden loud noise (revolver shot), it was found that many of the male infants, in addition to being startled, crying, etc., also showed a sexual response with genital tumescence. In 1872 Charles Darwin described the behavioral overflow of emotion in his classic work on the expression of emotion. The phenomenon illustrates the dynamic, energizing nature of emotion.

Peripheral Response and Expressive Behavior

Emotion is not limited to visceral reactions, but also involves the peripheral musculature under the control of the central nervous system. It is these easily observed peripheral responses which, as indicating certain internal or central events, are usually spoken of as *expressive behavior* in emotion. The attempt to find specific and predictable patterns of expressive behavior has attracted the research efforts of many psychologists.

Unfortunately, the results of their investigations have been both confusing and controversial. No clear and univocal expressive patterns have been found for the different emotions. Anger, it is true, seems to involve a general attitude of aggressive attack by the organism, but the specific behaviors by which such an attack is carried out are infinitely varied and change from situation to situation.

In part this variability arises from the fact that the peripheral musculature, unlike the visceral, is subject to voluntary control involving fewer reflexes. Thus a man can often inhibit and suppress his expressive behavior during emotion, and in different civilizations *sang froid* is cultivated in different degrees. When you are angry you cannot control your rapid pulse, nor your rising blood pressure; but you can repress hostile movement and you may even force a pleasant, disarming smile. The expressive peripheral behavior in emotion thus is not an immediate, involuntary, primitive reaction like the visceral response. It is complicated by voluntary control, the acquisition of learned modifications and the effects of social and cultural standards. No wonder that few clear, identifiable patterns of emotional expression have been discovered. Even those which are almost universal in meaning, like the smile, can, being voluntary, be used to deceive.

Facial Expression in Emotion

The difficulties of investigation and the conflicting findings of such research are seen most typically in the studies of facial expression. Most of the early work was undertaken under the assumption that specific facial expressions exist for the various emotions. Actors or other persons trained in mimicry were asked to pose, assuming the expressions representative of such emotions as anger, fear, surprise and disgust. Their faces were then photographed or drawn by an artist, and the pictures were presented to subjects who were asked to name the emotion portrayed.

That roughly typical facial expressions for certain emotions exist is demonstrated by the fact that subjects can identify these expressions when they are posed. The older and less subtle emotions are most consistently interpreted, whereas in other posed expressions there is a wide range of diverse interpretations. The ability of persons to interpret these expressions correctly improves with training, with increasing age and with increasing intelligence. What have we got in these uniformities: behavior that is instinctive and biologically determined, or behavior that is learned and adjusted to certain cultural conventions?

Since the pictures used in these experiments were deliberately posed and did not represent the features of an individual actually experiencing an emotion, they can only demonstrate the existence of stereotyped, socially accepted patterns of facial expression which can be assumed voluntarily by a man when he wishes to communicate his feelings to others about him. The behavior need not be instinctive but merely a culturally acquired means of social communication. Thus 'looking surprised' is not an immediate, necessary muscular response to certain stimulus situations, but rather a learned means of telling people how you feel under certain conditions. Facial expression substitutes for verbal expression in the communication of feeling. There are many anthropological findings on the differences of expressive movement in different cultures. For instance, in our culture round, wide-open eyes suggest surprise, but to the Chinese they mean anger.

One experimenter substituted for posed expressions photographs of the faces of people who were having actual laboratory-induced emotions. When the stimuli were weak, the classical expressions appeared as expected, but when strong stimuli were used to arouse strong emotions, the conventional facial patterns did not appear. The emotional situations were genuinely upsetting and included plunging the hand into a bucket of live frogs, decapitating a rat, looking at pornographic pictures and being suddenly given ammonia while smelling a pleasant perfume.

Instead of the conventional patterns there appeared a diverse mass of muscular response which varied from person to person. Each subject seemed to have his own characteristic pattern and there was little agreement among them. Nevertheless the amount of facial response varied significantly. Pain showed the most movement, anger less, disgust still less and revolting experiences very little.

This finding confirms the view that typical facial expressions exist as a tradition in our culture, and that people learn to use them as a means of social communication. In mild emotional situations where the reaction is largely intellectual, these cultural patterns predominate, but in strong emotion the social language is forgotten and varied expressions appear that have little relation to the classical patterns.

This interpretation is still further advanced by experiments which show that, in judging the feelings of people in actual emotional situations, observers rely more upon their knowledge of the stimulus conditions than upon the subjects' facial expression. A group of medical students were shown moving pictures of the responses of infants who were hungry, were dropped, were restrained by having their heads held and were stuck with a pin. With no knowledge of the stimulus conditions, the students had little success in identifying the emotions. With knowledge of the stimuli, the students could specify the proper emotions. But when the stimuli were associated with the wrong pictures of expressive behavior, the students became at once confused about the significance of the behavior.

The Startle Pattern

The one consistent exception to the general statement that there has been found no fixed, innate pattern of facial or bodily emotional reaction is sudden surprise or the *startle pattern.* If a person is suddenly stimulated by a loud sound or a flash of light, a very rapid response pattern occurs in him.

By means of high-speed motion-picture photography, the response to the sound of a pistol shot has been studied. Cameras running as fast as three thousand exposures per second have permitted the very exact analysis of this pattern. Figures 40 and 41 are schematic drawings showing the elements of this pattern in both the infant and the adult. The startle response consists of a sudden movement of the head, blinking of the eyes, a characteristic facial expression, raising and drawing forward of the shoulders, turning inward of the upper arms, bending of the elbows, turning downward of the forearms, flexion of the fingers, forward movement of the trunk, contraction of the abdomen and bending of the knees. Not all these elements occur in every person every time he is stimulated. Elements in the response which are opposed to any of these reactions, however, rarely if ever occur. Present evidence leads us to believe that, within limits, completeness of appearance of the pattern is closely related to the intensity of the stimulus; mild simuli may give only the eyeblink, but intense stimuli give the complete pattern.

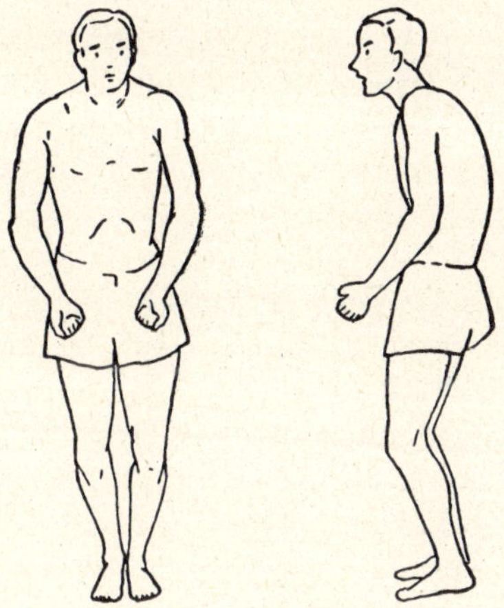

FIGURE 40. SCHEMATIC REPRESENTATION OF THE BODILY PATTERN IN STARTLE

[From C. Landis and W. A. Hunt, *The startle pattern,* Farrar and Rinehart, 1939, p. 22.]

It has also been shown that with repetition certain parts of the startle response die out—rapidly in some individuals and slowly in others. After a long series of stimuli, the eyeblink and certain elements of the facial contortion persist in practically everyone, although most other elements of the pattern will have dropped out. After a sufficient period of time, however, the appropriate stimulus will again elicit the total pattern.

The pattern, which can be evolved in very early infancy, does not change in its form throughout life. It appears in all the higher animals. In certain diseases it is exaggerated, whereas in epilepsy it is totally absent in about one-fifth of the patients.

The startle pattern is usually completed in less than half a second. Hence it cannot be adequately observed except by the temporal magnification of ultra-rapid photography. Few people are even aware that it has occurred in them.

The Emotional Consciousness

The question of whether or not the various emotions are accompanied by some sort of unique and specific conscious content has long bothered psychologists. While we would presume that the logical answer to this question would be found in a direct appeal to introspection (asking subjects undergoing emotion to report directly on how they feel), this method has not been used to any great extent. Most of the classical studies have *assumed* the existence of such distinguishing feelings and then proceeded to make hypotheses concerning their origin.

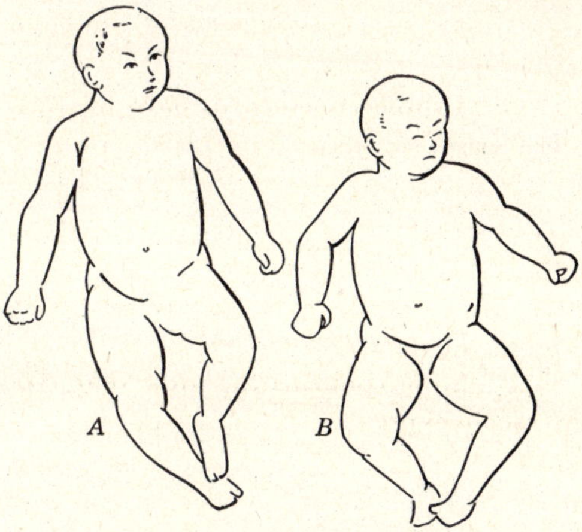

FIGURE 41. SCHEMATIC REPRESENTATION OF THE STARTLE PATTERN IN INFANTS

(*A*) resting posture. (*B*) startle pattern. [From C. Landis and W. A. Hunt, *The startle pattern,* Farrar and Rinehart, 1939, p. 61.]

In 1884 William James, the American

psychologist, and in 1885 C. G. Lange, the Danish physiologist, proposed independently what came presently to be called the *James-Lange theory of emotion.* This theory states that the conscious emotion consists of a man's awareness of his bodily changes as they occur in his emotion. There is a stimulus to emotion, the organism responds

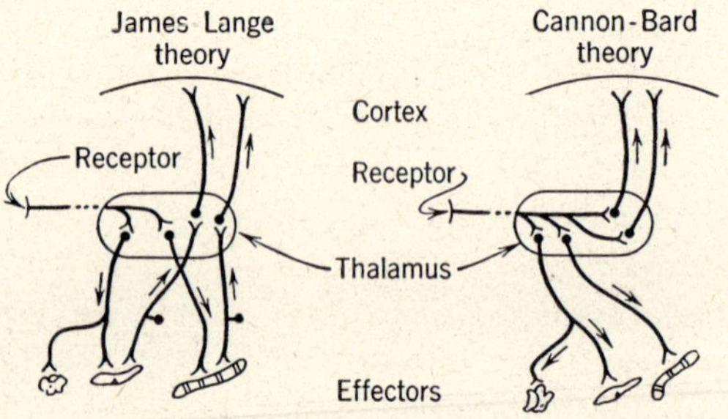

FIGURE 42. JAMES-LANGE AND CANNON-BARD THEORIES OF EMOTION

The James-Lange theory states that emotional experience in the cortex arises from autonomic reactions to the emotional stimulus. The impulses from the receptors go through the thalamus to the effectors and travel back through the thalamus to the cortex, giving rise to the consciousness of the emotion. The Cannon-Bard theory holds that both emotional experience and autonomic effects arise from the stimulus. The impulses from the receptors go to the thalamus and then both to the cortex and to the effectors. The responses of the effectors are an accompaniment of the emotional experience. [From C. T. Morgan, *Physiological psychology,* McGraw-Hill, 1943, p. 356.]

reflexly, and *then* the conscious awareness of these reflex changes gives the man his feeling of emotion. James said "the bodily changes follow directly the perception of the exciting fact, and . . . our feeling of the same changes as they occur *is* the emotion." We do not cry because we feel sorry, but feel sorry because we cry.

In some neurological disorders when the patient cannot feel these bodily changes, he may, nevertheless, report feeling an emotion. In other disorders, like pathological laughing or weeping, bodily responses typical of emotions take place and yet the patient may be without any experience that he would call an emotion. These facts and others have cast doubt upon any literal acceptance of the James-Lange theory.

The fact that the hypothalamus, a lower brain center, acts in mediating the reflex responses typical of emotion has led Cannon and Bard to posit this part of the brain as the seat of emotional consciousness. According to this theory, the action of this center adds the *quale* or distinguishing element of consciousness which gives emotion its typical characteristic feel. (See Fig. 42.)

All these interpretations, however, seem to rest upon an oversimplification of emotional behavior. There is little evidence that a peculiar, unique type of consciousness accompanies and identifies the different emotions. Different persons describe their emotional feelings in different ways. To one man conscious emotion may be his awareness of the bodily responses taking place; he may report that fear is typified by "an awful feeling in my stomach, and cold, clammy hands." Another man, however, may concentrate upon the cognitive, relational aspects of experience. He feels fear as the awareness of a threatening situation. "Something is present which I would like to avoid." We can only conclude that the conscious experiences in emotion are as complex and multiform as the behavioral items and that the existence of specific, unique, distinguishing conscious content in the various emotions has not been demonstrated.

Emotion and Learning

Emotional behavior, like much other behavior, is subject to learning. New responses may be attached to old stimuli, and new stimuli may be attached to old responses. Such learning results in a rapid complication of whatever stimulus-response patterns may be present innately in the human infant. Any universal patterns that may exist then are rapidly altered by learning in accordance with the unique life experiences of each individual.

A classic, early experiment in this field was performed in 1920 by John B. Watson. A nine months' infant showed no fear of a white rat, but showed evidence of fear when a loud sound was made by striking an iron bar. Striking the bar when the infant was reaching for the white rat resulted in fear behavior which later appeared when the rat was presented alone without the loud sound. The infant had now *learned* to be afraid of the white rat because of its association with the fearsome noise.

An important result of this experiment was the demonstration that the fear behavior not only became attached to the white rat as a new stimulus, but also spontaneously became attached to other stimuli resembling the rat, although these had not been present in the original learning situation. The infant now feared other furry animals, as well as fur coats and a teddy bear, which had never been associated with the loud noise. This generalization of learning shows how complicated our emotional behavior may become on the basis of a single emotional experience.

Such learning may explain the genesis of abnormally strong fears which become attached to specific stimuli or situations. During the war, an examination of Naval recruits who could not swim showed that many of them were nonswimmers because of a fear of water attributable to some emotional shock experienced during boyhood. One recruit had dived into a swimming hole shortly after a boy had been drowned there. He hit the corpse on the bottom and came up with it entangled in his arms. Since that one gruesome experience, he has been unable to force himself to enter the water.

Not only can emotions be altered by learning, but emotion itself may interfere with learning. Subjects attempting to solve problems under emotional stress do not do well. Their reasoning is inferior, and they tend to forget more recently learned responses and to fall back upon older habits which may no longer be applicable. Whether the emotional behavior directly affects the learning process or merely acts as a distraction to the individual attempting to learn is not clear, but the interference of emotion during learning has been demonstrated amply. It is hard to study when you are excited. It is also hard to think clearly when you are excited. The emergency aspect of emotion is right for running away or fighting or even for primitive love making, but civilization brings emotions and emergencies which need more brain than brawn. Man's emotions are still useful to him, but he is nowadays well advised to keep a cool head when emergencies arise.

The Genetic Development of Emotion

The preceding discussion has shown that, apart from the common element of visceral excitement attributable to the excitation of the sympathetic branch of the autonomic nervous system, there is very little uniformity and agreement in the specific behavior of different individuals during emotion with the exception of the startle response. To some scientists this finding means that no inherent emotional responses are provided for in the nervous system of the human being. Others believe that instinctive emotional patterns exist but that learning enters at so early an age as to confuse and complicate the original picture.

The appeal to studies of infant behavior has not clarified the problem. Smiling, laughing and crying, as we shall see later, seem to be fairly universal and predictable in infants, but even these behaviors are rapidly altered by learning and social pressure. Recent studies of these patterns show their occurrence in blind children in the same manner and under the same circumstances as in seeing children. In the seeing children, however, mimicry and social pressure produce behavioral changes which increase with age.

Watson, in an early study of the emotional behavior of infants, claimed to have found three basic patterns of response—*fear, anger* and *love.* The stimuli for fear were sudden loud sounds and the sudden loss of support (dropping the child and catching it); for anger, restraint of movement; and for love, cuddling and the stimulation of the erogenous zones. On this simple basis, through the various combinations obtainable by learning, he proposed to explain the entire complicated picture of adult emotion. Thus a student who fears loss of social prestige by dismissal from the football squad is afraid because, through learning and generalization, he has associated loss of social prestige with the loss of physical support which was the original fear stimulus in his infant environment. Fear of the dark, Watson thought, may also spring from a fear of loss of support, since in the darkness all the familiar orienting visual clues by which we habitually guide and steady ourselves in space are missing.

Later work has demonstrated that Watson's findings do not present the complete picture of infant emotion. Loud sounds, loss of support and restraint of movement are common and potent, but not universal, determiners of emotion. Not all infants cry when they are startled by a revolver shot. If they are already crying when the gun is fired, some may stop crying instead of crying harder. The truth is not so simple as Watson had believed.

The emotional response of the infant at birth, like all his other behavior, is limited by the relatively primitive state of his nervous system. As his nervous system develops, more complicated behavior becomes possible for him. Whether these changes are learned or not, it is hard to say. For instance, it was found that children under two had no fear of snakes. After two, caution in approach to snakes became evident in the children's behavior. Definite fear of snakes did not appear with any frequency until the age of four. Is this progressive development of the fear of snakes related to some innate reaction pattern which becomes operative as the nervous system matures, or is it a learned response acquired as the child becomes socialized? The complex nature of any emotional behavior shows that it must derive from both sources.

The emotional development of the child is characterized by a decreasing frequency of intense emotional response, by a progressive transfer of emotion to socially approved and experientially determined situations and by a change in the patterns of emotional behavior to accord with cultural pressures.

SPECIFIC EMOTIONS

Most of our consideration of emotion so far has been about the general characteristics common to all emotions. Now it is time to be more specific, to deal with individual characteristics associated with the different emotions.

Smiling, Laughing and Crying

Well-defined examples of emotional expression are smiling, laughing and crying. We habitually accept the occurrence of this sort of behavior as indicative of emotional experience. Although it is true that these behaviors may occur without attendant emotional experience, yet in the ordinary conduct of everyday life smiling, laughing and crying are by common consent regarded as truly emotional expressions.

The development of these patterns of response in the infant has long been a matter of interest to child psychologists. *Smiling* is exhibited at a very early age by most children. In the very young infant it is almost invariably brought about by specific stimulation, the response usually being evoked by other people, or at least exhibited only in their presence. Study of the development of smiling and laughing shows that originally several varieties of respiratory reactions or compensatory motor mechanisms are elicited by certain situations which the child has not met before and for which, consequently, he has ready no immediate appropriate pattern of response. On such occasions a response involving smiling or laughing is approved by the infant's mother or nurse, whereas other respiratory mechanisms may be disapproved. Smiling and laughing are thus quickly found to be socially acceptable and to lead to reward or comfort. They become learned reactions, selected as socially appropriate. Once incorporated in the reaction repertoire of the child, this original usage becomes widely generalized, blending into all the patterns of response which during most of our lives we call amusement. Already by the end of the first year of life, smiling has become a learned response to such an extent that the smile must be regarded as a communicative, adaptive, social reaction rather than a modified respiratory response.

Laughing appears much later in the child's life than smiling, usually not until after the twentieth week. During the first year of life it remains a stereotyped form of behavior. More differences between children occur in the frequency of smiling or laughing than in the actual form of these two behaviors.

Laughter presents us with more than one problem. We have laughter of joy, laughter of comedy, laughter as a form of social response, laughter as a release from tension and laughter under pathological, organic or mental conditions. All these laughters involve different psychological elements. The joyful laugh, a bubbling over of good humor, occurs in children or adults in a state of well-being. The comic laugh is directed *at* some joke or ludicrous situation. Laughter as a social response involves many principles of social psychology. We laugh more easily in a group than alone, for laughter is a variety of gesture language. The act of laughing may be used at times for a communication of good will and a spirit of fun, at others of pure joy and, at still other times, of embarrassment.

The laughter which is associated with a relief of tension has been explained on an evolutionary basis. Since the facial musculature is not primarily necessary to the active energetic preservation of life, it has been suggested that the excess energy, set up by emotional stimulation, is drained off by the activity of the facial and respiratory muscles in a way which does not interfere with any activity of the body essential to the emergency which induces the emotion. This drainage theory must not be taken too literally. The nervous system does not accumulate energy which has to be released by one channel, if not by another. Nevertheless, it is true that individuals often find themselves in states of emotional tension which can be relieved only by action—almost any relevant action. It is a problem of motivation, however, not of physics.

The behavior of infants during *crying* has been observed experimentally in a series of standard situations. Crying induced by the perception of strangers increases in frequency up to about ten months of age. Crying caused by fear or strange situations can, however, be distinguished from other types of the response. In the adult, crying, like laughing and smiling, is so bound up with the social reactions of the individual that it is impossible to be certain in a majority of cases whether the response is truly emotional, only partly so or an habituated response, devoid of emotion.

The observation of adults in situations which produce tears (funerals, for example) shows that tears are usually indicative of a mixed emotional state. Sorrow, dejection, joy and elation, when occurring alone, have but little effect in producing tears. Adult crying occurs in the main only when an otherwise depressing or unpleasant situation is partially redeemed by some pleasant or alleviating stimulation, or when there is a conflict in extreme frustration.

Fear

The most prominent feelings associated with fear are the bodily sensations attributable to the activation of the autonomic nervous system. Pounding of the blood, a sinking feeling in the stomach, trembling and shaking, weakness, faintness and tension all are common and prominent.

Present with these feelings is an insistent desire to get away from some threatening situation with which the individual does not feel able to deal adequately. Some form of withdrawal behavior usually results. Once the threatening stimulus has been removed or the threatening situation has been controlled, and the real or imagined danger has passed, fear disappears. If the danger increases rapidly, or if the fear strikes suddenly and severely, *terror* may result with a complete disintegration of the individual's behavior. Typical of terror are both the blind flight of panic and the occasional complete inhibition of activity with its attendant immobility and paralysis of volition. When fear is anticipatory, when it is aroused by something foreseen in the future rather than existing in the present, we may call it anxiety or apprehension.

The stimuli for fear are many and varied but they all involve some sudden change in the environment, some change which the individual regards as threatening and to which he is either unprepared or unable to respond. This fact has led one psychologist to speak of such situations as *catastrophic,* and fear behavior as *catastrophic behavior*. Once an adequate course of action develops, once the individual feels he is in control of the situation and doing something about it, fear disappears.

It is not the man who is successfully running away from a bear who is afraid. Fear comes when he realizes that the gap between him and the bear is decreasing instead of growing larger, or when he realizes that he is becoming exhausted and cannot run much farther. It is the soldier about to go into combat who most often experiences fear, rather than the one who is actually in combat, fighting desperately for his life.

Adequate action seems to be the antidote

for fear. Such action is more possible when the individual has full knowledge of the threatening situation. The existence of well-established habit patterns also helps. It is not the experienced big-game hunter who feels fear when faced by a lion. He has met the situation before, knows what to do and acts habitually and smoothly. It is the neophyte, hunting for the first time, who becomes frightened.

Knowing what to do *and doing it* is the best way to handle fear. As we have seen, it is possible that all the complicated response of the autonomic nervous system in emotion may be the body's way of organizing its reserves for action. To fight fear, use what the autonomic system has provided, the capacity for effective action.

Our understanding of fear has been confirmed by exhaustive questioning of men who have returned from battle. One study of 4504 flyers who had returned to this country after extensive tours of combat is particularly enlightening. These flyers reported the usual signs of fear when flying a combat mission. They experienced a rapid pulse rate, muscle tension, irritability, dryness of the mouth, sweating, stomach sensations and a feeling of unreality. Delayed symptoms which appeared later included fatigue, restlessness, depression, over-reaction to stimuli, loss of appetite, loss of zeal and even obsessive thoughts.

Their fear was greatest in danger when they were idle or unable to take counteraction. Fear was reduced by confidence in equipment and leadership, goal-directed activity and social stimulation. Organizational morale, sense of duty, hope of survival and personal pride were motivating factors which were much more successful in reducing fear than citations for bravery, pay, self-advancement and hatred of the enemy.

Anger

Anger is the normal response to frustration. When some situation or another person unduly limits the freedom of action of an individual, the restrained individual is likely to become angry. He may then attack the obstacle which is inhibiting his freedom.

Thus, the condition which arouses *anger* in young children is a situation which, instead of being a sudden call for action, is often a more or less sudden stoppage or *interference with action.* Interference with activity, especially activity motivated by the common urges or drives, is an essential characteristic of the anger-producing situation.

The anger responses in the child are outbursts of impulsive activity—kicking, stamping, slashing about with the arms and often a prolonged holding of the breath. With increasing age, the anger becomes more overtly focused upon a given end. Along with a decrease in the proportion of outbursts consisting of mere displays of undirected energy comes an increase in the frequency of retaliative behavior. The percentage of observable after-reactions, such as resentfulness and sulkiness, increases steadily with advancing age, perhaps in part because retaliation is not always practicable or carries with it its own penalties.

Mild anger, directed toward the legitimate removal of some barrier obstructing individual action, may well become an important motivator of behavior. Anger, however, is difficult to control and easily develops into disorganized rage. It may, moreover, call forth the same type of response from the object against which it is directed. In human affairs aggression tends to be met by aggression, and the results are disastrous for social intercourse.

Anger, like fear, is a primitive emergency response which energizes the individual. We may seriously question the general serviceability of such primitive responses in the complex social organization of contemporary life, in spite of the occasional good uses for righteous anger and moral indignation.

Anger can be misdirected. If the aggression aroused by frustration cannot be directed against the frustrating situation itself, it may be displaced and vented upon a substitute. If you are publicly embarrassed by some incident about which you can do nothing, you may suddenly become angry with an innocent witness of the affair. Majority groups may thus take out their aggressions against a minority group, and within the minority group aggression in turn may be directed against some poor individual selected as a scapegoat. Beyond the fact that such substitute reactions may offer emotional relief to the individual aroused, misdirected anger, being false, cannot be said to have any social value.

THE MEASUREMENT OF EMOTION

The importance of emotion, both as behavior itself and secondarily as an indicator of the conscious and unconscious vital concerns of the individual, has led to great interest in its measurement. The participation of the autonomic nervous system, with its attendant changes in pulse rate, blood pressure, breathing, etc., has held out to psychologists the hope that measures of such bodily changes might give a clear measure of emotion. Such hopes have not been fully realized. The autonomic nervous system is not exclusively concerned with emotion, and its complex organization adds further to the difficulty; still, measures of bodily processes are our best indicators of emotion.

The Galvanic Skin Response

In 1888 the French scientists, Vigouroux and Féré, called attention to the fact that, when electrodes are placed on the skin and attached to the proper electrical measuring instruments, variations in the electrical properties of the skin appear from time to time. During emotional excitement, they found, there is an increase in these electrical variations. The occurrence of these changes has been named the *galvanic skin response* or the *psychogalvanic reflex,* a phenomenon which has been extensively studied by many investigators. The response was first called prominently to the attention of psychologists by the work of C. G. Jung and his pupils, who came to the general conclusion that the galvanic skin response is associated with repressed emotional complexes. Whether this electrical response is associated with physiological and psychological occurrences other than emotion, they did not particularly consider. Their claim to have a measure of emotion was accepted more or less uncritically by many psychologists. More recent investigations show, however, that these electrical responses occur not only during emotional experience but also to some extent with practically every other variety of psychological experience. Furthermore, it appears that the degree of electrical change does not measure accurately the amount of emotion experienced by the individual.

Blood Pressure Changes

The amount of increase, decrease or variability in blood pressure has been used as a measure of emotionality. Perhaps the most extensive use of this type of measurement has been in the detection of falsehood, the so-called *lie detector* being an instrument to record changes in blood pressure. (Some lie detectors record the galvanic skin response and changes in respiration as well.) Under certain conditions it seems possible on the basis of the changes in the record of blood pressure to determine whether or not a person has told the truth or has lied, provided always that he is more moved when lying than when telling the truth. It has not been possible to standardize this procedure, since it depends upon so many variables and there are so many different factors which must be considered in the interpretation of the record. For instance, an habitual liar may be quite unmoved about his lies. There are, moreover, people who can convince themselves by their own lies to become sincere liars.

In a study of blood pressure, made on persons who had suffered severe injury in automobile accidents and upon friends and relatives who were called to the hospital to see them, interesting results were obtained. It was found that the injured individuals themselves, who had undoubtedly gone through profound physical and emotional shock, did not show very much alteration in blood pressure. Their friends or relatives, on the other hand, waiting to find out how severely the patients had been injured, showed a tremendous variability. Evidently, then, the rise in blood pressure frequently accompanies the apprehensive state preceding some possible emergency.

Rating Scales

The failure to establish good physiological measures of emotion has led to the development of new techniques. A common one is the rating scale. In this procedure, we ask the friends and acquaintances of some person to rate his emotionality or emotional expressiveness. By statistical manipulation of the data it is possible to obtain some idea of the probable emotional reactivity of an individual in comparison with that of his friends and associates.

Observational and Psychoanalytic Techniques

Several investigations of emotional reactions, particularly with children, have been made by the observational method. One observer watched a large group of children on the playground, following their behavior over a period of several months. All instances of anger, fighting, fear or other emotional reactions were noted. On the basis of such observational studies, we can obtain very good descriptions of actual emotional behavior, the stimuli or situations which produced the behavior and the results of the reactions. Although it has been found possible in this way to predict rather accurately the sort of situation which will evoke an emotional reaction in a particular individual, the evidence shows that the same situation is not uniformly effective in producing the same reaction in all individuals or even in the same individual every time.

Psychoanalysis provides a special situation under which emotion can often be observed in adults. In such an analysis, which consists essentially of talking in a free and uninhibited fashion about anything that comes into the mind, very marked emotional reactions sometimes take place. The subject may respond in an intense emotional fashion to his own descriptions of events long past and previously believed forgotten. By such methods we can acquire much knowledge concerning the emotional history of the person being analyzed.

Questionnaire Methods

An entirely different method of measurement and test makes use of the questionnaire, as, for example, the Pressey X-O test, Form B. This test consists of three lists of words. In the first, the individual is told to cross out everything he thinks is wrong; in the second list, everything about which he has ever worried; and in the third, everything he likes or is interested in. He is also told to encircle the crossed-out word in each line which he considers, respectively, to be the worst, the most worrisome or the most interesting. The total number of words crossed out is called the *score of emotionality,* since, theoretically, the more things a person dislikes, worries about or likes, the more generally emotional he is. The encircled words having been compared with a standard list that gives the most frequently encircled word for each line, the number of encircled words which deviate from this standard list is the *score of idiosyncrasy.* Various investigators have reported that students who obtain high scores of emotionality and idiosyncrasy tend to have more than the usual number of emotional conflicts in school.

DISORDERS OF EMOTION

Like the other bodily processes the emotional mechanisms sometimes fail to function correctly. The trouble may be some physiological or organic disorder, such as a wrong functioning of a gland or a disorder of the nervous system. Such disturbances can be classified as the *pathology* of emotion. On the other hand, if the cause is not organic but arises from faulty learning or poor habits of adjustment, we call the disturbances *functional* disorders. Often both functional and organic disabilities occur together in relation to each other, as in the problems of *psychosomatic medicine.*

Pathological Conditions

Since emotional behavior is mediated by the nervous system, it can be upset by any injury or disease which affects the pertinent parts of the nervous system. Tumorous growths in the thalamic or hypothalamic regions of the brain may produce uncontrollable weeping or laughing. The removal of large areas of cortical brain tissue has been known to result in an apparent lessening of social inhibitions with resulting inappropriate and embarrassing emotional behavior of a sort previously inhibited by the individual. Glandular disfunctions may also unbalance the emotional behavior. Feelings of anxiety, which may be accompanied by terror nightmares, are often found in advanced cases of hyperthyroidism.

Extreme emotional states are also prominent in the symptoms of the major mental disorders. Extreme euphoria, an abnormally strong sense of well-being, happiness, and exaggerated self-confidence, is found in the manic patient, and sometimes in general paresis. Both the depressive phases of manic-depressive psychosis and of involutional melancholia include persistent deep depressions which are accompanied by unhappiness, anxiety, apprehension and occasional thoughts of self-destruction.

In schizophrenia, or dementia praecox, we may find apathy, a relative dulling of emotional response. The patient does not show a normal emotional interest in and response to his environment. Such a patient might commit a crime, even murder, without the emotional conflict which such behavior would cause in the normal individual. We describe such emotional apathy as a *blunting of affect.*

Functional Disorders

Some emotional disorders are not due to physiological disorder but must be considered as inappropriate behavior produced by unusual experiences in the individual's past. *Phobias,* or unusually strong, persistent fear reactions, are an example. As we have already noted, the examination of Naval recruits who were nonswimmers showed that many of them had developed a phobia for water because of some traumatic experience with swimming or water in the past.

Phobias may appear to occur without reason and remain inexplicable to the individual suffering from them. They handicap his adjustment and limit his activities. They are often found in exaggerated form in the *psychoneuroses.*

Anxiety, which, as we have already noted, normally functions as a forerunner of some anticipated dangerous situation, may also get out of hand and may so dominate the individual's behavior that he is unable to take any logical action concerning the situation which produces the anxiety. Thus the student who is anxious and worried about an examination may become so upset as to be unable to study. His inability to study increases his feeling of unpreparedness which in turn increases his anxiety, and he is caught in a vicious circle. Next time he had better schedule his work so that he does not get caught so unprepared or he might make some other intelligent administrative changes in his life of study. In general, the best way to handle anxiety is by a frontal attack upon the problem causing it.

In many maladjusted individuals, however, the basic reasons for the anxiety may be repressed and unconscious. The person is then faced with a persistent worry or apprehension which colors all his emotional life and about which he is unable to do anything since he cannot understand its origin. In such cases, psychiatric counseling may be necessary to uncover the source of the basic insecurity or inferiority causing the anxiety.

Anxiety very frequently has a profound effect upon the *physiological functions* of the individual. Persistent respiratory, circulatory, digestive or muscular disturbances may occur. Chronic fatigue accompanied by insomnia is also common.

The effect of anxiety on psychological functions is to lower the general acuity and completeness of response. Although the individual still reacts, he does so either in a preoccupied fashion, paying attention to only part of what is going on around him, or inadequately, as though he were fatigued or had insufficient energy to meet the demands of the situation. Since anxiety is a rather common human experience, a great deal of medical work has been done in the attempt to control or alleviate it. Generally speaking, if in one way or another the anxious person can be made to discover the original connection between his anxiety and its primary or original cause, he will be able either to free himself of the anxiety or to control it in a satisfactory fashion. (For more on phobias and anxieties, see pp. 531–534.)

Psychosomatic Medicine

We have already seen that emotion involves activity of the autonomic nervous system and hence a profound change in the activity of the vital organs. Increased pulse rate, increased blood pressure, irregularities in respiration and interference with digestion may all result. Where the emotion perseveres over a period of time, as it does in chronic worry or anxiety, it may result in a persistent disturbance of vital function. Modern medicine has finally realized that many disorders of digestion, respiration and heart function are attributable, not to organic difficulties, but to emotional disorders. They must be treated by treating the individual's problems of psychological adjustment which are causing the emotional disturbance responsible for the physical symptoms. Thus a whole new branch of medicine, *psychosomatic medicine,* has arisen to handle these problems.

It must be remembered, however, that if such functional disorders continue they may in time result in organic damage to the bodily system involved. A chronic fear may produce the persistent diarrhea known as colitis, and, if such diarrhea persists, ulceration of the colon may result. After the ulcer has formed, psychological treatment alone has become insufficient.

HYGIENE OF EMOTION

In the preceding pages emotion has been pictured both as a helpful reinforcing agent which energizes and motivates man when he is faced with some threatening emergency and as a disrupting force which disorganizes his behavior and confuses his thinking at a moment of crisis. Actually it is both. The answer to whether emotion is helpful or harmful depends on whether the emotion is appropriate to the situation in which the individual finds himself.

The question of the appropriateness or inappropriateness of a specific emotional response must be settled by the individual himself after a consideration of all the important circumstances entering into the specific stimulus situation of the moment. Psychology can only offer us broad truths, but every man must apply them to his own particular needs at any specific time. The description of emotion which this chapter contains has in it much of value to govern us in understanding and controlling our emotions. We want to be able to have appropriate emotions, to dispense with the inappropriate ones. How can we tell the two apart; decide about appropriateness? Here are three principles which may help.

(1) *Emotion is inappropriate if it is harmful to the biology of the individual.* No intelligent person should allow himself the luxury of flying into a severe rage immediately after eating a full meal. Nor can fear or anxiety be considered desirable in an individual who is suffering from stomach ulcers, high blood pressure or a colitis of functional origin.

(2) *Emotion is inappropriate if it arouses conflicting motivations within the individual.* If we allow ourselves to become angry with those we love, we are plunged into a bitter and disrupting conflict within ourselves. The soldier who is possessed of an overwhelming fear of death while being driven at the same time by an equally strong desire not to let his comrades down may succumb to a mental breakdown during combat.

(3) *Emotion is inappropriate if it brings the individual in conflict with society.* There are innumerable social codes that control emotional behavior and they must be respected if the individual is to live in harmony with his neighbors. A frank expression of fear at an inappropriate time may result in a man's being branded a coward and subjected to the ridicule of his comrades. However strong the provocation, the enlisted man who strikes an officer must face severe disciplinary measures.

The overt demonstration of affection may not be considered proper in public.

Unfortunately, these principles do not always coincide. Anger in response to an insult may be considered socially acceptable, and the failure to exhibit it may result in the person's feeling he has lost caste and in being plunged into an unhappy personal conflict within himself. Nevertheless, such justifiable anger may be lethal to an individual afflicted with a severe heart disorder. The answer to such dilemmas is not an easy one, but on it rests the decision as to whether our emotions are beneficial or harmful, and on it rests in large part our chances for happiness.

REFERENCES

1. Bard, P. Emotion: I. The neuro-humoral basis of emotional reactions. In C. Murchison (Ed.), *A handbook of general experimental psychology.* Worcester, Mass.: Clark University Press, 1934. Chap. 6.

   In need of revision but still a standard technical reference on the neuro-humoral basis of emotion.

2. Beebe-Center, J. G. *The psychology of pleasantness and unpleasantness.* New York: D. Van Nostrand, 1932.

   The only adequate source book for the experimental literature in this field.

3. Cannon, W. B. *Bodily changes in pain, hunger, fear and rage.* (2nd ed.) New York: Appleton, 1929.

   An historical classic still very much worth reading as the basis of the emergency theory of emotion.

4. Jersild, A. T. Emotional development. In L. Carmichael (Ed.), *Manual of child psychology.* New York: Wiley, 1946.

   An excellent survey of the literature on the development of emotion in the child.

5. Landis, C. Emotion: II. The expressions of emotion. In C. Murchison (Ed.), *A handbook of general experimental psychology.* Worcester, Mass.: Clark University Press, 1934. Chap. 7.

   An excellent survey of the experimental findings on emotion up to 1934.

6. Landis, C., and Hunt, W. A. *The startle pattern.* New York: Farrar and Rinehart, 1939.

   An intensive study of the reflex response in startle based upon the use of ultra-rapid photography.

7. Ruckmick, C. A. *The psychology of feeling and emotion.* New York: McGraw-Hill, 1936.

   Somewhat outmoded as a survey of emotion, but valuable for its historical material.

8. Young, P. T. *Emotion in man and animal.* New York: Wiley, 1943.

   A treatment of emotion with particular stress on its relations to drive and motivation.

CHAPTER 6

Motivation

THIS chapter is concerned with what the layman usually considers the most important problem of psychology. The question which, above all others, he wants psychology to answer for him is, "Why do people act as they do?" Not satisfied with a mere description of man's behavior, he wants to know the motives back of it. The problem of motivation, narrowly conceived, is the problem of discovering the motives of human beings; but, broadly viewed, it is the problem of determining the forces which impel or incite all living organisms to action.

NEEDS

We cannot long study the behavior of living organisms without observing that they need things; and it is their wants, lacks or needs which have to be investigated if the reasons for their behavior are to be discovered. The things which they need, however, vary greatly, not only from species to species, but also from individual to individual within the same species. Oysters do not need automobiles and men do not need shells; but, if they are to continue to live, oysters and men, like all other living organisms, need to get from their environments a continuous supply of energy and materials. The needs of the amoeba are limited to these vital ones. The needs of man, on the other hand, are ever so much more numerous. He, too, has vital needs. He needs to breathe oxygen, to eat food, to drink water, to eliminate wastes from his body, to maintain a relatively constant body temperature. But, in addition to these, he has other needs which cannot be considered so vital or so universal. He may need to have more money than anyone else in his town, he may need to be loved by a particular person, he may need to be constantly praised and applauded.

Distinction among Needs

There are important respects in which *vital* and *nonvital* needs are different, though in other respects they have much in common.

The vital needs are *primary* and *innate* in the sense that they are the first needs of the organism. If they remain unsatisfied, the organism does not live to develop nonvital needs as a result of experience. In this sense, nonvital needs are *secondary* and *acquired*. This distinction does not mean, however, that secondary needs are necessarily weaker or less important than primary ones. The terms primary and secondary apply only to the origins of needs and imply nothing about their relative strengths. The need to possess great wealth

This chapter was prepared by Donald W. MacKinnon of the University of California.

may be so much stronger in a man than his needs for food and rest and exercise that, even though he succeeds in amassing great wealth, he may so break his health as to die. In such a case the secondary need for possessions is obviously stronger than the primary vital needs which are frustrated. Furthermore, the distinction between primary and secondary needs does not imply that the latter are always in the service of the former. The example just cited shows that such is not the case. The amassing of great wealth (a secondary need) may be an end in itself and not necessarily a means to the certain and more adequate satisfaction of the need for food or of any other primary need.

There is a sense, then, in which a secondary need may be more vital for the continued existence of an individual than a primary need. It is, for example, not uncommon for a man to commit suicide because he has lost his fortune in a crash of the stock market or because he has lost his honor through becoming involved in a public scandal. For such persons life without money or life without honor is impossible. In a very real sense their secondary needs have become vital ones.

The primary needs are sometimes called *physiological* needs and the secondary ones, *psychological* needs. This does not mean that the secondary psychological needs lack the physiological basis in the body which the primary physiological needs have, but merely that, in general, we know more about the specific physiological basis of primary than of secondary needs. We know, for example, that the physiological basis of the need for food is a matter, in part, of a reduction of the sugar concentration of the blood and consequent contractions of the smooth muscle of the stomach; and we know at least something about the physiological basis of the other so-called physiological needs. But what the physiological basis of a man's need for superiority may be, or of any other of his so-called psychological needs, we do not know. We assume, however, that they have a physiological basis even though we cannot demonstrate it.

On the other hand, the distinction between physiological and psychological needs does not mean that the psychological needs have a representation in consciousness which is absent in physiological needs. We may be just as much aware of our need for food as we are aware of our need to pass a crucial examination; and we may, at another time, be just as unaware of our need to get even with a person for a slight which he has given us as we are unaware of our need for vitamin B. Physiological and psychological needs are alike in that both may be at certain times known but at other times unrecognized.

The primary needs are sometimes referred to as *biological* needs because they have biological origins. The secondary needs are sometimes called, in contrast, *social* needs because they are the products of social life. Though this is a valid distinction among needs, we must not overlook the fact that social needs are also biological in the sense that they are needs of biological organisms and that biological needs are also social in that the expressions of these needs are to a large extent socially determined. All men need food, but the particular objects which will satisfy this need vary widely from one society or culture to another. Religious taboos and cultural prohibitions limit greatly the number of objects which will satisfy an individual's need for food.

We have seen that needs are of two kinds: first, needs which are *primary, vital, physiological* and *biological* and, second, needs which are *secondary, nonvital, psychological* and *social.* But we have seen also that, valid as these distinctions between the two classes of needs are, they are not rigid. All needs have much in common. It is this fact which makes it possible for psychologists to seek the general laws of need regardless of the particular need studied.

Needs, Structure and Environment

All organisms have the primary need for oxygen, but, although they have this need in common, they satisfy it in different ways. The fish supplied with gills and living in water gets oxygen in one way; man supplied with lungs and living on land gets his in a different manner. The ways in which an organism's needs may be satisfied are determined by its structure as well as by the nature of its environment. This relationship is no less valid for secondary needs. A common need in a highly competitive society is the need to be or to feel superior to others, but it may be satisfied in very different ways. A person skillful in athletics may gain his superiority by excelling in sports; a man of puny body but keen intellect may gain his feeling of superiority by scholastic excellence.

Behavior which is motivated by need depends then upon the following three factors.

(1) The *need* itself, conceived of as a want or lack in the organism, involving always a physiological disequilibrium or a tension which tends to discharge in behavior in such a way as to bring about a restoration of the equilibrium which was disturbed by the need. (See pp. 511–514 on tension reduction.) Such physiological disequilibria are to be considered the sources of the stimulation which drive the organism to action.

(2) The *structure* of the organism, which determines to an important degree not only the needs of the organism but also the manner in which they will be satisfied. Here are to be considered certain mechanisms—gills as against lungs, the claw of the lobster as against the hand of a man—as well as the sensory organs and nervous system which mediate the perception of needed objects and the muscles and glands which are organized into systems of response.

(3) The *environment* of the organism and the objects, present in the environment or absent from it, which are required for the satisfaction of any need. Here both the social and the physical environment have to be considered.

Any concrete case of behavior is determined by the interrelated functioning of all three of these factors; it is only by adopting an analytical attitude that they can be discussed separately. Later we shall consider them in their interrelation.

THE PHYSIOLOGICAL BASIS OF BEHAVIOR

The psychologist has long considered that one of his problems is the determination of the conditions in bodily tissues which release energy so as to stimulate the organism to overt activity. He has sought to determine the precise correlation between these known conditions and activity, both general and specific, and having found such correlations he has developed the concept of *drive,* which he defines as *an intraorganic activity or condition of tissue supplying stimulation for a particular type of behavior.*

Hunger Drive

The following facts are known about the physiology of the *hunger drive.* When the sugar concentration of the blood is reduced below a certain level, vigorous contractions of the stomach ensue. These contractions of the smooth muscles of the stomach wall are the physiological concomitants of the conscious pangs of hunger. This latter fact has been demonstrated by having subjects swallow a tube to the end of which a rubber balloon is attached. When the balloon is in the stomach, it is inflated and the tube connected to a recording apparatus so as to give a graphic record of the stomach contractions. If under these conditions subjects are instructed to press a signal key whenever a pang of hunger is experienced, it is found that their stomach contractions and hunger pangs coincide. These experiments have been carried further to determine the relation between stomach contractions and general bodily activity. Subjects were asked to recline on a bed so constructed as to yield a graphic record of their movements—even so slight a movement as that of a single finger. By taking simultaneous records of bodily activity and stomach contractions both when the subjects were asleep and when quietly reading, a very close correlation between the rhythmic contractions of the smooth muscle of the stomach and bodily activity was demonstrated.

Just as the altered chemical state of the blood consequent upon the reduction of its sugar concentration affects the stomach, setting up the vigorous contractions of the smooth muscle, so these contractions in turn set up nervous impulses which make for an increase of bodily activity. Hungry persons are restless.

Bodily conditions such as those just described are correlated, however, not only with an increase in general bodily activity but also with specific activity directed toward the satisfaction of the momentary need. The hungry person seeks food and eats it when he finds it. The thirsty one seeks water and drinks it if he gets it.

Although this activity, both general and specific, has been found to be associated with such specific internal conditions as stomach contractions, there are a number of experiments which have demonstrated that the activity may likewise occur in the absence of the usually associated physiological state. Rats in which practically all the contractile tissue of the stomach has been removed or in which the nerves between the stomach and the brain have been severed are still motivated, when deprived of food, to seek food and ingest it. A hungry hen placed before a heap of grain will eat a certain amount and stop, though there is still more food before her. Nevertheless, the hen can be motivated to eat again—this time in the absence of any stomach contractions—if the remaining food is removed and immediately replaced. With some hens this process can be repeated as many as eight times. In the light of such evidence we cannot assume that stomach contractions are always and necessarily the source of stimulation which motivates the hen to eat. In this case the perception of the food presented is alone sufficient to stimulate eating.

In another experiment the amount of grain that a hen will eat spontaneously after a twenty-four-hour fast was determined. The hen was then presented after a similar fast with a heap of grain larger than before. If ordinarily the hen eats fifty grains from a heap of one hundred grains of wheat, from a larger heap she will eat thirty-five to fifty grains more. Since presumably the chemical state of the blood and the condition of the tissues of the stomach are about the same under both conditions, the increase in eating must be determined by neither of these factors but by the increase in the size of the heap and by whatever physiological changes result from the perception of this fact.

Or again, if a hen eats until satisfied and remains motionless in front of a pile of grain, she will begin to eat once more if a hungry hen introduced into the situation starts to eat. And like hens we, too, will start to eat again if, having eaten our fill, we are joined by hungry friends.

Such observations as these indicate how necessary it is to consider, in addition to the internal sources of stimulation in the stomach wall, the environmental factors which may also stimulate the organism to eat. Objects which in the past have been present when physiological hunger has driven the organism to eat, or situations in which eating has occurred, may, because of their connection with previous eating, become adequate in their own right to stimulate the same behavior on later occasions. Thus, we eat when we see others eating; we eat more when more food is presented to us; and we eat, in everyday life, long before we are driven to do so by the goading pangs of hunger. Once we develop habits of eating certain things at certain times and in certain places, the appearance of these things, at these times and in these places, alone suffices to make us eat.

Sex Drive

Sexual desire waxes and wanes in cycles. There are life cycles: the specific desire for the sexual act does not characteristically arise until the animal is sexually mature or in man until puberty, and in old age the desire weakens. There are seasonal cycles for many animals: some mate only in the spring, others in the spring and fall. And there is also the estrus cycle in female mammals, the period of recurrent 'heat' when females are receptive to the advances of males. This sexual receptivity occurs at the time when the ova or female germ cells become mature and seems, indeed, to be dependent upon the process of their growth and development. The period of heat is also a period of increased activity. Female rats have been placed in cages with 'activity wheels,' like those provided for the exercise of squirrels, and the activity of the animals has been measured by the number of revolutions of the wheels per unit of time. Mechanical counters keep the record. Although a female rat ordinarily runs about a mile a day, it is not unusual for her, every fourth or fifth day at the peak of the estrus cycle, to run as much as fifteen miles in a day. Sexual drive, like the hunger drive, gives rise to general activity as well as specific.

In the absence of certain hormones—hormones secreted by the gonads or sex glands and by the pituitary gland—there is little sexual drive in the higher animals. The testes of the male, in addition to forming the male germ cells, the sperms, secrete hormones called *androgens,* and the ovaries of the female, besides producing the female germ cells or ova, secrete hormones that are known as *estrogens.* These hormones are most immediately responsible for sexual desire, but hormones secreted by the pituitary gland located at the base of the brain also determine the strength of the sex drive, since they in turn stimulate the secretion of the androgens and estrogens. In fact, the pituitary gland and the gonads act reciprocally. Pituitary secretion stimulates gonadal secretion, which in turn acts to diminish pituitary secretion, a process called *homeostasis,* by which the proper balance of the sex hormones is maintained in the body.

The role of the pituitary gland and the gonads in the sexual need and behavior of higher animals can be demonstrated in a number of ways. In female rats, for example, the increased activity at the time of the estrus cycle appears at puberty and disappears at menopause. Removal of the ovaries reduces general activity and abolishes the activity cycle. Injection of estrogens will, on the other hand, restore the cyclical behavior as will also replacement of the ovaries by grafting. Similarly, the removal from an animal of that part of the pituitary gland which secretes the gonad-stimulating hormones results in a loss of sexual drive unless gonadal hormones are artificially introduced into the animal's blood by injection. When the testes are removed from male rats and ovaries substituted for them, typically female cycles and levels of activity appear in the male.

The sex drive of the male rat, as well as that of other male mammals, does not appear until puberty. Castration after puberty reduces sexual desire as well as general activity and, although sexual behavior may not immediately cease, it is presently weakened and in most cases eventually disappears entirely. Injection of androgens into the blood stream of castrated rats not only revives their specifically sexual behavior but increases as well the amount of their general activity.

There is, then, no doubt that the sex drive of higher animals is in large measure dependent upon the presence of hormones in their blood. The hormonal origin of the sexual need of man is also clear. Though an infant or child may seek to gain through stimulation of certain erogenous zones of the body (for example, by masturbation of the genitals) a kind of pleasure which later would normally be gained in the act of sexual intercourse, a specific and strong sex drive is not observed in children prior to puberty. In fact, if ovaries are removed from a female child or fail to develop, she will never become pubescent; adult female characteristics will not appear and there will be a complete absence of sex drive. Similarly, early castration of a male child results in a person of neutral sex, lacking both sex drive and the male secondary sexual characteristics.

The mere fact that a person has reached or passed beyond the stage of puberty does not necessarily mean, however, that his sexual drive will find a normal and healthy outlet. Sexual maturation gives no guarantee of adequate psychosexual development. Unfortunate early experiences may so warp a man's attitudes toward sex that, although he may have a fully developed sexual mechanism and an adequate secretion of hormones in his blood, he may, nevertheless, find himself unable to perform the sexual act (impotency). A woman who has been made to fear her sexual impulses or has been led to think of sex as something dirty or sinful may find herself unable to experience any pleasure in the sexual act (frigidity), even though she is fully equipped physiologically and anatomically for such experience.

The hormonal basis of the sex drive can vary tremendously, but sexual need and behavior are not related in any simple manner to the amount of this variation. Just as frigidity is not always caused by a deficiency of hormones, so an abnormally strong sexual desire in women (nymphomania) is not always the result of an excessive secretion of hormones. In fact, nymphomania is often an attempt of a woman to compensate for a real or an imagined sexual inadequacy. Impotence in males, and its opposite, satyriasis, though sometimes correlated respectively with low and high levels of hormonal secretion, are in other cases entirely unrelated to physical and structural factors.

Man's sexual need and behavior are, then, no more completely determined by the level of hormones in his blood than is his eating determined solely by his stomach's hunger contractions. Both appetite and sexual desire also depend upon habits and attitudes that are learned and become, as derived needs, part of the personal adjustment of the individual. Herein lies the reason why love in man, with a better cerebral cortex than any other animal, can persist and even arise in the absence of adequate hormonal secretions.

The menstrual cycle in women is an estrus cycle, but a woman's sexual desire is not completely determined by the cycle. The peak of her desire has no fixed relation to the time of ovulation; it is usually reported to be greatest just before and just after menstruation, but it is often reached at other times. The fact that women do not lose their sexual desire or their ability to enjoy the sexual act after menopause is further evidence that sexual need and behavior are not entirely determined by hormonal secretions, once women have learned to enjoy sexual relations.

Androgens in men constitute an important basis for their sex drive, but the androgens do not alone explain the drive. Removal of the male gonads in mature individuals may have little effect upon sexual behavior, and old men who are impotent may still experience desire. This is not to say that androgens have no effect; they are important in the first stirring of desire, and beyond this they contribute to a man's energy and general efficiency. There is no doubt that castration impairs bodily vigor, and probably also intellectual verve and the power of creative thinking, but it does not necessarily destroy sexual desire or eliminate sexual behavior.

It can, then, be said of sex, as of hunger, that objects and situations associated with the arousal of the sex drive may, because of this association, become in themselves adequate to stimulate sexual behavior. Once an individual has developed habits of sexual behavior with a certain person or kind of person or at certain times and in certain places, the appearance of these established 'stimuli' alone may suffice to evoke again sexual need and behavior.

Other Drives

Many experiments have confirmed the drive character of other endocrine or ductless gland secretions. The removal of the pituitary, adrenal or thyroid glands in rats, as well as in other animals including men, has been shown to be followed by a reduction in general activity.

Other bodily conditions serving as drives to action are dryness of the mucous lining of the throat in thirst, distention of the bladder or large intestine, injury to the skin. Such examples could be many times multiplied, but these will suffice.

It is important to point out again, however, that while such physiological conditions as have just been described may be the primary drives to action, nevertheless, the environmental situation in which such action occurs may in itself become the effective stimulus for a similar form of behavior thereafter when the primary stimulus is lacking.

Behavior and Structure

As we have already seen, the way in which organisms satisfy their needs depends in part upon their structures. We cannot understand how an engine runs if we know only that there is steam in the boiler; we must also know the structure of the whole and the relationships among its parts. We have to know as much about living organisms if we are to understand their behavior. Needs and structures are related. The needs of a blind man are not the same as those of a man who sees, or those of a bed-ridden cripple the same as those of an athlete. Such individuals may and do have some needs in common, but they will have, in addition, unique needs.

One important respect in which organisms differ is in the extent to which they are able at birth to satisfy their needs. The human infant is absolutely dependent upon others for the gratification of many of his needs; not until years have passed is he able to care for himself alone. He must first learn how to get most of the things he requires. Many animals, such as spiders and the lower insects, on the other hand, are from the very first as capable of satisfying their needs as the adults of the same species. They do not have to learn how to take care of themselves, for they are born with mature structures organized for patterns of action adequate to meet all their needs. Such inborn patterns of response have been called *instincts,* and the behavior resulting from the activation of such patterns, *instinctive.* A fuller account of instinctive behavior has already been given (pp. 45–47). Here it is important only to note that, whereas man has to learn through years of experience how he may satisfy his needs, other animals start with behavior all ready to take care of most of their basic needs.

Needs for Particular Foods

Most animals are superior to man in the degree to which patterns of response activated by bodily needs operate unconsciously in the satisfaction of these needs. In one experiment hens were fed a diet almost entirely deficient in calcium carbonate. The omission of this important material from the diet soon resulted in a marked thinning of the shells of their eggs and, after four days, in a complete cessation of laying. After nine days of this diet deficient in calcium, the investigator divided the hens into two groups. To one group on one occasion he gave short pieces of macaroni within which shell had been placed, with the ends of the macaroni so closed that the shell could neither be seen nor tasted. These hens ate at that time an average of seventeen grains of shell. When he presented them plain shell a few hours later, each of these hens ate an average of only five grains more, making twenty-two grains of shell eaten in all. The other group he first gave plain macaroni, but, when later he presented them with plain shell, they ate on the average nineteen grains of shell. On the two occasions taken together the hens of the two sets ate approximately the same amount of shell, but that was because the hens who needed the calcium more on the second occasion ate more shell then. They were guided, it would seem, by physiochemical processes within their bodies. Being calcium hungry they kept on eating calcium when they got it.

In a similar experiment hens were offered a choice between three kinds of butter, one high in vitamins A and D, a second high in A but low in D, the third low in both A and D. They ate more of the first butter, the one most adequate for the satisfaction of nutritional needs, than of the others.

Rats have been shown to have the same ability to choose between suitable and unsuitable diets when presented with a variety of foods in so-called 'rat cafeterias.' Presented with two kinds of food, one containing sufficient and the other insufficient protein for normal growth, the rats ate both foods, but enough more of the former to maintain normal growth. Given foods varying in vitamin B content, they chose the foods with the richer vitamin content. The same results have been obtained with pigs and cows; these animals have demonstrated under controlled conditions their ability to select a diet adequate to their bodily needs.

These experiments have also demonstrated that hunger is not just an indiscriminate demand for any kind of food, but a complex of specific hungers or appetites, each for a particular nutritive substance, like protein, fat, carbohydrate, water, sodium, phosphorus, or calcium. (The desire for salt due to the removal or a disease of the adrenal glands is discussed on pp. 355 f.)

This discovery does not mean, however, that animals limit their eating to foodstuffs that satisfy specific nutritive needs. Like human beings, they may be tempted to eat whatever is appetizing to them rather than what is needed by their bodies.

In one experiment rats were allowed to choose between two different foods, a protein (casein) and a carbohydrate (sucrose), but they were required to make the choice in two different ways. In the first kind of choice, the protein and the carbohydrate had no fixed positions, but were shifted at random between the left and the right. The rats could see, smell and taste both these foods and made their choices on this immediate sensory basis. In the other kind of choice, the positions of the protein and carbohydrate were fixed, and the rat was required to make his choice in advance, after he had had enough experience to remember which food was where. When the rats had been deprived of protein for thirty days, they were allowed to select food under these two conditions. Their bodies then needed protein much more than carbohydrate. Were they wise? They were wise in advance, that is to say, when they had only the memories of the foods and their awareness of their own bodies in mind, they chose protein; but when they were close to the foods so that they could see, smell and taste them, they tended to take the carbohydrate, even though it was not so good for them.

This experiment was repeated with distilled water and powdered dog chow as the substances between which choice had to be made. The rats were deprived of both chow and water. When they had to choose in advance they all chose water, but, faced immediately with tasteless, odorless water versus smelly, tasty chow, they chose the chow.

The human analogy is apt. Motivation in rat or man is altered by immediate perception. The lure of the senses is strongest when sensation is actual and not merely remembered. In the days of the saloon and the drunkard, it was always a question as to whether the drunkard could get home with his pay without squandering it on drink. Starting home with high resolve, he could succeed if he did not pass the saloon, if he avoided the visual-olfactory perception that could so easily shift his motivation. The dinner table is replete with similar dilemmas. Do you eat what is good for you or what tastes good to you?

Since human adults so frequently and obviously eat an improper diet, it is interesting to note that newly weaned infants, if presented with a variety of foods and allowed complete freedom of choice, show an ability from the very first to select their food so that their bodily needs are adequately satisfied. To be sure, they also show preferences from time to time for different kinds of food, and these preferences change in unpredictable ways; yet records of food show from month to month that, in terms of protein, carbohydrate, fat, calories, acidity and alkalinity, the infants choose an adequate and balanced diet. With such self-feeding the infants gain in weight more than the average for this growth period.

Experiments of this sort, however, hardly justify the conclusion that infants and children should be allowed complete freedom in the choice of their food in the situations of everyday life. If a complete and adequate range of foods were always available to children—something which would be most uneconomical—and if the feeding habits of adults were unknown to them, and if, in addition, they were left absolutely free to choose, perhaps they would do as well. In the absence of such conditions, however, they seem to develop specific food preferences and habits of eating which make it difficult, if not impossible, for the infant to get along if such unconscious regulation of diet continues indefinitely.

Derived Needs

The greater plasticity of man means that he, more than any other animal, has to learn *how* to satisfy his needs. It also means that he learns to need more things than any other animal.

Learned skills and abilities and habits are important in the study of motivation not only because they enable the individual to satisfy his needs, but also because they may themselves become drives to action, constituting needs in their own right. The boy who learns boxing in self-defense may find that he wants to box, no longer in self-defense, but just for the fun of boxing; or the girl who learns to sew in order that she may have clothes as attractive as her friends may discover that she wants to sew, even though she needs no more clothes for her few social engagements. It might be argued that the boy who continues to box does so in order to feel superior instead of merely to protect himself, and that the girl who continues to sew does so in order to feel superior in the exercise of her skill rather than merely to be attractive. But even so it is in such ways that the number of our specific needs is multiplied many times over in the course of our lives. In general, the greater the patterning of the nervous processes underlying our actions, the greater will be the number of needs which we shall experience.

Such needs, resulting from mechanisms and habits which have become drives in their own right, are called *derived needs*. They are the clearest examples of what at the beginning of this chapter we called secondary needs. Their importance for everyday life lies in the fact that, through their development, objects and activities which earlier were *means* to an end now become *ends* in themselves. Their importance for any theory of motivation lies in the fact that they indicate the complexity of the physiological basis of the behavior which results from need and they reveal the inadequacy of conceiving of drive as simply a matter of a *specific* condition of the tissue in an organ or other restricted part of the body.

Because these secondary needs result from the patterning of the response mechanism, it follows that their physiological basis must be in large measure these neural patterns. Since even primary needs are satisfied only when the appropriate patterns of response are activated, and since, as we have seen, these primary needs may be aroused in the absence of the usually associated organic condition, it would seem no less true that their physiological basis is also in large part a matter of patterns in the nervous system. In other words, we are forced to conceive of the physiological basis of all needs, both primary and secondary, as being a matter both of certain organic stimulating conditions (for example, stomach contractions) and of certain neural states (for example, neural patterns).

BEHAVIOR AS DEPENDENT ON THE ENVIRONMENT

So important is the role of the environment in eliciting and determining behavior that it has been impossible not to mention it in connection with the other factors already discussed.

A rat confined in an activity cage shows an increase of activity as the time for feeding approaches. In that environment it is all he can do when driven by hunger. But if we take him from his cage and put food before him, he will no longer run; he will eat. If, on the other hand, we place him in a maze which he has learned, he will run directly to the food box and eat. We may assume in all three cases the existence of the same internal state of physiological disequilibrium or drive, so that the differences in behavior appear to be determined by differences in the rat's environment in the three situations.

Let us observe the same rat just after he has eaten to satiety. A satiated rat remains relatively quiet in his activity cage. If there is food before him, he ignores it. If placed in a maze, provided it is not a strange one, he shows no active seeking after food. Here, in the same three situations as described above and all quite different from each other, the behavior of the rat is practically identical—a quiet indifference to his environment. Are we, then, to draw from observation of a satiated rat a different conclusion from that we reached by observation of a hungry rat, namely, that the similarity of behavior in different environments is determined by the similar internal state of the rat in all three situations?

Relation of Environment to Needs

Neither conclusion is wholly right nor wholly wrong, and the conflict between them can be resolved if, instead of considering the internal and external factors separately, we see them in relation to each other. The point is that any situation as it exists psychologically for the organism—that is to say, as it is perceived and reacted to—is in large measure dependent upon the needs of the organism; and, since the needs of any organism are constantly changing, this fact means that the same physical environment and objects in it have at different times quite different meanings. When a child is hungry, an apple is something to eat; but when he is angry, it is something to throw at the provoking person. Similarly, a hungry rat is an alert rat, actively seeking in its environment anything that may serve as a means to the satisfaction of its need; but a satiated rat is a sleepy rat, indifferent to many aspects of its environment. Whether food is present or absent is a matter of no consequence to it. Environments *physically* unlike may all be the same *psychologically,* in that they are reacted to *as though* they were alike.

It is helpful in distinguishing the physical and psychological environment to call the former the *situation* and the latter the *field.* The physical *situation* is the environment considered as having independent real existence, whereas the psychological *field* is the situation as it exists psychologically for the individual. The psychological field is not to be equated merely to what is consciously perceived or known but rather to everything that at the moment determines the behavior of an individual.

Food in the situation may or may not be food in the field. If there is a need for it, food in the situation is likely to be perceived and reacted to. It then exists as food in the field and has a positive, attractive value, exciting the hungry person to eat. But the need for nourishment having been satisfied, the same food may be ignored. Although it may be perceived, it will not excite the individual to activity, for it now has a neutral quality, neither attracting nor repelling him. The presence of others who are hungry and eating may make the food seem slightly attractive so that it is nibbled at. An unpleasant story told at the table may make the food seem unpleasant so that it is pushed away. If, however, for any reason food has been eaten to the point of satiation, especially if this overeating has resulted in any degree of discomfort, the sight and smell of food cease to be neutral and acquire a negative character. The individual experiences a need to push the food out of sight or to remove himself from it.

Incentives

The existence of objects or activities in a person's field is thus seen to depend to an important degree upon his needs. It is for this reason that objects and activities in the field so often have to be described psychologically as having an attracting, repelling, exhorting, summoning, inviting or demanding character. Things possessing such characteristics are called incentives. An *incentive* may be defined as *an object, a situation or an activity which excites, maintains and directs behavior.* It must be clear, however, that a thing which is an incentive at one moment may not be an incentive at the next moment, or that a thing which is at one time a positive incentive attracting a person may subsequently be a negative incentive repelling the same individual.

Objects or activities offered to an individual may act as incentives to arouse his needs and stir him to action. When a need is very strong, he will actively seek objects to satisfy it if they are not present in his environment. But, under conditions of a lesser need, an individual may be relatively quiet and contented until something brought into his environment acts as an incentive to arouse that need more actively. A person may not be consciously hungry until he smells the pleasant aroma of food, or he may be little interested in stamp collecting until he hears a lecture on the fascinations of philately. As the advertiser knows, it is possible, within limits, to motivate people to action through a manipulation of their environments; but, if this activation is to be wholly successful, it is necessary to know something about the latent needs of those whom one seeks to influence. Otherwise what may seem the most attractive of incentives to the one who offers them may turn out to be no incentives at all for those to whom they are offered.

The social environment, no less than the

physical, influences the activities of individuals, causing things to lose or to acquire incentive value for them. It has already been pointed out that a hen which has eaten to satiation will begin to eat again if a hungry second hen is introduced into the situation; and she will eat more if two hungry hens, and still more if three, are brought in. This result occurs, however, only when the hungry hens have been accustomed to tyrannize over the satiated hen in other situations. If, instead, the satiated hen has habitually tyrannized over the hungry hens, she will attempt to keep them from eating by pecking at them or chasing them away. The converse experiment has likewise been performed, in which three hens eat to satiation and then are joined by a single hungry hen. Under these conditions the hungry hen begins to peck the grain, but her behavior has no effect upon the group of three, who remain passive or peck only a little. Evidently the satiated hens support one another in their indifference.

Other experiments have demonstrated comparable effects of social situations on eating in fishes, rats and monkeys, and the same effect is noticeable among persons. The child who does not want his oatmeal may nevertheless eat it eagerly when he sees his brother eating his with relish, just as, in the same way, the eating to excess at an old-fashioned Thanksgiving dinner is a function not only of the increased quantity of food (the same effect as seen in hens) but also of the *social facilitation* supplied by the sight of others eating. The presence of others may, of course, just as well cause objects or activities to become negative incentives as positive, as when, for example, the work we are doing ceases to be interesting because others gather for an evening of fun. (See also pp. 596 f.)

Cultural Determination of Needs

The importance of the environment in the behavior that is dependent on needs is, however, most clearly seen in the cultural determination of needs. The infant is born into a society in which there are certain social norms of behavior, certain customs which determine to a large extent not only the needs which the members of that society experience but also the particular means by which these needs may be satisfied. What the norms of his society are is one of the things the infant has to learn. The process of socialization in the developing child is in large measure the incorporation of these norms within himself in order that his general patterns of behavior may coincide with those of his group. In short, he learns that certain ends may be sought, but not others.

The specific nature of the means of satisfying primary needs no less than secondary ones is determined by social norms. The kind of food eaten by people of different cultures varies greatly. In many societies individuals are not permitted to eat the flesh of certain animals which are believed to be related to them, a relationship which thus renders the idea of eating such flesh abhorrent. In other societies fruits or plants are prohibited. There is no society in which the entire range of edible objects is included in the diet. Having learned to eat certain things and not others, and having learned to eat them only when prepared in certain ways, we find it difficult, if not impossible, to change our eating habits. It is known, for instance, that immigrants frequently find it easier to learn a new language than to learn to like the dishes of their new country. An American may demand a soft mattress and pillow if his need for rest is to be satisfied, a Japanese may demand a hard mat and pillow of wood and the African native may be able to rest only if he can lie upon the ground. Such differences as these are not racially determined but are rather the effect of social pressure on the needs of individuals in different cultures.

The young of the human species must be cared for if the species is to survive. This fact has led many persons to assume the existence in every mother of a need to care for her offspring, a need so fixed in its expression as to constitute a *maternal instinct*. Yet, actually, there is to be found among different peoples a wide range of norms of behavior in regard to the care and protection of infants. Among the Arapesh of the South Seas an infant is the object of great warmth and affection. Suckled whenever it cries, sleeping in close contact with its mother and carried by her wherever she goes, the Arapesh infant is almost continuously fondled and caressed. In contrast to the Arapesh, the Mundugumor treat their children with little love. The infant is kept in a hard uncomfortable basket, is not suckled unless clearly in need of milk, is not fondled or caressed, is made early to fend for itself and in general is so harshly treated that only the strongest survive. Among the Andaman Islanders adoption of children is so customary that it is rare to find a child of more than six or seven years of age living with its parents, for to adopt the child of a friend is an accepted form of expressing friendship and regard. On the Island of Mota, on the other hand, an infant may be sold at birth to the man who pays the midwife. Although this person is usually the father, it sometimes happens that, in the absence of the father or in the event that he lacks the necessary funds, another man buys the child and becomes its 'father.' In other societies infanticide, at least under certain conditions, is an accepted practice; and the Aztecs sold their children into slavery.

Another form of human behavior which has sometimes been regarded as instinctive is the *aggressive reaction* to frustration. Nevertheless conflict between individuals does not invariably or universally result in the same behavior. Instead of fighting with his fists, the Kwakiutl Indian fights with property in the institution of the "potlatch," in which the more property he can give away or destroy, the more superior he is to his opponent. Eskimos settle their conflicts in a public contest in which each sings abusive songs about the other. When two Indians of Santa Marta quarrel, instead of striking each other, they strike a tree or a rock with sticks, and the one first breaking his stick is considered the braver and hence the victor. In other societies aggression is expressed in still other ways; even within the same society there may be a wide range of different socially approved expressions of aggression.

It is now possible to demonstrate a wide range of behavior for any need. In the absence of crucial anthropological knowledge, it was formerly assumed that the needs were in all societies the same as in ours, and therefore instinctive. The fixedness and universality of forms of human behavior, however, turn out to be a myth. Instead, we find that the needs of the individual, as well as the ways in which he is permitted to satisfy them, are determined to a large extent by the social and cultural environment into which he is born and in which he is reared. (We shall learn more about social norms on pp. 560–562.)

DEFINITION OF NEED

The facts reviewed in the preceding sections of this chapter suggest the following definition of need. *A need is a tension within an organism which tends to organize the field of the organism with respect to certain incentives or goals and to incite activity directed toward their attainment.* For each need there are certain objects or activities—terminal situations—which, if they are obtained, satisfy the need, thus releasing the tension. It is for this reason that the fullest meaning of any behavior is described only when the final situation toward which it is leading is discovered.

At this point we must pause to note that a *need,* a *set* and an *attitude* are psychologically the same thing. The terms are merely being used in different contexts. When a subject is given pairs of digits and told to write down their sums, he is put in the adding attitude and is operating under a set for addition. Actually it would be just as reasonable to say that he has temporarily acquired a need for sums, a need which is derived from his need to do what the experimenter asks him to do and to do it well, which in turn is a phase of his need for approbation, which, of course, belongs properly to all gregarious animals like man. *Need, set, attitude*—these are all *dynamic* psychological concepts which express the fact that the organism can be set to pursue a given *end* or *purpose* consistently and without being put off the main track by every casual stimulation that comes along.

Needs have a qualitative aspect which makes it possible for us to distinguish such primary needs as those for food, sex, thermal constancy and elimination, and such secondary needs as those for superiority, submission, affiliation, freedom and inviolacy. Such terms as these are, of course, generalizations from the specific situations in which the concrete activities of needs end. We do not have a general need to be superior, but rather a need to be superior in a particular way in a specific situation, for example, to win this race, to get the highest mark on this examination, to know more about a certain field of study than any other person. Yet it is often helpful in the study of certain problems of personality and in the comparison of individuals to conceptualize general needs of which any given behavior or trait is but a specific and concrete expression.

MEASUREMENT OF NEEDS

Needs also have a quantitative aspect which makes it possible by the use of certain techniques to measure their strength. Although, of course, a need cannot be measured directly, an indirect estimate can be obtained by measuring its effect upon consciousness and behavior. Thus, by determining the work which the need will do, we get an indication of its intensity.

Obstruction Method

One technique for the measurement of needs is the obstruction method, by which the strength of a need is measured in terms of the magnitude of an obstacle or the number of times an obstacle of a given magnitude will be overcome in order to obtain a needed object. The obstruction method has been employed most often in the measurement of animal drive, rats having been the subjects most frequently studied.

A diagram of an obstruction box used in such investigations is shown in Fig. 43. To measure the sex need a female rat is placed in compartment *A*, a male rat (the incentive) in compartment *D*. In order to reach the incentive, the female rat must pass through the alley *B*. The floor of this section is covered with an electric grid which enables the experimenter to give the animal a shock. If she crosses the grid, she steps on *E* which releases door d_2, liberating the male from *D*. It has been found that when a female rat is in heat she crosses the charged grid frequently and with little hesitation, though at other times she scarcely ever crosses it.

Similar investigations of hunger, thirst and maternal need have demonstrated that a rat does not repeatedly cross the grid and take a shock in the absence either of a motivating need or of the appropriate incentive.

In the obstruction method not one need is measured, but two which are in conflict. There is the need for food, or water, or whatever other need is being investigated, but there is also the need for avoidance of pain, so that what is actually being measured is the relative strength of the two needs. If, for example, the need for food is stronger than the need for avoidance of pain, the animal will take the shock in order to get the food; and, presumably, the stronger the first need, the more often will the grid be crossed in a given period of time. Since every need is unstable, the measurement of one against another cannot be exact. In evaluating these results we must remember that the animal tends to become accustomed to the electric shock, so that the negative incentive of the physically constant shock decreases in time.

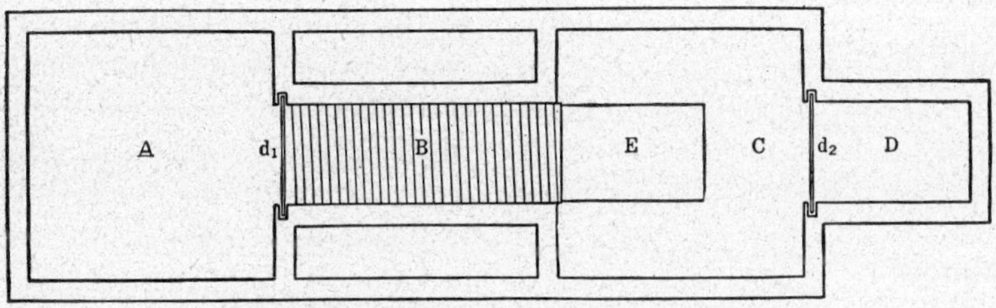

FIGURE 43. FLOOR PLAN OF OBSTRUCTION BOX

(*A*) Entrance compartment; (*B*) obstruction compartment (electric grid); (*C, D*) divided incentive compartment; (*E*) release plate; (d_1) manually operated door between entrance compartment *A* and grid *B;* (d_2) automatic door operated by animal's stepping on release plate *E*. [From T. N. Jenkins, L. H. Warner and C. J. Warden, *J. comp. Psychol.*, 1926, **6**, 366; reprinted by permission of the Williams and Wilkins Company.]

With the use of this method of obstruction attempts have been made to determine the relative strengths of various animal needs. In the most extensive investigations so far recorded, the maternal need has been found to be the strongest. The others in rank order of strength are thirst, hunger, sex and the exploratory need. This order depends, however, upon the degree of deprivation of the animal and upon the particular apparatus used as well as upon the comparison of one need at a time with the need for avoidance of pain.

Needs, however, are all interrelated. It has been shown that prolonged hunger both in man and in animals is accompanied by a lessening of sexual drive; that prolonged deprivation of water reduces materially the intake of food in rats; that the brooding of a hen reduces greatly the amount of food she eats; that an increase in the hunger of rats is accompanied by an increase in their need for exploration; and that, when sex need is strongest (at the time of estrus in the female rat), the need for food as measured by its intake is greatly reduced. A similar interrelation can be observed in persons. The need to get good grades may become much less when the student falls in love, the need for food may become secondary to the desire to have a slim figure, and the need of the mother to dress attractively may become negligible when the need to care for her child is great.

Learning Method

A second technique for the measurement of needs is the learning method, by which the strength of need is measured in terms of the readiness with which a task is learned under different conditions of motivation. It has long been known that for an organism to learn it must be motivated. This fact makes it possible to vary the factor of motivation and to measure its effect upon the rate of learning. Here again, because animal experimentation is simpler than human, most of the studies have been made with animals, but an analogue of the experimental findings can usually be found in the realm of human behavior.

It has been shown that, within limits, the stronger the motivation the faster the learning. In one experiment which demonstrated this relation, the rate of maze learning by three groups of rats differing only in their motivation was investigated. The first group was very hungry and very thirsty, the second was very hungry but only slightly thirsty and the third was very thirsty but only slightly hungry. During the first nine days of the experiment the rats were rewarded with bran mash; during the last nine days they were rewarded with water. In the first half of the experiment the rats motivated both by hunger and thirst learned slightly faster than the animals of the other two groups, a fact which indicates the superiority of two needs over one in motivating learning. In the second half of the experiment, with the shift to water as the reward, the very hungry and thirsty animals were temporarily disturbed by the change. They showed at first an increase in the number of their errors, but at the end of the experiment they were again superior to the other two groups. The effect of the shift in reward upon the other two groups, which had learned at the same rate during the first nine days, was striking. Now rewarded with water, the very thirsty animals speeded up their learning, whereas the very hungry rats showed very little improvement with the inappropriate reward. The second half of the experiment not only confirmed the finding of the first in demonstrating that two needs constitute a more effective condition for learning than one, but it also showed that learning is faster when the need serving as motive is appropriately rewarded.

The needs motivating children for their school work are numerous and varied. The arousing of more needs by presenting additional incentives has been shown to increase their accomplishment. In one investigation, the offer of a reward of a chocolate bar raised the performance fifty-two per cent above the usual level, whereas the introduction of a number of incentives, like candy, a definite goal, rivalry and praise, increased the performance sixty-five per cent. In human motivation, then, as in animal, it is easy to demonstrate that an increase in motivation leads to an increase of performance.

It has also been shown that the *amount* of reward offered influences the rate of learning. For instance, chicks who find six grains of boiled rice in the reward box at the end of a simple maze learn the maze more effectively than chicks who are rewarded with only one grain. That the amount of reward offered human beings is not without its effect upon performance is also clear. We work harder and better for more rather than for less pay. The student works harder for a large scholarship than for a small one.

Not only is the amount of reward important in determining the rate of learning but also the kind of reward. It has been shown, for example, that of two groups of rats learning a maze, the group rewarded with bran mash will learn the maze more rapidly than the group rewarded with less-preferred sunflower seeds. This finding also has its analogue in human behavior.

SOME EFFECTS OF NEED

Sensitivity, perception, imagination, thought, activity and persistence all depend on need and are affected by needs. Frustration often arises from a conflict of needs. To these effects we now turn.

Effect on Perception and Imagination

The investigations just reviewed have demonstrated the role of need in learning. They have also shown the effect of need on perception, for all learning involves a reorganization of a field. The maze which a rat has learned is *psychologically* quite different from what it was when first encountered. The keyboard of a typewriter is for the skilled typist quite a different field from what it is for the novice.

A simple example will illustrate that learning involves a *reorganization of a field* as a result of need. Let us take the case of a young child separated from an apple by a fence, as indicated in Fig. 44(*a*). If the child is not hungry, and is contentedly playing with some toys in the blind alley, he may not even see the apple; or, if he does, he will not be interested in it. If, on the other hand, he is restless, either because he is hungry or because he is tired of playing with his toys, the likelihood is greatly increased that he will see the apple.

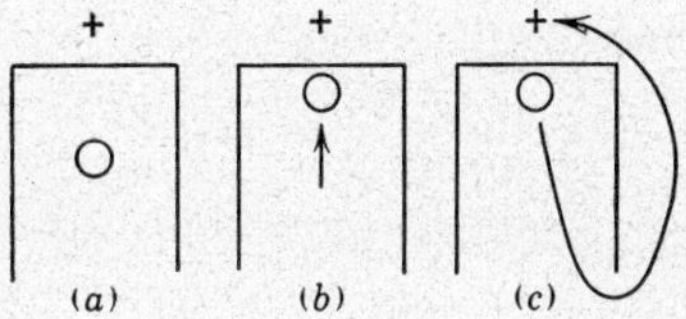

FIGURE 44. STEPS IN SOLUTION OF SIMPLE DETOUR PROBLEM

+ = apple. O = child. → = path taken by child.

Under two different conditions of need the field of the child is differently organized. Thus, whether the apple will become a positive incentive depends upon whether it can serve in any way to satisfy a need.

If it does become a positive incentive, the very young child will try to get it in the simplest and most direct manner, as indicated in Fig. 44(*b*). Since he cannot reach it, or crawl through the fence to it, his need is blocked and his field reorganized until what was previously for him a fence or a row of sticks now looms as a barrier. He may push against this barrier, try to crawl under or over it or reach through it as far as he can, all because the way to the apple is a straight line toward it. Then, blocked and frustrated, he may look around, see the opening and suddenly run to the apple in the roundabout direction indicated in Fig. 44(*c*). Again his field has been reorganized. What was previously either nonexistent as a way to the goal, or else a path away from the goal, now becomes the first phase of the path to the goal. If the child is again put back into the blind alley, he will at once take the roundabout way to obtain the apple. He has, in other words, learned the solution of what is called a *detour problem.* In this case it is clear that learning is the result of a need which reorganizes a field.

When there is no possible solution of a problem, the role of need in reorganizing the field may be even more marked. In an investigation of anger, subjects were given a task for which three different solutions were demanded, although there were only two possible ones. The subject was asked to step within a square outlined by long sticks laid upon the floor and, without leaving this area, to obtain a flower which was placed upon a sawhorse four feet outside the square. The two possible solutions were: (1) to place a chair which stood within the square between the square and the horse and, leaning with one hand on the chair, reach the flower with the other hand; and (2) to kneel down (keeping the feet within the square) and reach the flower. Both these solutions were possible only if the subject had perceived the field reorganized in these two ways. After the subjects had arrived at these two solutions, they were asked to demonstrate a third. Since there was no third solution and since the subjects were kept for hours at the task, the mounting tension resulting from the blocking of their need was expressed not only in anger but also in many new perceptual organizations of the field. As the experiment continued, all objects came to be seen in relation to the goal —as barriers, disturbances, tools, etc. The greater the tension, the more did objects offer themselves as possible means to the solution. Some rings which had been placed along the side of the square were seen again and again as having something to do with getting the flower. Although they were of no use, they were picked up repeatedly and juggled about in a vain attempt at use. Then they became disturbing factors which the subjects wanted to forget but could not. The subjects were also disturbed by the fact that the back of the square was made of two sticks rather than one, as though this, too, had something to do with the solution.

Such behavior clearly indicates that while a certain degree of need is necessary for that reorganization of a field which constitutes insight and learning, a need in excess of such an optimum may come so to distort the field that it no longer bears any resemblance to the situation. In this experiment, some of the subjects after long periods of frustration revealed momentary fantastic distortions of the field. One person began to act as though she had hypnotic power to draw the flower to her, while another, yielding to fantasy, saw the room filled with water and the horse and flower floating in her direction. Both subjects in their momentary fantasies forgot the harsh realities of their situation. Such a denial of the frustrating realities of a situation is, of course, characteristic of all *fantasy* and *wishful thinking.*

The behavior of these subjects was similar to that of a student who, having endured one frustration after another in his boyhood, was still in college being frustrated both in his scholastic work and in his social relations. Yet, if in reality his needs were frustrated, in fantasy his wishes were fulfilled. He confided that when he sat in a classroom he paid little attention to the lecture, for he found it easier and pleasanter to indulge in the fantasy that he was the head of a large office and that all the other members of the class (so industriously taking notes) were his secretaries and stenographers busily working for him. When he walked from one building to another on the campus, he thought of each as a separate city or town. To his mind he was not merely passing buildings on a campus; he was speeding over the highways from one city to another in a high-powered car. And when, one night, he was, in reality, walking along a country road with two of his friends, it seemed to him in his fantasy that they were a couple of the enemy whom he had captured in a lone raid into no man's land and whom he now was escorting back to his own lines—for which brave action he was soon to be decorated.

The fields of this student deviated far from the objective realities of his everyday situations. Since he found in them a pleasant, vicarious satisfaction of the needs which were in reality frustrated, his fantasies constituted escapes from this reality. We all indulge in such *flights from reality* from time to time, when our needs are excessively frustrated. We return from them frequently with renewed vigor and strength to force the satisfaction of our needs on the level of reality. As a matter of fact, the very distortion that our fields undergo at such times may suggest to us the way in which we can in reality satisfy our needs. There is always the danger, however, that such flights from reality will cease to be momentary or of relatively short duration and will become instead permanent. It is in this sense that the delusions characteristic of certain mental disorders are merely extreme and lasting distortions of the patients' fields by their needs. The poor man whose need for material things has been enduringly frustrated may end by living in a fantastically distorted field in which he is fabulously wealthy, although in reality he is an inmate of a mental hospital.

Less marked and less pathological examples of the organization of a field by a need can be seen in everyday life. When two persons behave differently in the same objective situation, they do so because the situation is for each a different field. Whereas one individual's need for attention may make him see a group of indifferent strangers as an appreciative audience before whom he must show off, another's need for inviolacy may cause him to perceive the members of the same group as hostile critics from whom he must shrink and withdraw. That Napoleon's need for superiority often determined the structure of his fields is revealed in his remark to an attendant prior to the meeting of an Austrian conference. "Carry that chair away before we begin. I have never been able to see a raised chair without wanting to sit in it."

Explorers who have been forced to live on short rations or whose food supplies have become exhausted have often reported their preoccupations at such times with thoughts of food. During the day their conversations have been mostly about the preparation of food; at night their dreams have been of sumptuous feasts.

In one investigation of the effects of abstinence from food upon imaginal processes, subjects were given, at various intervals after eating, a series of tests in which ambiguous or incomplete material had to be interpreted or completed. With all the tests it was found that, as the interval of time since the last meal increased, the number of interpretations or completions which referred to food also increased. When, for example, the subjects were given a word-association test in which they had to respond to a given word with the first word which came to mind, hungry subjects, more often than others, thought of such words as *spoon, fork, eat* and *food.* In another test the subjects were asked to tell what was going on in a series of pictures, parts of which had been cut away. In the case of one picture of a child pointing, subjects who were not hungry were likely to interpret this as a child about to strike a key of a typewriter or about to pick up a toy, whereas hungry subjects were inclined to see it as a child about to stick his finger in a pie or in some other way reacting to a food situation.

Tests comparable to those just described for hunger have been used to determine, by an analysis of subjects' responses, the relative strengths of other needs. Additional tests which have been used for the same purpose are a musical reverie test, in which, while a number of phonograph records are played, a subject allows a fantasy to develop which he later reports to the experimenter; an odor imagination test in which, as each of a number of odors is presented, a subject invents some episode or story from the first idea or image which comes to mind upon smelling the odor; and a thematic apperception test in which the subject is presented with a number of pictures and asked to make up a plot or story for which the picture might serve as an illustration. Such tests have been used for the measurement of needs on the assumption that the stronger a need the greater will be its effect in organizing the field. This means that in these tests the stronger needs of the individual determine the content of the fantasies which are evoked and the nature of the interpretations and completions of the material which are made.

Since, in thus reorganizing the perceptual field in accordance with his own needs, the subject is projecting his own needs into the situation which he faces, these means of assessing needs have been called *projective techniques,* procedures which have become important tools in the assessment of personality. (See pp. 495–497.)

Effect on Sensitivity

There is evidence that need may determine an increase in sensitivity. Fasting persons have frequently reported that they are more sensitive to odors and sounds during fasting than at other times, and for such statements there is some experimental confirmation in other sensory fields. In one case it was found that, as the fast was prolonged (it lasted altogether thirty-one days), the abilities to discriminate tactually between two adjacent points on the skin and visually two points on the retina were increased. Studies of animals and infants, in which the ease of evoking a response is taken as a measure of sensitivity, also indicate an increase of sensitivity to various kinds of stimulation under conditions of hunger.

In one investigation rats were allowed to choose between distilled water and weak solutions of salt. With concentrations of salt below the threshold of perception normal rats showed no preference, although, when the concentration of salt was increased to 0.055 per cent (about one part of salt to 2000 parts of water), they consistently preferred the salt solution. On the other hand, rats, whose need for salt had been increased by the removal of their adrenal glands, could distinguish much weaker solutions, for they chose, in preference to distilled water, concentrations of salt as low, on the average, as 0.003 per cent (about one part of salt to 33,000 parts of water). It seems clear that increased need increases sensitivity, although it is not so clear what the mechanism is. It is more likely that need heightens attention in these rats than that it sensitizes their taste receptors.

Effect on Persistence

If the activity of an individual is interrupted, we should expect, from the definition of need, that the residual tension remaining after the interruption would cause the individual to return to the interrupted activity and to attempt again to reach the original goal. A number of experiments have demonstrated precisely this effect.

In one experiment subjects, given a series of simple tasks to perform, were allowed to complete some of them but were interrupted before finishing the others. When, with both completed and interrupted tasks within reach, the subjects were left free to do whatever they desired, it was found that, whereas they almost never took up the completed tasks again, presumably because their corresponding tensions had been discharged, they resumed the interrupted tasks in about eighty per cent of the cases.

In another investigation subjects were asked to help the experimenter in thinking of words beginning with a certain letter. After writing down as many words as they could think of within the allotted time, some of the subjects were told that they had done unusually well, whereas others were told that they had done very poorly. The intention of the experiment was to create for some subjects an experience of success and for others an experience of failure. When, two weeks later, the subjects were questioned as to whether they had thought in the interim of words beginning with the assigned letter, there was considerable evidence that they had had difficulty in keeping their minds off the original task. One subject, who had experienced failure, reported:

"As soon as the experiment was over C-words came flooding into my mind. On my way home I felt that I should go insane if I continued to think of them, so I determined to banish them by thinking of other things. At intervals thereafter C-words would slip into my thoughts when I was not expecting them, but they gradually ceased coming."

In general the persistence of the activity was greater for those who had felt frustrated in the original experiment, presumably because of the greater unresolved tension which tended to continue the original activity until it was terminated by the fulfilment of the original purpose. We often experience in everyday life the persistence of activities which have failed to reach their goals. Having done poorly in an examination, we continue to think of all the things we should have written but did not. Worsted in an argument, we can think of nothing but the brilliant things we failed to say.

Experiments such as these, as well as the observation of persisting activities in everyday life, demonstrates that tasks which have been undertaken, like any purpose or intention, set up tendencies within the individual which keep him at work until the goals thus set are attained. It must be noted, however, that in the experiments reported above no conflicting purposes or intentions were aroused, as there might well have been and as there often are in everyday life. These experiments, therefore, offer no guarantee that all human beings will always complete their incompleted tasks if given an opportunity. In some individuals the need for initiating new action may be stronger than the need for finishing work already begun.

Since the residual tensions of incompleted tasks may cause preoccupation with these activities, we should expect to find that incompleted tasks tend to be better remembered than finished ones. This expectation is verified. If subjects are given a series of simple tasks to perform, are allowed to finish one half of them but are interrupted before they have completed the other half, and then are asked immediately after the experiment to recall all the tasks which they have attempted, they can recall incompleted tasks almost twice as often as finished ones.

Frustration Tolerance

The effects of need upon the behavior and consciousness of the individual depend to a large extent upon the degree of tension in the given case. Some degree of need is necessary for psychobiological adaptation, for otherwise the organism is inert. In order that learning may occur, there must be some degree of tension to reorganize a field, but we have already seen that an excess of tension resulting from a prolonged blocking of a strong need may cause a field to be so grossly distorted, as in the delusions of mental disorders, that it no longer bears any resemblance to the situation. Tension increased beyond a critical point results in a failure of adjustment of the organism to the requirements of the situation. These facts have suggested the fruitfulness of a concept of *frustration tolerance,* which has been defined as *the amount of frustration which can be borne without a resultant failure in psychobiological adjustment.* The frustration tolerance of an individual is, then, his capacity to stand frustration without distorting his field so that it no longer bears a valid resemblance to the real situation.

The frustration tolerance of an individual is exceeded in all cases in which the increased tension resulting from frustration causes the individual to react inadequately to the situation. If, instead of modifying his behavior in such a way as to effect a satisfaction of his frustrated needs, he reacts with crying, temper tantrums, regression to more primitive behavior or a breakdown of the personality in any of the various forms of mental disorder, the individual's tolerance for frustration has clearly been exceeded.

Just as there is a point beyond which the primary needs—for example, the need for oxygen—cannot be denied satisfaction without a collapse of the organism, so there is also a point beyond which the secondary needs—for example, the need for freedom—cannot be frustrated without a breakdown of the individual. One of the important problems of psychology is to discover the conditions which determine not only the general frustration tolerance of the individual but also his specific tolerance for the frustration of different needs.

INDIVIDUAL DIFFERENCES IN RESPECT OF NEEDS

The terms with which we characterize persons are often merely short statements about the need or needs which most often, or at least most obviously, motivate them. When we say of a man, "He is a show-off," we are, in effect, saying that he has a strong need for attention; and, when we say of another, "He's a go-getter," we are recognizing in him a strong need for superiority. Such characterizations point to the fact, which we have already noted, that not all the needs of an individual are equally strong, and that the differences among persons are at least in part determined by differences in the relative strengths of their needs.

Other differences in personality are determined by differences in the relationships of needs. It is important to know which of an individual's needs are regularly activated in the service of other more important needs. An individual may be motivated to collect rare antiques in order that he may show them off to his friends and thus gain a satisfaction of his needs for attention and superiority. If, however, he does not have the money with which to buy expensive antiques, he may be motivated to gain his goals of attention and superiority in some other way, perhaps by developing and exhibiting athletic skill. We may find at different times different particular needs serving the dominant need of a given individual. We know, however, a great deal about a person if we know, over a period of time, which needs primarily determine his behavior and which needs are more or less consistently subsidiary to these dominant needs. An important difference among persons occurs in respect of the subsidiary relationships which exist among their needs. One man may gain his superiority by cruelty to his subordinates; another man may gain his superiority by generosity to his subordinates. Both may get what they want—importance, recognition, prestige.

There are varying degrees with which one may be consciously aware of his own needs. At one extreme, a man may have no awareness at all of what he wants. He may not even be aware of any tension or uneasiness. At the other extreme, a man may know precisely what it is he is after. An intermediate degree of awareness is the case where a person recognizes that something is lacking, that he is uneasy and dissatisfied, and yet he cannot say exactly what it is he wants. No one is aware of all his needs at all times, but some persons have much more insight than others into their basic motivations.

A need may fail to be recognized because it is relatively weak in comparison with other needs, which for the moment dominate the consciousness and behavior of the individual. More important in its consequences for the personality, however, is the failure of a person to recognize a need because it is in conflict with his consciously recognized and accepted needs.

The consciously recognized and accepted needs of the person are often called his *ego needs,* since the *ego* is defined as that part of the person which is consciously knowing, desiring and willing. Needs which are recognized as one's own and for the satisfaction of which one takes responsibility are ego needs. Ideals which a man consciously sets for himself and for which he strives are ego ideals. The ego is an important factor in motivation. The need or needs which are most important to the ego are those which most clearly distinguish one person from another. They are the more enduring needs of the ego; yet needs, which at one time are central to the ego, absorbing all its energies, may at other times become quite unimportant.

In general, needs which are smoothly and silently satisfied do not involve the ego. Though the need for oxygen is one of man's most vital needs, the satisfaction of it does not involve his ego, since air is free and he ordinarily gets all he wants of it unconsciously and automatically. But, if air were not free, if getting it depended upon the cooperation of others or if one had to compete for it, the need for oxygen would become an ego need as the needs for sex, affection, recognition, superiority so often are.

Many of the effects of residual need tension described earlier in this chapter are more pronounced when they derive from ego needs, and, in the absence of ego involvement, they may not be observed at all. Interrupted tasks, for example, are more often resumed and better remembered than completed ones only if the tasks which have been undertaken have really involved the ego.

The typical shifts in a person's level of aspiration in attempting to solve tasks of varying degrees of difficulty, the raising of the level of his aspiration after success and the lowering of it after failure, occur most strikingly for those tasks in which a person is deeply egoistically involved. If the same set of tasks is given twice to the same persons, once as 'practice' and once as 'a test,' the shifting of the level of aspiration —up after success and down after failure— is greater when the tasks are understood to be a test measuring the ability of the individual and not merely practice. In other words, if, when setting our level of aspiration, there is something at stake for our ego, we behave more cautiously.

Other experiments as well as observations of everyday behavior suggest that ego motivation tends to be strong motivation. Ego needs are frequently selfish needs, but not always. Whether they are or not depends upon the person, for in so far as a person identifies himself with others and experiences their needs as his own, his motivation ceases to be narrowly egocentric, becoming instead sociocentric. Such common sociocentric motivation characterizes all successfully integrated groups which are held together by mutual loyalty—from the wedded pair up through many kinds of social groups to the nation itself. Those persons who hope for the democratization of the world and the achievement of international peace base their aspiration on this possibility of combatting egocentric aggression with this sociocentric identification. (For more on the ego, see pp. 567–570.)

REFERENCES

1. Katz, D. *Animals and men.* New York: Longmans, Green, 1937.

   A provocative discussion of problems of comparative psychology based upon the author's ingenious observations and experiments.

2. Kinsey, A. C., Pomeroy, W. B., Martin, C. E. *Sexual behavior in the human male.* Philadelphia: Saunders, 1948.

   A scientific account of sexual behavior written by leading authorities on the subject, from the point of view of biology, psychology and sociology.

3. Klineberg, O. *Race differences.* New York: Harper, 1935.

   A clear and simple survey of the findings of the biological, psychological and cultural approaches to the problem of race differences.

4. Köhler, W. *The mentality of apes.* New York: Harcourt, Brace, 1925.

   A Gestalt psychologist's report on the behavior of chimpanzees and the role of insight and intelligence in their solution of detour problems.

5. Lewin, K. *A dynamic theory of personality.* New York: McGraw-Hill, 1935.

   The beginnings of this author's dynamic psychology as illustrated in his early theoretical discussions and experimental findings.

6. Mead, M. *Sex and temperament in three primitive societies.* New York: William Morrow, 1935.

   An anthropologist's report of differences in culture and personality in three geographically closely situated primitive societies.

7. Muenzinger, K. F. *Psychology: the science of behavior.* New York: Harper, 1942.

   A systematic introductory text in psychology which gives a central position to the concept of motivation.

8. Murray, H. A., *et al.* *Explorations in personality.* New York: Oxford University Press, 1938.

The findings of a clinical and experimental study of fifty men of college age presented in conjunction with a dynamic theory of personality.

9. Sherif, M. *The psychology of social norms.* New York: Harper, 1936.

A clear and simple discussion of the ways in which individual frames of reference of experience and social norms of behavior become established.

10. Warden, C. J.: *Animal motivation.* New York: Columbia University Press, 1931.

Studies of various drives in the white rat by means of the obstruction method.

11. Young, P. T. *The motivation of behavior.* New York: Wiley, 1936.

A comprehensive review, presented in textbook form, of experimental investigations of the motivational bases of behavior.

12. Young, P. T. *Emotion in man and animal.* New York: Wiley, 1943.

A comprehensive review of experimental studies of emotion which stresses the role of emotions as motivating factors in behavior.

CHAPTER 7

Learning

OUR ability to profit from past experience is one of our most valuable assets. Learning—the process by which we do this—is the subject of this chapter. In it we shall analyze the conditions under which learning takes place. We shall discover that the same principles which account for our learning of desirable and appropriate reactions also explain our acquiring of undesirable bad habits.

We can best appreciate the important role which learning plays in our lives if we recall what a limited repertoire of responses a human infant possesses at birth. As we have seen, all learning depends upon maturation, which fits the organism for learning. On the other hand, all the increase in capacity and complexity which characterizes mature adult behavior must be attributed to learning. We learn, for instance, to eat the things we eat in the way we eat them, to respond as we do to other people and—the crowning achievement of the human being—to use language. We learn not only to use language for communication but to use it also to satisfy our needs and to control the behavior of other people. Nor is learning only intellectual. Likes and dislikes, emotional responses, most of the complex pattern of reactions which we call personality, all are learned. Most of this learning occurs informally in the give and take of daily life, for learning is by no means always intentional or formal.

The very fact that learning is so pervasive and bound into the warp and woof of our daily lives results in the process going almost unremarked. When we notice it at all, we think of it in rough, unanalytic terms; but, if we seek to understand it and its principles, detailed analysis is essential. As a consequence, much of our understanding of learning behavior is derived from controlled laboratory experiments. The careful laboratory analysis of learning requires the use of materials, methods and concepts which at first appear to be strange and divorced from the learning of everyday life. Nevertheless, learning in the laboratory is really the same in kind as the learning which pervades everyday life. What the laboratory does is simply to provide a better situation for analyzing the learning process.

ASSOCIATIVE LEARNING

Learning varies greatly in complexity. We shall begin our analysis with a very simple type, *associative learning*, which consists of the formation of associations between responses and the stimuli which are present when those responses are made.

This chapter was prepared by Carl I. Hovland of Yale University.

Association is a common phenomenon, exemplified by our 'being reminded of' an experience by stimuli which were present during the experience. The odor of a burning wood fire may recall a Christmas vacation in the north woods, or magnolia blossoms may remind us of a childhood trip to the South. Often, but by no means always, we have been aware of these stimuli in the original situation of which we are now reminded.

This phenomenon has, of course, been known for a long time, and philosophers for two centuries have called attention to the "association of ideas." Careful study of the conditions under which stimuli and responses are associated is, however, much more recent. It really begins about 1903 with the work of Pavlov, which we have already noted in a previous chapter. Pavlov, while studying problems in the physiology of digestion, made the observation that animals salivate not only to food but also in response to the various stimuli which in their experience invariably precede the introduction of food, like the clicking of a food release mechanism. Salivation to stimuli of this type, which were not originally effective, he called "psychic secretion."

Conditioning

This phenomenon fascinated Pavlov, and as a consequence he devised a series of experiments to determine the conditions under which it occurred. Mostly he used dogs as the experimental animals. He chose the salivary response for study because it provided a sensitive measure of the magnitude of response. (See Fig. 45.) He performed a simple surgical operation by which the flow of saliva from the dog's jowl is transmitted through a glass tubing to a measuring instrument.

To establish a connection between a response, like salivation, and an initially ineffective stimulus, like the sounding of a buzzer, Pavlov found that it was essential to pair the presentation of the new stimulus with the one which was originally effective. For example, he would sound the buzzer at the time he presented the food to

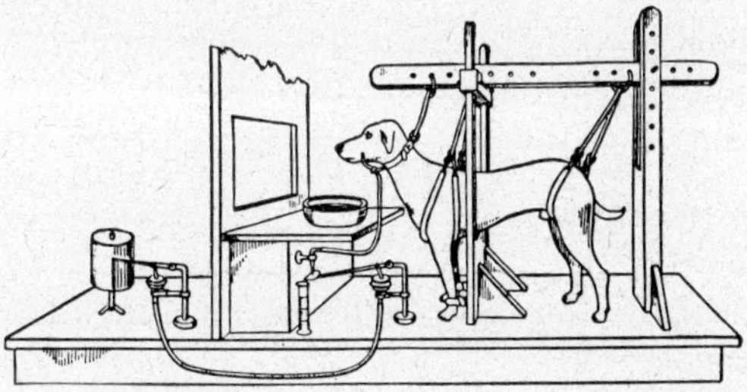

FIGURE 45. PAVLOV'S METHOD OF ESTABLISHING A CONDITIONED SALIVARY REFLEX

The unconditioned stimulus (food) is presented automatically in the small dish through the window. At the same time, or earlier, the conditioned stimulus (the ringing of a bell) is given. The saliva which flows through a tube from the dog's jowl is collected in the graduated class receptacle. As the saliva flows into the receptacle, it strikes a small disk which depresses the lever just in front of the animal. This downward movement is transmitted to the lever behind the screen, and an automatic tracing is thus secured upon a smoked drum or kymograph. The kymographic record tells the experimenter how many drops of saliva have been secreted and how regular the flow has been. [From R. M. Yerkes and S. Morgulis, The method of Pavlov in animal psychology, *Psychol. Bull.*, 1909, **6**, 264.]

the dog, or just before. The response which was thus learned he called a *conditioned* response because it was dependent upon conditions. The process is still referred to as *conditioning*. The stimulus which originally produced the response was called the *unconditioned stimulus,* and the new one with which the response was being connected by conditioning was called the *conditioned stimulus.* In Pavlov's laboratory food was customarily the original stimulus, and the sound of a bell or buzzer, the conditioned stimulus. After a number of trials the sound of the buzzer alone elicited some secretion of saliva. With more trials the amount of saliva secreted for the buzzer alone would increase until it finally became nearly as great as to the sight of food itself.

We can diagram this process quite simply.

Before Conditioning		After Conditioning	
	Response		*Response*
Conditioned Stimulus		*Conditioned Stimulus*	
Buzzer ——→	Listening, etc	Buzzer ——┐	
Unconditioned Stimulus		*Unconditioned Stimulus*	↓
Sight of Food →	Salivation	Sight of Food →	Salivation

At an earlier period of time, when the dog was a tiny puppy, the response of salivating to the sight of food was established through conditioning. Food in the mouth was at that time the unconditioned stimulus. This initial conditioning would be diagrammed as follows.

Before Conditioning		After Conditioning	
	Response		*Response*
Conditioned Stimulus		*Conditioned Stimulus*	
Sight of Food ——→	Looking at it, etc.	Sight of Food——┐	
Unconditioned Stimulus		*Unconditioned Stimulus*	↓
Food in Mouth →	Salivation	Food in Mouth →	Salivation

Factors Affecting Conditioning

Pavlov and his students kept careful records of some of the factors influencing the association formed between the conditioned and unconditioned response. These relationships have been further studied in American laboratories so that today we know a great deal about the phenomena of conditioning. Some of the more important conclusions follow.

(1) *Acquisition.* Repetition of the pairing of the conditioned and unconditioned stimuli increases the strength of the connection until a point is reached where no further observable gain is obtained. A sample acquisition curve is shown in Fig. 46. These results correspond to our everyday experience that learning is favored by repetition.

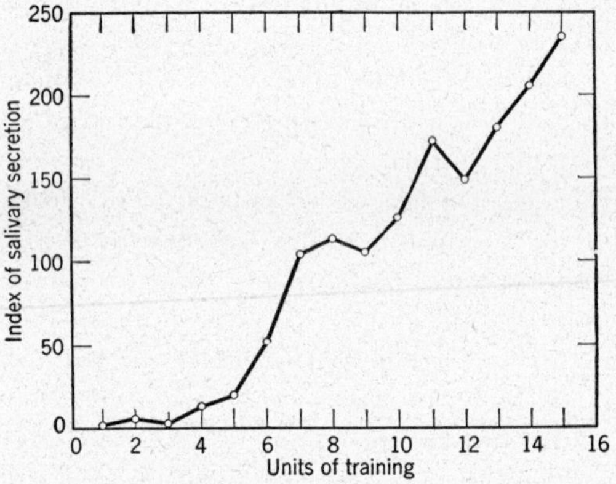

FIGURE 46. ACQUISITION OF A SALIVARY CONDITIONED RESPONSE

Composite curve of the data from four dogs. [As given by N. Kleitman and G. Crisler, and plotted by C. L. Hull in *Handbook of general experimental psychology,* 1934, p. 425; by permission of the Clark University Press.]

(2) *Time factors.* There is an optimal time between the presentation of the conditioned and unconditioned stimuli, and time intervals more remote from the latter are progressively less effective. The graph (Fig. 47) shows the percentage of conditioning at each of several different time intervals between the conditioned and unconditioned stimuli. The unconditioned stimulus in this experiment was an electric shock which produced finger withdrawal, and the conditioned stimulus was a sound signal which initially produced no finger response. In this case the optimal time interval was that in which the conditioned

stimulus was presented about a half-second before the unconditioned stimulus. The situation in which the conditioned stimulus comes *after* the unconditioned stimulus (called *backward conditioning*) produced some learning, but it was not nearly so effective as the situation where the conditioned stimulus was presented *before* the unconditioned stimulus.

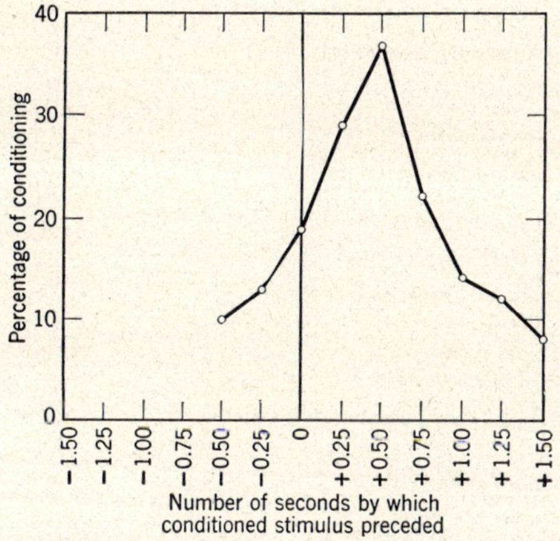

FIGURE 47. STRENGTH OF CONDITIONING AS DEPENDENT ON TIME RELATIONS BETWEEN CONDITIONED AND UNCONDITIONED STIMULUS

Graph shows greatest efficiency when conditioned stimulus precedes unconditioned stimulus by half a second. Negative times means that the unconditioned stimulus follows the conditioned stimulus. [After H. M. Wolfle, from C. L. Hull in *Handbook of general experimental psychology,* 1934, p. 420; by permission of the Clark University Press.]

(3) *Stimulus generalization.* In the initial phases of learning, the organism responds not only to the exact conditioned stimulus used in the original learning but also to a variety of stimuli similar to the one used. The response is generally greatest to the conditioned stimulus and progressively less to stimuli more and more dissimilar to the one originally used. If, for example, the conditioned stimulus is a tone with a pitch corresponding to 1000 cycles per second, the greatest response will be made to this frequency, a smaller response to a frequency of 800 cycles, and a still smaller response to 600 cycles. Figure 48 presents an experimentally derived curve of generalization.

(4) *Differentiation.* As learning proceeds, the range of stimuli which touch off the conditioned response becomes progressively reduced. This process is called *differentiation.* Thus after a while the animal conditioned to a tone of 1000 cycles no longer responds to tones of 600 or 800 cycles, but only to those nearer 1000 cycles. By giving food simultaneously with the conditioned stimulus and not giving food

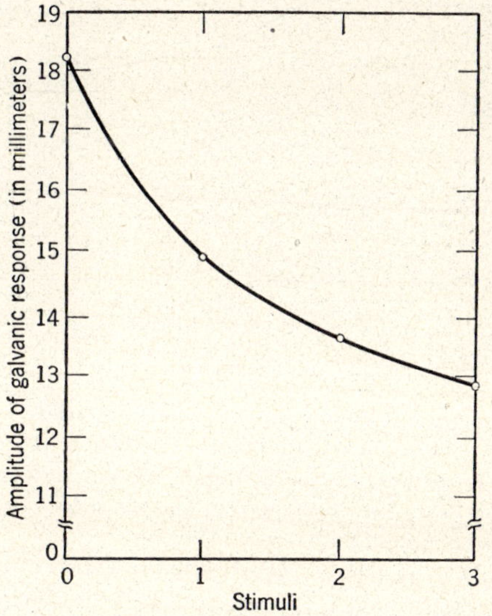

FIGURE 48. SENSORY GENERALIZATION: COMPOSITE CURVE

Shows amount of galvanic skin response, after conditioning to various standard tonal stimuli (0 in the graph), that is given for other tones removed from these standards by 25, 50 and 75 just discriminable differences (represented by 1, 2 and 3 in graph). [From C. I. Hovland, *J. gen. Psychol.*, 1937, 17, 136.]

with any other stimulus, you can finally produce very fine discrimination so that, for example, an animal will salivate to a tone of 1000 cycles but not to one of 1002 cycles. If you press discrimination too far, however, differentiation is broken down and disruption of behavior occurs, producing sometimes a pattern of nervous irritability which has been called 'experimental neurosis.' (See pp. 526 f.)

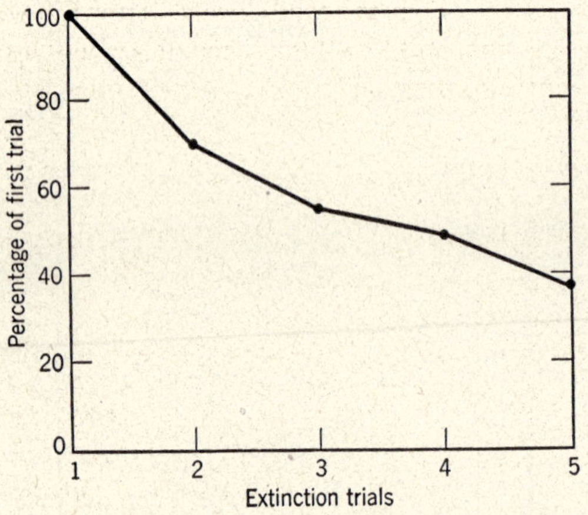

FIGURE 49. EXTINCTION CURVE

Diminution of response in successive trials without reinforcement. Response is plotted as per cent of the response in the first trial. [From C. I. Hovland, *Proc. Nat. Acad. Sci.*, 1936, 22, 431.]

(5) *External inhibition.* When stimuli other than those used in the conditioning are presented simultaneously with or just before the conditioned stimulus, they frequently serve to reduce the size of the response to the conditioned stimulus. Pavlov's students often found that, having set up a conditioned response in a dog, they could not exhibit it to Pavlov because his presence in the room inhibited it. This phenomenon is called *external inhibition.* We notice an analogous phenomenon in more complex types of behavior. For example, recently acquired acts of skill may be disintegrated by a distraction. When one has just mastered a difficult passage on the piano, the appearance of a stranger may prevent its execution.

(6) *Extinction.* Just as repetition of the pairing of the conditioned stimulus and the unconditioned stimulus strengthens the connection, presentation of the conditioned stimulus without its being followed by the unconditioned stimulus results in a progressive diminution of the response. The dog no longer salivates at the sound of the bell after the bell has been rung a certain number of times without food following it. The size of response on successive trials of this type is shown in Fig. 49. These laboratory extinctions of conditioned responses are, however, not necessarily permanent. A response that has been 'extinguished' may recur later, a phenomenon called *spontaneous recovery.*

(7) *Higher order conditioning.* We have seen how Pavlov chose as his unconditioned response the production of salivation in a dog by the dog's sight of food. We have remarked how this 'unconditioned response' is itself a conditioned response, for it had to be learned by the dog when a puppy. The original unconditioned response was the production of salivation by the feel and taste of food in the dog's mouth. That response was inherited and developed early in the course of maturation. Then, by conditioning, the sight of food was substituted for the feel and taste of food. Pavlov's substituting the sound of the buzzer for the sight of the food was conditioning at a second level. When conditioning is established to a new stimulus on the basis of a previously conditioned stimulus, we have what is called *higher order conditioning.* It is an extremely important aspect of conditioning in human beings because it permits learning by asso-

ciation to stimuli more and more remote from the one that was biologically adequate initially. Pavlov did find, however, that the farther this process is carried the more difficult the process of conditioning becomes.

Other investigators have studied a wide variety of stimuli and responses but have in the main supported Pavlov's original findings. Bechterev, a Russian neurologist who was a contemporary of Pavlov, devoted most of his studies to a type of conditioning called *conditioned withdrawal* in which a noxious stimulus producing withdrawal is used as the unconditioned stimulus.

Before Conditioning		After Conditioning	
	Response		*Response*
Conditioned Stimulus		*Conditioned Stimulus*	
Buzzer ——→	Listening, etc.	Buzzer ——┐	↓
Unconditioned Stimulus		*Unconditioned Stimulus*	
Shock to Forepaw →	Withdrawal of Limb	Shock to Forepaw →	Withdrawal of Limb

In other respects his experimental technique was essentially the same as Pavlov's, and it has been the method most widely used in America.

Conditioned Emotional Responses

The simple conditioned responses have been studied with care in the laboratory, but they are by no means just a laboratory phenomenon. They are a type of learning that we see all around us. Language is acquired to a large extent through this means. The infant has in his repertoire of responses a large number of random sounds. The selection of the appropriate sounds to signify objects and events is largely determined by adult behavior. When the child utters a meaningless sound, no consistent reaction on the parents' part is likely to ensue, and hence no learning occurs. But when a meaningful or near-meaningful sound is made, the adult repeats the sound after the child and may give the child the object named. In that way conditions are established for the child's learning the word. You have perhaps observed the behavior of a fond father when his child happens to say a word like "ted-di." The father repeats the sound after the child and hands him the teddy-bear. After a few trials the child will say "ted-di" when he wants it given to him. (For a fuller account of the acquisition of language, see pp. 594 f.)

We know from a previous discussion (pp. 101 f.) how experiments by Watson on infants showed that fears can be established by conditioning. It is well to repeat in more detail the observations of his experiments. He found, first of all, that a neutral object could be made frightening by the conditioning technique. The striking of a steel bar near the baby's ear originally elicited a strong fear response. He used this noise as the unconditioned stimulus. For a conditioned stimulus he used a white rat of which the child was initially not at all afraid. Then the white rat was shown to the child, and just as he reached for it the bar was struck. The child responded with symptoms of fear. This procedure was repeated several times. Presently the child showed fear of the previously neutral white rat. It was also afraid of a rabbit, a fur coat and even of cotton wool (*generalization*), but it did not fear building blocks (*differentiation*). Repeated exposure to the rat gradually reduced the fear when it was not followed by the sound of the struck steel bar (*extinction*).

A vast amount of clinical material indicates that many of the adult intense fears of objects and places (*phobias*) are traceable to an unfortunate pairing of a stimulus with an unpleasant experience. Often the person is unable to recall the specific conditioning experience which is, nevertheless, affecting him. Characteristically, such a fear response is *generalized* to include similar stimuli so that the affected person comes to fear a whole class of objects. Sometimes, but not often, such a phobia can be removed by *extinction,* once the relevant stimulus is discovered and isolated.

Anticipatory Function of Conditioned Responses

Although it is typical of conditioning that a new stimulus, becoming attached to a given response, has the power to call it forth, there is more to conditioning than this new stimulus-response connection. As the connection becomes established, the response to the conditioned stimulus occurs before the unconditioned stimulus. Salivation takes place before the food is eaten, the knee jerks before the hammer falls against the patellar tendon, the eyewink occurs before the puff of air strikes the eyeball, the finger is removed from the electrode before the shock is received. It will be recognized that here the conditioned response anticipates the unconditioned stimulus and in many cases prevents its occurrence.

This anticipatory character of the conditioned response pervades all learning. We are able, because of having learned, to respond in a way which looks to the future. We can learn to avoid harmful stimuli before they strike the sense organs. The child, once burned, avoids the stove. The cow, having been strongly shocked at the electric fence, never goes near it again. The results of such learning pyramid greatly. The word *danger* may be enough to warn us from a region where noxious stimuli are probable. Words of all kinds acquire the power to guide behavior anticipatorily. From the simplest forms of learning to the most complex, this anticipatory function, whereby we prepare for the future, is continuous.

The Law of Contiguity

From the studies of conditioning, certain authors have formulated what they believe to be a basic law of learning, the *law of contiguity,* which states that, when *two psychological processes occur together in time or in immediate succession, the probability increases that an associative connection between them will develop.* It seems clear that no learning takes place without fairly close psychological contiguity between the terms related in the learning. The extent to which this principle must be supplemented by others, especially by motivation, is a matter to which we shall come presently.

TRIAL-AND-ERROR LEARNING

Not all learning, however, is as simple as the conditioned response. More frequently our task is to learn complex sequences of responses or to select the correct response from a whole category of possible responses.

A good example of this type of learning is illustrated by an experiment of Thorndike's. A hungry cat is placed in a cage, called a problem box, with a small piece of fish lying just outside (Fig. 50). The box is designed in such a way that the door of the cage can be released by some simple act like depressing a lever inside the cage. At first we see a great deal of varied activity on the part of the cat: clawing at the wire, trying to squeeze between the bars, pawing and shaking movable parts of the apparatus. Such activity is often described as *random* or *trial-and-error.* After a time the animal succeeds in operating the lever by accident, and gets out. It is then allowed to eat a bit of the fish and is immediately returned to the box for another trial. The second trial may not differ much from the first with useless activity persisting until the cat happens again to operate the lever; but usually the time on the second trial is shorter than on the first, and on successive trials both the time and useless movements decrease until after enough practice the cat goes immediately to the lever and lets itself out. The course of its learning is not, of course, smooth and regular. On a trial after one in which it has performed the correct response quickly. it may go through so much trial-and-error activity that it would appear that it had not made any progress at all. With extensive practice, however, the cat makes the correct response directly with a minimum of activity irrelevant to the business of escaping from the box. It is interesting, nevertheless, to note instances in which escape is achieved by some clumsy maneuver which actually does release the animal. Often such clumsy behavior, having been successful, is continued, despite its inefficiency. On the other hand, if it is fatiguing or inconvenient, it may later be replaced by some more appropriate act.

It is not correct to say that the cat 'understands' *why* pressing the bar releases him. Thorndike found that causally irrelevant acts can be taught as the means of securing escape from the box, as when he taught cats to get out of the box by scratching themselves. Thorndike released the door as soon as the cat scratched himself, and before long the cat had learned to scratch itself immediately to escape from the box.

The animal's behavior sequence in the problem box situation may be analyzed into four basic elements: response, stimulus, motive and reward.

(1) *Response.* This is the center of reference in learning since the biological use of all learning is the making of new responses in new situations. The response

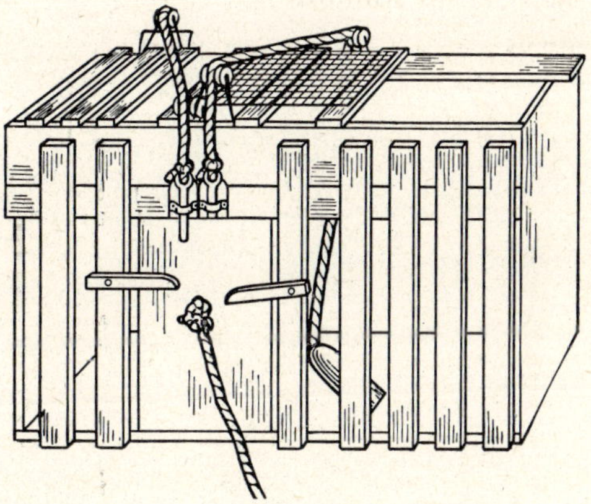

FIGURE 50. PUZZLE BOX USED BY THORNDIKE IN LEARNING EXPERIMENTS WITH CATS

[From H. E. Garrett, *Great experiments in psychology,* Appleton-Century, 1930, p. 107.]

may be simple or it may be a complex sequence. It must be one which the learner is able to perform. In Thorndike's experiment pushing the lever was a response the cat could make. If Thorndike had required the animal to insert a key in a lock to get out, the learning would not have occurred since cats cannot turn keys in locks.

(2) *Stimulus.* This is the causal factor which becomes associated with the response during learning and so becomes capable of evoking the response. There is initially a multiplicity of stimuli to which the learner is responsive, but the range becomes narrowed with learning. In Thorndike's experiment the cat originally looked about, sniffed and explored a host of stimuli.

With a high degree of learning, however, the cat singled out the essential stimulus of the lever and reacted to it alone.

(3) *Motive.* Although some learning occurs without obvious desire or intent to learn, it is true nevertheless that all learning depends on the individual's motives. They may be simple, like a need for food or a need to avoid the light, or they may be more complex, like a need to gain self-approval, the approval of others or to avoid criticism. Thorndike always used *hungry* cats. If animals are satiated (and hence without motive), learning does not occur.

(4) *Reward.* One generally learns those responses which are rewarded, the responses which lead to the satisfaction of motives. Often the rewards are not obvious, since they may consist of such things as self-approval, or the relief from anxiety or worry associated with fear of criticism or punishment. If Thorndike had not allowed his cats to get out of the box and eat the food after making the correct responses, if he had not rewarded them, they never would have learned how to get out.

Using these terms, we can describe trial-and-error behavior in simplest form as follows.

(1) The learner has a *motive* (in the case of the cat, to get out of the box and obtain food).

(2) The motive leads to varied types of activity in which the learner tries successively various *responses* in its behavior repertoire, beginning with the one which is most strongly established and then, successively, responses which are less and less well established.

(3) Some of these responses ultimately lead to a *reward* which satisfies the motive.

(4) The responses which lead to the reward become more strongly established (better learned) as a result of the satisfaction of the motive, being made more and more certainly on subsequent trials when the same *stimulus* situation is present.

(5) Responses not leading to the satisfaction of the motive tend to be eliminated after repeated trials.

Thus we see that trial-and-error behavior is regular and predictable in that it depends upon the motives of the learner and the responses in his repertory of behaviors. Such learning is random only in the sense that the learner has a problem to solve and cannot solve it by insight or foresight. He has to test out possible actions by random behavior until he hits upon the one that brings success. Then success succeeds. It would really be better to speak of this kind of learning as *trial-and-success,* for the errors retard learning, whereas success is what establishes it finally.

In *trial-and-error* learning we find again all the characteristics which belong to associative learning. When a subject has learned by trial and error a response which leads to a reward, the omission of the reward results in the gradual disappearance of the response—*extinction.* An extinguished habit may, however, reappear after the passage of time—*spontaneous recovery.* Situations similar to the one in which the original learning took place will also elicit the newly learned behavior and, the more similar the situation to the original, the greater the transfer of learning to it. That is *generalization.* If, however, reward is not forthcoming in the new situation, the generalized response will presently be extinguished, while the primary rewarded response continues. That is *differentiation.* Last, time relations are as critical for trial-and-error learning as for associative learning. The shorter the interval between the response and the reward, the greater the strengthening of the response.

The Law of Effect

The important principle which emerges from our discussion of trial-and-error learning is the importance of reward in fixating learning. This result is so universally obtained that it has become a law of learning, the *law of effect.* The name stresses the importance of the *effect* or consequence of an act on its acquisition. This law was first formulated by Thorndike in terms of the satisfaction or dissatisfaction which follows the making of a given response. He said: "When a modifiable connection between a situation and response is made and is accompanied or followed by a satisfying state of affairs, that connection's strength is increased. When made and accompanied or followed by an annoying state of affairs, its strength is decreased."

The terms *satisfying state* and *annoying state* were defined by him as follows: "By a satisfying state of affairs is meant one which the animal does nothing to avoid, often doing things which maintain or renew it. By an annoying state of affairs is meant one which the animal does nothing to preserve, often doing things which put an end to it."

Learning and 'satisfaction' are so closely related that it is difficult to measure satisfaction independently of learning; but that difficulty can be avoided if we discover what is satisfying or rewarding in one situation and then apply this knowledge in predicting the strengthening of other stimulus-response connections. If a certain kind of food is an effective reward for learning one task, it can be used to induce the learning of other tasks.

Experiments have established the generalization that the greater the reward, the more it facilitates learning. This rule is closely related to what has been called by Thorndike the *law of intensity.* All evidence points to the fact that the greater the size of the reward, the stronger the motivation; and the stronger the motivation, the faster and surer the learning. (See p. 129.)

As we have already seen, the time interval between the response and the reward

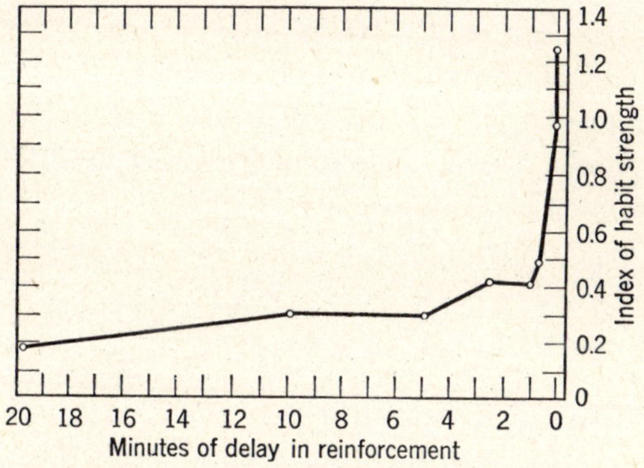

FIGURE 51. DELAY-OF-REINFORCEMENT GRADIENT

The circles show the amount of learning for constant numbers of reinforcements plotted as a function of the delay in the occurrence of the reinforcement. [From data published by J. B. Wolfe, and plotted by C. L. Hull, *Principles of behavior,* Appleton-Century, 1943, p. 137.]

is an important factor to consider in predicting the effect of reward. The strength of learning is greater, the shorter the time between the response and the reward. Thorndike said: "The closeness of connection between the satisfying state of affairs and the bond it affects may be due to close temporal sequence. Other things being equal, the same degree of satisfyingness will act more strongly on a bond made two seconds previously than on one made two minutes previously." Verification of Thorndike's principle is shown in Fig. 51. Eight groups of white rats learned to find food in a simple maze with varying delays between the correct choice and the food. A clear tendency is seen for learning to be most efficient when a short time elapses between the response and the reward.

These results have considerable importance in practical learning situations, particularly in child training. Very often too long a period is allowed to elapse between the act which a parent is attempting to strengthen or weaken and the reward or punishment. If the time is much too long, the reward or punishment may even get attached to the incorrect act merely because it has immediately preceded the reward or punishment.

THE ROLE OF MOTIVATION IN LEARNING

Now that it is clear that the concepts of *learning* and *motivation* cannot be dissociated, let us examine their relationship in greater detail.

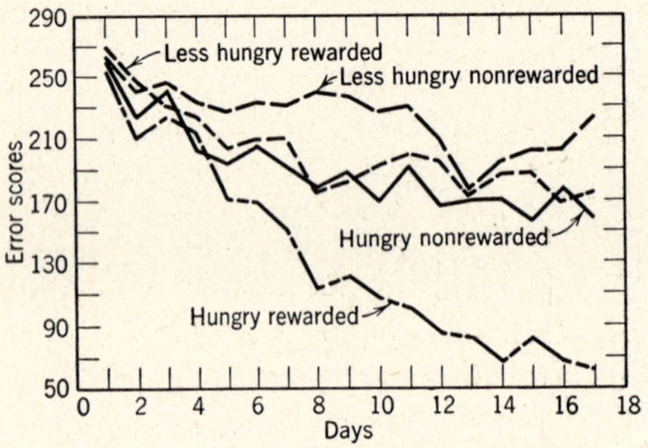

FIGURE 52. EFFECT OF FOOD REWARD ON MAZE LEARNING IN RATS

[From E. C. Tolman and E. H. Honzik, *University of California Publications in Psychology,* 1930, 4, 246.]

As we have seen in the preceding chapter, motives are forces which impel to action, and the simplest are physiological, like thirst, hunger and pain. They are the motives most frequently used in laboratory experiments on animal learning because they are most universal and easy to control. In human learning, however, much more complex motives are usually involved, motives which are derived from the simple ones. Desire for prestige, money, approval, all such motives are built upon earlier simpler ones.

Rewards may be thought of as events which satisfy motives. Thus in Thorndike's problem-box experiment the reward was food which reduced the cat's hunger drive. When an experimenter controls strength of motive by controlling amount of reward, it is not necessary for us to distinguish between motive and reward. On the other hand, motive and reward can vary separately. The following experiment shows the relationship between the two.

Rats were taught to follow a complex pattern of runs and turns through a maze to reach food. One group of rats was *not hungry* and was *not given any food* at the end of a trial; a second group was *hungry* but was *not given food;* the third was *hungry* and *given food* at the end of a trial. The results are shown in Fig. 52. Only the group that was hungry (had a motive) and was given food (was rewarded) learned appreciably. To be motivated and unrewarded is to have before you nothing worth learning. Nor is it worth while to work for a prize you do not want. It is the motive that gives the reward its value, and the satisfaction of reward that fixes the learning of which it is the effect.

Motivation is equally important in human learning, but here the motives are not usually the simple physiological needs. There is no doubt that human beings learn effectively when motivated by primary drives like hunger, thirst or pain, but these drives are rarely intense in present-day life.

The motives which are involved are what are called *learned* or *derived motives.* That is to say, they have been associated with the biological needs and now operate in the same way as the original needs (pp. 121 f.). An anxious parent praises a stubborn child every time it takes a spoonful of food. Eventually the child, even though not feeling hungry, will eat merely to obtain the reward of its parent's praise or approval.

The way these learned motives operate may be illustrated by several experiments. In one, students were instructed to add columns as rapidly and accurately as possible. One group worked without any particular incentive. In the second group the children were praised in front of the class for their performance, while the members of the third group were reproved for their careless and inferior work. The performance on successive days for the three groups is shown in Table II. The control group

TABLE II

EFFECT OF PRAISE AND REPROOF ON LEARNING SCORES

[Data from E. B. Hurlock, *J. educ. Psychol.*, 1925, **16**, 149.]

	Average Scores in Addition				
	Day 1	*Day 2*	*Day 3*	*Day 4*	*Day 5*
"Praised"	11.81	16.59	18.85	18.81	20.22
"Reproved"	11.85	16.59	14.30	13.26	14.19
"Ignored"	11.84	14.19	13.30	12.92	12.38
Control	11.81	12.34	11.65	10.50	11.35

shows no consistent gain from practice. The reproved group shows an initial improvement, but the improvement is not maintained. The most effective incentive is shown here to be praise, which results in consistent improvement.

Rivalry or competition is another motive which has long been effectively used in learning, particularly in school situations. The competition can be either between individuals or between groups. A study in which these two types of competition were compared is presented in Table III. In

TABLE III

EFFECT OF INDIVIDUAL AND GROUP RIVALRY ON VARIOUS TASKS

[After V. M. Sims, *J. educ. Psychol.*, 1928, **19**, 481, 483.]

	Per Cent Gain in Substitution Task	*Per Cent Gain in Reading*
Group rivalry	109.9	14.5
Individual rivalry	157.7	34.7
Control: No rivalry	102.2	8.7

the first experiment one group competed against another in a substitution test; in the second matched pairs of children competed with each other in reading. The latter condition was found to be the more effective.

THE EFFECT OF PRACTICE

In learning anything of even moderate complexity, several repetitions are required. It is impossible to master a complex or elaborate task in a single try, no matter what the degree of motivation or what the value of the reward. You could not learn the Constitution of the United States in one reading, even though your life depended on it, even though the prize were a million dollars. A great deal of research has, therefore, been done on the effect of repetition on learning, that is to say, on *practice.*

The clearest way to bring out the effect of practice is to graph learning on successive trials. Learning may be measured in a number of ways. One way with which we are all familiar is in terms of the speed with which we can do a task. In learning to type, for example, at first we can do only a few words per minute but with practice greater and greater speed is attained. *Speed* may be measured in terms of how much work is done in a given time or how rapidly a single task is performed. A second way in which improvement is shown is in *accuracy*. In the typing there is a reduction in the number of errors as practice continues. More difficult to measure but very important is reduction in *effort*, the

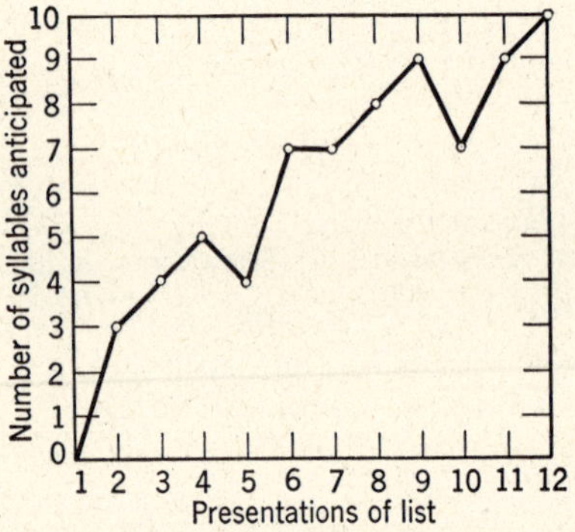

FIGURE 53. MEMORIZATION CURVE FOR LIST OF NONSENSE SYLLABLES

Learning is shown by the increase in the number of syllables that are anticipated in the tests for recall. This curve is for one subject.

energy cost in performing a task. At first, a task is difficult and fatiguing, but with further practice it becomes smoother and requires less effort.

A typical record showing improvement with practice is given in Fig. 53. Here is shown the number of syllables in a list of ten which a subject was able to recite correctly after twelve successive repetitions. The curve shows an upward course of improvement, but with marked up-and-down fluctuations. Such variations are characteristic of all individual learning curves and are the result of chance conditions which the experimenter has not controlled, such factors as distraction and fluctuation of motivation.

When the curves of a number of individuals who learned the same material are averaged, we can see the course of improvement more clearly. We find, however, that there is no single type of learning curve but that the type depends upon the nature of the task and the conditions under which the learning is done. The three most common types are shown in Fig. 54. The first type (*A*) is the one in which improvement is rapid at first but then progressively slower toward the end. It is called a *negatively accelerated* learning curve. It is the type most often obtained when motivation is high at first but decreases as practice continues, or when the subject has had previous practice on a similar task so that the learning is not really 'from scratch.'

The second type (*B*) is called a *positively accelerated* curve. Here the increments are relatively small during the early part of practice but increase in magnitude with

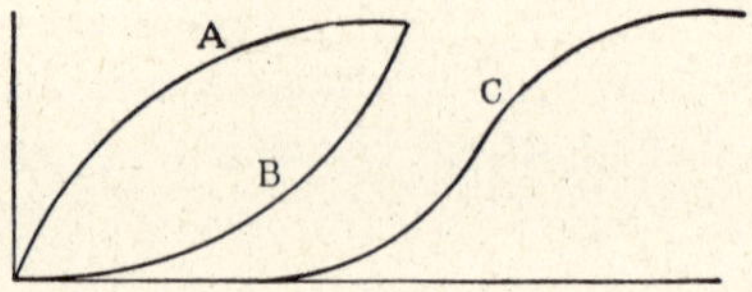

FIGURE 54. REPRESENTATIVE LEARNING CURVES

[Curves *A* and *B* are from H. A. Carr, *Psychology: a study of mental activity*, 1925, p. 218; reprinted by permission of Longmans, Green.]

continued practice. Curves cannot, of course, be positively accelerated throughout, since, at the end, as perfect learning is approached, they necessarily level off.

In the third type of curve there is an initial period of positive acceleration followed by negative acceleration. In this case, the total curve is S-shaped (type *C*). All initially positively accelerated learning curves, if carried through to the leveling-off stage, become S-shaped.

Curves of types *B* and *C* are most often obtained when the subject has had very little prior practice, particularly when the acts learned are relatively difficult for the learner. The manner in which the difficulty of the material affects the type of learning curve obtained is shown in Fig. 55. With the easy material a negatively accelerated learning curve is obtained; with hard items a positively accelerated learning curve is found.

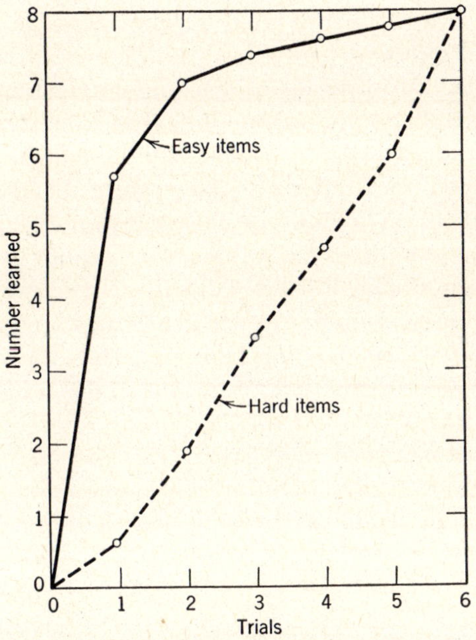

FIGURE 55. MEMORIZATION CURVES FOR EASY AND HARD ITEMS

[From J. A. McGeoch, *The psychology of human learning,* Longmans, Green, 1942, p. 56.]

Wherever the entire learning of a task from zero performance to masterly is studied, the third type of curve (S-shaped) is most likely to be obtained. With difficult material we are more likely to be starting near 'scratch' with initial positive acceleration, whereas with easy material we are more likely to be beginning further along toward mastery, where negative acceleration is obtained. As learning progresses, what began as hard is becoming easier, and acceleration may therefore change from positive to negative—the S-curve.

Plateaus

Sometimes there occurs in learning a long period of practice in which no improvement is apparent, where the trend for a period of time is toward a relatively constant level of performance. Periods of this sort in which no improvement takes place are called *plateaus.* This phenomenon was first noticed in certain experiments on the learning of telegraphy (Fig. 56). In the the curve for receiving telegraphic signals there is a period of arrested progress in the midposition of the graph. The hypothesis formulated by the experimenters for this result was that plateaus occur in the region of transition from one type of habit to another. In the early stages, they thought, learning is by letters. Later it would proceed by words, and then still

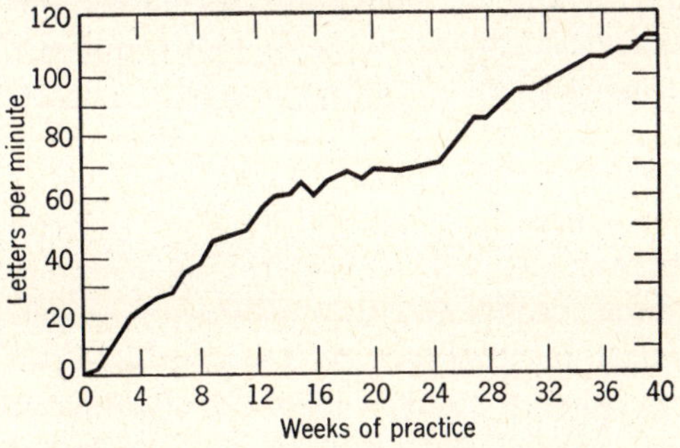

FIGURE 56. PLATEAU IN A LEARNING CURVE

Curve for one subject's learning to receive in the telegraphic language. "This is a curve of sample performance. The region of very little or no progress toward the middle of the curve is a plateau." [From W. L. Bryan and N. Harter, *Psychol. Rev.*, 1897, **4**, 49.]

later by phrases, and thus on to the largest units which a skilled telegrapher can receive as a whole. They thought that the change-over from one type of learning to the next introduced a plateau, and indeed that may sometimes be true when plateaus occur. Learning telegraphy does not, however, usually go by jumps, nor do its learning curves always show plateaus. Certainly other factors enter into the production of plateaus. Any long-drawn-out S-curve would be said to have a plateau in the middle of it. Sometimes plateaus are caused by loss of interest and motivation, by discouragement with the slow progress which the difficult nature of the task makes necessary. The important thing for a learner to remember is that plateaus are natural phenomena in learning, can be overcome and do not last forever. If the learner allows a plateau to discourage him, the plateau by reducing his motivation will prolong itself.

Insight

A curve strikingly different from the ones we have been considering is sometimes found when the fully learned response makes its appearance suddenly, as is the case when a problem is solved by the grasp of a single general principle or method. This type of learning is called learning by *insight*. In a famous experiment with chimpanzees one of the animals, which had already learned to pull a banana through a fence by using a stick, was given two sticks, each one alone too short to reach the banana. The two sticks, however, were constructed in such a way that the end of one would fit into the other. Playing with the two sticks in another part of his cage, the chimpanzee casually fitted the two together and then, suddenly realizing that he had now a long stick, rushed to the other side of the cage and raked in the banana. This 'seeing' that the two together made a stick long enough to get the banana is an instance of insight. The learning, moreover, stuck. Thereafter the chimpanzee always knew how to use the two sticks together. (See Fig. 73, p. 203.)

Physiological Limits

A consideration of learning curves leads directly to the question whether—or how rapidly—learners reach a physiological limit, the level of performance beyond which, by reason of the physical limitations of their organisms, they cannot go. Since under ordinary laboratory conditions subjects seldom approach such an extreme limit of performance, one must rely for an answer to this question upon fragmentary evidence.

It has been found that years of practice at such skills as telegraphy or typesetting do not commonly bring a man to his maximal performance. Even among workers with many years of experience, the introduction of special incentives may greatly improve performance. In a printing house, for example, where hand compositors had been working at their trade for an average of about ten years, performance rose steadily for at least twenty weeks when a special bonus was introduced for output beyond a certain level. The increased output resulted from elimination of stabilized ineffective habits of work and the acquisition of better ones. Analogous results have been obtained with other kinds of work.

The fact that in athletics and in other skills records are repeatedly broken under standard conditions is best interpreted as an indication of the practical remoteness of a physiological limit. It has, likewise, been found repeatedly in the laboratory that, after a subject has reached a relatively high level of performance, increased motivation or better methods will produce further substantial increments. It thus appears that a physiological limit is not reached in normal persons by ordinary amounts of practice and, indeed, may not be reached even by prolonged practice under favorable conditions. On the other hand, there are physiological limits to the *speed* of human reaction which no degree of practice, insight or motivation will enable the learner to transcend.

The Law of Frequency

The results which have been presented above clearly indicate that repetition is usually required for mastery in learning. This fact has led to the belief that frequency is the basic determiner of learning, a generalization often called the *law of frequency*. The law of frequency (or *law of exercise*) states that the connection between a stimulus and a response is strengthened by its recurrence, its exercise, its use.

Experiments have conclusively demonstrated that mere repetition is itself not a sufficient condition for learning. If we set a man the task of hitting the bull's-eye with a rifle but do not tell him how close to the bull's-eye he comes, no amount of repetition results in his learning to shoot straight. Similarly, if a learner is not trying to learn, repetition becomes ineffective. This fact has been demonstrated in one study by presenting students with a series of cards, each bearing a printed word, a number and a strip of colored paper. The subjects were instructed to learn the word-number pairs, so that, when the word was given, the accompanying number could be recited. No mention was made of the colors accompanying the words. After several presentations the subjects were asked to name the color that went with the given word. Few of them had learned any of the colors. They knew the numbers, but not the colors, although they had seen the colors with the words as often as the numbers. In the same way a man can be driven frequently over a route without learning how to go. The best way for him to learn is to drive the car himself; then he will remember.

The motive to learn is tied up with good attention. People can remember events when they have paid good attention to them without intending to learn them or expecting to have to report on them. The witness of an accident will recall certain details. Such learning is called *incidental learning* and is not very reliable. Although the man who stumbles in the dark over what turns out to be a corpse will not at once forget what it was he found so unexpectedly, it is difficult on the witness stand to get an accurate report of the details of such an important, exciting event. If you witness an accident or a crime, you had better invoke the intent to learn at once. Commit to memory what seem to be the important factual items which you observed, and then write them down later so that you can go to court and be a good witness.

There are certain schools of psychology today which believe that all learning is basically instantaneous, like the flash of insight which gives the solution to the problem and once seen is not forgotten, or like the emotional experience (the corpse in the dark) which leads to instant permanent learning of a simple interesting fact. These psychologists argue that repetition is necessary only because tasks are too large to come all at once within reach of the conditions for learning. You learn most on the first experience. If you learn a third of the material the first time, perhaps you can learn a third of the remaining two-thirds the second time, and so on. Frequency is necessary, they argue, merely in order that all portions of the learning should eventually get their full opportunity to be realized.

Certainly the repetition of practice is necessary to most learning, even though there is this doubt that the same associative connections need repeated reinforcement before they become fixed for the use of the learned man.

OTHER FACTORS AFFECTING THE EFFICIENCY OF LEARNING

We have seen how learning is affected by practice and by motivation. In this section we shall discuss some of the more specific factors affecting the speed and efficiency with which learning takes place, considering successively the importance of (1) the learner, (2) the material learned and (3) the methods of learning used.

The Learner

Great individual differences between people learning the same task are invariably found. The influence of such factors as age, intelligence and previous training have been studied, but even when all are controlled pronounced variation still exists. In one study made with subjects of the same age, sex, year in college and equivalent previous practice at the activity being learned, the fastest learners required 8 trials to learn, perfectly and in the same order, a list of 8 nonsense syllables, whereas the slowest learners required 37 trials, more than four times as many. Similarly, the fastest learner mastered a maze of considerable difficulty in 19 trials, whereas the slowest took 78. When the records of a large group of subjects are examined, they are found to be distributed after the fashion of many large populations, with medium speed most frequent and the frequency of instances diminishing for slower and faster learning.

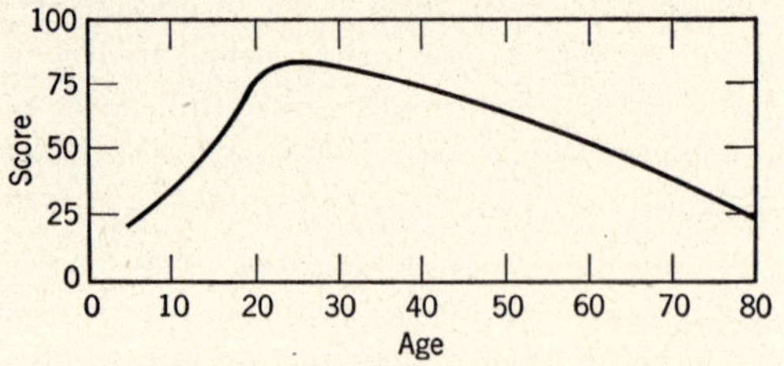

FIGURE 57. DEPENDENCE OF LEARNING ABILITY ON AGE

The trend of mean performance in digit-symbol substitution with age. (See Figs. 37 and 38, p. 85.) [From R. R. Willoughby, *J. educ. Psychol.*, 1929, 20, 678; reprinted by permission of Warwick and York.]

Differences between the sexes in speed of learning are only rarely found, and then they are due to sex differences in interest and motivation with respect to the material being learned.

A variable affecting learning, one which has great practical importance, is *age*. The curve of learning improves as one grows older, at least until the late teens. After the early twenties a gradual decline with increasing age is found. A sample of performance in a simple learning task at various ages is shown in Fig. 57.

An interesting experiment on the effect of age on learning is the following. Three groups were studied. The young group was 12 to 17 years of age; the middle group 34 to 59; the oldest group 60 to 82 years. The three groups were comparable in social background, native ability and willingness to cooperate in the experiment. The five different tasks learned by the subjects were chosen to represent different degrees of dependence upon previous habits.

The investigator found only moderate decline with age in the tasks which involved the perfecting of previously learned habits, but extremely marked decline with age when the new learning was in conflict with previously learned coordinations, as in a task like learning false multiplication tables, $2 \times 4 = 9$, $5 \times 4 = 14$.

These results suggest a reason for the greater conservatism of older individuals. Being less able to learn new materials, particularly of the type involving tearing down old habits of response, they are limited in their thinking to experiences acquired in the past. The further a proposed change deviates from their past experience, the harder it is for them to learn the new relationships and implications which they must substitute for old knowledge if they are to appreciate the need for change.

Kind of Material

We are all aware that some kinds of material are much easier to learn than others. What accounts for the difference in ease of learning?

Probably the most important factor is the *meaningfulness* of the material to be learned. It is possible to rank a large number of verbal materials from low to high with respect to their meaningfulness. On such a scale, nonsense syllables (artificial syllables like ROP, BAV, GEX; see p. 161) are placed well toward the lower end, single words are higher, poetry and prose are still higher. An almost perfect relationship is found between meaningfulness and ease of learning, so that it may be said that, over a wide range of materials, rate of learning is a direct function of the meaningfulness of the material, provided everything else remains constant. The results of an illustrative research on this point are given in Table IV.

TABLE IV

EFFECT OF MEANINGFULNESS IN LEARNING EQUAL NUMBER OF UNITS OF DIFFERENT MATERIALS

[After Lyon, *J. educ. Psychol.*, 1914, **5**, 85–91.]

Material	*Minutes Required for Learning 200 Units*
Nonsense syllables	93
Digits	85
Words (prose)	24
Words (poetry)	10

A closely related factor is the one which Thorndike has called *belongingness.* He demonstrated this principle in an experiment in which he read a series of twenty-four unrelated sentences several times to a group of students. The students were then asked to name the word that had followed the word now read by the experimenter. In 42 per cent of the cases the students were able to give the second word of a sentence when the first was read, but in less than 1 per cent were they able to give the first word of the following sentence when the last word of the preceding sentence had been read. The difference was attributed to the fact that words in a sentence 'belong' together in a way that the words in different sentences do not.

Another way in which the importance of relationship as belongingness can be demonstrated is in the learning of pairs of words. If we make up pairs like *table-chair, green-grass,* they will be learned much more rapidly than combinations like *book-dog, candle-rose.* In the first type of pair the relationship is familiar and meaningful with a high degree of belongingness. In the latter type of pair the words are unrelated and more difficult to associate.

It seems probable that both meaningfulness and belongingness help learning because they indicate previous familiarity with the terms or their relations or both and are seen thus to depend on the fact that a certain amount of learning has already taken place.

Closely related to the factor of meaningfulness is the type of learning activity required for mastery. It is well known that it is a great deal easier to learn the ideas in a passage than the exact phrasing used. The former is often called *logical* learning and the latter *verbatim*. In a recent experiment it was shown that logical learning can be three times as rapid as verbatim learning. It is further significant that telling the subject to try to find meaningful relations in the material speeds up his learning. And there are also the ingenious learners who perpetually see meaning in nonsense, who perceive at once a belongingness between WED and NAG in a list of words to be learned, who remember the sequence BOS–BEN because of Boston (baked) beans and who, because of their skill at punning meaningful insights, always rank high in learning nonsensical stuff.

Distribution of Practice

Given a particular material how is it most efficient for an individual to proceed in learning it? Should he try to learn the material in a single sitting or distribute his practice over a period of time, learn it in large units or small? Research has given the answers to many of these questions.

When a period of time separates each trial in learning, the method is called *distributed practice*. When trials are given without a break, the method is called *massed practice*. Results indicate that for almost all situations some form of distributed practice is more effective than massed. A sample study is shown in Fig. 58, where rate of learning nonsense syllables continuously without a break is compared with the rate when a short rest interval of two minutes was introduced between successive trials. We see a marked difference favoring distributed practice. This statement refers, of course, to comparisons of amounts of time actually spent in practice. Total elapsed time will almost always be greater under distribution because the time for the rest periods has to be added. As a consequence it is sometimes necessary to use massed practice under high pressure for time despite its relative inefficiency.

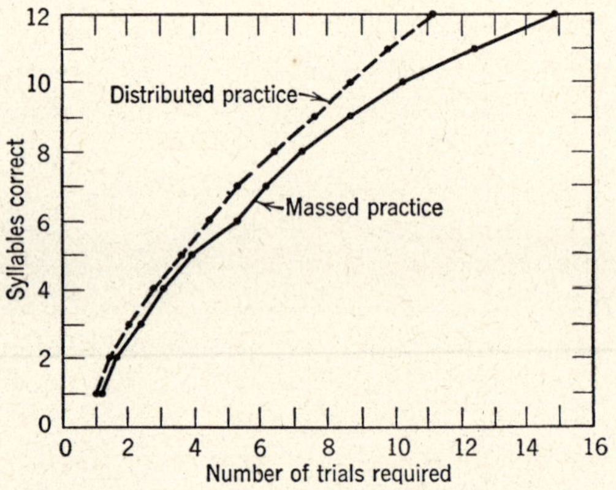

FIGURE 58. MASSED VS. DISTRIBUTED PRACTICE

Curves show average number of trials to reach successive levels of performance by massed and distributed practice. For example, it takes only about 11 trials to get all 12 syllables correct by distributed practice, but nearly 15 by massed practice. [From C. I. Hovland, *J. exper. psychol.*, 1938, **23**, 176.]

The length of the time interval between trials is a critical factor in the relative effectiveness of massed and distributed practice. If the time is very short or of zero duration, learning is likely to suffer because of reduced motivation, interference and fatigue. If, on the other hand, the interval is too long, considerable forgetting will occur between trials, and hence the efficiency of learning will be reduced. In practice, however, because we are more likely to err in the direction of too much massing than in too wide separation of trials, the admonition to distribute learning trials is usually correct.

For many activities a variation in the length of the interval between trials as learning progresses is beneficial. For certain activities massing in the early stages of learning, with distributed practice later, is best. For others the pattern of distributed practice at first, followed by shorter and shorter intervals between trials, is optimal.

The advantages of distribution of practice are greater when the learning is less meaningful and rote in character. Material high in meaningfulness benefits less from spaced practice. This difference is probably at least partly due to the greater ease in maintaining a high degree of interest in material that is meaningful or in which the learner sees significance.

A number of studies have indicated that the longer and more difficult the task, the more effective is distributed practice. In Fig. 59 results are reported showing that the longer the list of syllables learned, the greater the advantage brought about by distribution of practice.

Several factors appear to be involved in the explanation of the superiority of distributed over massed practice. An important one is fatigue. In certain learning tasks continuous practice produces fatigue; then rest periods between trials benefit the learning. But in many situations we obtain the favorable results of distribution without fatigue's being a likely factor. In these cases we often find evidence of the formation of conflicting connections which adversely affect further learning. These conflicts appear to subside quite rapidly during a rest period, so that the positive effects of repetition can presently become more apparent. Motivation is also an important factor to consider in the effectiveness of spaced practice. Prolonged practice often results in reduced interest in the task, so that the learner does not work so effectively. Following a rest pause the learner may return to his task with increased vigor and interest.

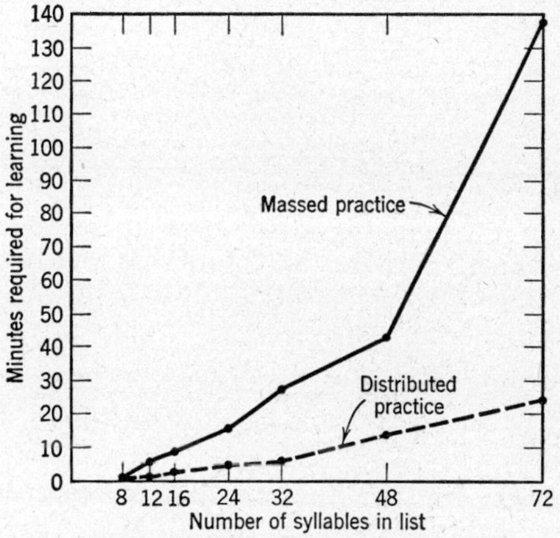

FIGURE 59. MASSED VS. DISTRIBUTED PRACTICE IN RELATION TO LENGTH OF LIST LEARNED

Mean number of minutes required for learning by massed and distributed practice with varying lengths of lists of nonsense syllables. It is especially important to distribute practice with long lists. [Data from D. L. Lyon, The relation of length of material to time taken for learning, and the optimum distribution of time, *J. educ. psychol.*, 1914, V, 1–9; 85–91; 155–163, published by Warwick & York, Inc. Summarized by C. L. Hull, *Massed vs. distributed practice,* from *Mathematico-deductive theory of rote learning,* Yale University Press, 1940, p. 131.]

Whole or Part Learning

In attacking a learning problem is it better to try to learn it by going all the way through it on each trial or by breaking it into small portions and learning each in turn? The former is usually called the *whole method* and the latter the *part method.*

The majority of studies have found it to be more efficient to learn by the whole method than by the part, but, as in the case of distributed practice, the relative efficiency is to a large extent a function of the special conditions of learning. Some of the factors affecting the relative effectiveness of the two procedures are these.

(1) *The age of the subjects.* Children tend to learn faster with the part method, adults with the whole method.

(2) *The ability of the learner.* Brighter children tend to learn better with the whole method, less bright ones with the part method.

(3) *The stage of practice.* At first better results are obtained with the part method, but later on, after practice, the whole method usually proves to be more effective.

(4) *The length of the material to be learned.* If the assignment is of moderate size the whole method has been found superior, but if it is lengthy the part method is superior.

These apparently conflicting results can perhaps all be placed under one generalization: Learn units as large in size as can be grasped at one time. If material is difficult in relation to the learner's ability, smaller units will have to be employed, but they should still be as large wholes as the learner can manage efficiently.

Verbalization

Often in the acquisition of a complex motor task learning is facilitated by reducing it to a verbal formula. It has been observed, for example, that this is what many adults do in learning the route through a maze. They repeat to themselves: "One to the right, then two to the left, and then one right again," and so on.

The importance of verbalization in the learning of skills is supported by a recent experiment in the learning of mechanical puzzles. The task was the assembly of a mechanical puzzle. With one group of children the teacher demonstrated the puzzle silently, but the child was required to engage in counting, an activity calculated to interfere with the child's inner verbalization of the steps in solving the puzzle. In a second group the teacher assembled the puzzle silently while the child was instructed to describe the procedure used by the teacher. In two other groups the teacher described the procedure of assembly while the child watched silently. In still another group the teacher corrected the child's verbal formulation of the procedure, and in the final group the same procedure was followed except that the process of describing the assembly was facilitated by having numbers pasted on the parts in the order of assembly. The six groups can be seen thus to differ in the degree to which the child was aided in verbalizing the procedure for assembly. It was found that the greater the verbalization, the more rapid the learning. The results are shown in Table V.

Data from another study of this type are given in Table VI. Subjects who had learned the correct path through a maze were asked to describe their modes of attack and the subjective means which they used in learning. The means reported fall into three categories. (1) In verbal methods the turns and other moves are remembered in words, so that the subject guides himself through the maze by saying, "First turn to the right, then straight ahead," etc. (2) In motor methods the sensory cues employed are predominantly the feelings of movement; the subject 'follows the lead of his hand' without consciously organizing his movements. (3) In visual methods attempts are made to construct visual images of the maze pattern. The frequencies with which the three methods

TABLE V

EFFECT OF VERBALIZATION ON LEARNING

Number of trials required for children to learn to assemble a mechanical puzzle. The amount of the child's verbalization increases from item 1 to item 6. [From Louise Thompson, *The role of verbalization in learning from demonstration*, unpublished dissertation, Yale University, 1944.]

Group	*Procedure*	*Number Subjects Learning*	*Average Number Trials Required*
1	Silent demonstration. Child required to count so as to prevent verbalization.	3	25+
2	Silent demonstration. Child describes proceedings orally.	22	22.00
3	Demonstrator describes partly. Child watches and may verbalize silently	25	16.16
4	Demonstrator describes fully. Child watches and may verbalize silently.	25	14.12
5	Teacher watches but makes corrections when child's description is in error.	25	12.44
6	Same as 5, except that blocks are numbered in the order in which they are to be assembled.	25	9.52

are used decrease in the order just given, with the visual methods appearing but infrequently. The learning curves of subjects using the different methods show the clear superiority for the verbal method over the other two and, usually, a superiority of visual over motor cues. Table VI gives a sample set of results for one section of a high-relief finger maze on which the subject, without the use of vision, learns to trace a raised line with one finger. Similar results have been found with stylus mazes (the maze is made of grooves and the path is traced with a stylus while vision is excluded) where the more intelligent subjects are likely to adopt the verbal method.

TABLE VI

PERFORMANCE SCORES MADE BY SUBJECTS USING DIFFERENT MODES OF ATTACK

[Data from R. W. Husband, *J. genet. Psychol.*, 1931, **39**, 261, 269.]

Mode of Attack	*Average Number Trials*	*Score (Errors)*	*Time (Seconds)*
Verbal method	10.1	20	358
Visual method	15.0	29	505
Motor method	25.8	23	802

The pronounced superiority of the verbal method over the motor in the learning of a motor problem is significant. It shows that the motor skill as actually acquired by most subjects is learned as a pattern with both verbal and motor constituents. The so-called motor learning is not limited to the learner's perception of his own movements, for the trials, errors and successes are often ideationally controlled. Learning, furthermore, proceeds much more rapidly when the ideational factors are employed. These facts also show that there is no clean-cut division between different kinds of materials with respect to the activities they require.

Active Participation

The more the learner enters into his task, the more effective is his learning. Many times active participation is insured by the nature of the task, as in learning to pilot a plane. On the other hand, in a great deal of instruction in school and college, material is *presented to* the learner, as in lectures, while the learner fails to participate in the learning process, merely sitting back and reacting passively. In these cases the teacher can improve instruction significantly by devising means of insuring active participation by the learner.

An experiment from the training of soldiers in the Army illustrates the difference between active and passive learning. The objective was to teach the soldiers the phonetic alphabet, in which word equivalents are learned for letters, like *Able* for A, *Baker* for B, *Charlie* for C, etc. This system increases the clarity and accuracy of material transmitted over telephone communication systems.

The standard method of instruction was to employ a film in which the letter, presented on the screen, was followed by the equivalent word. After a number of individual letters had been presented, a portion of the list was repeated by the narrator.

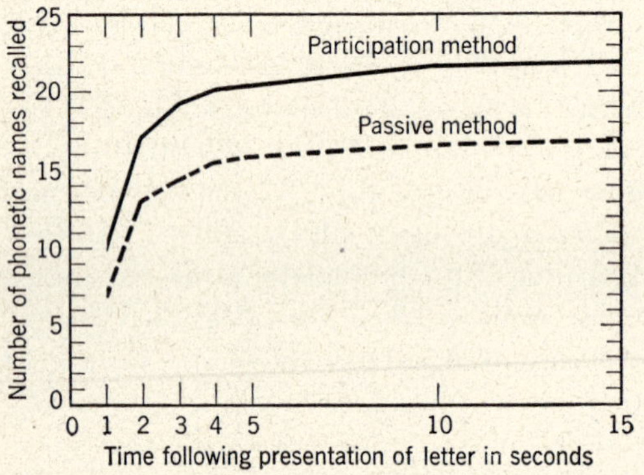

FIGURE 60. ACTIVE PARTICIPATION AS AN AID TO LEARNING

The subjects learned phonetic names for letters, like *Able* for A, (*a*) by a passive method (listening to the narrator repeat the letter-word combinations) and (*b*) by a participation method (reciting aloud the combinations). The graphs show the number of items recalled in different periods of time after the presentation of the letter. The active participation method is more efficient. [Adapted from the forthcoming *Experimental studies of Army educational films.*]

In the participation method the same film was used, but, instead of the narrator's repeating the words in groups, the trainees were instructed to recite aloud the word equivalent when each letter was presented, thus insuring active rehearsal. The effectiveness of this procedure is shown in Fig. 60.

Since learning depends on motivation, active participation is basic to learning. Teaching does not compel learning, for the learner must himself participate. The best that teaching can do for learning is to provide optimal conditions for its achievement. The teacher makes the materials to be learned available to the student, he gives instruction as to the best methods of learning and in some cases requires by periodic examinations a favorable distribution of practice, and then he resorts to all the conventional devices and the other means that his own ingenuity supplies to induce the students—to 'motivate' them—to participate actively in the learning process. The ultimate responsibility, however, is the learner's. It is he who must accept participation if he is to learn.

Recitation

One way actively to participate in learning is to begin using the material learned before the learning is complete. A man learning a maze may rehearse verbally to himself the turns which he has just made, while at the same time he is going forward through other sections. When he has to memorize a list of words he may try to repeat the list without the copy before he has fully learned it. In one experiment, the learning of lists of nonsense syllables and of short biographies was practiced, sometimes by repeated readings until they were learned, and at other times by reading followed by recitations with prompting given whenever necessary. The relative effectiveness of recitation in varying proportions is shown in Table VII, where the percentages of material recalled immediately at the close of the learning period are presented.

These results show that direct repetition-plus-recitation yields larger increments of learning than time spent only in direct repetition, and that the increments increase when the proportion of the total learning time spent in recitation increases. The advantage of recitation is greater with

TABLE VII

INFLUENCE OF DIFFERENT AMOUNTS OF RECITATION UPON LEARNING

The figures are for subjects in Grade VIII and have been obtained by computing the percentage which the amount learned by each method is of the average of all methods. [From A. I. Gates, *Arch. Psychol.*, 1917, 6, 36, 41.]

Per Cent of Total Time Spent		*Materials Learned*	
In Reading	*In Recitation*	*Syllables*	*Biographies*
100	0	65.4	87.8
80	20	92.2	94.6
60	40	99.7	105.0
40	60	105.5	105.5
20	80	137.3	106.8

the nonsense syllables than with the biographies, probably because the biographies invite more active organization of the material during its repetition than the nonsense syllables. Other investigators have found that more favorable results are obtained when readings and recitations are interspersed than when they are grouped together.

The superiority of reading-plus-recitation over reading alone results from several independent conditions. (1) The recitation arouses more active participation by the subject. (2) During recitation the subject is practicing the recall of the material in the way he is to use it later when tested. (3) The recitation yields progressive information about errors and right responses, thereby permitting the correction of errors through prompting from the copy and providing increased motivation for improvement.

ACQUISITION OF SKILLS

When we acquire through learning a coordinated series of responses which are performed with proficiency, we speak of the accomplishment as *skill*. Playing the piano, piloting a plane and reciting a poem are all skills. Characteristically, they involve a *serial* organization of responses. The name *serial learning* is applied to the process of learning such a sequence of responses.

One of the commonest types of serial learning is the learning of verbal material, like a poem, so that we can recite it all the way through. The process of learning poems has been analyzed, but for the careful study the use of poetry presents certain difficulties. For one thing some poems are easy and others hard, and it is difficult to know how much previous experience the subject has had with the particular poems. Even the separate words will not be uniform in their associations from person to person. To overcome these difficulties many studies have used materials devoid of much meaning so that all learners can start learning with an equal degree of unfamiliarity with the material. The method of achieving this end we owe to the German psychologist, Ebbinghaus, who developed the system of nonsense syllables for use in memory experiments. They are usually three-letter units of two consonants with a vowel between them. Lists of these syllables of equivalent difficulty can be readily prepared. In the laboratory the syllables are usually presented by an automatic machine, and the experimenter records the subject's progress in learning the list.

Often a motor skill also involves learning in serial order. A device frequently used for studying this type of learning in its simplest form is a *maze*. The maze, a sample of which is shown in Fig. 61, can be used to study both animal and human learning. In animal studies white rats have been used most frequently with mazes similar to the one illustrated and with more complicated ones. A hungry rat is put at one end and required to learn the path to the food box, where it is fed. It

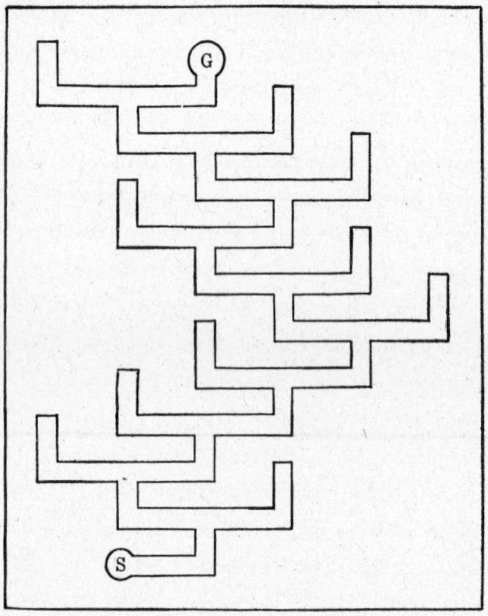

FIGURE 61. TYPICAL STYLUS-MAZE PATTERN

The subject learns to trace with a stylus the correct path from the start (*S*) to the goal (*G*). He is blindfolded or else prevented from seeing the maze and his own hand by a screen. [From C. J. Warden, *J. exper. Psychol.*, 1924, 7, 101.]

will be observed that this learning is similar to that studied by Thorndike with his cats, except that it involves a sequence of acts, rather than a single one, to achieve the goal.

Mazes have also been used with human subjects. Sometimes a large maze is constructed through which the subject must learn to walk to find the goal. More frequently, however, the same task can be arranged by using a stylus maze in which the maze pattern is cut into the surface and the subject traces the path (constantly blindfolded, of course) with a stylus (Fig. 61).

In the learning of many acts of skill the task continually changes as greater skill is achieved. This type of learning has been studied most extensively in telegraph sending and receiving, but an identical problem is involved in learning to type. At low speeds we learn to make an appropriate movement for each letter required, for example, to press the *a,* then the *n* and finally the *d* in *and.* As greater skill is achieved we respond with an integrated act of successively pressing the three keys to the total word *and.* With still greater

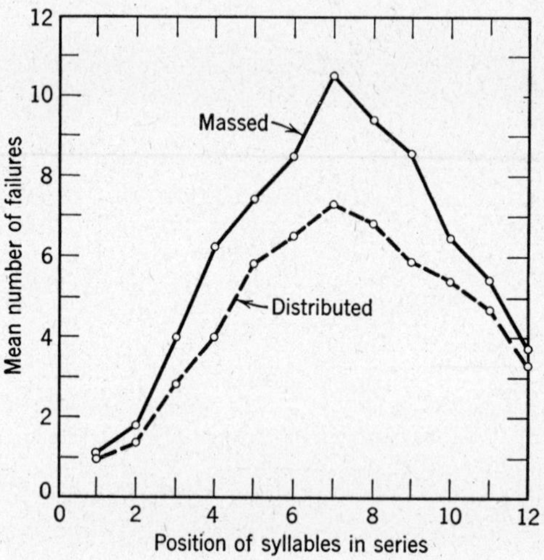

FIGURE 62. EFFECT OF SERIAL POSITION ON LEARNING

Composite curves showing mean number of failures in recall at various syllable positions involved in the series when the subject learns the lists to complete mastery by massed and by distributed practice with a 2-second rate of presentation. The beginning is learned best, the middle least. Distributed practice is better than massed. [From C. I. Hovland, J. *exper. Psychol.*, 1938, 23, 178.]

practice, phrases and even complete sentences are learned as units.

From studies of serial learning we find that the various portions of a sequence are not equally difficult to learn. The first responses and the last responses are easiest, and the middle ones the most difficult. A typical curve of difficulty is presented in Fig. 62. These results have sometimes been explained by the principles of *primacy* and *recency*. The first principle states that, other things being equal, the first experience is most readily learned. The principle of recency is that recent experiences are remembered more vividly than earlier ones. Current studies indicate that the first and last responses are usually easiest to learn because of a minimum of interference. Maximum interference is in the central portion of a series.

When a rat learns a maze, the law of effect enters into serial learning. The rat learns first the goal end of the maze where the food lies. As learning progresses his skill extends farther and farther backward from the goal, being least at the very start of the maze which, of course, lies farthest away from the satisfying goal. This increasing familiarity with the maze as the goal is approached is called the *goal gradient,* which thus constitutes a striking example of the operation of the law of effect.

It is clear that serial learning involves many different factors. A rat learning to run a maze is not like a person learning a poem. The person remembers the poem by its first line and can find it again through an index of first lines, but the rat must remember the maze by its last line, as it were, by the food to which it led.

Basic Principles in the Acquisition of Skills

All the principles of learning bear on the problem of obtaining efficiency in the acquisition of skills, but there are certain practical rules, based upon these principles, which may be set down. Here they are.

(1) *Stress the correct performance from the start.* In other words, do not let wrong habits get established. This rule may seem obvious enough, stated in this general way, yet you often try to learn skills in the hope that you can discover the correct way by trial and error. Then it is that practice may not make perfect. Practice makes perfect only when practice is restricted to the correct performance. Use trial-and-error if you must, but not when available information will enable you to avoid error. Never practice errors when truth can be had for the asking.

In skills, like golf or typing, you, as the learner, often keep practicing without improvement. Guidance may be necessary to bring about improvement. A skilled teacher or coach can often demonstrate the exact form of the correct response, thus enabling you to discriminate between correct and incorrect procedures. For example, one of the reasons it is so difficult to stop slicing in golf is that the difference between the correct drive and the slice is not sufficiently obvious to you. If you felt a jab in the back when you took up the position which results in slicing, only a few trials would suffice to abolish your incorrect movements. Since there is no such dramatic differentiation, you may never by yourself develop the proper drive. What the 'pro' does is to show you the specific respects in which the right and the wrong methods differ, and he shows you just when you are about to make the response.

(2) *Concentrate on the actual task to be learned.* This principle is closely related to the first. To be most effective, learning should be directed to the actual operations you want to perform. Training by transfer from a similar skill always gives performance inferior to direct practice. This rule means that you should practice on a

full-sized standard typewriter, a full-sized piano keyboard, with real golf clubs. Do not attempt to practice tennis by playing squash. Anyone who has learned to type by the touch system after having originally learned by the 'hunt-and-peck' system can attest to the fact that just having had experience in operating a typewriter is not enough; you have to practice the identical motions involved in the finished performance, for otherwise old habits are always interfering with the new. (That is, negative transfer; see p. 180.)

(3) *Learn in natural units, not piecemeal.* You have seen that learning in large units is ordinarily more efficient than piecemeal learning. Too often practice is directed to small details instead of to the entire performance. This neglect of the larger units results in the learner's being able to perform the detailed acts, while remaining unable to coordinate them in a finished performance. The natural rhythm of the entire operation is broken by the concentration on minute details. You sometimes see people learning to play golf by learning first the up stroke and then the down stroke; they should learn the total pattern into which both these two parts must fit smoohly.

This rule does not mean that learning should not sometimes be broken down into convenient units, but merely that the units must be natural rather than artificial. The unit of practice must involve the entire sequence or pattern which is essential for correct performance. Thus, in learning to drive a car, practice may be profitably broken up, with separate practice on starting a car from rest, but the principle would be violated if the learner were to concentrate first on operating the clutch, then on the gearshift, then on the accelerator, since the finished pattern for this operation always involves simultaneous movements of the accelerator, clutch and gearshift, and practice on the separate movements will not bring about a smooth integration of motions.

Learning to type is greatly accelerated by applying this principle. In typing, the natural unit is the word; yet for years students were taught to practice the individual letters first (the well-known *r-t-y-u* method), coming to words later. Learning the general layout of the keyboard and then beginning at once to practice whole words instead of letters have reduced the number of trials required for learning by more than half.

(4) *Space learning trials.* The experiment cited earlier concerning the advantages of distributed over massed practice is relevant to the acquisition of skills. Two rounds of golf on one day are likely to be less effective training than one round on each of two days. Materials learned by speed-up processes are also likely to be more rapidly forgotten, as you will recall if you have ever tried 'cramming.' Determine for the skill you are learning the period which is short enough to avoid fatigue, boredom and interference effects, but long enough to avoid wasting time in getting warmed-up for the task.

(5) *Overlearn; do not count on barely learning the task.* For a performance to be skilled it must be a smooth flawless coordination of responses. To achieve such integration, it is not nearly enough that learning should continue until a single correct performance is reached. Any such minimally learned performance will be quickly forgotten and easily disrupted by even slight distraction. The armed forces in the late war were well aware of the importance of this principle in teaching complex military skills. Men were given prac-

tice long after they thought they 'knew all about it.' This overlearning was designed to take care of the needed performance of these skills under battle conditions where fatigue, fear and confusion would have a disrupting influence on any but the best-learned habits. You will find that any skill you wish to perform in public must be similarly overlearned to prevent its being broken up by stage fright or distraction.

(6) *Speed or accuracy?* From these specific principles and the earlier analysis of learning in this chapter you should yourself be able to deduce the answers to many specific problems that arise in acquiring skills. Should you, for example, stress accuracy or speed first in learning manual skills? You know that the correct pattern must be practiced from the very start, if that is at all possible. You must, therefore, analyze the operations to determine whether the performance at a slow speed is the same as that at a high speed. If it is, you should start your learning with emphasis upon accuracy, so that the exactly correct performance is carried out from the very beginning. This relationship certainly holds in learning typing. No fundamental change in the nature of the movement occurs as greater speed is achieved. If, on the other hand, the operation changes significantly between low and high speeds, you should strive toward the form of the finally correct performance even if some accuracy must be sacrificed. This type of learning exists in bricklaying. An entirely different method is involved when the job is done slowly, one which hardly resembles the form used when the work is performed rapidly. Speed would, therefore, have to be stressed from the start, even if the learner's work would have later to be redone by an experienced bricklayer. Thus the paradox as to whether to stress speed or accuracy first can be best resolved in the particular situation.

(7) *How much guidance?* This is another puzzling problem. How much help or guidance should you have at the beginning of learning? Analysis of this problem indicates that some guidance is usually needed at the start to help establish the correct pattern and avoid practicing errors. But it is also true that the learner must learn the task in the manner in which it will have to be performed later. He will not, then, want to become dependent upon someone else for help and guidance, not for very long. An intermediate procedure works best. Let the learner get help when he thinks he needs it but cultivate self-reliance in his learning.

(8) *Motivation.* Attention to these practical rules must not lead you to forget the great importance of motivation in the learning of skills and all other tasks. Knowledge of results, competition with yourself and other persons are useful motivating devices. Enthusiasm and real desire to progress are factors which distinguish the mediocre from the exceptional learner of skills. The man who can bring zest to his learning has a great advantage, but the zest must be controlled by wisdom. Errors too can be quickly learned zestfully.

REFERENCES

1. Bird, C., and Bird, D. M. *Learning more by effective study.* New York: Appleton-Century, 1945.

   An analysis of factors affecting efficiency in study and a description of the effects of programs designed to improve efficiency.

2. Garrett, H. E. *Great experiments in psychology.* (Rev. ed.) New York: Appleton-Century, 1941. Chaps. 3 to 7.

   Interesting accounts of the experimental contributions to the study of learning by Ebbinghaus, Pavlov, Thorndike, Woodworth and Watson.

3. Guthrie, E. R. *The psychology of learning.* New York: Harper, 1935.

   A provocative attempt to cover all the major aspects of learning in terms of the principle of association. Quite readable.

4. Hilgard, E. R., and Marquis, D. G. *Conditioning and learning.* New York: Appleton-Century, 1940.

   A systematic coverage of the empirical studies of conditioned response learning and the implication of these studies for the general analysis of all types of learning.

5. Hull, C. L. Learning: the factor of the conditioned reflex. In C. Murchison (Ed.), *A handbook of general experimental psychology.* Worcester, Mass.: Clark University Press, 1934.

   A comprehensive review of the most significant experimental studies of the phenomena of conditioning published from 1902 to 1934.

6. Hull, C. L. *Principles of behavior.* New York: Appleton-Century, 1943.

   An analysis of the fundamental principles of behavior derived from numerous conditioned response experiments. Not easy reading.

7. Hunter, W. S. Learning: experimental studies of learning. In C. Murchison (Ed.), *A handbook of general experimental psychology.* Worcester, Mass.: Clark University Press, 1934.

   A good summary of experimental studies of the acquisition and retention of learning up to 1934.

8. Kingsley, H. L. *The nature and conditions of learning.* New York: Prentice-Hall, 1946.

   The most recent coverage of the facts of learning with a good discussion of the relevance of these facts to the educative process.

9. McGeoch, J. A. *The psychology of human learning.* New York: Longmans, Green, 1942.

   The most authoritative and comprehensive summary of present evidence concerning factors affecting human learning.

10. Miller, N. E., and Dollard, J. *Social learning and imitation.* New Haven: Yale University Press, 1941.

   In these chapters there is a clear and interesting analysis of learning from the point of view of stimulus and response, applied later to problems in social psychology.

CHAPTER 8

Retention and Transfer of Learning

IN the preceding chapter we studied learning, the way learning is accomplished, the fundamental conditions which favor and hinder learning. Now we must consider, first, *retention* of learning, and its opposite, which is *forgetting*. When do we remember and when forget? How fast does forgetting go on? And what makes us forget?

In answering these questions we shall find ourselves studying the interactions between different learnings. Sometimes learning one thing means unlearning another. Sometimes learning one thing makes it easier to learn another. There is a *transfer* effect from the learning of one thing to the learning of another, a transfer which may in some cases help and in other cases hinder the new learning.

With these complex principles and their use in the formation of efficient habits of *study*, the present chapter is concerned.

RETENTION AND FORGETTING

One phenomenon with which we are all familiar, often to our regret, is forgetting. We can learn the meanings of a thousand French words, but, unless we use them, the new knowledge gradually disappears until only a few meanings can be correctly given.

The earliest systematic study of forgetting was made by Ebbinghaus. He himself learned lists of nonsense syllables until he could recite a list of them without error. Then he tried to repeat the recitation after

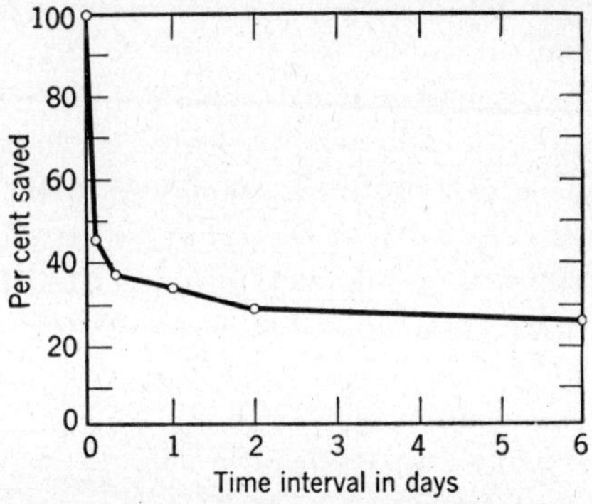

FIGURE 63. EBBINGHAUS' CURVE OF RETENTION AS MEASURED BY THE METHOD OF SAVINGS

Shows decrease in savings when original material is relearned after different periods of elapsed time up to 6 days. [Data from H. Ebbinghaus, *Memory*, Teachers College, Columbia University, trans. 1913, p. 76.]

allowing various periods of time to elapse. Figure 63 is his curve that shows the decrease in retention with time—the forgetting curve. The figure indicates that he found a continuous loss in retention with increases in the length of time during the first six days after the original learning.

This chapter was prepared by Carl I. Hovland of Yale University.

The rate of loss was rapid at first and then much less rapid as time went on.

How Retention Is Measured

The simplest way to measure retention is to determine the amount we can recall of the material originally learned. This is usually called the method of *recall,* or sometimes the method of *reproduction. Recall scores* are usually given as the percentage of the original material that can be recalled at a later time. If, for example, we learn the meaning of twenty French words today but can recall only thirteen tomorrow our recall score would be $^{13}/_{20}$ or 65 per cent.

Sometimes, after several years have elapsed, we cannot recall a single line of a poem we had learned earlier; yet, if we attempt to memorize it again, we find it comes back rapidly as compared with the original learning of the same poem. This fact suggests another way of measuring how much we retain of what we have learned, the method of *relearning* or *saving* which was first employed by Ebbinghaus and has been widely used since. The subject is asked to *relearn* the material after a time interval, and his performance is compared with the amount of time, number of trials or number of errors required to learn it in the first place. If, for example, it took Ebbinghaus 33 trials to learn a list of 15 nonsense syllables to the point where he could repeat them once without error, and after six days it took him only 11 trials to relearn them to the same standard of performance, we would say he had made a saving of 22 trials (33 minus 11.) These results are often expressed as a *savings score* in which the numerator is the number of trials saved and the denominator the original number of trials. In the present example Ebbinghaus would have had a savings score of $^{22}/_{33}$ or 67 per cent. The curve of Fig. 63 was determined by the method of savings.

A third method is the method of *recognition.* Here the subject is shown the material which he formerly learned together with other items which had not been shown him initially, and he is asked to identify the items which were in the original material. In one memory test, pictures of a number of persons are studied by the subject, and he is asked later to say which ones he has seen before. This procedure is, of course, the well-known method used by the police for identifying suspects.

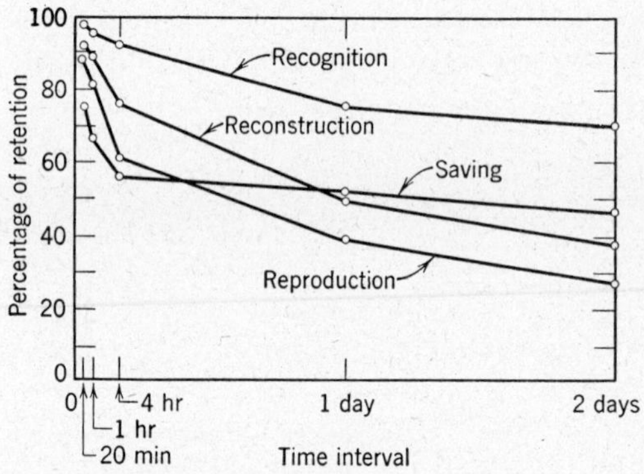

FIGURE 64. RETENTION CURVES OBTAINED BY DIFFERENT METHODS OF MEASUREMENT

[From C. W. Luh, *Psychol. Monogr.,* 1922, **31,** No. 142, 22.]

When material has been learned in serial order, a fourth procedure is often used in which the learner is given the original items all mixed up and is then required to arrange them in the original order. This is called the method of *reconstruction.* The learner recalls the relationships but not the terms related. As a matter of fact a subject who can reconstruct a series can nearly always also identify the terms. The method is useful for studying the learning of series of unreproducible terms, like odors or photographs.

The type of forgetting curve obtained is to some extent a function of the type of measurement used to determine it. As you might expect, forgetting is greatest when the learner must reproduce material verbatim. The ability merely to recognize what was and what was not originally studied (method of recognition) is retained longest after learning. The methods of saving and reconstruction show intermediate amounts of retention. Retention measured in these four ways is shown in Fig. 64.

Individual Differences in Retention

As we should expect from the close relationship between learning and retention, wide individual differences exist in the amount of material retained over an interval. Retention plotted against age gives a curve closely similar to that presented in the last chapter for the learning ability of various age groups (Fig. 57, p. 154). By and large, we find that more intelligent persons retain more than those less intelligent. Closely related is the general finding that the rapid learner is more likely to be the good retainer than the slow learner. The slow learner gains no advantages in retention from his slowness, and the fast learner suffers no disadvantage from his fastness. There is here between individuals no benign law of compensation, as there is between speed and accuracy for the single individual.

The Exceptional Memorizer

Occasionally, because of remarkable performance in memorizing and retaining, a person attracts popular attention and sometimes even scientific study. Persons who can learn a list of two hundred digits in nine minutes and retain it for some time or who can repeat the numbers of every car in a long freight train to a total which fills several pages in the conductor's notebook are cases in point. The question at once arises whether such performances are a result of some special native ability or of intensive practice. Certainly these performances do not require high intelligence. One man, for example, who could give the populations of any of our larger cities, had an IQ of only 74. The conclusion which emerges from the available data on these exceptional memorizers is that their performances are a result of special practice. Their abilities are usually limited to narrow classes of materials, such as dates, numbers and similar disparate items.

The exceptional memorizer is highly motivated to put into relation and recall the materials with which he works. He groups the items, uses them whenever possible and utilizes many of the basic methods of learning and recalling. With sufficient motivation almost anyone could do as well. In one experiment the feat of a memory expert was duplicated with relatively little practice by a group of college students. This expert could recall the order of a 52-card deck of shuffled cards after twenty minutes of study. The college students were able to duplicate this performance after an average of 5.25 practice periods of twenty minutes each. Two students did it at the first sitting and twelve at the third.

Retention of Different Types of Material

A number of generalizations can be made about the effect of the type of material learned upon retention.

(1) Meaningful materials are better retained than meaningless. A comparison of Figs. 63 and 65 illustrates this fact. We

retain better the material that we understand than the material that we do not.

(2) The more extensive the amount of material learned, the better the retention. When materials of varying length are learned to the same level of performance, the longer series are better retained. The greater effort expended in learning the longer lists is, therefore, rewarded with a

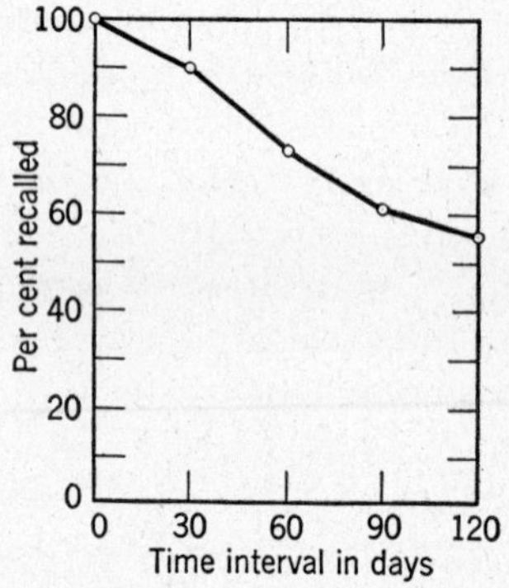

FIGURE 65. RETENTION CURVE FOR MEANINGFUL MATERIAL (OBJECTS OBSERVED BRIEFLY)

[From J. A. McGeoch and P. L. Whitely, *J. educ. Psychol.*, 1926, **17**, 422; reprinted by permission of Warwick and York.]

higher degree of retention. Results on this problem are shown in Table VIII.

TABLE VIII

RETENTION FOR LISTS DIFFERING IN LENGTH

Method of recall and method of savings. The longer lists, which require more work in learning, are retained better. [From E. S. Robinson and W. T. Heron, *J. exper. Psychol.*, 1922, **5**, 443, and E. S. Robinson and C. W. Darrow, *Amer. J. Psychol.*, 1924, **35**, 241.]

Number of Items in List	*Nonsense Syllables*	
	% Recalled	*% Saved*
6	71.3	68.7
9	78.3	78.8
12	78.7	78.1
15	77.0	80.7
18	81.7	86.3

Number of Items in List	*Three-Place Numbers*	
	% Recalled	*% Saved*
4	60.0	25.0
6	66.5	72.5
8	66.6	69.4
10	70.8	78.9

(3) Materials which have pleasant emotional tone tend to be better recalled than those which are unpleasant. Most of us can find in our own experience how much easier it is to remember a pleasant engagement than one which we expect to be unpleasant. And how much oftener we recall our greatest triumph than our most embarrassing moment.

In one experimental study the investigator asked his students on the first day after Christmas vacation to write out the experiences which they had during the vacation period, and then to indicate which of the items were pleasant and which were unpleasant. Six weeks later, without anything having been said about the experiment, the students were again asked to describe their vacation experiences. Of the experiences which they had initially described as pleasant they recalled after six weeks fifty-three per cent, whereas less than forty per cent of those initially described as unpleasant were recalled on the second occasion.

Freud and the other psychoanalysts have explained such results in terms of the concept of *repression*. They believe that memories which are painful tend to be ejected from consciousness although still present in the 'unconscious.'

It is likely that some of the factors accounting for the differential recall of pleasant and unpleasant material can be analyzed without recourse to the concept of the unconscious. One important factor is the greater tendency to rehearse our pleasurable experiences, a repetition which, under the law of frequency, results in their better recall on later occasions. If, moreover, we analyze the initial unpleasant experience, we shall usually notice that pain, shame or guilt are associated with some aspects of the unpleasant situation. Not remembering in these instances is a case of avoidance conditioning. Just as a man learns to avoid people who are unpleasant, so he learns to avoid activity (in this case remembering) which is unpleasant. It is also true that we learn to make other responses to the clues which originally aroused the feelings of shame or guilt. These responses serve as distractions and help us to inhibit the recall of unpleasant events.

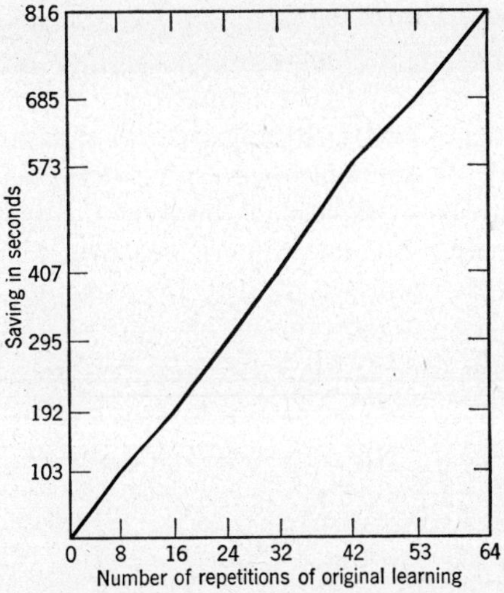

FIGURE 67. RETENTION AS A FUNCTION OF DEGREE OF ORIGINAL LEARNING

The graph shows the savings after 24 hours for different numbers of repetitions in the original learning. [From J. A. McGeoch, *The psychology of human learning,* Longmans, Green, 1942, p. 377.]

Retention as Affected by Original Learning

The amount of material retained is influenced to a considerable extent by the method used in learning it initially.

(1) The set with which a material is studied affects the degree to which it is remembered. Retention is greater when the material to be learned is studied with the intent to remember it over a long period than when it is studied with the set to learn it only for immediate recall.

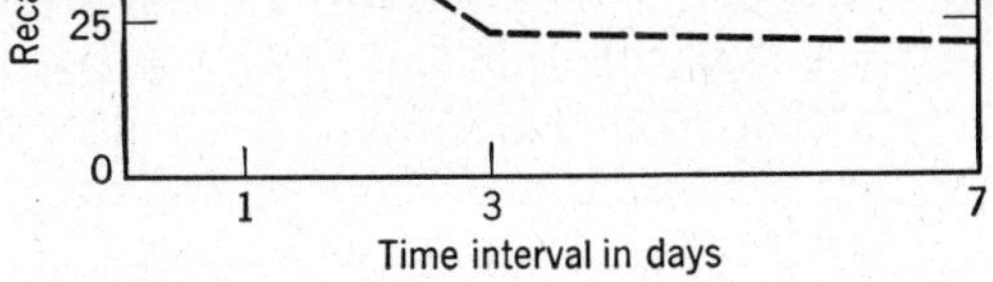

FIGURE 66. RETENTION CURVES FOR DISTRIBUTED AND MASSED PRACTICE

Shows mean recall scores at intervals of 1, 3 and 7 days following the memorization of 12 nonsense syllables by distributed and massed practice. [From J. A. McGeoch, *The psychology of human learning,* Longmans, Green, 1942, p. 130.]

(2) Recitation of material during learning increases the amount which will be retained.

(3) Material learned by distributed practice is better retained than material learned by massed practice, when both are learned to the same level initially. Retention curves obtained under these two conditions are shown in Fig. 66.

(4) The greater the degree of original learning, the greater the retention. This relationship is illustrated in Fig. 67.

(5) Degree of retention depends upon whether the original learning task is completed or whether it is discontinued before completion. (See pp. 133 f.)

Reminiscence

Although rapid initial forgetting is the rule, there are some interesting exceptions. Sometimes we find that, when we have been studying material for a while, we do better if we lay it aside and come back again to it later. The psychologist, William James, called attention to this phenomenon in striking fashion when he said that "we learn to skate in the summer and learn to swim in the winter." This phenomenon of improvement in performance without intervening practice is called *reminiscence*. A retention curve showing reminiscence is shown in Fig. 68.

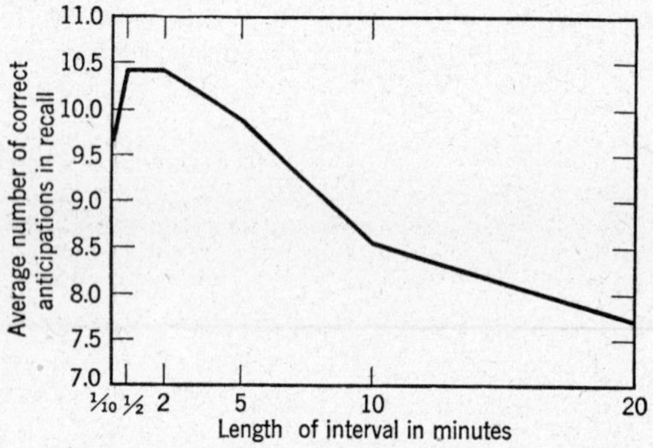

FIGURE 68. REMINISCENCE

The graph shows retention (correct anticipations in recall) as a function of elapsed time up to 20 minutes after learning. Lists of nonsense syllables were the material. Retention is greater at 30 seconds and at 2 minutes than it was at 6 seconds or than it will be at 5 minutes or thereafter. Reminiscence is this increase shortly after learning. [From L. B. Ward, Reminiscence and rote learning, *Psychol. Monogr.*, 1937, **49**, No. 220, 17.]

The conditions under which reminiscence rather than forgetting is obtained are not completely known. It appears at present that reminiscence indicates that there is some interference which operates at the end of practice and which disappears with the passage of time. If this explanation is valid it would be reasonable to expect that, if we gave short rest intervals after each practice trial, the interferences would not accumulate and reminiscence would, therefore, not occur. This result has indeed been found and is shown in Table IX.

TABLE IX

REMINISCENCE AFTER MASSED AND AFTER DISTRIBUTED PRACTICE

[From C. I. Hovland, *J. exper. Psychol.*, 1938, **22**, 212.]

	After Massed Practice	*After Distributed Practice*
(*a*) Number of syllables recalled on trial *immediately* after learning has reached the level of 7 correct syllables out of 12	6.96	8.00
(*b*) Number of syllables recalled on trial *2 minutes* after learning has reached the level of 7 correct syllables out of 12	7.49	8.04
Reminiscence = (*b*) − (*a*)	0.53	0.04

The general conclusion is that both reminiscence and distributed practice gain their advantage for recall by the removal or avoidance of some inhibiting factor rather than by the introduction of a special reinforcing agent.

CAUSE OF FORGETTING

It was once thought that forgetting is due merely to the lapse of time, that an impression made on nervous tissue would naturally fade out. There is now considerable evidence to show that this simple explanation is inadequate. Both laboratory experiments and common sense support the view that the rate of forgetting during a time interval must be dependent upon what is going on during that time rather than upon time itself.

This conclusion receives support from the fact that retention during active waking hours is poorer than retention during sleep. Ordinarily, on waking up we can recall what we did before retiring better than we can recall in the evening what we did that morning.

The results of an interesting laboratory experiment on this topic are shown in Fig. 69. Two subjects were tested after varying amounts of sleep, and again after varying amounts of interpolated work. The curves for the subjects when they remained awake fall with negative acceleration in a manner not unlike the forgetting curve obtained by Ebbinghaus (Fig. 63). The curves for the subjects tested after various amounts of sleep fall less rapidly during the first two hours, and then not at all. The authors of this study concluded that "forgetting is not so much a matter of the decay of old impressions and associations as it is a matter of interference or obliteration of the old by the new." The old impressions fade because they are blotted out by the new impressions of an active waking life.

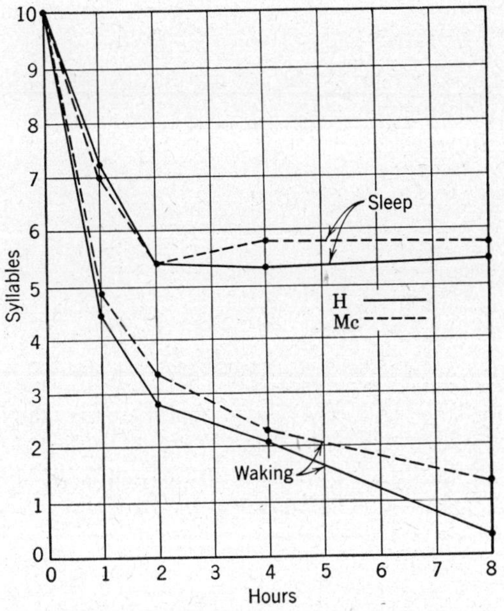

FIGURE 69. FORGETTING AS A FUNCTION OF RETROACTIVE INHIBITION

Two subjects learned 10 nonsense syllables. The graphs show for each subject the number of syllables recalled after 1, 2, 4 and 8 hours when the subjects remained awake, and when they went to sleep. Forgetting is less during sleep and almost nonexistent when sleep has become sound 2 hours after learning. [From J. G. Jenkins and K. M. Dallenbach, *Amer. J. Psychol.*, 1924, **35**, 610.]

Retroactive Inhibition

Considerable research has been devoted to finding out more about this problem of how intervening activities affect retention. Usually it is found that learning another sample of the same material during the interval between the end of practice and the measurement of retention produces a decrement in retention. Such interference is called *retroactive inhibition.*

The experimental procedure employed in studying retroactive inhibition is of the general form shown in Table X, where the

TABLE X

EXPERIMENTAL PROCEDURE FOR STUDYING RETROACTIVE INHIBITION

Condition	*Original Activity*	*Interpolated Activity*	*Final Test*
(1) *Rest*	Learn (*A*)	Rest	Measure retention of (*A*)
(2) *Work*	Learn (*A*)	Learn (*B*)	Measure retention of (*A*)

letters *A* and *B* stand for two different learning materials. The difference between retention under these two conditions—(1) rest and (2) work—is the gross amount of inhibition.

If a subject recalls ten words of list *A* after rest and only six words of *A* after the work of learning *B,* he shows a gross interference effect of four words and a relative interference of forty per cent owing to the interpolated activity *B.* The two conditions must be arranged so that they differ importantly only with respect to the interpolated activity (rest or learning) between the original learning and the measurement of its retention.

The experimentally obtained decrements from interpolated learning vary in amount from nearly zero to almost one hundred per cent. The amounts which appear are a function of several conditions. (1) Over a considerable range of similarity, degree of inhibition varies directly with the degree of similarity between the orginal and the interpolated activities. When, for example, the original material consists of lists of adjectives and the interpolated material of lists of synonyms of these adjectives, the amount of inhibition is maximal and decreases when antonyms, unrelated adjectives, nonsense syllables and three-place numbers are interpolated. (2) Meaningful material is less susceptible to retroactive inhibition than unrelated disconnected material. (3) The longer the material and the more difficult to learn, the less susceptible it is to inhibition. (4) The amount of practice with the original and interpolated materials affects the amount of inhibition. If the learning of the interpolated activity is held constant, inhibition decreases with increased learning of the original activity. When, on the other hand, the degree of original learning is kept constant, inhibition increases at first with degree of interpolated learning. As complete mastery is approached, however, additional increments of interpolated learning cease to increase the amount of inhibition and may finally even decrease it.

Alteration of Stimulating Conditions

Retroactive inhibition brought about by the interpolation of new learning accounts for a large share of forgetting, but another important factor is the alteration of the stimulating conditions between the time of learning and the time of the measurement of retention. Forgetting will occur because some of the stimuli present during the original learning are missing during recall, or it will occur when new stimuli are present which evoke competing responses sufficiently strong to block the originally learned ones. These stimuli are both external (like the furniture in the room, the apparatus, the experimenter) and internal (like sensations resulting from posture, responses made during learning). Recall may be reduced merely because the learning has taken place in one classroom, whereas the testing of retention is conducted in a different room.

Similarly, when words are learned with one color of background, recall is reduced when the color is changed. A language learned in one setting may be poorly retained in a different setting. One person, for example, lived for several years in China and acquired considerable fluency in Chinese. Upon his return to the United States for a couple of years' vacation, he found that by the end of the time his ability to speak and understand Chinese had practically disappeared. Upon his return to China, however, he was astonished to discover that he was again able to speak the language fluently. This is a dramatic example of the familiar phenomenon of being unable to recall material in a changed context, as when we are not able to remember the name of a person who is met in a new environment, although his name comes readily enough in the usual environment.

Change of Set

It is probable, although the experimental evidence in support of it is not yet conclusive, that forgetting also depends upon our *set*. That interest or set in a given direction has a selective influence on recall is well known; if the set is in an incorrect direction, recall may fail, even though with a correct set it may occur. Thus, if in seeking to recall a name we insist incorrectly that the name is Scotch, the search may be confined to Scotch names to the neglect of others, and it will seem that the name has been forgotten. When the correct set is established, the name may be quickly recalled.

There is no lack of evidence that set helps recall. In the reaction experiment we remember to press the key when we see the green light, provided we are set to make this reaction. We start to the theater at eight o'clock because we perceive the time and a set—a special set for this particular evening—operates. Posthypnotic suggestion also shows how set affects recall. But, if set can make us remember something, it can also make us forget something else, because the range of human attention is limited; and remembering one thing is necessarily, at least at the moment, a forgetting of everything else.

The psychoanalysts argue that forgetting may be wishful, that we forget what we prefer not to remember. Jones is talking to a girl whom he is courting. Smith appears. Jones dislikes Smith and is jealous of him. Jones knows Smith very well, indeed had called him by name only that same morning. But now, strangely, Jones is at a loss to recall Smith's name. Try as he will the name will not come. He is embarrassed and blushes, muffs the proper introduction to the girl. Was not Jones' abnormal forgetting an intentional one? Did he not want to forget Smith's name, and succeed? It is very hard to arrange a test case to prove or disprove this kind of unconscious intentional forgetting, for there are always other possible ways in which the forgetting might have occurred. It is, moreover, possible that Jones actually did remember Smith's name momentarily, put it out of his mind and then forgot that he remembered. Nevertheless such determined forgetting is consistent with many other phenomena—with the facts of hypnosis and with the adjustive mechanisms of the personality (pp. 520 f.).

UNLEARNING

Forgetting is the natural dropping out of one habit owing to interference by new learning. On some occasions, however, we wish to reduce the strength of a habit deliberately, to forget by design. This process of 'unlearning' assumes particular importance when bad habits need breaking.

Overcoming Fears

One of the earliest studies of unlearning was an attempt to teach children to get over their fears of being alone or in a dark room and their fears of snakes, rabbits and other animals.

It is often suggested that fears will disappear spontaneously if no further contact with the feared object occurs. In this experiment no diminution in the strength of fear occurred by simply not exercising the fear. Verbal appeal, in which the experimenter talked about the feared object, connecting it with pleasant experiences, was likewise quite ineffective.

The method of 'negative adaptation' was also tried, a method in which the child was exposed to the feared object repetitively. In one case this procedure led to considerable improvement, but in other cases the children actually became more frightened. Ridicule of the fear caused the children to hide or repress their fear without actually feeling less afraid.

Under certain conditions distraction was effective. When toys and playthings which the child wanted were placed near the frightful animal the child was, in some cases, so eager to get the toys that he would ignore the animal. But this method requires the constant presence of an adult to arrange the distractions, and the effects seemed temporary.

The two ways which were found most effective in overcoming the children's fears were (1) reconditioning and (2) social imitation.

In the first method, direct conditioning was used to associate the feared object with a stimulus capable of arousing positive reactions of acceptance and pleasantness. For example, when hungry, a child was placed in a high chair and given something to eat. Then the feared object was brought in and placed some distance away. Gradually the object was moved closer and closer to the child as he ate. In this manner tolerance would be gradually built up until the child became indifferent to the feared object and in some cases finally responded positively to the object with acceptance and interest. That is *reconditioning*. This method must, however, be very carefully applied. If the child fears the object intensely and the object is introduced too rapidly, the treatment may 'boomerang,' so that the child learns to be afraid of eating instead of learning to like the rabbit or snake or whatever the feared object is.

The method of reconditioning was used by the British during the Second World War as their 'battle conditioning.' The training was directed at reducing soldiers' initial fear of artillery. The British used the method of gradual increase in exposure, starting with the discharge of a gun at a great distance from the training ground, and then each day bringing discharges of ammunition closer and closer, until the soldiers could at least tolerate quite intense artillery fire without signs of fear.

The method of *social imitation* is to allow the children to participate in the activity of other children who react to the critical object without fear. When the social group in which the child is placed has great prestige for the child, he behaves the way the group behaves. When the other children approach the object without fear, the child who was afraid accepts the suggestion from the others and loses his fear.

Breaking Habits

A novel method of breaking habits has been described by Knight Dunlap. In his procedure the individual is taught to practice the very error he wishes to eliminate. For example, Dunlap had the 'bad' habit of typing *"h t e"* for *"t h e."* By deliberately practicing the writing of *"h t e"* he became more fully aware of his movements, brought the misspelling under control and thus broke the habit. If we are not fully aware of the undesirable movements we are making it is hard to stop making them. Stuttering, nail biting and other undesirable habits have sometimes been curbed by practicing them with the set to break them. This method may at first glance appear contradictory to the principle learned earlier that practice fixates a habit (law of frequency, p. 153). We shall realize, however, that deliberately practicing a habit we know to be bad is punishing rather than rewarding, and hence would be expected to result in extinction of the habit (law of effect, p. 147). The important factor in Dunlap's method is, however, the having of insight into the nature of the habit.

Another effective procedure is to recondition the subject by attaching new but incompatible responses to the old stimulus which originally produced the undesired response. We are told to "Reach for a Lucky instead of a sweet." We can break the habit of eating too much candy if we can substitute for candy eating the incompatible response of cigarette smoking whenever we have a craving for candy. After that we can break the smoking habit with chewing gum.

Punishment is sometimes useful in breaking up habits, but it must be carefully timed. If applied too long after the act which is to be corrected, the unpleasantness is likely to be associated with the events just preceding the punishment rather than with the act to be extinguished. (See p. 148.) Furthermore, punishment is unreliable in its effects, and particularly so with children. It is likely either not to be severe enough or distracting enough really to break up the habit. Instead it may reinforce the habit by making its performance exciting. Excitement usually facilitates the learning of habits. In this way the 'naughty' behavior of children may be encouraged by mild punishment or by moderate parental opposition. Once again we may note that reward is better than punishment, praise is better than reproof, for the facilitation of training.

TRANSFER OF LEARNING

It is seldom that the situation in which we learn is identical with the situation in which we use the learning. For example, we learn arithmetic at school and use it in the grocery store. To what extent does learning transfer from one situation to another? In a common-sense way we know that old learning is useful in new situations. A man who has learned to drive one car can drive a similar car almost as well without additional practice. That we call *positive transfer.* On the other hand, previous learning often interferes with new learning. If, for example, a man learns to type with a special kind of keyboard, he has a much more difficult time learning to use a standard keyboard than if he had started with the standard one in the first place. It is for this same reason that initial learning with the 'hunt-and-peck' method of typing may make it actually harder to learn with the touch system. When learning one task makes learning a second task harder, we speak of *negative transfer.* Would you expect that it would be more difficult, less difficult or about equally difficult to teach golf to a person who was expert at tennis than to teach golf to an equally competent person who had not learned tennis? That is the kind of problem with which we are concerned in studies on the transfer of training.

Formal Discipline

Not so long ago educators had a clear-cut answer to these problems. They believed that the mind was composed of a number of faculties which could be improved through exercise, just as a muscle is strengthened by use. Consequently they believed that certain subjects should be taught in school primarily for their disciplinary value, especially Latin, Greek and mathematics. This theory is now called the doctrine of *formal discipline,* the theory that what is hard is good for us because it makes us strong. Such a statement carries with it a specious tone of morality of which we must beware. Learning higher mathematics would benefit an astronomer but would scarcely improve the art of a glamour girl. Transfer may be positive or missing or even negative. Learning is not good just because it is hard.

The first experimental attack on this problem was made by the American psychologist, William James. He determined to find out whether practicing the memorization of poetry really improved memorizing ability. First he learned 158 lines of Victor Hugo's *Satyr* and recorded his time. Then he spent more than a month committing to memory Milton's *Paradise Lost.* When he had finished with it he returned to the *Satyr* and memorized another 158 lines. He found that these 158 lines actually took longer than the first 158, and he concluded that all the work on *Paradise Lost* had not improved his ability in memorizing.

James' study was not ideally set up as an experiment and was therefore not conclusive, although it did set other investigators to studying the problem. We question whether James' learning was representative of all learning. We do not know that the first 158 lines were equal in difficulty to the second. We wonder whether James' physical condition was the same at the two times. (He himself says he was fagged out by other work at the time of the second learning.) We note that the effect of practice itself was not separated from transfer of training proper.

A Transfer Experiment

Later experiments have corrected these procedural defects. A large number of subjects has been used. To rule out practice effects, two equivalent groups have been employed, of which one was given the practice and the other (the control group) was not given any practice. This gives the following experimental design.

Experimental Group

(1) Given test on activity (*A*)
(2) Then given training on activity (*B*)
(3) Then retested on activity (*A*)

Control Group

(1) Given test on activity (*A*)
(2) Then given no further training
(3) Then retested on activity (*A*)

The amount of transfer—the effect of learning (*B*) on skill in (*A*)—is measured by the amount of improvement—(3) minus (1)—made by the experimental group as compared with the improvement made by the control group which did not get any practice. (See Table X, p. 173.)

These later experiments have greatly extended our knowledge of the conditions under which transfer of training occurs. Several types of transfer can be distinguished.

Transfer within the Same Class

Practice upon one sample of a given kind of material—mazes, word lists, poetry, etc.—usually affects favorably the learning of other samples of the same kind of material.

TABLE XI

POSITIVE TRANSFER

EFFECT OF LEARNING MAZE *A* UPON SUBSEQUENT LEARNING OF MAZE *B*.

The number of trials, the number of errors and the time are all averaged. The time is in seconds. [From L. W. Webb, *Psychol. Monogr.*, 1917, **24,** No. 104, 18.]

	Measure of Performance in Maze B					
	Trials		*Errors*		*Time*	
	Mean	*A.D.**	*Mean*	*A.D.*	*Mean*	*A.D.*
(1) Maze *B* (control)	33.6	14.3	285.2	205.4	1166.0	514.2
(2) Maze *B* preceded by Maze *A* (experimental)	10.8	5.9	32.4	13.7	149.4	54.7
Number of units saved: (1) minus (2)	22.8		252.8		1016.6	

* Average deviation from the mean

A sample of such positive transfer is shown in Table XI, where the learning of one maze is seen to reduce the time required to learn a second maze. Under certain conditions, however, negative instead of positive transfer may be found.

Bilateral Transfer

Bilateral transfer, or *cross-education,* another form of the positive transfer of learning, is the facilitation of the learning of responses on one side of the body by the previous learning of responses made on the other side. When we practice a task with the left hand for a number of trials, we usually find that we can learn to do the same task with the right hand in many fewer trials than if we had not initially practiced with the left hand.

Bilateral transfer has been found in a large number of acts, among them mirror drawing (tracing a diagram when we can see only it and our pencil reflected in a mirror), rapid tapping on a tapping board, tossing a ball at a target, finding and learning the correct path through a maze. The amount of transfer varies from a small amount to as much as fifty per cent. Tactual discrimination of the Braille alphabet for the blind by subjects with normal vision has been found to transfer completely from one hand to the other. That is a positive transfer of one hundred per cent. Conditioned responses established on one side of the body have been found to appear on the other side with a consistency almost equal to that shown on the side used in training.

Bilateral transfer is common enough when great motor precision is not required, as in learning to shift automobile gears, to manipulate the knobs on a radio, to handle a telephone transfer readily from one hand to the other. Such transfer is seldom complete at the beginning, but the learning on the new side is so rapid that it very quickly reaches the level of performance which the first-trained side required long practice to attain.

Transfer from One Class to Another

The next question, the one which is basic in the problem of *formal discipline,* is whether practice upon one or more samples of one class will facilitate the learning of samples of a different class. Will practice at maze learning facilitate card sorting? Will practice at learning nonsense syllables transfer to learning poetry? Will studying Latin help in writing better English? Will it help in learning calculus? Will it help in learning golf? Would the formal discipline in learning to make discriminations help a rat to find the goals in mazes?

One of the most important studies of transfer of academic training was made by Thorndike. He studied the effect of a year's work in such high school studies as Latin, mathematics and history. All students used in his study were first given a test of "selective and relational thinking." An equivalent form of the same test was given again at the end of the year. During the year some of these students took a program which included Latin, mathematics, history and other subjects, while others instead took subjects like shop work and bookkeeping. Thorndike then compared the relative effects of different school subjects on performance in the test. The effects were so small that Thorndike concluded that there is no marked balance in favor of one rather than another school subject in its effect on "selective and relational thinking."

Numerous other experiments have tended to confirm these findings. The evidence indicates that the most effective way to achieve a desired educational objective is to train directly for it rather than to hope to attain it as a by-product of training in other subjects which have been taught for their disciplinary value. These results support the trend in modern education to teach things for their own values—social, esthetic, recreational or utilitarian, as the case may be—rather than for a general training of the mind, a kind of training which is not known to be possible.

On the other hand, there are all sorts of ways in which having learned one thing may help a student to learn another. Learning Latin may help the formation of the habit of sitting still and paying attention to the contents of books, so that the Latin does make the learning of mathematics easier. If a student with a poor scholastic record should do brilliantly in Latin, because it is easy for him, his pride in his success might motivate him to work harder with his algebra, which is hard for him, and thus unexpectedly to do well in algebra. For studying one thing he may have to hunt up a quiet place so that he can concentrate on his work. Then that place will remain available for studying other things. So situations transfer, fundamental habits of study transfer, motivation and pride transfer from one study to another. Formal discipline often, not always, has positive transfer effects of these kinds. Yet even then formal discipline is inefficient.

Positive versus Negative Transfer

We have seen that while positive transfer is very common, negative transfer also occurs. What determines whether the transfer is positive or negative? Research indicates that the most important factor is whether the new learning involves making an old response to a new stimulus or making a new response to an old stimulus. In the former case, where we are learning to make an old response to a new stimulus, positive transfer is the rule. We shall see that this phenomenon is similar to that of generalization in conditioning (p. 141). The general principle is that *each new stimulus situation tends to elicit the response which has been connected with similar stimulus conditions in the past.*

On the other hand, when a new response must be made to an old stimulus, transfer is usually negative. This result has been generalized as the *law of associative inhibition,* which states that *when any two items, like a stimulus* A *and a response* B, *have been associated, it is more difficult to form an association between the initial item,* A, *and a third item,* K. If, for example, you are accustomed to carry your cigarettes in your right pocket but shift them over to the left, you will observe numerous errors and false movements in learning to reach automatically to the new location. The stimulus, desire for a smoke, which has been connected with the response *reach-to-the-right-pocket,* must now become connected with the response *reach-to-the-left-pocket.* The formation of this new association is interfered with in its early stages by the appearance of the old response, now wrong, or by delay and fumbling.

In general, it is clear why this difference between positive and negative transfer occurs in these cases. If we have learned the sequence stimulus-*A*-to-response-*B,* and want then to learn the sequence stimulus-*J*-to-response-*B,* we have positive transfer. When *J* occurs, *A* is not there to interfere, and *B* is attached to *J* easily because we got familiar with *B* and made it more meaningful when we were learning *A*-to-*B*. On the other hand, when we wish to substitute for *A*-to-*B* the new association *A*-to-*K,* we find

B making trouble for *K*. When *A* occurs, *B* is likely to appear and prevent or delay the appearance of *A's* new partner, *K*. It is this conflict that makes the transfer negative.

EFFICIENT STUDY

All the general principles that apply to learning and retention are applicable to the student's daily work and study habits. We shall, therefore, consider here use of these basic principles in laying down rules for the improvement of efficiency in studying.

Motivation

One well-known textbook advises students: "Be motivated!" Although we cannot, of course, turn motivation on and off on demand as this advice implies, the importance of motivation in learning cannot be overemphasized. The best motive for learning is a strong desire to achieve certain results by learning. When you want to drive the family car, you don't have to be bribed to take driving lessons. Are you equally interested in the outcome of your school learning? It is worth while to review every now and then your ultimate goals to remind yourself of why you are studying at all. But ultimate goals are often too remote to provide effective motivation. We saw in the preceding chapter (p. 147) that the more immediate the reward, the greater the learning. One way of taking advantage of this fact is to set for yourself intermediate goals short of the final one.

These subgoals enable you to see how you are doing and thus to guide your future improvement. Try to make the goals as concrete as possible and keep accurate tab of your progress in achieving them. Some students find it helpful to make up a chart in which they record their progress (such as how many foreign words they are able to translate, or the number of errors they make on successive examinations). The United States Army found this technique extremely helpful in improving performance. In some cases men had been instructed in learning to operate complex weapons merely by being told to "practice for a while." When a system of informing them exactly how well they did on each trial was introduced, their performance improved rapidly. Plotting your own performance as you go along is a way of competing with yourself. Another good motivation booster is to compete with others in your class or with your roommate's performance.

Although it is helpful to maintain a high level of motivation, you should not attempt tasks beyond your ability. You must set your level of aspiration at a level commensurate with your ability. Otherwise you will experience constant frustration, and the consequent absence of reward will reduce the efficiency of your learning.

Planning

Even with the best of motivation, study cannot be efficient unless it is carefully planned. Most students find it helpful to draw up a schedule in which are listed all their daily activities with a specific time reserved for each type of activity. Such a schedule, to be realistic, must include time for recreation and even for 'wasting.' Scheduling helps to separate work sharply from play, increasing the efficiency of each. A loose mixture of 'fiddling around' and work is likely to be inefficient for work and not much fun as play. To have duty watching while you play cuts down the joy of playing.

In planning a work schedule of this sort,

it is well to bear in mind the facts about distribution of practice (pp. 156 f.). You should determine for each topic the optimum length for your uninterrupted study. You have to hit near the happy medium between barely getting warmed up before you shift to the next topic and keeping on with interference, boredom and fatigue working against you.

In arranging a program, avoid 'cramming' just before examinations. Hurriedly learned is hurriedly forgotten. Careful initial learning with periodic review insures the best retention.

In laying out your plans it is well for you to provide for a constant place in which to study. Such a place will come to provide cues for study and will lack the distraction which a changing environment is likely to have upon performance. Even if the place is noisy, it is better to have a constant noise than a variable, unpredictable, imperfect quiet. You can get accustomed to the same old noise, and then it will not distract you, may, in fact, even spur you on to work a little harder, in the way that the continuous jumble of a radio can help some students to study better.

Reading Habits

Since learning in college deals so largely with verbal material, it is extremely important that the individual be able to read efficiently. For efficiency, it is of first importance that your reading instruments, your eyes, should be up to their peak performance. A check-up on your eyes by a competent eye doctor will guard you against defects which can be corrected by exercise of the eyes or suitable glasses. Headaches and tension around the eyes are often attributable to poor vision. Also important for maximal visual efficiency is adequate illumination. Arrange for enough light to fall directly on the material you are reading. (For the specification of the best intensity and distribution of illumination, see pages 475–477.)

Efficient readers differ markedly from inefficient in the way they read. Study of eye movements may help you to improve your efficiency in reading and learning. If you will take a page of reading material and cut a small hole in it, about the size of a dime, and will ask a friend of yours to read the page while you watch his eyes through the opening, you will be able to make some interesting observations. You will see that his eyes do not move continuously along the lines as he reads but jump a few words, then pause, then jump again. Between the end of the last pause on one line and the first on the next there is a long sweeping movement. During this time the eyes are not able to see. At each pause, or fixation, the reader takes in several words. The more words which he can take in per fixation, the fewer fixations he needs and hence the more rapid his reading. Slow readers not only take in very small numbers of words at a time but often will be observed to go back and reread, a shift called *regression in reading*. Regression, of course, greatly reduces reading speed.

Considerable increase in reading speed can be achieved through practice. In one experiment a poor reader was able to reduce his pauses from 15.5 to 6.1 by practicing only twenty minutes a day for twenty days. He was able to comprehend just as much at the increased speed. Practice should consist primarily of forcing yourself to read as rapidly as you can without sacrificing the meaning of what is being read. All of us can benefit by this practice, since nearly everyone reads less rapidly than his capacity permits.

Slow readers also tend to vocalize the

words as they read them, often using actual tongue and lip movements. This unnecessary extra work further slows down reading speed. Silent reading increases reading speed, and with practice you can learn to read swiftly and silently without loss of the significance and meaning of the text.

One of the most common reasons for slow reading and eye movement regression is lack of adequate vocabulary. A shortage of familiar words can be readily overcome by a systematic use of the dictionary. Making a habit of looking up in the dictionary every word which is unfamiliar to you will save you time later, and, as your vocabulary increases, your reading rate will also improve.

Meaningfulness

Learning the definition of all unfamiliar words will also help learning by increasing its meaningfulness. Another way in which we can take advantage of this important factor is by getting a bird's-eye view of the entire material to be learned before concentrating on the individual parts to be learned. Such a perspective increases interest in the details and makes the entire task more significant.

In learning new material always try to relate it to material you already know. It is much easier to add a new fact when you already have a background for it than to learn a new isolated fact related to nothing else in your repertoire. Translating a material into your own words is also helpful in guaranteeing that material will be meaningful, as well as in adding the favorable circumstance of more active participation to the learning. When you do not paraphrase a material as you learn it, you may find that you have it in fairly good shape for verbatim reproduction but that you can recall the words better than the sense. Usually what you want to remember is the sense. One good way to get more sense than words is to study material from more than one source. Reading the same topic in several different textbooks will give you a better knowledge of the topic than a single coverage, even if the same points are covered. Approaching the same material from different points of view also aids in retention. It may seem confusing to read two books that appear to contradict each other, but if you put into your learning the activity necessary to resolve the confusion and make the sense consistent, you will know more than you would if you had had only a single clear consistent but unchallenging book to read.

Active Participation

There are many ways in which learning can be favored by making participation more active. When material is studied with the intent to remember, it is better retained than when read without intent to remember. Just studying with the book in front of you never insures learning. You have actively to practice what you are trying to learn. You can, for instance, attempt to recite the material in whatever way you wish to learn it, words or sense. Close your book and see how much of the material you can recall. If you are studying for quizzes, think up questions for yourself and undertake to answer them. Keep putting your book down to see how much of the material you can recite after you have read it.

Active participation in learning also implies paying close attention to the material you wish to acquire. Various *memory systems* attempt to guarantee this close attention by elaborate devices, memory 'crutches.' If you will spend the same time and effort directly on the material that is required to learn the system, you will usually be ahead of the game.

And do not forget the importance of *overlearning,* if you want the material to stick. Never be satisfied with bare mastery. Always learn your material well enough so that distractions and excitement will not interfere with your recall.

REFERENCES

See the references cited for *Learning* at the end of Chapter 7, pp. 165 f.

CHAPTER 9

Recollecting, Imagining and Thinking

ALL the topics to be dealt with in this chapter are frequently referred to by the layman as *thinking*. When he says, "I am thinking about the time my car skidded into the ditch," he probably means that he is going once more through the experiences of that accident, recalling the visual scene of the road, the snow and ice, reproducing the 'feel' of the car as it went out of control and re-experiencing the fear which accompanied the event. This kind of 'thinking-about' in which we bring back the past and recognize it as belonging to the past we shall call *recollecting*.

When a person says that he is 'thinking about' a plan for remodeling his house, his activity is probably what we shall call *imagining*. He is creating new pictures or scenes which are neither present nor past. Sometimes these imagined events are regarded as future, as things which the individual *expects* to occur. At other times, imagining has no definite reference to time at all. The imagined scenes are not past, or present, or future; they are simply unreal.

The term *thinking* usually includes more, however, than the 'thinking-about' which is labeled recollecting or imagining. It is a complicated process and requires more of an introduction than recollecting or imagining. The kind of thinking which leads to the solution of important problems of personal decision, of political theory or of science is more than a creation of pictures or images. For the sake of clarity we had better use the term *thinking* only when we refer to this more complicated activity with recollecting and imagining recognized as important tools for this kind of thinking. It is easier, as a matter of fact, to state what is *not* thinking than it is to give a clear and useful definition of the term. For the time being we can be content with a rough characterization and a few examples. Later in the chapter we shall give a fuller description.

Thinking is directed toward the solution of a problem. It is not automatic. It requires effort. It frequently uses symbolic short cuts and signs. And it takes us beyond the immediate concrete situation by the use of concepts. A man regards his thinking as successful when it provides him with new knowledge, with better understanding of a situation, with a decision which he believes to be correct, or when it leads to an action which is successful in overcoming the obstacles in his path.

Suppose, for example, that you are told that the sum of the first N integers is equal to $N(N + 1)/2$ and that you are unable to understand *why* this is true. Your search for an understanding is an example of what

This chapter was prepared by T. A. Ryan of Cornell University.

we mean by thinking. It is not thinking if you are satisfied with the recollection that you once learned this formula in an algebra class in high school. It is not thinking if you have already worked out an understanding of the relationships involved, so that you simply recall the results of your earlier thinking.

When you accept this problem and there is no ready-made answer available, you start on a course of thinking. The problem engages your attention. You 'work hard' (effort) trying to find the point of view which will make the relationships clear. You consider the various meanings which may be attached to numbers (signs, symbols and concepts). Your thinking ceases when you believe that you at last understand *why* the formula works or when you are interrupted by other affairs. It is not necessary that you arrive at a solution (to say nothing of finding a correct solution) in order to call the process *thinking,* for the process has its characteristic features whether it is successful or unsuccessful. The applied psychology of thinking is, of course, interested in the correctness of the result; but, before we can control thinking and direct it toward correct solutions, it is necessary to understand thinking in general, both correct and incorrect.

Although all the above characteristics appear typically in thinking, they also appear separately in many other kinds of activity as well. Suppose we ask someone to tell us which of two weights is heavier. We have given him a problem, but we would not say that his solution ordinarily requires thinking. Similarly when we read a description of a landscape we are dealing with symbols, but it does not require thinking to understand the description and to translate it into an imagined scene.

RECOLLECTING

Recollection is a process by which events and situations from the past are recreated by the individual and *recognized by him as coming from his past.* It is in the emphasis on recognition that recollection differs from recall as that term is used in the more general study of learning. The test for recall in an experiment upon memorizing is whether the individual is able to reproduce the words in the memorized list. It is immaterial whether he remembers having seen the words before. In learning a motor skill, recall is also measured by the accuracy of performance. Recall may or may not involve recollection. For example, when you multiply you are demonstrating recall of the multiplication table, but seldom do you *recollect* the occasion of your original learning of the tables.

In other situations, however, recall may *depend* upon recollection. To describe the details of a picture seen in the past, we usually re-view the picture, reading (recalling) the details from the visualized (recollected) picture.

As a part of his act, one vaudeville prodigy used to learn a 10-by-10 square of numbers—100 digits in all. The numbers were called out at random by the audience at the beginning of the act. After writing the numbers down, the prodigy turned the blackboard over and performed other numerical tricks. Half an hour later he would repeat the whole set of digits, writing them down in an order different from that in which they had been originally placed upon the board. The stunt might have been managed by tricks of memorizing, but in this case it was found to depend upon a detailed visual recollection. In general, a subject's ability to reproduce in different order the items of a material is evidence of visual recollection.

Recollection, of course, is by no means limited to visual scenes. Any of the sense departments may be involved, singly or in combination, with each showing special development in certain individuals. The prodigious feats of musical memorization exhibited by some musicans would be likely to be instances of unusually accurate auditory recollection.

Eidetic Images

At times recollected and imagined objects can appear in extremely complex and clear detail, resembling ordinary perceptions. Such images are known as *eidetic images.* They are more frequently found in young children than in adults. They can be definitely localized and 'projected' upon a screen.

Figure 70 is a picture that was shown to English school children in an investigation of eidetic imagery. Some of the children could recollect the picture in such detail that they were able to spell the strange German word on the house at the left. Three out of thirty children could spell the word correctly forward or backward, whereas seven could spell it either way with only two mistakes—the same mistakes in either direction.

This is an example of an eidetic recollection, but similar clear images can also occur without reference to the past. An eidetic image is an experience which lies

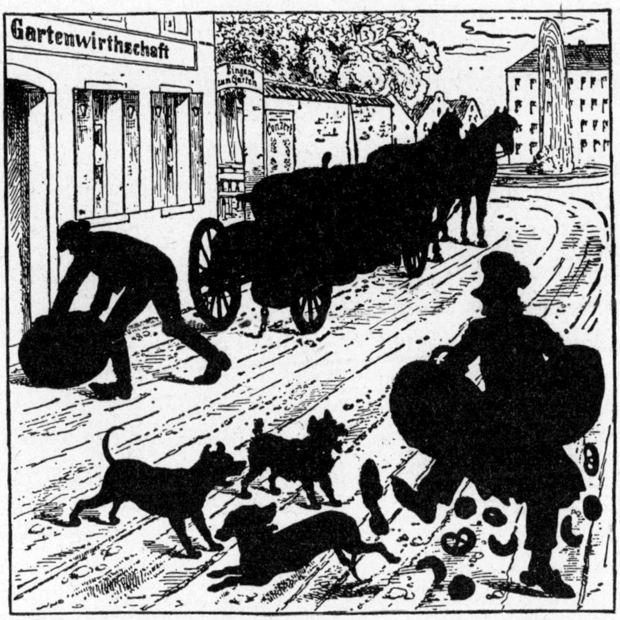

FIGURE 70. EIDETIC IMAGERY

This picture was shown to a number of English school children for 35 seconds. From an image of the picture the children were later able to describe accurately a very great many details, including, in some cases, the long German word over the entrance of the building. [Used by G. W. Allport, *Brit. J. Psychol.*, 1924, **15**, 99–120.]

on the borderline between a perception and an image.

Although adults do not often report having eidetic images, they may experience them under special circumstances. After a long and concentrated day of visual study of some particular material, like microscopic slides or blueprint drawings, images of the material may insist on floating in front of the eyes later when the tired observer is falling asleep. A haunting tune may be made of auditory eidetic imagery.

Recollection and Perception

Recollected events are describable in terms of color, shape, sound, warmth, feelings of movements and the like. We describe them in the same terms we use for perceived objects and events themselves. A question arises, therefore, as to how recollected objects differ from perceived objects, a question which has troubled a great many psychologists in the past. Almost any criterion of differentiation upon a descriptive basis is faulty because of the exceptions which occur. Recollections are usually less clear, less definite and less detailed than perceptions, but that is not always the case. Some recollections, especially the recollections of certain gifted individuals (like the 'prodigy' mentioned above) and eidetic recollections, are extremely clear and detailed, whereas an object seen briefly out of the corner of the eye or in a mist is anything but clear, definite and detailed.

The question is: How do we tell the difference between a bit of melody which has come back from the past and the snatch of melody heard as being played right now on the neighbor's piano? How can we distinguish, when either or both may be clear or unclear, loud or soft, have the same pitches and so on? The fact is that we *do* usually distinguish perceived objects from recollected objects, even when the recollected objects are clear and detailed. The difference lies in the *meaning* of the experience, rather than in the pattern of colors, sounds, shapes or movements. We can say that we 'just know' fact from memory, perception from recollection.

What really happens is that there are two worlds—the world of perception and the world of imagery. To the experienced adult the world of perception is a complex but unitary whole. A thing is 'there,' is 'real' and not imaginary, if you can see it, touch it, handle it, find it there whenever you turn to it, discover that what you perceive of it depends on what you do to put your sense organs in relation to it. The hard yellow floor of your room, the blue walls, the uncomfortable chair with the too soft cushion, the brown radio with the swing music coming out of it, the smell of fresh paint from the next room mixed with the smell of magnolias through the open window, all these items of experience together with hundreds of others make up a consistent systematic whole which we think of as reality. Other items that fit into the system are necessarily 'real,' have the meaning of reality given them.

All is, however, not so simple. A woman enters your room and takes a chair. Thus she fits into the system, is presumably 'real.' But she might be a delusion. So might the magnolias, the music and the whole room. The only proof of reality you have is that the items of it all fit together and are consistent with the host of your recollections about them and about the relations of things in general. If the woman is transparent, if she walked in through the door without opening it, perhaps she is not 'real,' for she does not fit past experience with 'real, live' women.

You have only to feel that the consistency of the system is destroyed to doubt the reality of perception. Starting off to work in the morning when there is really no work because it is a holiday soon shows you how the system fits together. The streets are half empty, the other people are not hurrying to work, and you get first a feeling of unreality, until you find out what is wrong. You had forgotten about Washington's birthday.

Recollection and imagination make up the experience that comes into your life without fitting the basic perceptual pattern as do perceptions. You are recollecting when what you experience fits into a past perceptual system, is dated and placed in relation to past places and events. If there is no such specification upon the experience, presumably it is an imagination, a vision, an inspiration.

RELIABILITY OF RECOLLECTION

There are ways of measuring the reliability of recollection and of studying how a recollection changes with the lapse of time.

Reliability of Testimony

If you follow the accounts of a criminal trial in a newspaper or if you read detective stories, you may have been impressed by the amount and accuracy of detail which the witnesses to the crime are asked to recollect. Actual testimony is, however, frequently conflicting and is often changed under cross-examination.

Prompted by the practical problems of the law, psychologists have performed a number of experiments to determine the accuracy of testimony and the conditions under which recollection is accurate. Their method is to stage a scene or event for a 'witness' or to show him a moving picture. Sometimes the witness knows in advance that he will be required to recall the details later. In other experiments the crucial event is introduced casually and apparently accidentally, so that the witness is not prepared for his later examination. The examination of the witness takes place later after various periods of time have been allowed to elapse.

Even when subjects have no 'axe to grind' and are merely collaborating in an experiment, their errors of recollection are many. Errors occur even though the subject is instructed in advance to be ready for a later test of his accuracy. They increase markedly when the original event occurred 'accidentally' and without the subject's expecting it. Thus perception with the intention to recall the event later is an important factor in the accuracy of recollection, a factor seldom operative in courtroom testimony.

Another factor that can affect the accuracy of recollection is questioning or cross-examination at the time of recall. If a witness is allowed to report what he can, without questioning, his reports may be fairly accurate, although still not perfect. Cross-examination may, however, double or triple the proportion of incorrect information which is given by witnesses. The leading question is very effective in inducing witnesses to recall something that did not appear in the original event at all. The leading question in the form, "Wasn't there a horse in the street?" will often receive the reply "yes" if it is at all reasonable to suppose that a horse could have been there. Once such a false recollection has been reported under cross-examination, it tends to become fixed and to reappear later, even spontaneously. Perhaps the witness did not really recollect the horse when the question was asked, but later, under pressure to be consistent, he becomes convinced that he is actually recollecting something he truly saw.

These experiments differ from the real-life situation involved in testimony in three ways. First, the laboratory or classroom situation is relatively calm and unemotional. Emotion is likely to decrease accuracy of perception and recollection. Second, the experimental situation is not so intensely interesting as a real accident, robbery or similar dramatic event. Interest favors accuracy but is likely to be coupled with emotion, which favors inaccuracy. Often psychologists have introduced both interest and emotion into their experiments by staging dramatic episodes in the classroom with some success in convincing the students of their authenticity. In one case, for example, the instructor had an argument with a man who interrupted his class. The event was carefully rehearsed and staged so that the accuracy of testimony could be checked. The amount of error was found to be extremely high. Descriptions of the man ranged from tall to short, dark to blond, fat to thin and so on.

A third difference between the experiment and the courtroom lies in the fact that errors of recollection become much more important in the courtroom. In the experiment the subject may be willing to report something of which he is not certain, largely because error will not matter much. Often the subjects are asked to distinguish between those things which they are willing to swear to and the things of which they are only moderately sure. See Table XII for the results of one experiment. Although the accuracy was higher

TABLE XII

Errors of Recollection

Showing the errors in an experiment upon testimony. Subjects were shown a picture, then answered a questionnaire about the contents of the picture at each of the time intervals listed. Each answer was labeled according to the degree of certainty of the subject. "Report" refers to an answer which was "just a little better than a mere guess." "Fairly certain" is the description given to the next degree of certainty. The last column shows percentage of errors in answers where the subject was "willing to give his sworn oath." [From K. M. Dallenbach, *Psychol. Rev.*, 1913, **20**, 323.]

	Percentage Error		
Time of Recall	*Report*	*Fairly Certain*	*Sworn to*
Immediate	48.2	28.3	6.7
5 days	66.6	30.7	10.0
15 days	64.5	25.3	15.4
45 days	55.0	31.4	19.5
Average of errors	58.6	28.9	12.9

for those reports of which the subjects were very sure, the percentage of error was still substantial.

Changes in Recollection with Lapse of Time

In addition to these practical experiments upon the reliability of testimony, the way the recollection of an object changes with lapse of time has been investigated. We need to know what happens to the memory of an object or event as time passes and whether the memory of an object simply fades out, gradually becoming more and more fuzzy and indefinite, or whether it undergoes other changes.

The experimental procedure is as follows. An observer is shown an object, a series of objects or a story. Later he is asked to redraw the object or retell the story as he recalls it. (See Fig. 71.) In some of the experiments the observers reproduce each object just once, with the time intervals between initial observation and reproduction varying. In other experiments the observers are asked to reproduce the same material over and over again, thus getting at the effects of repeated recollection.

Both these experimental conditions have their counterparts in everyday life. Sometimes your first recollection of an event occurs only after a considerable lapse of time. You have not thought of the event

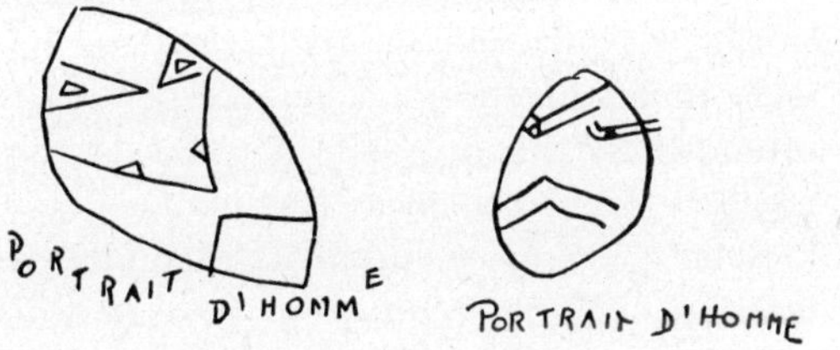

FIGURE 71. PERCEPTION AND IMAGE

The drawing at the left was observed by a person and reproduced by him 15 to 30 minutes later as on the right. Thus the figure at the left represents the stimulus, and the figure on the right the recollection of it. [From F. C. Bartlett, *Remembering*, Cambridge University Press, 1932, p. 178.]

or reviewed it between the original perception and the recall much later. More frequently, however, a striking event in your life is recollected over and over again at intervals for many years. When you recall an important event of your childhood, you have probably recollected it many times before. Your present recollection is, therefore, a result of many previous rehearsals. In part this recall is a recollection of a recollection of a recollection, but it also may refer to the original observations. It is, moreover, impossible to be sure that the period of time between the original perception and the recollection is ever entirely free of spontaneous rehearsals by the subject, and it is certainly not improbable that we never recall an event after a long time span without there having been intervening rehearsals.

When the experimenter has collected a great many reproductions—drawings or reports—he is likely to be impressed by the great variety of things which can happen to a recollection. To describe the memory merely as indefinite and unclear does not, however, do justice to the findings. Some aspects of a design or a story may become *more* clear as time passes. To be sure, these clear aspects are not necessarily correct, even though the observer believes that they are.

Some of the changes which frequently occur are these:

(1) Details are omitted; only the general pattern is reproduced.

(2) New details are added; for example, eyebrows were added to a drawing of a face which originally had none.

(3) Certain peculiarities of the original figure may become exaggerated in the reproduction; for example, slanting eyes become more slanted in recollection.

(4) The resemblance between the figure and some familiar object is increased; for example, a conventional drawing of a cat becomes more catlike.

(5) Different figures in the same experiment come to resemble one another more than they did originally.

(6) Under repeated recollection, errors and changes may finally become stabilized.

(7) Stories, and sometimes figures, may be made more 'logical' or made to fit a more familiar pattern. (See Fig. 71.)

Nature of Errors in Recollection

The factors which bring about these changes in recollection operate both during

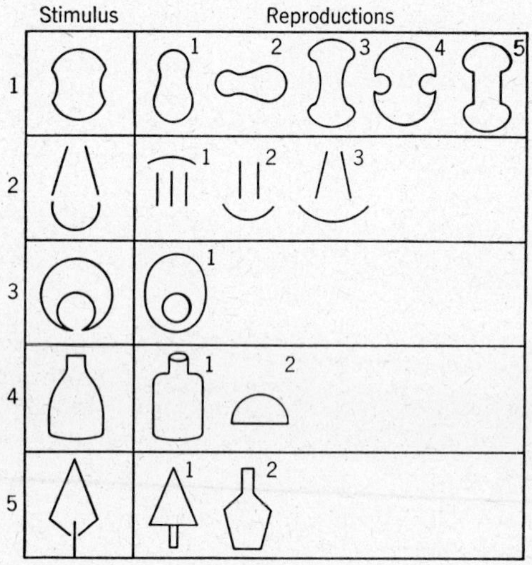

FIGURE 72. DEPENDENCE OF RECOLLECTION ON MEANING

The figures in the stimulus column were shown, among a number of others, to a group of subjects for a short time. Their reproductions of these stimuli, made from memory, varied according to the meaning suggested by the figures. Thus stimulus 1 suggested (1) a woman's torso; (2) a "footprint on the sands of time"; (3) a dumb-bell; (4) a violin; (5) a dumb-bell. Stimulus 2 received the names (1) pillars with curve; (2) pillars with curve; (3) megaphone in a bowl. Stimulus 3 was named (1) one circle inside another. The experimenter gave different names to stimulus 4 as he showed it to different individuals. Their reproductions varied according to the name: (1) bottle; (2) stirrup. Stimulus 5 was treated like stimulus 4. The names were (1) pine tree; (2) trowel. [After J. J. Gibson, *J. exper. Psychol.*, 1929, **12**, 15 and 19; and L. Carmichael, H. P. Hogan and A. A. Walter, *J. exper. Psychol.*, 1932, **15**, 75 and 80.]

the original perception and afterward. If the original object is seen as resembling something familiar, if it is given a name or if certain special features of it are noticed, these characteristics tend to become more marked in the reproduction. Figure 72 shows some examples of this effect of the original mode of perception. Such characteristics are likely to appear in the very first reproduction, immediately after the perception. As time goes on, the effect may become more exaggerated. Sometimes it appears that the observer recalls only the verbal identification or the general resemblance to a familiar object, and reconstructs his recollection from it.

We have noted that forms as well as stories may become more 'logical' or sensible in recollection. That happens most often when the original material is fragmentary or perceived as fragmentary, as it may be if perceived hurriedly or under distraction. Then recollection goes to work to make a whole out of the parts, to complete and unify the event or form or whatever it is that is being recalled. It is not easy to describe disconnected scraps. Recollection needs to have a total structure if it is to represent adequately the original perception. The same thing happens in recollecting dreams. There we piece the seemingly silly fragments together into a sensible story.

These laboratory experiments on recollection are concerned with impersonal material. They differ from the recall of events in our own past lives, events involving emotional relationships to other persons, success and failure in work or sport. The emotional context of most of our ordinary recollections is another factor which modifies our recollections and frequently falsifies them.

The psychoanalysts have collected examples from clinical practice showing the falsification of memories of emotional situations and conflicts. (See pp. 175 and 520 f.) The experimental results we have described represent changes in recollection which are but mild and slight compared to the changes which occur in normal personal recollections. Autobiographies and memoirs, unless they are carefully authenticated, must be full of these personalized distortions.

Some investigators have sought to study recollection of events into which an emotional flavor has been injected. In one experiment a subject was given various problems to solve. He succeeded in solving some of them. Others, however, were too difficult for him and he was disturbed at failing. Later he was asked to recall the problems upon which he had worked, and the experimenter compared his accuracy in recall of those problems in which he experienced failure with those which he solved. It was found that as a rule he recalled with greater accuracy the problems he solved than those in which he failed.

Another way of showing how personal factors influence recollection is to use for perception and recall material which either accords with the attitudes and opinions of the subject or contradicts them. Here follows the account of such an experiment.

Two groups of students—one group strongly pro-Communist, the other strongly anti-Communist—were chosen as the subjects. Each subject was asked to study two brief excerpts from books. One of these passages was a strong anti-Soviet argument; the other was moderately pro-Soviet. The materials were studied repeatedly; hence there was more learning than recollecting going on. Nevertheless, the biases entered in. The anti-Communist subjects recalled the points of the anti-Soviet argument better than the pro-Communist subjects did. The converse held for the pro-Communist passage. These differences appeared after each of the repeated periods of study of the materials. After four such periods of study, the tests were continued for five weeks without further opportunity to review the printed materials, and the two biases became more and more effective during the series of repeated recollections.

Failures of Recollection

Often recollection fails. The conditions seem to be right for its occurrence, yet it is blocked, temporarily or even permanently. Emotional factors are often to blame, for they may lead to a forgetting which is called *repression,* a blocking of recollection which can be overcome only by treatment, such as psychoanalysis. (See p. 541.)

When forgetting is complete and persistent it is called *amnesia.* Amnesia may occur after a bad shock like an accident or after an intensely emotional experience. The person affected may lose his memory for a period either before or after the event. In extreme cases, he may lose his memory for his whole past life, including his knowledge of his identity, of where he lives and so on.

Amnesia illustrates clearly the distinction between learning and recollection. It is a characteristic of amnesia that the individual loses *recollection* alone. He does not forget how to walk, how to speak his native language or even other skills acquired later in life such as typing, or his other occupational skills. Recollection is the recall of experiences in the *personal* past, and it is these experiences which are lost in amnesia.

There is, however, a certain selectivity in recollection which does not seem to follow strictly from the laws of learning. Only a few past events come back out of the many which association might bring. The selection is doubtless due to the sets and motives that are operating.

A more complete analysis of the problem of amnesia requires an understanding of the general problems of abnormal psychology. (See pp. 531–535.)

TYPES OF RECOLLECTION

Accurate recollection of the same object or event does not necessarily always take the same form. There are different kinds of recollection. One man may differ from another in the kind of recollection he uses most of the time. One task may differ from another in the type of recollection that is best suited to it. These differences are found between persons and also between recollections by the same person.

One of the two most important distinctions of this sort is the difference that occurs according to the sense departments used. We can recall events in *visual* imagery, or *auditory* imagery, or in *motor* processes. The other important distinction lies in the difference between *verbal* recollection and recollection in terms of *concrete* imagery. Take the recollection of a particular hammer. A man may recall in imagery (1) the look of the hammer, (2) the feeling of swinging the hammer in his hand, (3) the sound of the blows of the hammer, (4) the look of the word *hammer,* (5) the sound of the word *hammer,* (6) the voice-feeling of what saying the word *hammer* is like. The first three recollections are made of concrete imagery, visual, kinesthetic and auditory. (*Kinesthetic* means pertaining to the feeling of the movement of your own body and its parts.) The last three are verbal imagery, visual, auditory and kinesthetic. There are different combinations of these types of verbal imagery. For instance, auditory-kinesthetic-verbal imagery is much more common than pure auditory-verbal imagery. If you hear the sound of a word in imagery, you are likely also to feel how it is to pronounce it.

Are there differences among persons in respect of these imagery types? Do some people prefer visual imagery, others kinesthetic, others auditory-kinesthetic? Yes, there are such persons but they are exceptional. Occasionally you find a person who seems never to have visual imagery, who recollects entirely in terms of kinesthetic and auditory-kinesthetic imagery, both verbal and concrete. He will tell you what the colors of the rocks in the Grand Canyon of the Colorado look like, but he will be recollecting words, not actual colors. Occasionally you find a person who does nearly all his thinking in visual terms, even in his verbal thinking. Most persons, however, use all the types on different occasions. Versatility is the rule.

Versatility is also more efficient. As we have already seen in the discussion of eidetic imagery, recollection of great detail of an object is easiest if it occurs in visual terms. If you can see the *Mona Lisa* in your 'mind's eye,' you can do a good job at recollecting it. If you have to depend on kinesthesis, you will be likely to get only the words with which you originally described it. On the other hand, if you are remembering the *Ninth Symphony,* auditory imagery is more fun, even though visual recollection of the looks of the score may be quite accurate. Kinesthesis, of course, fails, since you cannot sing or play a symphony by yourself. The best you could do with kinesthesis would be to remember descriptive words. The stroke in golf which you have at last mastered; how do you recollect that? Kinesthesis is best there, though you might have a visual image of how the 'pro' swings his club. Sometimes imagery type is thus related to efficiency in recollecting.

On the other hand, it is surprising how often type does not matter. Verbal recollection fits into any of the common types, and most recollection can be made verbal. Musicians do not necessarily recall music in auditory terms. Geometricians do not necessarily use visual terms. Persons who have been blind and deaf from birth and have no visual and auditory imagery are capable of learning language and of doing any of the abstract thinking which is normal to a person without sensory defect. They are shut off from certain perceptions and from such direct recollections, but they are able to substitute kinesthetic imagery. Blind persons learn to perceive in auditory and kinesthetic terms with remarkable accuracy, and their recollections take place in similar terms.

One reason why type of imagery makes so little difference in human life is to be found in the fact that the most important recollections for civilized adults are general and abstract, not concrete and objective. Most recollecting of this sort, and indeed most thinking, can be done in words, and any of the three main kinds of imagery will work with words.

Verbal recollection is commoner than concrete recollection, less accurate as a rule, but more efficient in the sense that the telescoping of a complex object or event into a verbal formula is so compact that it gets out of the way of other recollections. Any important business of living is likely to include the making of judgments. You can recollect the judgment you previously made of an observation in words and do it fairly easily. More difficult and less common is it to recollect the observation itself, as you might be able to do quite accurately in eidetic imagery, and then to make your judgment of the recollection. The witness on the stand is asked to recollect the event and to let the court or jury pass judgment. More often he recollects his past judgment of the event and reports it or tries to reconstruct the fading event from it. It is easier for a witness to remember that he thought the driver who hit the pedestrian was at fault than it is for him to recollect just what it was that made him blame the driver. Accuracy and scope are here inversely related. You can remember best if you remember details of an event; but you can remember more events if you condense each into your assessment of it and remember merely the assessment. How often a man says: "I know that's a fallacy, but I can't remember why."

IMAGINING

Like recollection, imagining creates objects without benefit of the sense organs. A person who is blinded during his childhood can continue to imagine colors and shapes. A person who becomes deaf can still imagine sounds and melodies. Beethoven composed and conducted great music after he was stone deaf.

There is no essential difference between the kinds of experience—colors, shapes, sounds—that make up perceptions, recollections and imaginations. As we have already seen, these experiences differ only in their meaning. The perceived object is there-now-in-front-of-me, belonging to the system of present reality. The recollected object is something-I-once-saw, belonging to some system of past reality. The imagined object is the thing which is about-to-happen or which might happen, and it is either isolated without fitting any established system or else it fits temporarily and insecurely into a reality system, as is the case when I look at my empty garage and imagine a splendid car in it.

Imagination and Perception

Since imagination is free and not tied to reality, there is no problem of the reliability of imagination. There are, however, the cases in which imagination occurs together with a perception, the cases in which imagination gets confused with perception, the cases in which the imagination is mistaken for a perception and the contrary cases in which a perception seems strange and is taken for an imagination.

Synesthesia. There are a few persons (perhaps five per cent of the population) who report that they experience colors whenever they hear sounds; that is to say, there is a definite color or color pattern which regularly appears when a certain sound is heard. This phenomenon is known as *chromesthesia* or *colored hearing. Synesthesia* is the general term for relations of this kind between sense qualities. Thus we may have colored odors or tastes as well as colored hearing.

Colored hearing can be very stable and dependable. Table XIII is a record of the colors associated with notes of the musical scale for one person with colored hearing. The two records, taken seven years apart, show remarkable consistency.

TABLE XIII

A CASE OF CHROMESTHESIA INVESTIGATED IN 1905 AND AGAIN IN 1912

The notes of the musical scale are associated with images of very constant colors. [From H. S. Langfeld, *Psychol. Bull.*, 1914, **11**, 113.]

	1905	*1912*
c	Red	Red
d♭	Purple	Lavender
d	Violet	Violet
e♭	Soft blue	Thick blue
e	Golden yellow	Sunlight
f	Pink	Pink, apple blossoms
f♯	Green blue	Blue green
g♭	Greener blue	Greener blue
g	Clear blue	Clear sky blue
a	Cold yellow	Clear yellow, hard, not warm
b♭	Orange	Verges on orange
b	Very brilliant coppery	Very brilliant coppery

Synesthesia is a special form of imagining—apparently not imagining of objects but of abstract sensory qualities. It differs from other forms of imagining in being so closely tied to the perceptive situation.

How synesthesia develops is not certain, but it is probably learned early in childhood. When colored patterns are perceived in colored hearing they are likely to be familiar kinds of designs, like wallpaper patterns. Closely resembling synesthesia are *number forms,* in which the person sees any number fitted into a geometrical schema, and *date forms,* which are similar. A number form is likely to have corners in it at 'important' numbers, like 5, 10, 12, 25, 50, 100, 1000, and 10,000. A common academic date form for the year is a closed ellipse, with the spaces for June, July and August much longer than the spaces for any other month. Such forms must certainly be learned and cannot be innate.

Dreams are the most familiar events in which imagination plays the role of perception. Since dreams are bizarre and fragmentary and do not fit in well with any total reality system, why do they seem real? The answer to that question is that dreams do not, as a rule, seem real. They do not seem unreal; that is all. Dreams occur under some strong tension or set—sometimes in partial fulfillment of a suppressed wish, the psychoanalysts think. They are vivid and usually emotionally toned, but limited in scope and not fitted into any reality system at all.

The *hallucinations* of persons with mental disease are like dreams. The schizophrenic who tells us what his voices are saying to him, the mean, ugly, abusive things they say, is accepting uncritically imagery which does not fit in with reality; but then that is what schizophrenia is, the splitting up of the integrated personality and its reality systems.

These instances show that the kinds of stuff of which perception and imagination are made are so much alike that without a label imagination may be identified as perception or at least not distinguished from it.

False imagination. There is also the converse case in which perception is thought to be imagination. That is what happened in a well-known experiment in which the observers were instructed to look at a screen, fitted into a window in a wall, and to imagine a specified object projected upon the screen. Unknown to the observers, a projector behind this translucent screen projected upon the screen a very dim image of the object called for. The observers were quite pleased that they were able to get their images of imagination so clearly. They did not guess that they were actually being provided with a visual stimulus. Even when the projected image failed to correspond exactly with the character of the thing they were trying to imagine, they still regarded the object as 'imagined.' "I can see that knife standing up on end," one observer said. "I should have thought I would have imagined it as lying down." It is important to note that the image remained even after the projector was turned off. The imagination, which the stimulus helped to start, continued independently afterward.

Creative imagination also sometimes works in a similar way. An author, artist or musician creates his work of art—his story, his poem, his melody. His pride in it tells him that his work is new, his own creation; and then someone comes who tells him that what he has done is a close copy of what someone else has done. Sure enough, he really did know the work which he copied unconsciously, but his recollection was separated from its proper past reality system and the composer—doubtless reinforced by his own wishes—mistook his old memory for new imagination. Many cases of plagiarism are unintentional and to be accounted for in this simple manner.

THINKING

The psychology of thinking is not, of course, the same thing as *logic*. Logic analyzes the correctness and incorrectness of thinking or, more generally, the drawing of conclusions from premises. Thinking, however, may be quite illogical, even when it gets to the right conclusion. Often important creative thinking goes on by trial-and-error. You form an hypothesis as a hunch. You test it out in thought, and find it wrong. You make up another hypothesis. Finally you get one that seems to work where you need it and you accept it. It may be an hypothesis in such form that you can test it by logic, but the trial-test-error-trial-test-success method is not the procedure of logic.

We have already noted that the term *thinking* is often applied indiscriminately to a great many different kinds of psychological activity—recollecting the past, imagining the future or even deciding what to do now. The kind of thinking which requires special and separate treatment is a more complex kind of performance. It starts with a problem which cannot be solved by methods which come readily to hand. We have to invent new methods for it or grasp new relationships; at least they are new to the thinker. Sometimes this kind of thinking is called *elaborative thinking* to distinguish it from recollective and imaginative processes.

Starting with the acceptance of the problem, elaborative thinking progresses through a series of phases, reversing direction, discovering new problems, dealing with concepts and symbols, recollecting, imagining, applying memorized formulas and so on. In other words, the progress of thinking consists of a series of manipulations of objects and of other *tools of thinking.* These tools exist in great variety. Before we can understand the total process of thinking, we must examine them and try to describe them accurately.

Important Tools of Thinking

Here we may list and discuss the more important tools of thinking—objects, concepts and symbols.

(1) *Perceived, recollected and imagined objects.*

(*a*) *Concrete or specific objects.* You understand the word 'ancestor' by imagining your own grandfather. In testing the truth of a general statement, you look for concrete exceptions. In understanding the word 'friction,' you imagine rubbing your hands together.

(*b*) *Objects as examples; generalized objects.* In solving a geometrical problem you imagine a triangle but do not consider it as this particular imagined triangle; that is to say, in the geometric operation you do not consider it as obtuse, acute or as any other particular kind of triangle. It is just an object of 'that general kind.' Geometry always discusses the general but illustrates with the particular.

(*c*) *Objects with dynamic properties.* In solving many concrete problems, objects are seen as tools for doing certain things. A stone is seen only as something heavy, something you can pound with. An object may be seen as about-to-fall, as instable on its base, as easily broken. Through past experience the object takes on a significance beyond that immediately given in the stimulus pattern. You *see* that ice is cold and heavy.

(2) *Concepts.* A very important tool for thinking is the concept. A concept is a 'general idea,' an item in thinking that stands for a general class. As an experience the concept may seem to be nothing more than an ordinary image, but as a concept it has acquired, through learning, various potentialities which give it much more general meaning. In other words the concept implies the state in which there is a broadly generalized response.

Consider the word *dog,* and also the concept dog which may enter into thought. If you read in a story the sentence, "He called his dog," you may have a visual image of a particular dog, you get the meaning of the sentence, but you are not then using a concept. If, on the other hand, you read the title of an article in a journal, "Conditioned Responses in the Dog," this dog is the concept dog, for it means any dog and every dog, the class of dogs. How do these two experienced dogs, the particular and the general, differ psychologically? In both cases you may have the same visual image, an image of a dog, and every image is in itself particular. In the case of the concept, however, the particular image is associatively connected through learning with all sorts of other images, which have in common whatever learning has taught you to believe are the essential characteristics of dogginess. Given a chance, a pause in the thinking process, a challenge as to whether you understand the concept, and many of these alternative images will actually arise, attesting the conceptual nature of the item of thinking which is represented consciously at the moment only by the particular image of the dog.

The main thing to remember in this context is that thinking needs to use generalized concepts, that the concept is necessarily represented in conscious thinking by some particular item, like an image, but that the concept is nevertheless more than a particular image because in thinking this image plays the role of a generalized abstraction. Thinking, as we shall see, could not go on without the great economy which generalization makes possible.

(3) *Symbols and signs.* Thinking also gains economy by making use of both symbols and signs. Since every symbol is potentially a sign, and every sign potentially a symbol, the two conceptions must be considered together.

A *symbol* is a concrete particular item in thinking that stands for something more general. A particular dog—seen, imaged or pictured—can be the symbol for the general concept dog. Concepts are usually represented in thinking by symbols. The word *two* is a symbol for the concept of duality, and *2* is another symbol for the same concept. A traffic light, perceived or imagined, may be a symbol of police power. The symbol is simpler and more easily used than the generality for which it stands, and the employment of symbols for thinking also contributes enormously to the economy of thinking.

Symbols tend to become *signs.* They act as signals for thinking or action, as stimuli for conscious or motor response. The traffic light is a sign; it tells us what to do. The symbol for multiplication is a sign; it also tells us what to do. Thinking progresses because symbols act as signs and carry the thinking process along.

Symbols and signs are thus seen to be the pawns and pieces with which the great game of thinking is played. It could not be such a remarkable and successful game without them. As it is, by letting a little symbol act for a large, complex and clumsy concept, we can think quickly and efficiently. We can also avoid starting our thinking from scratch. The original understanding of a concept and the attachment of a symbol to represent it is in itself often an elaborate job of thinking, but once done and the symbol given its proper powers as a sign, the thinking does not have to be done again. We use the symbol without stopping to recollect for what it stands, and we use it as a sign to indicate the processes which we have learned belong to it.

Take the algebraic symbol of involution, x^n, the raising of x to the nth power. The exponent, n, written as a superscript, is the symbol. It stands for a generalization. We learn the processes of squaring and cubing and then of raising numbers to other powers. Thus we get the meaning of involution attached to the symbol. We must grant the symbol the greatest generality. It means that x could be raised to the power of 2, 3, 510, $\frac{1}{2}$, $1\frac{1}{2}$, $\sqrt{2}$ or π. After we understand the symbol, we no longer need to recall the various processes by which it acquired its meaning. Instead we need to recognize it as a sign, knowing what operations it indicates in the process of thinking. Mathematics constantly builds up symbols for the relations of symbols, creating new signs and proceeding ever at a level more and more remote from the particular objects whose relationships it investigates.

Mathematics is, of course, a highly symbolic form of language, but in principle it does not differ from any other form of language.

Language

Language, because it uses symbols, is the best medium for thinking. Ordinarily the symbols are words, which, of course, have meaning and readily act as signs. The words can be spoken, written or printed, or fingered in the manual alphabet that the stone deaf use. There are languages in which the symbols are gestures, the gesture languages of the Neapolitans and of the North American Indians. It is not true that man alone among the animals has language. Every animal with a conditioned response is reacting to a symbol, for the conditioned stimulus is a symbol of the unconditioned stimulus. The dog who salivates when he hears the dinner bell understands the meaning of the bell, which has become for him a symbol for food. When that little bit of language has been built up between a scientist and a dog, it becomes possible for the dog to tell the scientist whether long-continued loud noise deafens the dog, for the dog can say "I hear the bell" simply by salivating, or "I do not hear any bell" by not salivating. Human language is nothing else than a high development of such symbolic responses.

Human language has four chief functions. (1) It serves to *communicate* ideas from one person to another. That is its chief social function. It is not, however, its only function. (2) It serves to *persuade* or to incite others to action. That is another social function. Persuasion *per se* is not communication. Yelling "Fire!" when there is no fire may incite a stampede without directly communicating thought. (3) Language serves also to relieve tension in the speaker. That is its *cathartic function*. Exclamations and profanity may have this purpose, but so also does a great deal of unilateral talk. The hypochondriac who wants to tell everyone his symptoms is trying less to get understanding or action in his vis-à-vis than he is to relieve his own frustration. An exclamation can be used to communicate, to let others know how you feel. However, Robinson Crusoe doubtless used expletives before he had his man Friday to talk to, because the conditioned response of talking does not become easily extinguished, and some action is needed in emotional situations.

Those are three functions of language most usually cited, two of them social and one of them individual. There is, however, a fourth and more basic function. (4) Language is used as a tool in *thinking*. It is the system of symbols which makes thinking efficient. Men think to themselves in words. An argument, a discussion, an exposition is developed verbally, whether an audience is present or not. The words and phrases are symbols, and as such they carry with them meanings which have become implicit and do not have to be expressed. They are also signs, and as such they indicate, because of much past conditioning, the proper course of thought. Often a verbal argument, written or spoken, seems to develop of itself. Even its author does not know how it is coming out. He lets his mouth talk while he listens, or he lets his fingers work his typewriter while he perceives the sentences as they form. The final result is a conclusion, one that is quite satisfactory to the author, and valid as far as he can see. That automatic factor in language is possible because so much learning precedes its acquisition.

It is a fact that thinking is, for the most part, unconscious. The symbols, acting as signs, carry on from symbol to symbol without the things to which the symbols refer getting themselves represented in imagery. We can see how abbreviated the conscious processes of language are if we consider the nature of *reading*.

Reading

The child at first reads slowly and laboriously. He does not, if he is well taught, read letter by letter; he reads word by word or phrase by phrase. That is what you too do in learning German or French. At first the word *cat* will evoke its referent, that is to say, the child will perceive the word and then see the visual image of a cat. Soon, however, as learning progresses, the symbol comes to work alone. There is not time in reading for imagery of the referent to arise. The word *cat* acts properly as a sign without arousing any conscious associates at all. And the word *Katz,* which at first you translated into the English word *cat,* comes, as your German improves, similarly to act alone without this extra addition of translation.

In short, you know much more than you are conscious of. You can read a simple clear prose passage of five hundred words through quickly and understand it perfectly. Perhaps the preposition *by* occurred in the first sentence, and the passage would have been altered throughout in its meanings if the word had been *to* instead of *by*. If quizzed, you have the meanings correct. So you must have perceived *by*. Yet you do not remember the word, you did not pause to pronounce it or to let any imagery arise to indicate its meaning. You just went on and let your brain take care of the sense for you. If you had allowed as little as a second to become conscious of the meaning of each of those five hundred words, you would have had to spend about eight more minutes on the passage, and that is exactly what does not happen. You can read without pausing because the symbols are safe substitutes for their referents.

Since children learn to read aloud, pronouncing the seen word when reading becomes for them a much overlearned conditioned response. Many adults who can get rid of all other associations for read words, still pronounce them or at least form the words with their vocimotor organs as they read. After much reading their tongues get tired! This translation of sight into movement and kinesthesis is just as unnecessary for effective understanding as is the translation of every German word into English for the understanding of German. Skill in language means that both kinds of translation are dispensed with. An adult with a tired reading tongue can learn visual reading and gain enormously in efficiency. He may prefer to read more slowly and pronounce the words when he wishes to appreciate the esthetic beauty of prose or poetry; yet for the tough practical business of getting as much sense as possible as quickly and accurately as possible, visual reading is the correct method.

This same principle applies, of course, to the use of arithmetic. How many people can set themselves to add, and then, seeing a 4 below an 8, can at once image a 12, without wasting time to say "four and eight are twelve"? Yet that way of adding is extremely inefficient. A good adder, an expert accountant, can perceive an 8, perceive a 4, image a 12, perceive a 9, image a 21 and so run his eye down the column with partial sums popping out in imagery as he goes along, and he could even learn to whistle while he adds.

A visual reader ought not to be able to

see sense in the sentence: "Two beer knot tube bee thought is thick west shun." The slow-pronouncing reader will, however, detect a familiarity in the sound as he forms it, and, if he repeats the sound, with his eyes shut or his attention off the looks of the words, he will discover the sense. So too with "Pas de la Rhône que nous."

The first step in the development of the understanding in reading is the stripping off of these conscious contexts from words. The second is for the words themselves to become obscure, and the imagery for which they are signs to occupy attention. Not only can you understand a text when the meanings of the words do not arise in consciousness, but you also can understand it when the words do not have time to become clear in detail. What happens is that symbolization goes farther. A part of a word becomes an adequate symbol for the whole word. That is why errors in printed matter are so hard to catch. We do not always see the whole word. *Psycology* seems to be what this book is about.

The Problem and the Set

The problem determines the course of thinking. Thinking is aimed at a goal, a solution, a conclusion. It gets somewhere or attempts to. We have said that it is the symbols-become-signs which determine the course of thinking, but there is no inconsistency here, because the problem is the overlord which chooses the signs that operate. The problem has this effect because it is represented by a set or attitude that it induces in the thinker.

This matter becomes clearer if we go back to the experiments on set and attitude which were described in connection with reaction (pp. 60–62). Reaction closely resembles thought and often cannot be distinguished from it. If you are set the problem to press a key when you see a green light and not when you see a red light, and you press for the green light, you are *reacting* in accordance with the set that you have taken on from our instruction. If you are set the problem to decide whether a statement is true or false and are given the statement, "To give every man his due were to will justice and achieve chaos," and you decide that the statement is true (or false), you have done some *thinking* in accordance with the set which you have accepted from our instruction. But if someone flashes this statement at you on a card in a stimulus-exposure apparatus, and you call out *True* or *False* as your decision is, and he measures the reaction time, why then surely your thinking *is* reacting.

A famous experiment on set was performed by Ach in 1905. He showed his subjects pairs of digits, one below the other. Sometimes he asked them to tell him the sums of each pair, sometimes the differences and sometimes the products. Those operations depend on three different sets or attitudes which his subjects could take on at his behest. It was not for them a matter of learning. They already knew all the sums, differences and products perfectly. The discovery in Ach's experiment was that any one of the three kinds of answer could be obtained from an *unconscious set.* Asked for sums, the subjects gave sums without even remembering consciously that it was sums they were to think of and not differences or products. Set for sums, they got no differences or products. Then, with the very same pairs of digits, the subject at a word could be reset for differences, or for products, and get only what the set called for. As a matter of fact Ach held that his experiments were actually an investigation of thought, and these arithmetical reactions are indeed simple thinkings.

Ach called the set a determining tendency and he said that progress of thought is set by a determining tendency toward the ideated goal. Since *set, attitude, need* and *determining tendency* are similar concepts, this book gets along by using the first three terms but omitting Ach's.

The notion of set as determining action and thought is further illustrated by examples. In the morning you decide that you need a certain book from the library and that you will stop for it on the way downtown. Then you forget all about this decision. Yet as you pass the library you find yourself turning in, and you wonder for a moment why you are entering the library. Presently you recollect your original decision. In thinking the same sort of phenomenon occurs continually. Many scientists and inventors have described this phenomenon of 'incubation' in thinking. The solution of a baffling problem suddenly occurs to the thinker when he is thinking about something else.

Trial-and-Error and Insight

We have already seen how animals solve problems by trial-and-error and by insight. Thorndike's cat in the puzzle box (p. 145) escaped to get food by trying this and trying that, and finally hitting upon the right movement. A rat in an alley maze cannot possibly get to his food by insight. He does not know where the food is and he has to try and try again until he finds it. On the other hand, a rat that can see before him the paths of an elevated maze may solve his problem by insight and without trials that end in errors. He examines the situation and picks the correct path to the food, provided the maze is very simple. The chimpanzee that tries to get the banana from beyond the fence (p. 152) tries and errs, tries and errs, and then, when he realizes that the two sticks will fit together to make a long one, a flash of insight gives him the solution. (See Fig. 73.)

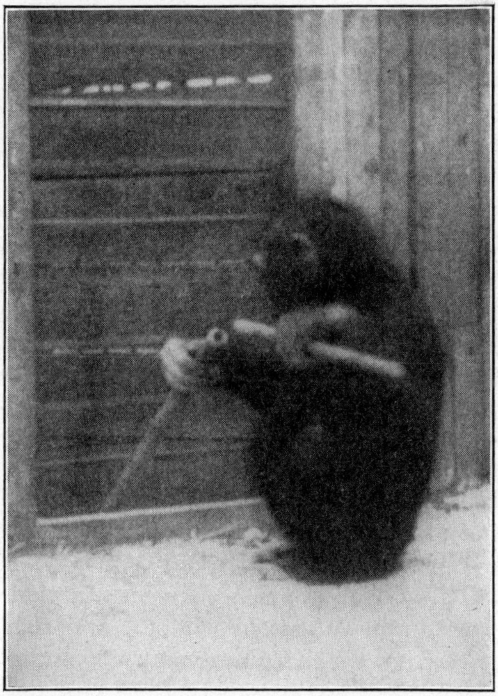

FIGURE 73. INSIGHT: CHIMPANZEE PUTTING TOGETHER A DOUBLE STICK

Having discovered that the two sticks would go together to make one long stick, the ape took the long stick at once to the other side of his cage and secured a banana outside the bars and too far away to be got by either short stick alone. [Courtesy of W. Köhler.]

Human thinking is not different. The thinker, faced with a problem, tries for a solution. He keeps on until a trial is successful. Many of his errors are errors of insight, false insights that come as inspirations and do not solve the problem. His final success may be an act of true insight, or it may be a blind success, as when the puzzle finally comes apart in your hands and you have no idea what it was you did to get it apart.

If the problem is simple and the solution has already been learned, then there need be no errors and no insight. You want to know the sum of 4 and 8; you appeal under the set for addition to past learning; and the answer is before you, 12.

You want to decide whether a novel proposition is true or false. Past learning is not going to be enough to decide the issue for you without insight. This is a brand new proposition and you need a little time, perhaps several seconds, to think. Images come up, and then presently some insight into the relations of the concepts decides you, and you make your judgment.

You have a puzzle to solve. The block at the upper right corner must be moved to the lower left corner. You can work blindly with trial-and-error, and you may indeed solve the problem thus, though you will not have learned it and cannot do it again. Or you may study the situation, form an hypothesis, try it out, find that it does not work, try out another hypothesis and continue in this fashion until one hypothesis or a series of partial hypotheses give the required solution. This is trial-and-error thinking, but it is also insightful thinking because the hypotheses are formed by insight and abandoned when found inadequate.

Here is a simple example that shows how problems get solved. Suppose that your alarm clock has stopped. You may first use blind trial-and-error. You shake it, try to wind it some more, shake it again, turn it upside down, change the setting and so on. So far you have used methods which sometimes work, but you have shown little insight into the problem. Finally, having exhausted these possibilities, you open the case. You notice that the hair spring has been tangled, apparently because the clock has been dropped. At that point, believing that you have the solution of the difficulty, you untangle the hair spring, and the clock begins to run. You put it back together again, and the clock stops again. Your first insight may have been correct, but it was inadequate. You need to know something more. So you reopen the clock, find that the shaft of the balance wheel is out of place and replace it—another insightful trial. You put the clock together, and it runs. Success stops your thinking, just as satisfaction stops a need.

Trial-and-error without insight would be the case if your clock stops, you take it apart, see nothing the matter with it, put it together again and find that it runs.

There are problems in which trial-and-error does not help and in which one correct act of insight is enough. For instance, there is a ring problem, with two rings, each on a loop of cord. The ends of the cord are fastened permanently to a stick, and the cord is also looped about the stick through a hole in a special manner. The problem is to get the two rings on the same loop. Blind trial-and-error seldom helps. It gets the puzzle tangled up and makes solution difficult or impossible. Inspection of the situation shows that you must pass the ring along the cord, through a hole in the stick, around a loop of the cord and then back through the same hole; but the hole is smaller than the ring, and the ring cannot go through it. Able scientists have worked for hours on this problem, but the solution comes in a single flash of insight. You cannot put the ring through the hole to pass it around the loop, but you can pull the loop through the hole to the ring, pass the ring around it and then push the loop back. The necessary insight is as simple as that; if you cannot get the ring to the loop, you must bring the loop to the ring.

Insight is not always either false or adequate. Sometimes it is imperfectly adequate. The chimpanzees of Fig. 74 were solving the problem of getting the banana, suspended near the top of their cage, by piling boxes on top of one another and climbing up on the pile. As the figure shows, they could solve the problem when three boxes were necessary in the pile, but they never learned the mechanics of equilibrium. Their rickety piles often fell over, or else the apes balanced perilously on them as they tottered.

When a rat begins to know the correct path through a maze, he may come to a place where he must choose, look down the wrong alley and then abandon it for the correct path. This behavior, since it is not actually an error, has been called *vicarious trial-and-error*. Human thinking makes liberal use of vicarious trial-and-error. You form your hypothesis, examine it and then abandon it as inadequate, without trying it out on the actual problem.

Sometimes it has been said that solving a problem by trial-and-error and by insight are different and opposed methods of thinking. Such a statement is obviously false. Trial-and-error is what happens in certain kinds of learning and certain kinds of thinking; but we learn by trial and success, and we solve problems by trial and insight.

What is the way to solve a problem? (*a*) Inspect the situation, study it carefully, examine it. (*b*) If you find you know the answer, the problem is solved. (*c*) If you do not know the solution, you continue your examination, hoping for an adequate insight. (*d*) If the insight comes and is adequate, the problem is solved. If it is inadequate, you continue hoping. (*e*) When it becomes apparent that the data necessary for insight are not available to your inspection, you begin with trials, random trials if you have no insight at all to

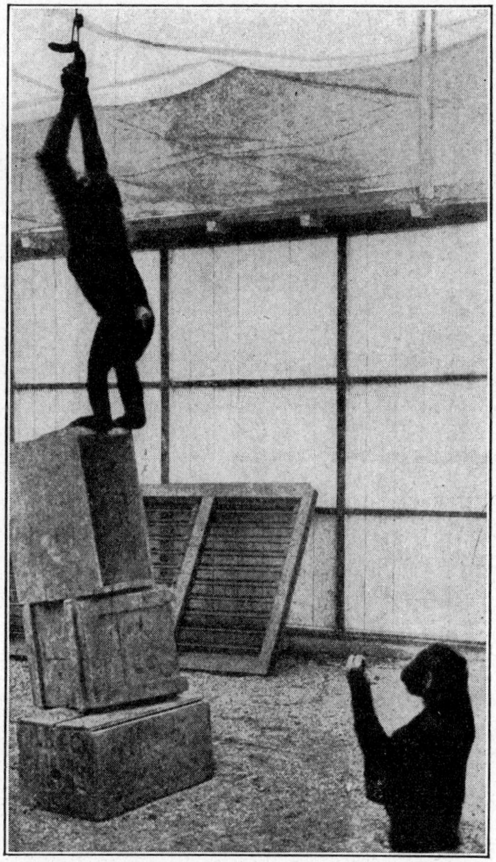

FIGURE 74. PROBLEM-SOLVING: CHIMPANZEE STACKS BOXES TO REACH THE BANANA SUSPENDED ALOFT

The ape solves this problem but does not learn to pile the boxes securely on top of one another. The other ape, watching, makes a sympathetic gesture with his left hand. [From W. Köhler, *Mentality of apes,* Harcourt, Brace, 1927, Plate IV.]

guide you, like a cat in a box with escape dependent on her touching an object which the experimenter has selected. The cat does not know the experimenter's secret, which is arbitrary and not open to insight.

Blind trial is the only possible method. (*f*) As trials alter the situation, insight may become possible, and the problem, partly solved, may then be attacked at stage (*c*) or even stage (*a*).

Blind trying is inferior to insight, but it is better than nothing; and insight is not always possible. Most complex thinking makes use of actual trials, vicarious trials, insights, successes and partial solutions, as thinking continues to the final solution.

INCORRECT THINKING

Thinking may completely fail to solve its problem. That is the safe kind of failure, because, since it does not give satisfaction, the frustrated thinker continues to address himself to the task of finding a solution or else abandons the problem with no false belief that he has solved it.

Thinking may, however, fail by being incorrect, and the thinker may accept a false conclusion as true, experiencing the relief of resolved frustration. That is a dangerous event in thinking, for it lulls the thinker into a false sense of security.

In this section we consider some of the ways in which incorrect thinking takes place and some of the reasons why it occurs.

Fallacies

Textbooks of logic expound the nature of fallacies. Although logic is not psychology, correct thinking must not contravene the logical canons. Everyone ought to know the nature of the common fallacies of thinking, but this book is not the place to set them forth. We must content ourselves with a single example from science, the failure to 'control' conclusions.

A personnel expert in a factory writes: "We have been trying out a new means for reducing absenteeism in the plant. It has turned out to be very good. Absenteeism has dropped twenty per cent during the six weeks the new method has been in use." That sounds right, doesn't it? You vary x (the method) and you get a concomitant change in y (absenteeism), so y is a function of x. Perhaps. Life in a factory is, however, a very complex affair, and a personnel expert, if he is an expert, would want better evidence before he reached that conclusion. Absenteeism varies for many different reasons. How does this expert know that it is the new method which is reducing absenteeism? Some other factor might be at work—the weather, the season, the fading out of an epidemic, a factor that arises from within the factory itself. He should have had a *control* (p. 14). Perhaps he could have divided his workers into two groups, using the new method for the test group and the old method (or lack of method) for the control group. If the test group and the control group showed the same decrease in absenteeism, he would know that the new method was not working, or conversely.

The fallacious thinking that arises from lack of control is similar to what is called *the fallacy of the single instance.* Thinkers not trained in scientific research, often men in public affairs, accept this fallacy easily. You can never safely draw a general conclusion from a single instance. Any observed concomitance of events could happen for many different reasons or by chance. You must repeat the concurrence again and again, keeping what you think is important the same and letting everything else vary. Only in that way do you at last become secure in concluding that a generalization holds. If rats always have been found to speed up toward the end of a maze, you can begin to talk about a goal gradient. A great economic depression followed the election of Hoover as President of the United States. That is a single instance. Did Hoover cause the depression? It is quite impossible to say until you have tried electing Hoover under a number of different economic conditions.

Wishful Thinking

Opinions and attitudes are affected by wishes and prejudices and tend to accord with what the thinker desires. The course of thinking is biased by desire and need. (This matter is discussed more fully on pp. 603–613.)

You find wishful thinking in politics, in courts of law, in science, in everyday social relations. Wherever controversy exists, there men try to prove themselves right, instead of trying to find out the truth. Wishful thinking is so insistent when important human needs are involved that the law makes a virtue of necessity and lets the opposing lawyers show how good their contradictory biases can make their cases, while the judge tries to transcend bias and remain impartial. Scientists try to be impartial judges, but scientific controversy, the unwillingness to accept the possibility of their own past mistakes, shows that egotism may control the scientists too. We take pride so much for granted that we hardly expect a man to think correctly if the right conclusion to his thought would be humiliating to him.

Hunches

A hunch is an imperfect insight. Your guess that a relationship might be true seems right to you, and yet you lack the evidence to validate your guess. That is a hunch. The hypotheses and insights of trial-and-error thinking are often such hunches. A hunch should always be used as a tentative conclusion to be tested out. It becomes a form of incorrect thinking only when it is accepted without subsequent validation.

On the other hand, it may be said that human action is based on a very large number of incorrect conclusions, conclusions that may never, during the lifetime of the person who uses them, be recognized as incorrect. The history of thought about diseases and their cures is full of such incorrect beliefs. Every day every man makes hundreds of decisions that are based upon inadequately validated opinions which he holds to be facts. When a hunch is held to firmly and we are sure that it is incorrect, we name it a *superstition*. People who bet on horse races have to use hunches (or superstitions) because they have not enough else to use; they are taking action in the absence of adequate information.

Word Fallacies

The commonest trouble into which language can get your thinking arises from the same word's having several different meanings. The meaning shifts as thought progresses from one sense in the premise to another in the conclusion. Said one newly naturalized immigrant: "Of course I'll vote Democratic. This country's a democracy, isn't it? They told me so when I was studying to be a citizen." And then there is the old joke from the Victorian era: "A piece of bread is better than nothing; nothing is better than Heaven; therefore a piece of bread is better than Heaven."

These are crude examples. The modern science of *semantics* studies the meanings of words, showing how often thought is falsified because the meaning of a word shifts without the thinker's knowing that it has. We are advised always to be aware of the referents which a word has as defining its meaning, but that advice must not, of course, be taken too literally. Language gets its efficiency from the fact that it uses words without their meanings having to become explicit. We have to trust language, in spite of the ways in which it betrays us, becoming critical only when we find that our thinking is not working accurately.

There is also *word magic,* the belief that when an unknown thing or event is named it is understood. Labeling tends to allay thinking. The lazy thinker is content with a name or with a classification which naming establishes. Such naming is useful and safe when the object named is understood. "That noise is a burglar." There is a classification of a noise that could properly incite to action. But naming, when it adds no new information except the name, is a delusion if it is mistaken for thinking. "Why," says someone, "do you notice details so much better than I? I suppose your perceptive faculty must be better." Noticing detail *is* perceiving better. Yet many a would-be thinker gets satisfaction from such redundant thinking.

Motivation

One of the most potent causes of failure and error in thinking is so obvious that it is usually overlooked. Thinking takes time, and it requires effort; the thinker has to be strongly motivated. Errors occur because he does not have time or inclination for complete and careful analysis of the problem. He takes short-cuts and jumps to conclusions. He gives up as soon as he comes to a point of serious difficulty.

This state of affairs is especially marked in our thinking upon political and social affairs. Careful assessment of the relative merits of political parties requires an analysis of a mass of information which must be sought out from books, periodicals and newspapers. Some of the essential information may not even exist. Political propaganda, moreover, is so phrased that it never suggests the possibility of thinking out political problems. No wonder thinking upon these topics is so rare.

Tacit Assumptions

The set or attitude under which a thinker undertakes to solve a problem may involve certain tacit assumptions of which the thinker is wholly unaware. Very often these assumptions prevent him from solving the problem, because they exclude from his consideration the hypothesis which is necessary for his success.

For example, consider this laboratory study of thinking. The experimenter gave the subjects a string of beads, on which two small white beads were alternated with one large yellow one. In the middle portion, however, there were five white beads separating two yellow ones. The instructions were: "Make a single regularly repeated pattern without either unstringing or restringing the beads, and without knotting or breaking the thread." On the table were many assorted objects, including a bottle of glue, a saw, pliers, and needles. Most of the subjects took some time to reach a solution of the problem, and some failed altogether to solve it. The only possible solution available was to break the extra beads with the pliers. It did not occur to the subjects who failed that the beads might be destroyed, even though the instructions did not explicitly forbid it.

Figure 75 is the horse-and-rider puzzle. The thinker is given two pieces of paper or cardboard, one square with the two horses printed on it, the other a strip with the two riders printed on it. He is told to put the riders on the horses without injuring the two pieces in any way. At first solution seems impossible. The riders would be upside down on the horses and not adjusted to the horses' bodies. Solution is, however, possible, and it may come by blind trial, error and success or by insight. In Fig. 76

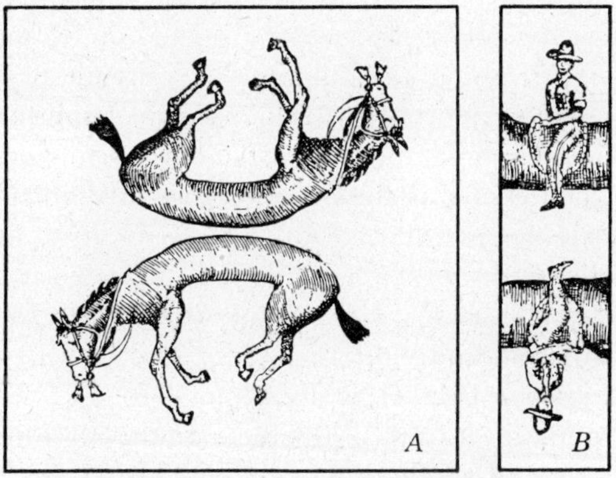

FIGURE 75. HORSE-AND-RIDER PUZZLE

The strip with the two riders on it, *B,* must be superposed on the square with the two horses on it, *A,* so that the riders will appear in proper positions, each astride a horse. (Do not break, bend or tear the two pieces.) [From *Amer. J. Psychol.,* 1941, **54,** 437 f, by M. Scheerer, K. Goldstein and E. G. Boring.]

the two pieces are shown together, with the strip, *B,* superposed upon the square, *A.* How is that possible? You turn the square through 90 degrees, so that one rider rides the head and forelegs of one horse and the tail and hind legs of the other. That is an utterly unexpected kind of a solution. All your tacit assumptions are against it.

Some of these results may be a function of the experimental setting. If the problem had arisen in the course of everyday events, the tacit assumption might never have arisen. Nevertheless, these examples are important because similar unrecognized assumptions occur constantly in the everyday course of thinking. In industrial production, for example, there are numerous situations in which tacit assumptions prevent the development of better methods of doing a job. Operation *A* has always preceded operation *B,* so everyone assumes that the order cannot be changed. The workers make this assumption without ever considering the need for it. To combat such mistaken assumptions it has been necessary to develop special techniques like time and motion studies, which locate the accepted but inefficient procedures. (See pp. 470–472.)

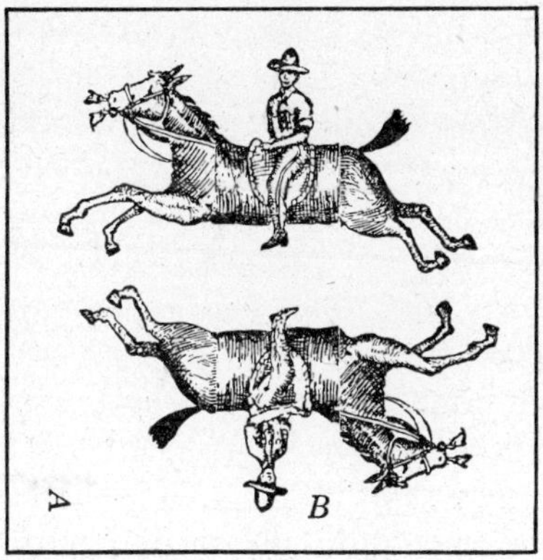

FIGURE 76. HORSE-AND-RIDER PUZZLE: SOLUTION

This figure was made by photographing the strip, *B,* of Fig. 75 lying on top of the square, *A,* of Fig. 75. Can you see how it was done?

Atmosphere Effect

Sometimes mistakes in thinking occur because unrecognized and unconscious factors attach the sense of conviction to a false conclusion which convinces the thinker that his problem is solved—when it is not. In the case of the problem of absenteeism mentioned above, the personnel expert could have said correctly (and it was probably unconsciously in his mind): "If the new method is a good one, its use will be followed by a reduction in absenteeism." What he did say is the converse of this statement, a converse that is not necessarily true: "If the new method is followed by a reduction in absenteeism, it is a good one." The one statement creates an atmosphere in which the second statement appears to be equivalent and, therefore, as true as the first.

The atmosphere effect is sometimes present in syllogistic reasoning. When you reason from a major and minor premise to a conclusion, a conclusion containing the word *all* tends to be accepted as correct when both premises also contain *all*. Thus: "All X's are Y's. All X's are Z's. Therefore all Y's are Z's." The conclusion is a *non sequitur,* but it will be accepted by many. It is easy to see the fallacy when it asserts a conclusion that we know to be wrong. Thus: "All dogs are mammals. All dogs have four legs. Therefore all mammals have four legs; [or] all four-legged animals are mammals." Atmosphere does not stifle knowledge, but it does seduce ignorance.

Atmosphere also affects opinions and attitudes. That fact becomes clear in the questionnaire studies of the values which people hold. The effects are very subtle. The way a question is worded may change utterly the frequencies of the different answers to it in a public opinion poll. (See pp. 580–584.)

Habitual Methods of Attack

Correct thinking is limited by the habitual methods of attack that the thinker employs. That these methods are arbitrary and may not be the only possible methods, the thinker is usually not aware. Like tacit assumptions and atmosphere they constitute for his thinking a limitation of which he is usually unconscious and which he is therefore not likely easily to change.

One kind of a problem will be translated almost at once by one person into an algebraic equation. Another person will try to solve the same problem by a diagram. Problems in plane geometry call for diagrams and construction figures, but multidimensional geometries seem to require algebraic expressions. A detective problem can be solved by systematic logic or by insight. Some psychologists like to put psychological problems into terms of stimulus and response and always to envision human phenomena as they would exist in animals or even in robots. Others like to stick to the terms of experience and the data of consciousness. Methods of attack differ for different individuals.

If the thinker is accustomed to use one method, it is not likely to occur to him that the method may be inefficient in a given case or even inapplicable. He will go ahead with the old familiar method instead of looking for a new one. The most successful problem solvers are those persons who are constantly on the lookout for new methods and on guard against the inefficient use of habitual action in novel situations.

A famous psychologist who investigated the nature of thinking—his name was Max Wertheimer—once posed this problem. We have a simple organism—an amoeba—which multiplies by division into two once every three minutes. Every new organism redivides every three minutes. We place a single amoeba in a jar and we find that the jar is filled with amoebae in one hour. How long will it take to fill the jar if we start with two amoebae instead of one? Wertheimer found that his friends who were accustomed to the use of mathematical procedures would start in at once to work out geometrical progressions in undertaking to answer this question. It requires a great deal of work to reach the answer in this way, but not much work or time by a simple insight. The student with this admonition and a little thought, with no formulas and no paper and pencil, should be able to give the answer with assurance, provided only he can subtract and knows how many minutes there are in an hour.

Faulty Transfer of Method

A frequent source of error or failure in thinking is the use of a method which is not adapted to the problem at hand. There is also the tendency to take over for a new problem some superficial aspect of a method successful in a different problem, while overlooking its fundamentally important feature. Another example of Wertheimer's will make this matter clear.

In one case children had been previously taught to prove a theorem about the area of a rectangle by dividing the rectangle into unit squares. By this process they found, of course, that the area was the product of the two sides. Then the children were given the problem of finding the area of a parallelogram. Some of them applied the method used before in a completely blind manner. They divided the parallelogram up into smaller parallelograms—which did not help them at all. They had transferred to a new problem a feature of the old method, but it was only a superficial aspect. They had failed to grasp the important part of the original method for finding the area of a rectangle, having learned to use the method mechanically without really understanding it.

Wertheimer blames conventional and unimaginative teaching for the fact that many children rely on this blind and superficial transfer. He complains that the schools stress drill too much and insight not enough. The child, after being shown how to do one kind of problem, practices by using the method upon essentially the same problem. Little is changed but the numbers and arithmetic involved. This kind of drill may blind the pupil to the essential principles involved in the procedure. At any rate drill is not the way to learn to be alert for novel relationships. Too drilled a child may lose the fun of learning to think.

Individual Differences

Certainly some persons are better thinkers than others. They are more alert to the perception of novel relations, to getting insight. They follow habitual procedures less inflexibly when insight—or a hunch—shows an alternative, possibly better way. They like problems, accepting the unsolved as a challenge. Their motivation to carry on to a solution is high; an unresolved dilemma keeps coming back into their field of attention, compelling them to work at it. Some men of genius fit these specifications, but not all who are proclaimed geniuses by the world.

Some people think that the intelligence tests could be used to measure thinking ability, but it is doubtful if such tests are good indicators of a person's insight.

HOW TO THINK

Thinking is not easy, and there is no easy substitute for thinking other than accepting your solutions and beliefs ready-made from others without troubling to check their adequacy for yourself. You can, however, reduce the effort of thinking by eliminating false starts, by avoiding unnecessary errors and stumbling blocks or by taking pains not to repeat the same error. There remains, however, a process which takes time and which those persons who have not learned to enjoy it regard as 'work.'

The fundamental problem of the applied psychology of thinking is the improvement of the adequacy of thinking. For the individual thinker this means improving his 'batting average' in the solution of the problems which he meets from day to day. For society at large it means reducing the gullibility of the voter, the radio listener and the reader. Thought in our culture will be improved if we better the quality of thinking which is broadcast, printed and spoken by writers, editors, speakers, commentators and men of public affairs.

The partners in that undertaking are logic, education, psychology and all the sciences, social and natural. Logic provides tests of the validity of thinking. Psychology furnishes knowledge about the actual thinking process and the causes of bad thinking. Education and the sciences provide the factual background which the individual needs in his thinking, and also training and practice in this difficult art.

It is not possible to print a dozen or a hundred practical rules guaranteed to make anyone an effective thinker. Good thinking depends upon (1) strong motivation for the particular problem in hand, (2) constant general interest in problem solving, (3) the alertness and flexibility that favor insight over the continued use of stereotyped procedures and (4) the wide range of wisdom that gives insight—the perception of novel relationships—something to work on.

In addition to these general dimensions of good thinking, not all of which lie under voluntary control and many of which it is too late for the mature adult to acquire, this chapter suggests many rules that can be applied in favor of correctness and efficiency. Here are a few of them.

(1) Because thinking takes time, best results cannot be obtained with rigid time limits. When a problem is intrinsically and strongly interesting there is no need for a time pressure. If the problem is less interesting, a time limit may serve as a convenient device for maintaining motivation. Too short and too rigid a time limit is likely to reduce the quality of thinking.

(2) Although the phenomenon is not well understood, *incubation* can be put to practical use. When thinking appears to be 'getting nowhere' and failure after failure occurs, put the problem aside for a time. When you return to it fresh, it will often progress well. You may even experience the sudden insight which comes unexpectedly 'out of the blue.'

Incubation is not effective if you have not really tried to solve the problem before resting. The success of incubation depends upon the previous labor you have devoted to the problem and the level of your motivation. Incubation cannot be used to avoid work upon the problem, and it is not a substitute for factual information. You will hatch nothing if there is not something already there to incubate.

(3) Tacit assumptions and unrecognized sets are such frequent causes of failure that we must continually watch for them. Perhaps one reason for the incubation effect is that the interval permits us to lose some of these wrong sets. At any rate, when you are 'stuck,' start looking over your assumptions and the conditions of the problem. It may be helpful to write down all the conditions of the problem and those assumptions which are *necessary*. Then examine your procedure to see if you have missed some possibilities which are not explicitly forbidden by the nature of the problem.

(4) Check the logical pattern of your reasoning. If you have had no training in logic, try to obtain it. In any case, make sure all the steps of your reasoning are explicitly stated. Frequently you will have taken for granted one or more important steps. If all the steps were explicitly stated, you might not accept them as readily as you do in their vague unformulated state.

As a check upon the validity of reasoning it is frequently useful to follow through a parallel argument in another field where the correct solution is known. For example, in discussing the syllogism (p. 210), we used first an example of a formal argument with X's and Y's, and then we took a look at the same form of argument with animals instead of the letters. In the second case we found that the conclusion was contrary to known facts. This kind of parallel check with familiar materials does not prove that the original logic was sound. The parallel might be right by accident. But when the parallel is patently wrong, the original logic does, indeed, need careful scrutiny.

Always suspect yourself when you are inclined to accept a conclusion while the details of the argument remain unclear. Let your knowledge of atmosphere effect warn you that conviction of correctness is not necessarily valid. Intuition and hunch are extremely valuable in thinking, but they are means for getting to a sound conclusion and they are not necessarily self-validating. Sometimes an insight is as self-validating as a geometrical axiom, but there is still the danger that habit or atmosphere or wishful thinking may have deceived you.

(5) A final word has to do with motivation in thinking. Thinking itself, regardless of its practical outcome, does not have to be 'work'; it can be intrinsically interesting. The modern occidental culture is an aggressive culture. We like competition. A fight is always news. In America competitive sports interest almost everyone, at least as onlookers, most of whom like the indoor contests that are waged with cards or comparable weapons. Thinking is just such a game. Mostly it is solitaire, but in it you compete, not against chance, but against nature which yields up its truth only to those who are deft, wise, alert and eager to be right.

REFERENCES

1. Allport, G. W., and Postman, L. J. *The psychology of rumor.* New York: Holt, 1947.

The how and why of the spread of rumor in relation to the psychology of perceiving, remembering and reporting with the results of experiments.

2. Bartlett, F. C. *Remembering.* Cambridge, England: University Press, 1932.

Descriptions of the author's own researches upon recollection of form, using both pictures and stories as materials.

3. Bentley, M. *The new field of psychology.* New York: D. Appleton-Century, 1934. Chaps. 14 and 15.

A careful survey of all the psychological processes. The chapters on recollecting, comprehending and thinking stress primarily the descriptive approach.

4. Duncker, K. On problem-solving. *Psychol. Monogr.,* No. 270, 1945.

Descriptive experiments upon problem solving, interpreted from the point of view of Gestalt psychology.

5. Hayakawa, S. I. *Language in action.* New York: Harcourt, Brace, 1946.

As the subtitle states, the book is "a guide to accurate thinking, reading and writing."

6. Kasner, E., and Newman, J. *Mathematics and the imagination.* New York: Simon and Schuster, 1940.

An entertaining account of some of the important concepts used in mathematical thinking; mathematical rather than psychological in its orientation, but holding many implications for the psychologist.

7. Köhler, W. *The mentality of apes.* New York: Harcourt, Brace, 1925.

An interesting and detailed report of Köhler's experiments upon insightful behavior in chimpanzees, and their use of simple tools and constructions in solving problems.

8. Stern, W. *General psychology.* New York: Macmillan, trans. 1938. Part 4. Chaps. 15 to 19.

Good chapters on recollecting, imagining and thinking, in a descriptive survey of psychology from the personalistic point of view.

9. Thouless, R. H. *How to think straight.* New York: Simon and Schuster, 1939.

The technique of using logic instead of emotion in thinking.

10. Wertheimer, M. *Productive thinking.* New York: Harper, 1945.

The approach of Gestalt psychology to thinking is summarized and illustrated by the author's own experiments with children and adults, as well as by certain instances of scientific thinking (for example, Einstein's).

11. Woodworth, R. S. *Experimental psychology.* New York: Holt, 1938. Chaps. 25, 29 and 30.

Excellent chapters on memory for form, problem solving and thinking in an advanced but clearly written survey of experimental psychology.

CHAPTER 10

Perception

IN the first chapters of this book we have studied men doing, acting and learning; but before men act they usually perceive, they sense, they note what things and events are about them. Perception is the first event in the chain which leads from the stimulus to action. To understand perception we must find out just what it is in the world that we respond to. What things are important for us, and why?

In the simplest sense, a stimulus is any sort of energy change, that is to say *event,* which can set off a response. Heat or pressure on the skin, light falling into the eye, chemical particles carried into the nose, these are all stimuli in this simple sense. For many of the simplest organisms they are all that matter. The immediate physical agent is all important. It is the water, as hot or cold, acid or neutral, which makes the amoeba swim forward or back. In the same way, the initial response of our sense organs depends upon these proximal stimuli.

As organisms become more complex, they no longer react just to the stimulus which touches the skin. They acquire also an ability to know something about what lies at a distance. The 'eyes' of starfish and the octopus can tell the direction from which light comes. The 'ears' of insects permit them to hear sounds made by their distant mates.

The receiving equipment of mammals and of men is made far more complex by the addition of a nervous system. The physical and chemical stimuli, of course, still pass through the skin, but man's reactions are gauged to objects and events often quite far away. It is the steak sizzling in the pan, the friend walking by his side, the ball flying through the air which directs what he does. For the simple animal it is only the proximal events in his physical environment, the events that come into actual contact with him, which set the pattern of his action; for higher animals the more distant occurrences are of great importance. To describe these remote stimuli a more complete inventory of the human environment is necessary. We have to go farther afield to find just what it is that, corresponding with our experience, is represented by that experience. Just what are, we ask, the more distant things in the world around man to which he responds.

It is not easy to understand fully the problem of perception. Reality, the objects and events around us, seems so tangible, so concrete that we believe the world exists just as we perceive it. Our experi-

This chapter was prepared by Edwin B. Newman of Harvard University.

ence mirrors what is out there. Or, at its worst, experience is but a slightly tarnished copy of the world. More thoughtful people realize that this view is too simple. The physicist tells us, for instance, that this hard, smooth, solid object which I hold in my hand is actually not solid at all. In his view it is many tiny bits of matter spinning in orbits like the moon's about the earth with relatively large spaces between the particles. He may call attention to other 'errors' in our perceptions. White to the eye is a simple color; to the physicist it is a most complicated mixture of many kinds of light. Consider musical tones. In our experience they are smooth and continuous. Physically they consist of a rapidly alternating series of sound waves striking our ears. Clearly then, the object out there, as a physical object, and our experience of it are two quite different things.

There are philosophers who are so impressed by the difficulty of relating our experience on the one hand to the physical world on the other, that they give up the problem altogether. Experience, they say, is the only thing which we can know with assurance. There is no proof of the existence of the physical world; hence it is only an illusion. These philosophers are the *idealists.*

Today most people reject philosophical idealism. We believe there is a real world apart from our experience of it. We accept both the fact that there is a world out there and that we as organisms respond to it. The way in which an organism responds to the world is a problem which is on a par with any other scientific problem. What happens when we perceive, and what is it that makes it happen? That is the problem of perception.

THE DEFINITION OF PERCEPTION

It will perhaps be well to set out clearly the meaning of a few of the words which we are going to use. *Perception* is the experience of objects and events which are here now. It excludes those things which are somewhere else, things about which we may think clearly but do not sense directly. Furthermore, it is convenient to use the term perception for the more general aspects of this activity, reserving the term *sensation* for those facts in our experience which depend upon how the sense organ acts.

Some perceptions seem to us to be in error. If one perception does not agree with another, we call the unusual one an *illusion.* Everyone knows, for instance, that the movement seen in the movies is an illusion. A series of still pictures is shown in rapid succession. Each picture, projected alone, is quite stationary, but when the series is shown at a proper rate we see movement. It is not true in an illusion that one perception is 'wrong' while the other is 'right.' Actually *each is just as normal as the other.* It is no easier to explain why slow projection is seen as a series of objects displaced discontinuously than it is to explain why faster projection shows the same objects moving continuously. Both kinds of seeing are complicated and need a great deal of explaining. The word *illusion* is a convenient handle for designating these unusual perceptions, but we must remember that naming a phenomenon does not explain it.

Hallucinations are clearly abnormal. They are perceptions which are unique for one person alone. If nine people in a room see nothing while the tenth sees a black cat, the tenth is probably hallucinated. Hallucinations occur occasionally for everyone. When frequent and persistent, they are almost always in our society regarded as a symptom of mental disorder. We send the person who has them to an institution for special care.

CHANGE IS THE BASIS OF PERCEPTION

Many of the facts about perception are so simple that they almost escape notice. Let us start out, however, with some of these simple facts because they are very general and apply to almost all cases of perception. One such fact is that *perception is always a response to some change or difference in the environment.* If the world were perfectly homogeneous and we were in equilibrium with it, we should experience nothing. Let some condition change *suddenly,* or one receptor be stimulated and another not, and we sense the fact at once.

Take as an example our experience of pressure. At the surface of the earth there is a pressure of 15 pounds on *each* square inch of the surface of our bodies. Yet we feel nothing. Let 15 pounds more press on a *single* square inch, and we feel it very clearly. Proof that we do not feel a uniform pressure comes from aviators who go up to an altitude of 35,000 or 40,000 feet in the air. At this altitude the pressure on the surface of the body is but 3 pounds per square inch. Still they do not feel any pressure. The same is true of the diver or the sand hog who works in a caisson under the river. These men may be subjected to pressures as great as 50 or 60 pounds per square inch. Of the pressure itself, they feel nothing.

Rapid change of pressure is a different story. Sound which stimulates our ears is just such a rapid change. Tactual stimulation is a difference in pressure between one part of the body and another. A nice demonstration of these facts may be made by a very simple experiment. Place your

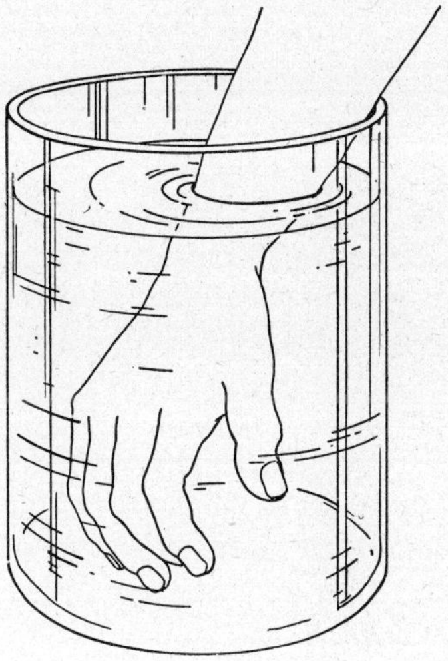

FIGURE 77. CHANGE IN PRESSURE DETERMINES PERCEPTION

When the hand is held under water, only the ring around the wrist is felt. Neither the uniform pressure of the air nor of the water is sensed by the subject.

hand in a deep basin of lukewarm water. So long as you hold your hand still, you feel pressure neither from the water nor from the air. All that you feel is the ring where the water joins the air, where there is a sharp change of pressure due to the surface tension. (See Fig. 77.)

Temperature is another familiar illustration of this same fact. What we perceive as hot or cold depends largely upon what has just gone before. If the temperature is lowered we perceive cold; if it is raised we perceive warm. This is probably all that counts. It has been said that a frog, a cold-blooded animal, may be heated up gradually while sitting in a pan of water until killed by the heat without feeling anything, at least without jumping out. The problem is somewhat more complex in man who possesses a special temperature-regulating mechanism and the means for getting ill with fever when the blood gets too warm.

The visual perceptions, white and black, are notoriously dependent upon differences. The intensity of light given off by the darkest black object in sunlight may be greater than the intensity of the brightest white object in a dim light. And yet the white object looks white and the black object black, even though the white object reflects less light than the black. What is most important is the *relative* amount of light from each part of the visual field, from the object and from its surroundings. Black is not just the absence of any visual experience. It is a definite something which is not-white. The person born blind, whose optic nerve is destroyed, sees neither white nor black; he sees nothing.

PERCEPTION IS SELECTIVE

A second general characteristic of perceiving is that it is *selective*. At any given moment hundreds of stimuli are reaching our sense organs. Out of this welter of forces acting from outside, the organism has to select the particular one to which it will attend, the one to which it will respond in some unified, coherent way. Simplicity, or singleness of response, is part of the basic biological nature of living matter.

This selectivity of perception amounts to giving one sense impression a clear track. The one impression captures or preempts the reacting machine, momentarily shutting out all other sense impressions. For the moment the favored sense impression holds sway. Later, of course, some other sense impression will take over.

In our experience we speak of these facts by saying that we *attend* to something. Only a small number of items can fall within the *span of attention*. Our experience is said to have a *focus* and a *margin*. Those items which are clearest in experience lie within the focus of attention. Mixed in with them or off to one side are many less clear items which make up the margin. Still other things, which we might be experiencing and are not, lie entirely outside the field of attention.

Your experience at this moment will make this matter quite clear. The focus of your attention is occupied by the words you are reading on this page. The margin of your experience is filled with such things as the table on which this book is lying, the sound of people moving near by, perhaps a pressure from your stomach which reminds you of lunch or a slight pain in your foot from an ill-fitting shoe. You have been quite unaware as you read this of the touch of your clothes, of slight strains in your eyes as they move back and forth over the lines of print, of the sounds of your own breathing, of the color of the paper on which this is printed. You *were* unaware of them, that is, until reading the preceding sentence made you attend to them!

Attention may indeed be selective, but it seems to be fickle in its choices. The stream of consciousness is rarely smooth and placid. It seems rather to dart here and there, never continuing for long in a single direction. Some modern writers, such as James Joyce and Eugene O'Neill, have made much of this jumpiness of experience. They try to portray the kaleidoscopic character of experience in actual words and thoughts. Carefully studied, however, the kaleidoscope turns out to be an orderly machine. Our attention may fluctuate from one thing to another but it is not really capricious. There are rules which help to predict what will gain attention and what will hold it. Here are six of the rules.

(1) The *intensity* of the stimulus is obviously the most important single factor in determining response. A loud sound, a bright light, a hard slap, an intense pain, each of these demand action, and they usually get it. Of course the basic rule that *change* is the stimulus for perception still holds. It is the sudden loud sound, the flash of bright light that gets attention and action. When it persists an intense stimulus can usually be neglected. We work under bright lights, or ride on the subway train without serious results. Severe pain may even go unnoticed. On the other hand, a sudden decrease in intensity may also get attention. When suddenly the din of a steel mill stops, the silence seems almost to shout at you. Alone in a quiet room with a ticking clock, you do not hear the clock until it stops. Then again the silence is noticeable. Nevertheless a racket is more compelling than a silence. If a whisper does not get a reply, a shout nearly always will.

(2) *Novelty* is a factor scarcely less important than intensity. Any mode of perception loses its effectiveness as it grows older. The new sight, the new sound gains relatively in strength because it is different from the old ones, contrasts with them. When we want something to be noticed, we give it a new color, a new shape, perhaps a new odor or taste, and see to it that it contrasts with what precedes it and accompanies it. Just as perceiving cannot take place at all without there being difference or change, so there must be difference or change in the factor novelty. A strange object grouped with ninety-nine other strange objects does not get attention, because there is no reason for the choice of one object more than another. On the other hand, one familiar object placed among ninety-nine novel objects does stand out and catch the eye. Paradoxical as the statement is, here familiarity is novel, or at least rare, and strange objects are too common to seem novel.

(3) The *repetition* of a stimulus helps in several ways to evoke action. First of all, a repeated stimulus is in some senses a more intense stimulus. Two shots in succession are more likely to attract our attention than one; three are perhaps more effective than two. Sometimes regular repetition helps attract attention because the first few instances sensitize us to the later ones. How often do we start to count the strokes of a clock after two or three have gone by. We hear a new song two or three times over before we really seem to hear it. Finally, the regular repetition of a stimulus often produces a set or expectation so strong that later members of the series are perceived the same way even when they have in fact been changed. An example is the 'proofreader's illusion,' the failure to see a misspelled word because of expectation of the correct form (see p. 202). The movies trade on this factor when they use 'doubles' and 'stand-ins' which the uncritical person readily accepts as if the principal actor were continuously present. Repetition also multiplies the chances of a stimulus' getting attention: if it misses on the first two tries, it may succeed on the third. Nevertheless, the effect of repetition is not primarily due to the operation of chance. There can be no doubt that the marginal occur-

rence of stimulation helps eventually to bring it into the focus of attention.

(4) *Intention*—the effect of set or attitude—is a very important factor in determining what experience is selected for attention. When we intend to speak to a particular person, he stands out quite clearly as we meet him in a crowd. When we decide to get the hammer from the shop, we see it at once even though it is out of place on the bench. The bird lover at once hears the thrush's song, while the business man remains unperturbed, examining the woods as possible pulp for making paper. Intention is in a way a rehearsal of an expected experience. When the experience comes, it is like meeting an old friend.

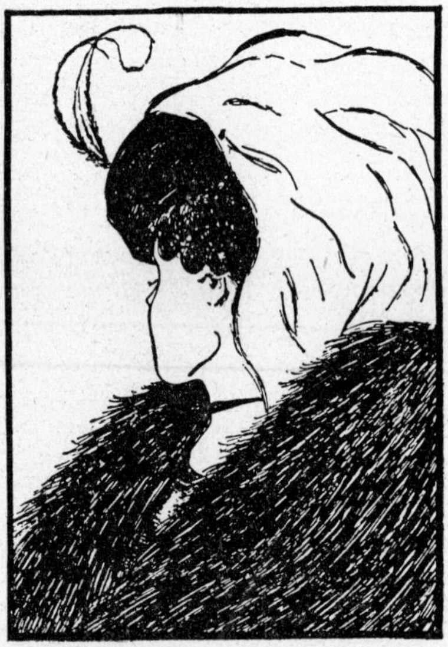

FIGURE 78. THE WIFE—AND THE MOTHER-IN-LAW

There are two equally 'good' faces shown in this picture. You can see one. Can you see the other? [Adapted from W. E. Hill.]

(5) All those forces within the individual which are lumped together as *motivation* act as a powerful selective agent in perception. The familiar example is the pretty girl of any advertisement. Senseless though it seems, 'leg art' and 'cheese cake' are basic principles of advertising. Sex appeal gets attention more quickly than any other factor. For a half-starved man the values are quite different. The odor of food is far sweeter to his nostrils than the finest perfume. Sex, food, water, need for shelter, parental love, operate both in animals and men to determine perception. Other needs, for social approval and security, for play and activity and order, may have less evident although perhaps no less real effects.

(6) Finally, selection is determined by *the part which the particular stimulus plays in the whole pattern of perception.* Each part by itself, in a figure such as Fig. 78, stands little chance of being selected. But when it is given an important role in the scheme of things, it suddenly stands out. Note how this happens as you discover the mother-in-law. An unimportant shadow becomes her eye, and an inconspicuous band her mouth. At the same time the pert nose of the wife becomes only a slip of the artist's pen.

The parts of the hidden figure were there all the time waiting for you to discover the object or to have it pointed out to you. Once the object is seen it directs attention to its own parts, makes them significant and important. At the same time, of course, it makes other details unimportant, makes them just members of the crowd as background for the star actor.

PERCEIVING IS ORGANIZED

The task of selecting among the many stimuli presented to our senses would be almost impossible were it not for teamwork among the individual sense organs. Each element of the eye does not report to the brain upon what happens to it alone; rather, a group of receptors sees a square or circle, a moving figure or patterns with more complex structure. The eyes and the brain are able to group or to organize a number of stimuli into a larger unit to which the organism now may respond in a simple fashion. This unifying activity of perception makes it possible for a person to respond to a far more complicated environment than he could without it.

The way grouping works can best be illustrated by a number of simple examples chosen to illustrate the more important principles.

(1) If there are various objects in a field, those things will be grouped which are *similar*. Look, for instance, at Fig. 79. In the left-hand part of this figure, which are the obvious series of objects? In what direction do the sets run? Up and down? right and left? diagonally? What do you see in the right-hand part of the figure?

In both parts it is the *similar* figures which appear linked together. In the left part of the figure they mark out five horizontal lines, three longer and two shorter. In the right-hand part the three cubes stand out while the small figures form a closely knit background for the cubes. It would indeed be unusual if you saw one of the tiny figures, such as the *A*, forming a pair with one of the cubes, while the other cubes formed some other figure with other parts of the background. (Can you find the *A* among the other small figures?) Similarity may be similarity of shape, similarity of size, similarity of color or, for that matter, similarity in any property of an object which can readily be distinguished.

(2) The second principle of grouping is nearness or *proximity*. How would you describe the lines at the left in Fig. 80? Everyone would say of the figures at the right that there were two people followed by a single person. The relative nearness of the two lines or of the two people makes them seem obviously a pair. Proximity is a relative matter, to be sure. Two objects might be separated by quite a distance and still form a pair if no other object of the same kind were in the vicinity.

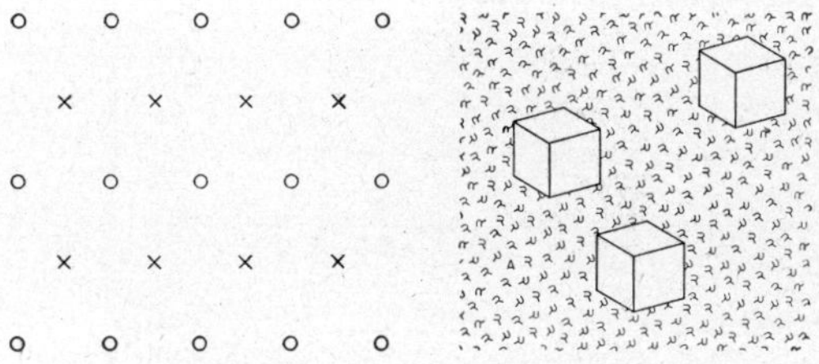

FIGURE 79. SIMILARITY FAVORS GROUPING

In the left-hand figure one sees five horizontal lines. The circles, or the crosses, are grouped together. Three figures stand out easily on the right. The small similar figures of the background form such a firm pattern that the letter A among them can be found only with difficulty.

(3) The factor of proximity may be modified to some extent by the *symmetry* of the entire figure. Compare the two sets of lines in Fig. 81. In the upper set, *A*, proximity operates so that you see three pairs of parallel lines. In the lower set, *B*, a person usually sees two sets of parallel lines with a single line on each end which forms a disturbing remainder. Set *B* may, however, be seen almost as well as three sets of broadly spaced parallel lines. Thus the pairing favored by proximity may be broken down in favor of a pairing which uses up the entire set of six lines. It is much more difficult to see this pairing across the broad space in the set *A* because this would in turn leave a remainder on either end. It is as if the organism abhorred something left over.

FIGURE 80. NEARER OBJECTS FORM A PAIR

To the left, one sees two lines, plus one. How would you describe the grouping of the three men to the right?

(4) The principles of grouping determine not only the way separate items are linked together but also how a number of parts fit together to form a figure. The choice of parts to be grouped would seem to be especially difficult if one figure is

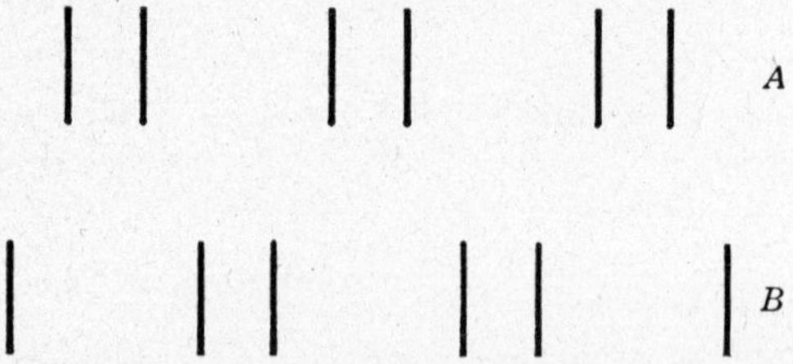

FIGURE 81. PAIRS LEAVE NO REMAINDER WHEN POSSIBLE

In *A,* the pairs favored by proximity take in all the lines. In *B,* the end lines work to favor a pairing across the longer distance.

drawn over the other one as, for instance, in Fig. 82. Here there appear to be two lines. One is a wavy line, the other is like the edge of a wall with its square corners. In terms of the detail, *a* belongs with *c* and *b* with *d.* But proximity would favor the linking of *a* and *d* or *c* and *d.* In this figure, however, the *good continuation* is the straight or continuous line, and such a grouping is favored over other possible groupings.

(5) The forces which group visual elements into a stationary figure are multiplied in a sense many times over when that figure moves. The significant links among the parts of the figure itself remain constant while the relations between parts of the figure and parts of the background are constantly changing, and getting lost in the process. A familiar example is looking through a dirty or spotted window. If the person looking holds his head quite still, it is not easy for him to know whether the spots are on the window or on the object seen through the window. If, now, he moves his head ever so slightly, all the spots on the window move in one direction while the object seen through the window moves in the other. What was unclear a moment before is now neatly divided between window and object. Elements are linked which have a *common movement.* The same things occurs to spoil camouflage. The grouse or partridge with its protective coloration will remain invisible so long as he remains still. Just as soon as all the spots of his checkered plumage move together, they are grouped in perception, and the bird is seen to be a single object.

(6) Moving figures illustrate still another principle of considerable importance. This principle is that when a figure moves, the parts of the figure will hold constant their relation to one another. The parts of the

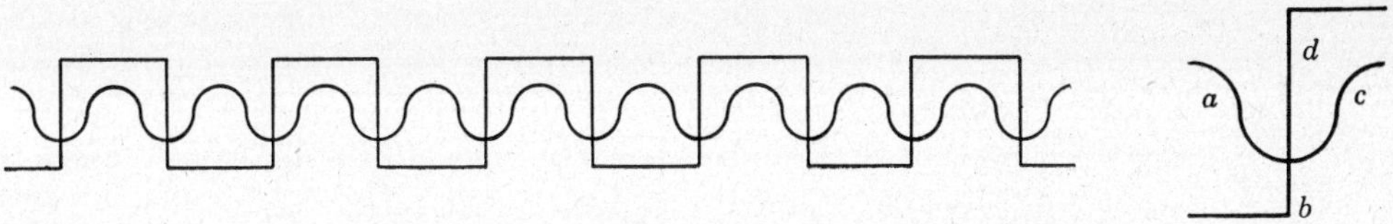

FIGURE 82. LINES ARE GROUPED INTO CONTINUOUS FIGURES

A wavy line is drawn over the square-cornered, straight line. In terms of the detail to the right, *a* is paired with *c* and *b* is paired with *d*. [After Wertheimer (1923).]

figure keep in formation as they march along, and the role which each plays will determine what points are linked from one moment to the next. A single example will show what is meant. Imagine that you have put before you nine white spots arranged in a diamond-shaped pattern as shown by the circles of Fig. 83. Let these spots disappear and a moment later let nine similar spots appear in the places marked by the crosses in this figure. Notice that four of the spots are exactly the same when they are shown the first time and the second time. If these four spots were shown alone each time, they would of course not move at all. We might suppose that the four spots would do the same when all nine were present, and the other five would have to move around them from left to right. What happens is quite different. Everyone sees a diamond-shaped pattern which moves *as a whole* over to the right. The spot which was the right-hand corner in the first presentation is linked or grouped with the spot which is the right-hand corner in the second showing. 'Right-hand-corneredness' has more to do with what is linked together than the actual stimulation of the identical spot in the eye in the first and second showing.

All the examples which we have chosen have been visual figures, largely because vision is our most complex and highly developed sense. Grouping occurs in the other sense departments as well. In hearing, for instance, the appreciation of a rhythm depends upon the linking together of the proper notes or beats in a series. It turns out in this case that the principle

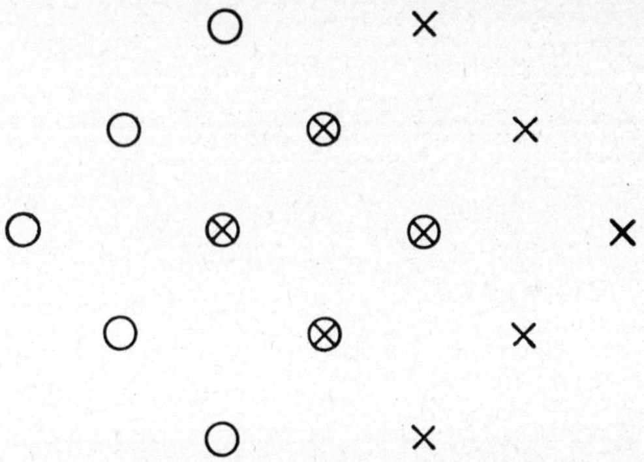

FIGURE 83. PARTS OF A FIGURE RETAIN THEIR RELATIVE IDENTITY WHEN THE FIGURE MOVES

The circles indicate the initial position of nine points of light. These disappear and are followed by nine lights in the positions marked by X's. All nine lights move equally to the right, even though the four center lights are identical in the first and second exposures. [After J. Ternus (1926).]

of proximity, expressed in time, is very compulsory. Pairs of beats, dit-dit, dit-dit, dit-dit, are invariably grouped into pairs that follow closely on one another. Regrouping across a longer interval, such as we had in Fig. 81, does not occur in hearing.

An interesting instance of grouping occurs in the skin in what has been called the *tau* effect. Try this one on a friend, as it is very easy to demonstrate. Mark out three equidistant points on his forearm or the back of his hand. They should be sufficiently separated to give a clear impression of distance. When his eyes are closed, touch the three points in succession but with your timing unequal. For instance, try 1-2-pause-3, or the reverse, 1-pause-2-3. Ask him which distance is the longer. It will be evident at once that the distances which are felt on the skin depend very much upon the grouping of the successive stimuli in time.

WHAT IS IT THAT WE PERCEIVE?

At the beginning of this chapter we noted that to understand perception we must find out just what it is in the world around us to which we respond. Before trying to answer that question, we took time to describe three important characteristics of the act of perceiving itself. It was found first that, in perceiving, the organism always responds to some change or difference in the environment. Second, the organism selects the particular stimulus or group of stimuli to which it will respond. Third, the organism links together a number of stimuli into a group so that a single simple response may be made to a complex pattern.

It is time now to return to the original question. Let us examine some of our simple perceptions to see if they help to tell us what aspects of the world are important as the stimuli for these perceptions.

THE SIMPLEST PERCEPTION: FIGURE ON A GROUND

The simplest perception is a single figure which appears against a uniform background. Imagine, for instance, that the cross of Fig. 84 is a white figure on a perfectly uniform gray background which extends out beyond the limits of vision. The experience of such a figure represents very nearly the absolute minimum of complexity that can be obtained. Nevertheless, several things can be stated about such a figure.

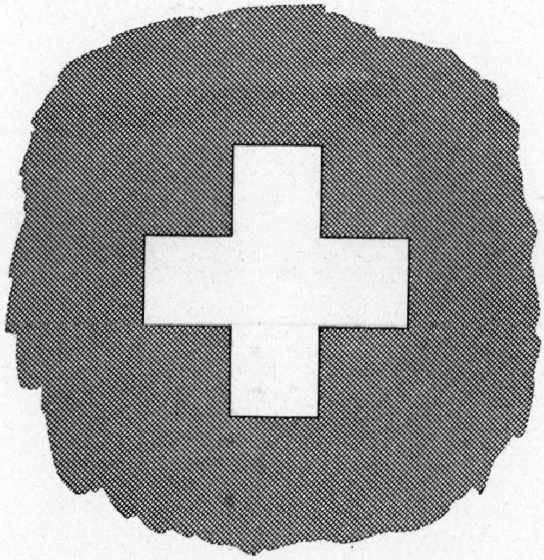

FIGURE 84. SIMPLE FIGURE ON UNIFORM BACKGROUND

Imagine that the cross is a white figure on a uniform dark gray background that extends out beyond the limits of the visual field.

First of all, the figure is seen as a single unitary thing. It has some sort of shape, it is spread out in space, and it is bounded by edges or contours. Characteristically, the figure seems to stand out slightly in front of its background. It has a color, and this color is usually seen as a surface; it is dense and opaque, seen on the face of the figure, spread out and at a definite distance away. In contrast, the ground is less well localized and has neither a well-defined surface nor bounding edges.

A simple perception such as this lies within the scope of animals which have a nervous system like man's. They respond as if they 'see' a figure on a ground. Such animals include birds and certainly all mammals. If you wish to train a cat or dog or monkey to respond to some stimulus, it is necessary that the stimulus be set off from its surroundings so that it is a clear signal.

An experiment will help make this matter clear. Figure 85 shows a pattern which was used in testing a raven. The bird was first taught to look for food under an inverted flower pot. After he had learned to find food under a pot, he watched while one of these thirteen pots was baited. If the food was placed under the pot *A*, the bird flew to this outstanding object at once and found the morsel left for him. If, however, the food was placed under the pot *B* or any of the eleven other pots in the circle, the bird was uncertain and confused and made many errors before finding the right pot.

Human memory also depends upon man's perception of a figure. In a way, this is a matter of common observation. What is not seen as a figure cannot be recalled later. In one famous experiment a series of odd-shaped patterns were shown, each of which could be seen in two different ways, having a duplicity like that of Fig. 88. Later on, the subjects were tested to see if they recognized the patterns as being the same ones they had seen before. If they succeeded, it was always because they saw the same figure in the test that they had seen originally in the stimulus. But if the alternative figure was perceived on the second showing of the stimulus, the pattern seemed strange and unfamiliar. It is the figure, not the stimulus, we recognize.

Actually, very few figures are as simple as the cross or the flower-pot pattern. Most figures are more complex and exhibit quite a number of properties, some of which we shall study in more detail when we come to the subject of vision. A few of the more important properties of figures should, however, be mentioned here.

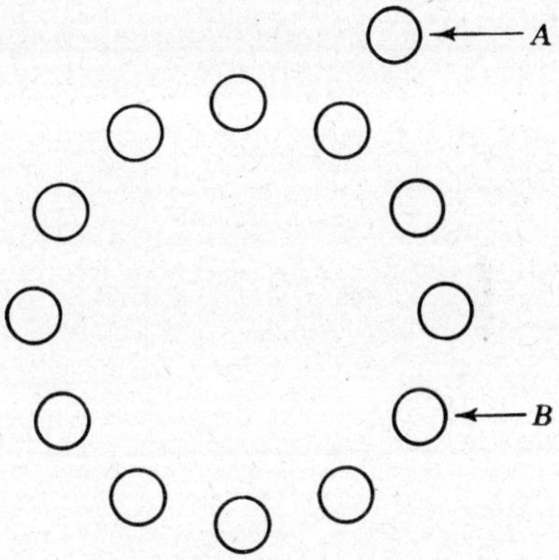

FIGURE 85. FIGURE-GROUND PATTERN USED TO TEST BIRDS

A raven could be taught to find food under the isolated flowerpot *A*. It was unable to distinguish *B*, or any other pot in the circle. [After M. Hertz (1929).]

(1) All figures have some kind of *shape*. If nothing else, they are vaguely round or extended. Usually they have a very definite form set by a sharp outline. But it is not enough simply to name and to describe the shape. Shapes can be smooth or rough, flowing, angular, compact, regularly stepped, etc. These properties represent something which the organism is doing about shape, something which goes beyond the simple geometry of the stimulus. Ernst Mach, a famous physicist, made this clear by a simple example which is shown in Fig. 86. He drew the four-sided figure in the two positions shown. Looking at the two figures, we call the one a diamond, the other a square. The diamond and the

square have quite different 'dynamics,' if we may use the word to describe something of the feeling we have in looking at them. The important difference lies in what is regarded as the axis of symmetry of each figure. In the square the axis runs parallel with the sides; the top is opposite to the bottom, and the left side is paired with the right side. In the diamond, on the other hand, the axis runs from one corner to the opposite one, and the sides which are paired are always the ones next to each other.

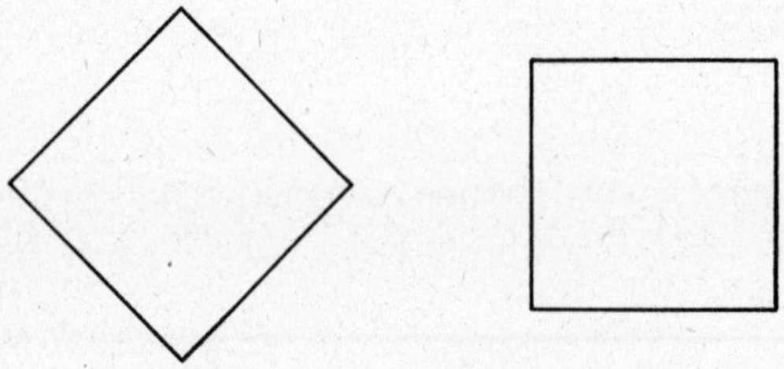

FIGURE 86. A DIAMOND AND A SQUARE

The two figures are identical geometrically, but they are perceived as two quite different shapes. [After E. Mach (1886).]

Shape makes a difference in other ways. Some shapes seem to be preferred over others and may be more readily or more frequently perceived. If a simple closed figure like a square or a circle is broken or blurred, it tends nevertheless to be seen perfect and completed. A very small brightness difference on a screen will be much easier to see if a thin line sets off a figure at the point where the difference is supposed to appear. A very faint figure will be seen more readily if it is anchored in our field of view by an index or by reference marks.

(2) Simple figures appear to have a surface which is only just evident. Objects in perception, on the other hand, seem to possess a surface which is very hard and close and definite. The difference between the two lies principally in a special sort of detail which is present in complex figures and which is called *microstructure* or texture. Microstructure is present when there is a very fine detail which is repeated continuously from one boundary of a figure to the other. There are certainly other things which contribute to our appreciation of a surface, but microstructure is probably the most important.

(3) Just as surface is enhanced in complex figures, so may the impressions of *depth* and *solidity* be somewhat greater than they are in the simplest figure. The impression of depth increases from the simplest to the most complex figures as more lines, more surfaces and planes and more figures are added. Figure 87 helps to make this clear. These outline shapes no longer appear flat and thin, as indeed they really are when printed on this page. They appear to extend back into space and to be thick and solid. In the case of the cubes we can readily imagine that there is a fourth cube behind and beneath the others filling out the unseen corner. In the other case, we see just two bars, one in front and one behind. The one behind appears, of course, to be continuous.

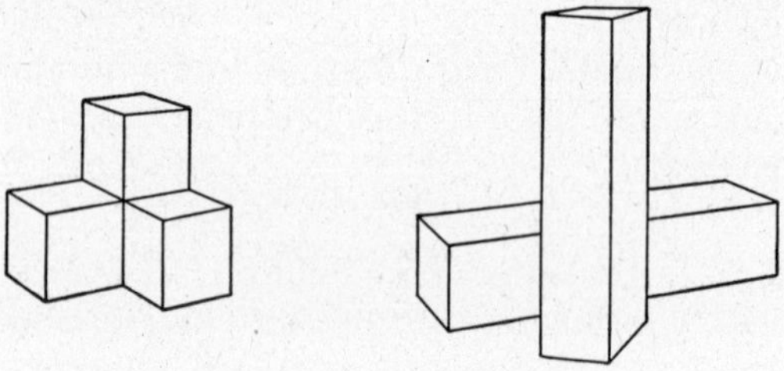

FIGURE 87. CUBES AND BARS

Line drawings frequently appear to be solid, three-dimensional objects. How many bars are there? How many might there be?

The perception of depth is the result of the common action of many factors. Some contribute largely to the appreciation of distance; they tell us how far away things are. Others have more to say about the thickness and solidity of objects. The factors governing depth perception will be taken up in detail later (pp. 298–304). What is important here is to point out that all perceptions of objects involve depth in some small degree and that a strong impression of depth or solidity can be created with patterns whose stimuli are actually flat and two-dimensional.

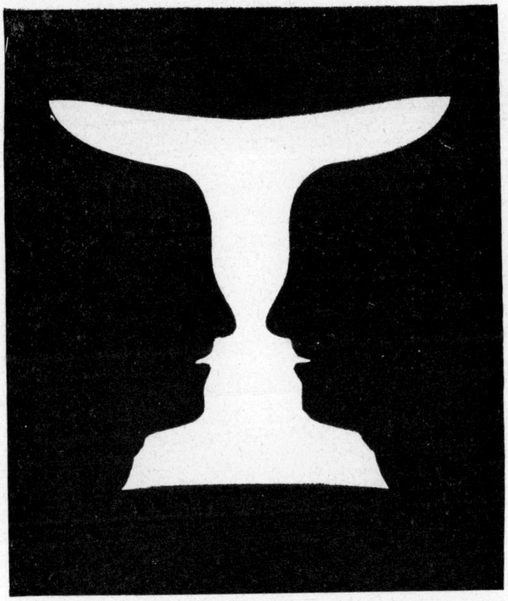

FIGURE 88. THE PETER-PAUL GOBLET

What do you see, the goblet or the famous twins? Whichever you see, try to find the other. Then, when you have found the other, try to turn the perception back to what it was at first. [After E. Rubin (1915).]

(4) Often lines are arranged so that not one but two or three or several figures can be picked out. Everyone at some time or other has puzzled over the mosaic of lines in a tile floor or in a wallpaper design. He combines first one set of lines and then another to form constantly changing figures. Such patterns, when reduced to a simple form, bring out a quite basic principle in the perception of figures. For this purpose the psychologist commonly uses a *reversible figure,* that is to say, one in which there are two equally good ways of seeing a figure, so that a person looking at it sees first one and then the other. Figure 88 and Fig. 89 illustrate two common instances. Figure 78 (p. 220) is another instance. Figure 88 is the picture of a famous goblet which outlines two human profiles. Can you find the two faces? When you have found them, what has happened to the goblet? Or examine Fig. 89. Keep your gaze as steadily in the center of the figure as possible. Do you see an × or a + as the figure? If you think you can change the figure at will, just see how long you can continue to see the × or the +.

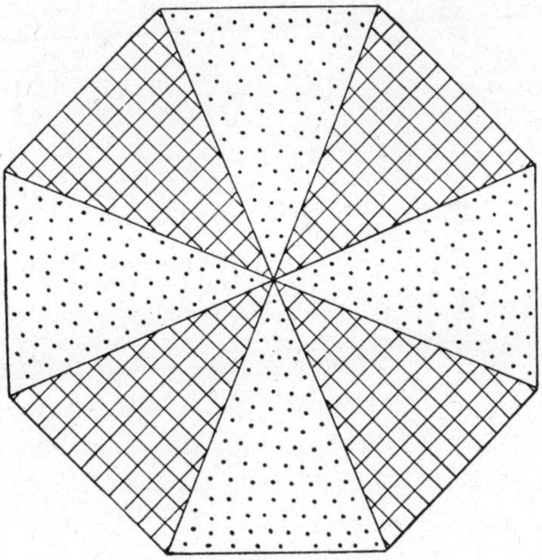

FIGURE 89. A REVERSIBLE CROSS

Keep your eyes fixed near the center of the figure, and note whether you see an × or a +. Maintain your fixation and see how long the cross at which you are looking lasts.

Once it has started to reverse, nothing can keep it fixed for long.

The principle underlying these fluctuations can be understood from an easy experiment. Gaze steadily at one of the figures in Fig. 90 while you count slowly to 25. Then turn quickly back to page 227 and glance at the center of Fig. 89. Which do you now see, the $\times$ or the $+$? Repeat the test using the other part of Fig. 90. What do you see now? Try the experiment before reading further.

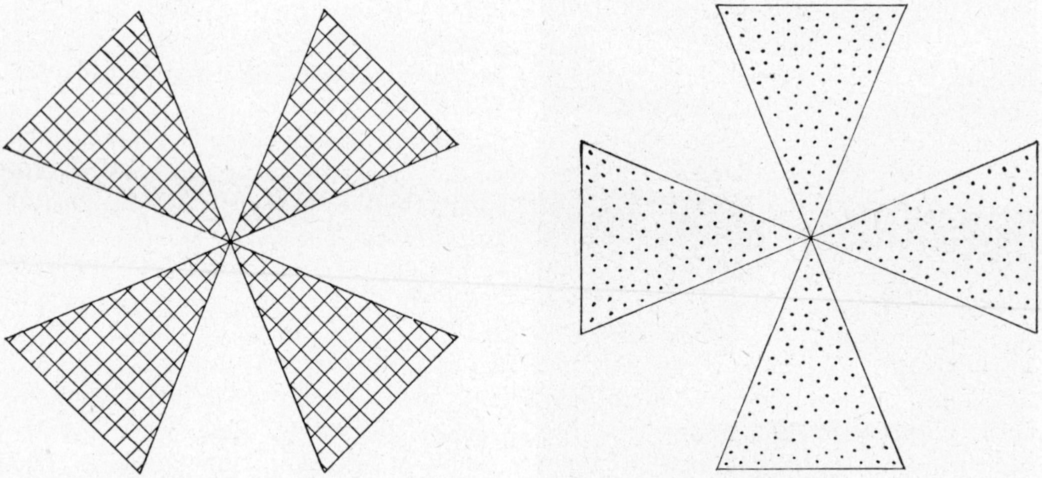

FIGURE 90. ADAPTATION STIMULI FOR FIG. 89

Keep your eyes fixed near the center of either figure for about 25 seconds. Then glance quickly at the reversible figure in Fig. 89. Is the cross you see the same one as you have just been fixating? Repeat the experiment with the other cross.

What has happened in this experiment is exactly what happens all the time in a reversible figure. Any figure process gradually weakens itself as it continues. We say that it becomes *satiated.* In Fig. 90 you do not notice this satiation because it is possible to see only one figure. In Fig. 88, however, you see one figure which gradually weakens itself until suddenly, flip, the other figure is there. Then the second figure gradually weakens itself while the first one recovers. Finally, flip, and the first one is back again.

This process of satiation affects many characteristics of a figure. Size, shape, depth, perspective, direction and mode of movement all become weakened or altered through continued observation. Under proper conditions, the changes can be measured directly, but that is rather hard as it requires very close observation. More frequently, the satiation is noted only as it leads to reversals when, as we saw above, the stimulus can be made ambiguous.

OBJECTS ARE OUR COMMONEST PERCEPTIONS

In reading the past few pages you may have had the thought, "All this discussion of simple figures is well enough in a textbook and in the laboratory, but it has nothing to do with my everyday experience." You may say that your world is full of people and chairs and tables, shoes and books and automobiles. The psychologist can explain trick figures and odd happenings, but does psychology deal with the flesh and blood of what we see and hear and feel?

Science, of course, always deals with abstractions, and the abstractions are, indeed, less 'real,' less palpable, than the actual observed things and events from which the abstractions were derived and which they are now prepared to predict. Nevertheless people, chairs, tables, shoes, books and automobiles are objects, and psychology has a great deal to say about *objects*. Just what does it say?

(1) First of all, *objects are figures*, figures in the particular sense we have been using the term. An object is something which fills a certain part of my visual field and is set off sharply from the background, and from other objects, by a well-defined *contour*. Within the contour, the object, like a good figure, is coherent and continuous. What happens to one bit of an object also happens to the neighboring bit. A perceived object acts as a unit. It is usually so constructed that the forces underlying grouping can have their strongest effect. When a drawing or a picture is designed so that it is strongly organized, it usually turns out to be such a good figure that it looks as if it ought to be an object!

(2) In the second place, objects usually present the eye with a stimulus pattern which produces *good surfaces* and *depth* and *solidity*. Under conditions which are suitable for their perception, the surfaces of objects almost always possess *microstructure*. The lines and planes of an object give rise to light and shade and perspective, which are powerful determinants of the perception of depth. Objects are commonly separated from one another in three-dimensional space. All these factors contribute to the impression of an object as a separate, space-filling thing.

(3) In the third place, objects almost always involve *cooperation among the senses*. Rarely do we receive information about an object from one sense alone. There is a rustle beside us, we look down, and there is the cat. You are looking at the pages of this book; in a moment you will reach out and turn the page, touching and pushing it in the act. A good deal of the mutual aid which one sense gives to another depends on timing. Sight and sound happen at the same moment. Sometimes this results from what the objects themselves do. The cat moves, your friend speaks; such events themselves provide you with multiple clues. In other cases the perceiving organism itself provides half the information. If you move your head or eyes a bit to one side, muscles and joints tell you about the movement. At the same time there are changes in what you see. Whenever what happens to an object is sensed in more than one way, the resulting perception is likely to be more complete and more sharply set off.

The contribution of the senses other than vision and hearing is often so subtle that it goes unnoticed. There is a tendency for the more highly developed senses of vision and hearing to 'see' or 'hear' everything, even though some of the information may have come from a simpler sense. Try this experiment. Turn the stem of your watch backward with your hands behind your back. Notice how clearly you can *feel* the clicks of the ratchet. Now hold the watch near your ear and turn the stem again. What does the *sound* of the click do to the feeling in your fingers?

(4) The fourth important characteristic of objects is that they have *meaning.* Every common object in your view is thoroughly familiar to you. You not only see it but you also recognize it as being such and such an object. Your pencil, the crumpled sheets of paper, the door, the books you wish you were reading, none of these is just an indifferent object. Even something quite new and unfamiliar has a little meaning. It is made of a familiar material. It can be used for some purpose. It does or does not belong here. Later it may have a different or richer meaning, but it is at least not a complete unknown. Ebbinghaus' nonsense syllables had this kind of meaning. They were not meaningless. They had some meaning, and their great advantage was that this slight meaning was about the same for different syllables.

Meaning in this sense, it should be pointed out, is not the same as a dictionary definition, although the two are not unrelated. Psychological meaning includes much more. Much of it is personal and individual. What some picture means to you can be quite different from what it means to me. Furthermore, psychological meaning includes shades and nuances which are expressed with difficulty in words.

Specifically, *what an object means to us is first of all what we do about it.* This object is something to drink from. That object we use to make marks on paper. Almost every object is dealt with in some way. One of the commonest things we do about an object is to give it a name. A child picks up something and quickly learns to say "book" or "shoe" or "doll." Many objects have meanings not so much because of what is done with them *now* but because of something which happened in the past. So fundamental is this dependence of *meaning* on *doing* that it has become an important principle of education.

Objects also have meanings because they are *related to other objects.* That is the rug which lies by the door. A chair is something which stands at a table. Horses pull wagons. Frequently the relations among objects are not just indifferent links but are directed in some way. This handle is a *part of* a machine. This spoon *belongs to* a set of silver. That is a leaf *from* the tree in the yard. *Part of, belonging to, necessary for,* these are samples of the many kinds of relations which objects may have to one another.

Meaning is, of course, a much larger subject than has been outlined in the last few paragraphs. A full discussion takes us into the problems of language, thinking and concept formation. The point to be established here is simply that what we see and what we hear depend in some measure on what the things we see or hear mean to us. Especially is meaning a help when we are faced with something that is confused or overcomplicated. A student's first view through a microscope is usually confused and unclear; to the skilled biologist each small detail fits into place. In contrast, meaning contributes very little at the simplest level; complication provides an opportunity for its development.

We have been discussing how objects are perceived. The question might, however, be asked with propriety: Why do we need all this explanation of how an object is perceived? Is it not obvious that there are all kinds of things in the world, and we simply perceive what is there? The answer is *no;* it is not obvious. In fact, it is not true. Here are the reasons.

To see an object is to have something happen within you. The *object* is something that you *do,* an event in your brain. It is the result of a long series of physiological events, in your eye, in your nerves, in your brain. These internal events have, in turn, been set off by proximal physical events, complex patterns of light waves and movements and pressures.

The near-by physical event usually, but not always, starts from some single region out in space, from the 'physical object' that you see, and hear and feel. That thing out there is a red book with color and solidity and weight, or at least it seems to be. Actually that is not true. The red book, the puffing engine, the crying baby, they are events within you which are about to cause you to read, to step back, to pick up the child. The 'object out there' is a physical and chemical process. You know it only indirectly. It is but one of the causes, several times removed, of the event in your brain.

That the object exists out there is something that you take for granted. That is proper, since many of the formal properties of the objects are mirrored in your experience of them. Man's adjustment to the world is aided by the fact that his brain creates an acceptable copy of what goes on outside himself. He sees squares as square. He perceives the longer of two times as the longer. There is a reasonable correspondence between stimuli and perceptions, but it is, nevertheless, contradicted by many exceptions. In perception, for example, white is simple. In light, the stimulus, white is a mixture of colors, that is to say, a mixture of many wave lengths. But seen white is known directly in experience. The wave lengths you get at only by scientific inference.

THE CONSTANCY OF OBJECTS

It would be ever so much easier if objects we once perceived stayed fixed and constant in relation to us. They do not, of course, and man is faced with the necessity of adjusting his behavior to the changing aspects of objects around him. One of the major difficulties is that, having seen an object, we move about, towards it, away from it, to the one side or the other. As we move, the proximal stimulus (the light entering the eye) changes. The image on the retina grows smaller or larger or changes in shape. There is the same trouble when the object itself moves. Or again, the colors and brightnesses of objects change as the sun rises or sets, as we pass from the sunlight into the shadow, or as we add man-made light to that provided by nature.

To the simplest organism all changes must appear alike, whatever may have been the *cause.* One thing, the immediate stimulus, is altered and for all it knows the world itself around it is changing in its very nature. To man, to us, the world is quite different. We move around among *fixed* and *constant* objects. Our point of view may change but the things at which we are looking do not. This important aspect of perceiving is called *object constancy.*

It is convenient to divide the total problem of object constancy into constancies of the various aspects of the object itself. Thus we speak of size constancy, shape constancy, whiteness (brightness) constancy, color constancy, velocity constancy, etc.

Size Constancy

Constancy of size is both one of the most perfect constancies and one of the easiest to understand. Let us take it as an example.

But first of all let us review some simple geometry.

Everyone knows that the eye acts like a simple camera. The lens in the front of the eye throws a picture of what is outside on the sensitive retina which lines the back of the eyeball. The size of the image on the retina may be determined by drawing a straight line from any point on the object out in space through a crossing point just behind the lens and extending it until it meets the retina. Such lines are shown in Fig. 91. Notice that the near arrow throws a large image on the retina, indicated by the letters *N–N*. If the same arrow were twice as far away, it would produce the smaller image *F–F*. Actually, the change in the linear size of the retinal image is exactly proportional to the change in the distance. Only, of course, the changes are reversed. The farther the object is from the eye, the smaller will be the image. If the distance is doubled, the size of the image is halved. But it is more important for our present purpose to notice that the smaller image might just as well have been formed by a smaller object such as the arrow marked *S–S*. In other words, a given change in size of the retinal image might equally well be produced by a change in the size of the object itself *or* by a change in the distance away of a constant object.

It is clear that a physical *object* of fixed size produces in the eye a series of constantly changing images as the object comes closer or goes farther away. What about our experience under these conditions? Does the size of a person's head grow larger as he comes toward us? Of course not. Only if he is very far off and we are not clearly aware of the distance, as happens when we look down from a tall building, does he seem to become abnormally small. Try the experiment of setting up a series of cards of graded size across the room as shown in Fig. 92. Hold another card in your hand and see if you can pick out the card in the series having the same size. Usually we find that the judgment is almost perfect—perfect on the assumption that there is a constancy! If the card in the hand is four inches wide and the distance of the observer from the table is twelve feet, the observer is matching the image of the card in hand to the image of the card in the series, when one image is

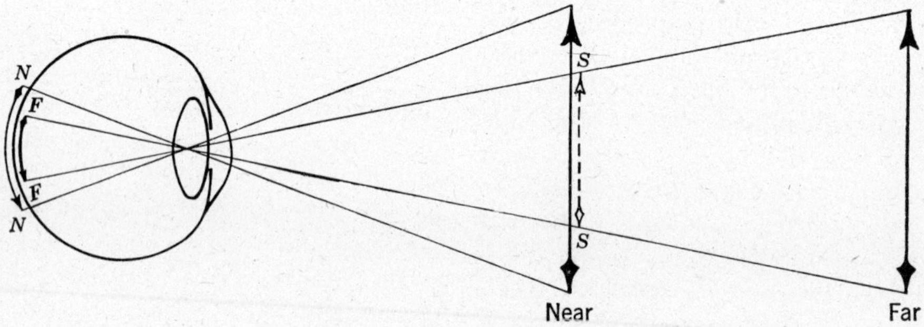

FIGURE 91. GEOMETRY OF THE EYE

The diagram shows how an object, represented by an arrow, throws an image on the sensitive retina in the back of the eye. Note particularly that the smaller image *F–F* may be produced either by the short arrow at the near distance or the large arrow at the far distance.

actually thirty-six times as wide as the other.

The secret of these amazing judgments lies largely in our ability to judge distance correctly. We know that the card across the room which throws a small image on our retina is at a much greater distance than the one we hold in our hand. Size is always judged as a function of distance.

So compulsory is constancy in the perception of size that even an artist cannot always overcome it. The drawings of children illustrate the problem in the extreme. A child is likely to draw a man the same size wherever he may be. It is not clear to the child that the drawing of a man is something which should change constantly in actual size. The child does not care too much, for his drawings are really a way of telling us about something, a kind of sign language, rather than a picture of the world.

The formal art of some Eastern peoples shows this same carry-over of size constancy into their representation of landscapes. In old Chinese and Japanese paintings in particular, objects supposed to be at different distances from the observer still have the same size in the drawing. An example of this, in exaggerated form, is shown in Fig. 93. Note how the men drawn in the background to the left are as large, or actually a little larger, than those in the foreground. It is wrong to suppose that the Japanese artist did not know better. This same artist, using a different style, might have pictured the sizes of objects correctly, but he was bound by a tradition which made it improper for him to draw figures with photographic precision. It is only that his tradition is different from ours. Even we of the Occident did not fully develop the use of perspective in art until the fifteenth century, although the general principles were understood, though not always used, by the ancient Greeks and Romans.

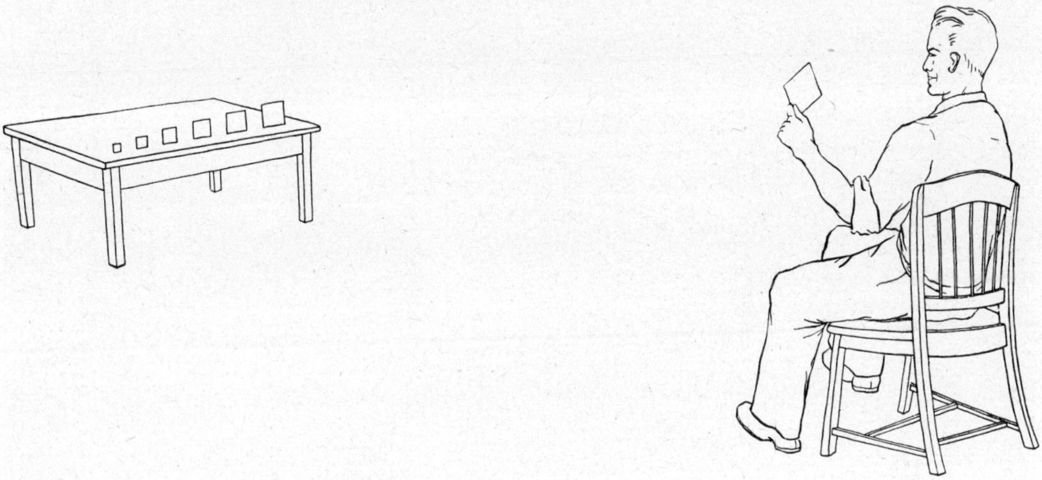

FIGURE 92. TEST OF SIZE CONSTANCY

The problem is to designate the card on the table which is the same size as the one held in the hand. The task is accomplished easily and correctly, although the retinal image of the one in the hand is at least 36 times as large as the retinal image of its match on the table.

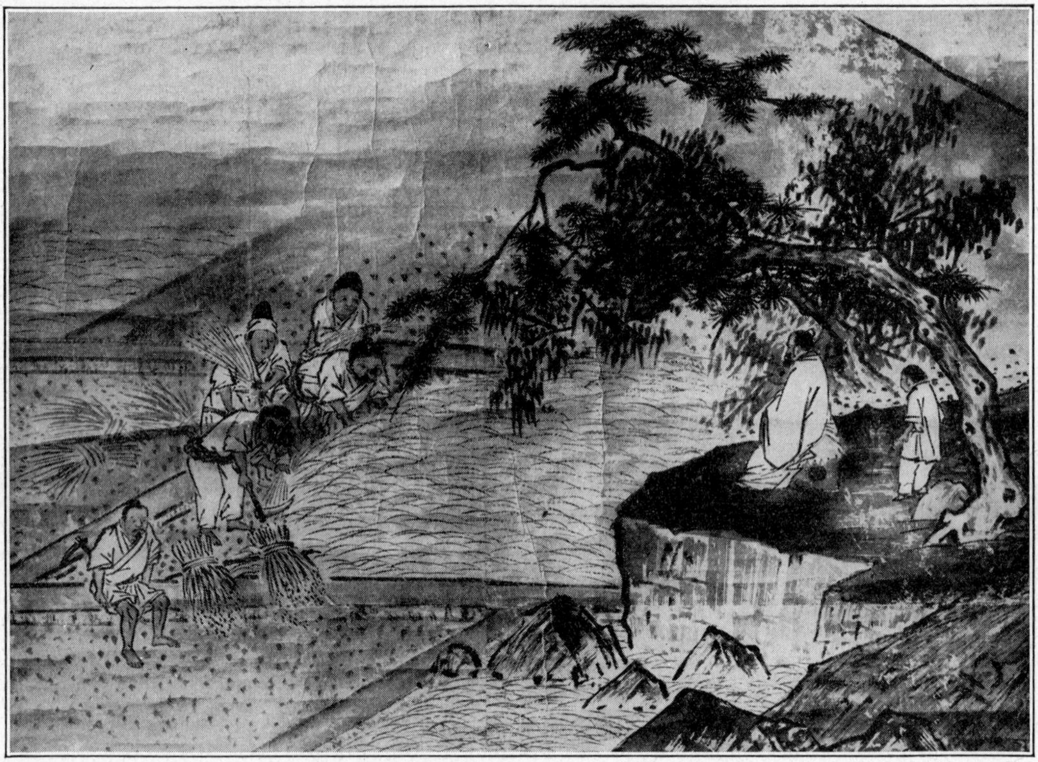

FIGURE 93. JAPANESE HISTORICAL SCENE OF THE FIFTEENTH CENTURY

A drawing by Sesshu in which the artist followed a style which did not allow for size constancy. Note the distorted linear perspective and the large size of the more remote figures. [From J. C. Conell, *Under the seal of Sesshu,* De Pamphilis, 1941.]

(Further information about size constancy appears in the chapter on visual space perception, pp. 304 f.)

Whiteness Constancy

The instance of constancy which has been most widely investigated is whiteness constancy. This visual characteristic has been in many ways more interesting than size because, since we commonly experience something less than perfect whiteness constancy, it has been possible to discover more readily which factors help the effect and which hinder it and also to measure the relative importance of these factors.

Whiteness constancy is familiar to everyone. Our scale of blacks and whites remains quite stable even though the level of illumination changes a great deal. The most common change in illumination is the result of shadows. There is less light in a shadow, and a piece of white paper, for instance, will reflect much less light when it is in shadow than when it is in full illumination. It seems, nevertheless, almost as white in shadow as in bright light, provided we know that the object we are looking at really is a piece of white paper.

To measure the effect of shadows on whiteness constancy an experiment can be set up as shown in the plans of Fig. 94. Two spinning cardboard disks, *A* and *B*, are set up in one end of a room. The light comes in from the window *W* at one side. The light falls directly on disk *B*, while a screen *S* cuts off the light from disk *A* and casts a shadow over it. A person, who is standing at *O*, compares the two disks, judging their relative whitenesses.

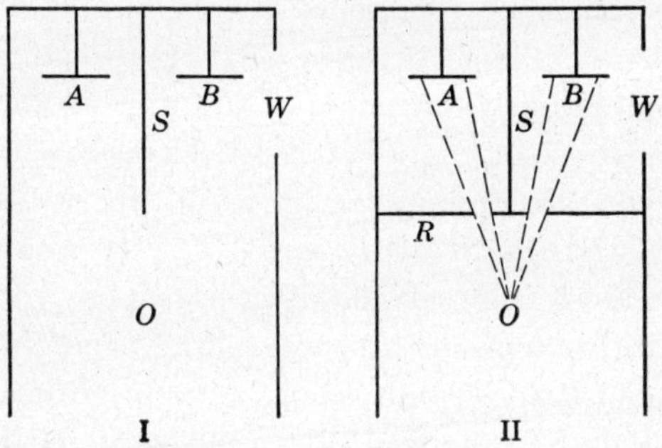

FIGURE 94. PLAN OF EXPERIMENT TO MEASURE WHITENESS CONSTANCY

Plan I shows the arrangement for measuring constancy. Plan II shows the arrangement for the 'reduction' equation. *A* and *B* are the disks to be matched. *W* is a window, the source of light. *S* is a screen casting a shadow on disk *A*. *O* is the observer who makes the judgments. *R* is a reduction screen cutting off all the field except small patches of *A* and *B*.

Each disk consists of a black and a white sector which fuse, when the disks are spun rapidly by motor, to give a uniform gray. Let us assume that disk *A* which is in the shadow is made up of 320 degrees of white and 40 degrees of black. The experimenter now adjusts the proportions of white and black in disk *B* until the observer says the two disks are equal in whiteness.

What proportions of white and black might we expect to find in disk *B*? Table XIV makes clear the various possibilities. If

TABLE XIV

RESULTS OF WHITENESS-CONSTANCY EXPERIMENT

	Disk A (in shadow)	*Disk B (in light)*	*Percentage Constancy*
Perfect constancy	320° white	320° white	100
Actual constancy	320° white	152° white	40
No constancy (reduction equation)	320° white	40° white	0

there were perfect constancy, that is to say, if the observer could discount completely the darkening produced by the shadow, disk *B* would also have 320 degrees of white.

The other end of the scale, an equation which would reveal no constancy, requires that we make a special measurement as in plan II of Fig. 94. Here a second screen *R* with two holes in it, a *reduction screen,* has been placed in front of the observer so that all he can see is a small section of each disk. No longer can he see that there is a shadow and he has to judge the brightness of each disk *reduced* to the common conditions of proximal stimulation by the reduction screen. Under a given set of conditions, conditions which vary widely from one experimental setup to another, he might find that only 40 degrees of white in disk *B* would be required in the second equation.

Now if the reduction screen is removed and an equation is made with the arrangement shown by plan I of Fig. 94, we shall be measuring the actual amount of 'constancy' achieved. Such a measurement will tell us how well the shadow has been discounted. A typical result is shown by the second line of Table XIV. Disk *B* will be 152 degrees white, a value which lies $^{112}/_{280}$ of the way from no constancy to perfect constancy.

From the result of experiments which have followed this general plan it is possible to formulate the following rules.

(1) The most important single condition of whiteness constancy is the background against which the disks are seen. In fact, it has recently been shown that almost perfect constancy can be achieved if each disk is close to its background, and the two sets of disk-plus-background are well separated. In other instances the background is effective only as fixing a general level in terms of which each item in a given part of the field is evaluated.

(2) Second in importance, particularly if the background is placed so far away from the disk that it can no longer play an important part, is the clear perception of the shadow. That there is a shadow may be seen from several details. For instance, the edge of the shadow may fall across the top of the table on which the screen and the disks are sitting. Or the screen may cast a shadow on some more remote object in the background. One way of showing how strong is the effect of the shadow is to move the screen so that the edge of the shadow falls across disk *A*. Almost perfect constancy will be the result. Shadows are recognized as such because they usually have a *penumbra,* which is the fuzzy edge that most shadows have.

(3) If there is light from some special source or if neither the background nor the edge of the shadow gives sufficient clues, constancy may be improved by putting any small object in the field of view around disk *A*. These small objects serve as tiny guideposts to give the observer information about the amount of light on disk *A*.

(4) Objects in their natural surroundings are helped out considerably by the perception of the whole pattern of illumination in a room. There will be gradual falling off of brightness as one goes away from the window or other source of illumination. Furthermore, there will be the lines of shadows all pointing away from the place from which the light is coming. Often this sort of general information about the lighting of the room helps out constancy a great deal.

General Explanation of Constancy

The general problem of constancy may be formulated without difficulty from these two examples. Let us say that each case of constancy represents a *problem of two systems.* The organism is trying to handle a situation in which the stimulus is constantly changing. For practical reasons we prefer to operate in a world in which *objects appear to be constant.* It would be most inconvenient if objects were constantly shrinking and expanding, changing their shapes and color and brightness. What the organism does is to split its information about the world into two systems, one of which it can maintain steady and constant.

In Table XV we can see just what pairs of systems are operating in the more familiar constancies. The first two columns

TABLE XV

THE PERCEPTUAL CONSTANCIES

Proximal Stimulus: Variable	*Situation of Stimulus Object: Variable*	*Property of Perceived Object: Constant*
Size of image in eye	Distance of seen object	Size of seen object
Shape of image in eye	Angle of object to the line of regard	Shape of seen object
Intensity of light in eye	Illumination on surface	Whiteness of surface
Spectral composition of light	Color of illuminant	Color of surface
Intensity of sound at ears	Distance of sound from listener	Loudness of sound at its source

Proximal Stimulus: Variable	*Condition of Observation: Variable*	*Property of Perceived Object: Constant*
Displacement of image in eye	Turning of head or eyes	Location of seen object in space
Binaural difference in time or intensity	Turning of head or body	Location of sound in space

show the two variables which the organism integrates to achieve the constancy which is noted in the third column. In size constancy, for example, the proximal stimulus (changing size of the image on the retina) works concurrently with the situation of the stimulus object (changing distance of the seen object) to effect size constancy of the perceived object. Thus perceived object size becomes the system in which things remain constant, whereas distance is the system in which they vary. In whiteness constancy, the two systems are whiteness and illumination. The former is constant, the latter varied.

The great utility of this arrangement to the organism is evident. By and large, physical objects in the world *are* constant, whereas conditions of observation are variable. The mechanism of object constancy goes a long way towards enabling the organism to deal with the physical world in a manner suited to the world's actual construction.

THE FRAMEWORK OF PERCEPTION: SPACE

Up to this time we have centered our attention on objects and have said little about the space they occupy. The objects themselves may be short, long, wide or thin, but in addition they may be located to the right, left, behind, above, around other objects in the field. Distance between two objects is just as real as the distance on the surface of one object. Space is a dimension of experience, a characteristic about which we have to ask the questions *how far? what direction? where does it start and stop?*

Space does not belong to one sense alone. It is common to several senses. Distance felt on the skin is related to the distance through which you feel your finger moving, and the size of an object held in your hand is like the size you see with your eyes. The space perceived is the joint creation of several senses and is richer for the contribution of each.

The dimensions of perceived space must be chosen with reference to the problems to be studied. The real world of objects is fitted into three dimensions—up-down, north-south, east-west or else some other system of three coordinates. The world of visual perception similarly has three dimensions—up-down, right-left, near-far. Perceived up-down may approximate the geographical vertical or it may differ from it. Near-far is not perceived so precisely as up-down and right-left; its mechanism is more complex, its correspondence with reality not so sure. In the field of auditory space perception the primary dimension is right-left, determined by the spatial relation of the two ears. Direction up-and-down is less accurately perceived, and near-far is so uncertain in heard space as sometimes not to figure at all in the localization of sound (see p. 337). Kinesthetic space—for instance, the space that an animal experiences in a maze or an automobilist in old Boston—is something else again. It is a space of connections and may have nothing at all to do with the points of the compass (see pp. 380–384).

Because there is a fair degree of correspondence between the geometry of physical space and the dimensions of visually perceived space, it is tempting to believe that there is some necessary relationship between them. It is so easy to think that we see this object near by and that object far off simply "because that is the way they are." Yet most people can realize that this statement is not true. When you look at the stars, for instance, you see them all roughly the same distance away. Actually, one star may be thousands of times as far away as another which looks to you equally distant. On the other hand, you may perceive depth where there is none. Two flat photographs when viewed properly in a stereoscope produce an impression of depth which cannot be overcome. There is no escape from the conclusion that perceived space, like other perceived qualities, is something which exists within each of us.

How then shall we account for *perceived* space? What takes place in the eye, in the brain, in order that the perceiving organism can usually respond so neatly to actual places and things? Let us consider first a few general points that answer these questions, filling in some of the details later.

(1) First of all the organism must have sense organs which are able to respond to the appropriate physical stimulus that is received from the object. The eye must be sensitive to light, the skin to contact, the ear to sound. Furthermore, each of these sense organs must be able to give a different response when a different space is occupied by the stimulus object. Thus the eye must respond differently to a large object than it does to a small one; the ears must act differently when a sound comes from the right or from the left. Patterns of stimulation are set up in the sense organs which correspond in some degree with the properties of the world we are perceiving.

(2) The brain and the nerve pathways leading from the sense organs to the brain must be constructed so that the information from the sense organs is properly transmitted and registered in the brain. It was once supposed that this effect was managed by means of a set of fixed connections, single nerve fibers running from a receptor to a fixed point in the brain. The brain was thought to be like a large electric sign with thousands of lights, each light connected by a single wire to a single switch or photocell so that a pattern of light and dark falling on the bank of photocells is reproduced point by point on the electric sign.

Modern physiology has made it quite clear that this picture of the nervous system is in error. True, there must be available a number of nerve fibers and nerve cells sufficiently large to copy the pattern of stimulation. But order is maintained among the many impulses passing to the brain only by *functional relations* among the messages in the nerves and centers along the line.

As an analogy we may think of the nervous system as a football team making a particular play. Where the play goes, the pattern of the moving men, depends neither upon exact distance nor upon particular men. *Off-tackle* means inside the end man and outside the rest of the line. Perhaps a better example would be a well-trained army as it moves forward. Each man in the skirmish and supporting line must guide his movements in terms of the men on either side of him. Once given a pattern or order of attack, that order is maintained as the entire group moves forward. Pattern is transmitted to the brain by such team play. The physiological mechanisms by which one fiber works with its neighbor include summation, inhibition, thresholds and proper timing. Order may also be maintained by electrical or chemical factors which serve to unify the actions of many individual nerve cells.

(3) Once the information received by the sense organs has been relayed to the brain, the brain takes charge of the job of interpreting this material. Each item must be located with reference to other items being perceived at that moment or to points sup-

plied by memory. Each item will be located or *anchored* with respect to a total *frame of reference.*

If a person looks at a single small spot of light in the dark, its location is a very unstable affair. The spot wanders first in one direction and then in another; it pauses and speeds up, stops and reverses, but the extent of the movement is seldom seen to be more than 40 degrees. Such seen movement is called *autokinetic.*

If a second spot of light is now introduced at a fixed distance from the first, two things happen. First of all the two spots together will undergo autokinetic movement, but the speed and extent of this two-spot movement will be less than it was with one spot alone. Second, the distance and direction of the spots from each other will undergo some change. It is as if each of the dots were trying to move as it would were it alone; yet each is constrained by the presence of the other spot in the field.

The introduction of a third spot, or a fourth or fifth, increases the effects noted when the second spot was added. With each further spot the movement of the total pattern is gradually reduced, and the relations of the spots to one another become more and more stable. From these experiments it appears that the position of a figure in the visual field depends in some measure on its anchorage to the other figures in the field. For any given item, the rest of the items in the field constitute its *frame of reference.* Autokinetic movement does not occur if there is a fixed frame of reference.

Let us look briefly at another experiment which extends this conclusion. Suppose that we are looking at two spots of light in a completely darkened room. One of the spots is much larger than the other, or, better, the larger is an outline of a square or circle. Let one of the stimuli actually move back and forth. We shall discover at once that it makes no difference which stimulus actually moves, for the small figure will always be seen to move while the large one remains at rest. Particularly is this true when the large outlined figure moves back and forth with the small figure located within it, as shown in Fig. 95.

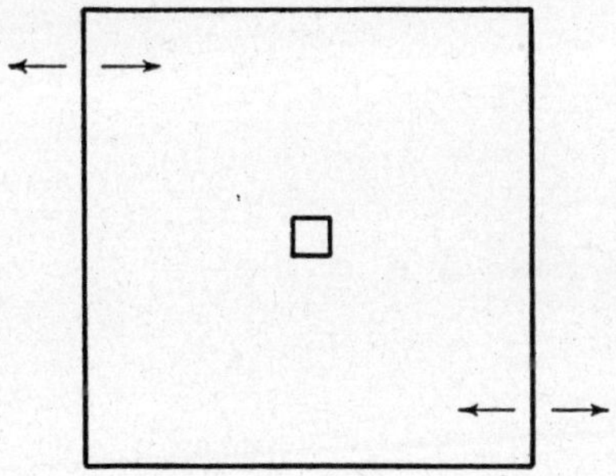

FIGURE 95. EXPERIMENT TO SHOW INDUCED MOVEMENT

An observer, sitting in the dark, sees two dimly lighted squares. The large square is moved to and fro. The small square remains stationary. The observer, however, sees the small stationary square moving, not the large square which actually is moving. [After K. Duncker (1929).]

Then the small enclosed figure will appear to do all the moving. We call this phenomenon *induced movement.* Do you remember marveling as a child upon the fact that the moon seemed to race across the sky when it was the clouds which were drifting over it? Induced movement shows us that a larger, enclosing figure forms a more stable frame of reference than a small isolated figure.

Even the rate of any movement is judged in terms of its particular frame of reference. A set of dots is arranged to move behind each of two windows, as shown in Fig. 96. The dots will have to be moved *twice* as fast physically in the *larger* window as they are moving in the smaller in order to appear to have the same velocity.

The frame of reference in which places and positions are anchored is not a matter of the present alone. Our memory of what has been seen in the past can serve us just as well. A carpenter, for instance, knows the size of each nail at a glance. The plumber picks out the right size of pipe or fitting unerringly. The skilled salesman picks the right shoe from the shelf or coat from the rack without measuring the customer. Such standards or anchors may be accumulated over a long period of time and carried unconsciously. Since there is no easy way to wipe them out, it is hard to estimate how much effect they have upon present perception.

(4) Perceived space depends on the joint contribution of several senses to a much greater degree than we ordinarily realize. A good many of the things which seem to be so natural and fundamental about space actually take form only when what we see is brought into line with what we hear, and with our feelings of movement. It is quite correct to say, for instance, that the hand is guided by the eye when you throw a ball, or that when you thread your way through a crowd, it is the eye which helps you to pick out the correct movements. On the other hand, what your eye sees would have no meaning were it not for your hand. If you were to be paralyzed all your life, and what happened around you rolled off like a movie on a screen, what you would see would have a dreamlike quality indeed. The real, substantial quality of space comes from your walking and moving in it, your doing something with it. Several well-known facts help to make this fact clear.

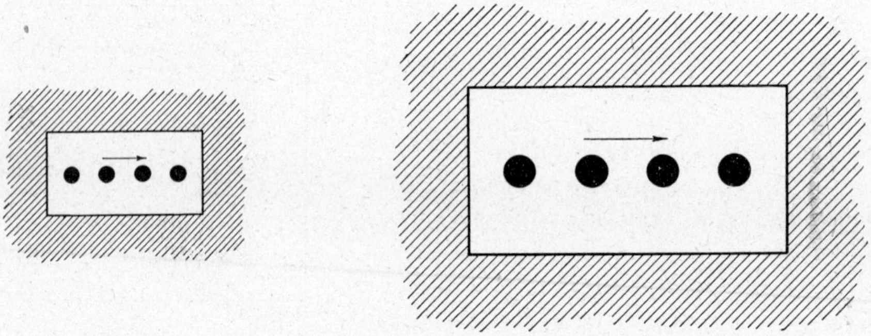

FIGURE 96. FRAME OF REFERENCE DETERMINES RATE OF MOVEMENT

The large dots moving behind the large opening must have twice the physical velocity of the small dots behind the small opening if the two sets are to appear to move at the same speed. [After J. F. Brown (1931).]

Suppose that you are looking at a movie on a screen directly before you. Let the picture jump quickly and violently to one side or up and down, and the experience is most unpleasant. Nothing is so disturbing as to watch amateur movies made by a cameraman with an unsteady hand. Now consider that the eye is far more unsteady than the worst of such movies. You glance about the room and the images projected on your retina will shift in bewildering succession. Yet in this case you see the world standing still! The difference lies in the fact that when your eyes move you have full and precise information about their movements; when the camera moves you do not. The brain is able, by a process which seems almost miraculous, to put together these two sets of facts, the moving visual pictures, on the one hand, and the knowledge of eye movements, on the other, and to come out with a stable stationary view of the world.

The adjustments of this mechanism are not always quite perfect. When you are dizzy you are no longer able to discount the movements which your eyes make, and in consequence the world 'out there' seems to move. Ear infections and diseases of the nervous system can produce unwanted movements of the eyes with the same result. Another familiar experience is that of a person who puts on strong glasses for the first time. His eyes make the accustomed movements to bring a new object into focus, but the field of view shifts too far or too little because of the strong lens. Consequently he sees everything jump each time his eyes move. Fortunately experience and practice gradually correct this state of affairs, and things eventually stay put the way they normally do.

This same kind of coordination is present when you hear a sound coming from a particular direction. Hearing the sound, you expect to be able to look for it 'there' or to put out your hand and touch it if it is near by. A psychologist once upset this relation by wearing a device he called a *pseudophone*. The pseudophone is constructed as shown in Fig. 97. It has one horn and a tube to lead to the right ear the sound which is ordinarily heard by the left, and another horn and tube to lead to the left ear the sound ordinarily heard by the right.

Wearing the pseudophone was at first a most upsetting experience. There was almost complete reversal of sounds, right and left. When the device was worn out on the street the wearer bumped into people because he would move in the wrong direction when he heard them approaching. Automobiles at a busy intersection created a real hazard. If, while he was eating, a waiter addressed him on his right, he

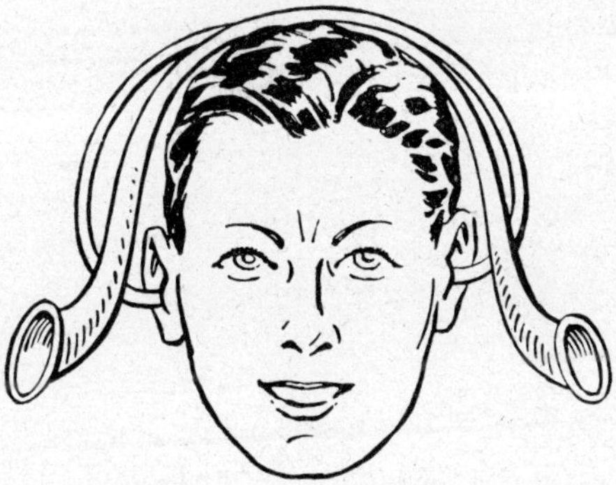

FIGURE 97. THE PSEUDOPHONE

Sound from the left is picked up by the horn and led through the tube to the right ear. Sound from the right goes to the left ear. The subject therefore looks for the source of the sound on the wrong side until he has adjusted himself to this novel artificial situation. [After P. T. Young (1928).]

would turn to the left in answering him. If, however, he saw the lips of the person who was speaking to him move, he located the sound correctly. But more interesting was the fact that, after some time, the wearer began to get used to the new locations which sound had. Unfortunately a long experiment was not possible. If the experiment could be continued long enough, a new set of coordinations between sound and sight, and between sound and movement, would probably be developed.

Two related experiments have been done in vision. In one, a set of glasses was invented which tipped everything over at an angle. Naturally, a good deal of difficulty was encountered when these glasses were first worn, but very soon everything began to straighten up. What had seemed tipped when the glasses were first put on now became vertical. The person wearing the glasses could walk about without tending to fall over. This experiment seemed to show that, when vision is distorted in this simple way, we can gradually readjust the relation between what is seen and our movement.

The other visual experiment went even farther. The glasses were constructed so that everything in the visual field was turned upside down. The subject had a great deal of difficulty when the glasses were first worn. After several days of continuous wear, adjustments were gradually made to the new appearance of the visual environment. And as the subject learned to carry out the necessary movements in this new world, the visual scene lost its character of being upside down. As a matter of fact, right side up and upside down probably have little meaning except in terms of what we do about them. *Down* is a direction we move our heads when we bend over; *up* is a direction we move our feet when we lift them from the floor.

THE FRAMEWORK OF PERCEPTION: TIME

Time, as we experience it, is a good deal like space; it is something that most people just take for granted. We are usually so occupied with what is happening that we pay no heed to the temporal frame in which our experiences are set. Only occasionally does time become the specific object of our attention, while we are waiting for a friend to keep an appointment, when we suddenly realize that the hour has grown late, in the few minutes we have left for last-minute preparations. Thus, although all our experiences are, of course, stretched out in time, it is only when some importance attaches to time that we particularly notice it.

Perceived time is also like perceived space in that it is easy to confuse physical time and psychological time. What we try so hard to judge correctly and what counts when we are making a train is clock time. Sometimes we succeed quite well in getting our personal internal clocks regulated so that they agree with physical clocks. But any person who has to 'kill' time is convinced that the physical clock runs much too slowly. Clearly, our personal clocks do not always keep the best of time. The kind of time they do keep is a matter of perception and must be explained by the psychologists.

A couple of distinctions are in order before we begin our more detailed inquiry. First of all we must distinguish between time which we can know directly and time about which we have knowledge. *Knowledge about time* is greatly aided by having elaborate means of keeping time. We are beset on every side by clocks and calendars. Our getting up in the morning, our going to class, our meals, our entertainment, all these events are regulated by clocks with elaborate means to insure their synchronization. Furthermore our lives for weeks and months and years ahead will be regulated by calendars. In the absence of such formal things as hours and dates, men have controlled their lives by the rhythms of natural events, the rising and setting of the sun, the phases of the moon, the seasons of the year. So elaborate are the schemes of marking off time that we make use of long periods extending frequently beyond the life time of any one person. In this way we know collectively a great deal about spans of time which no one can ever apprehend directly. This kind of time is important for the sociologists or anthropologists, but it is not part of our present problem.

Within the range of time which we apprehend directly a second distinction is important. In this case we distinguish between short intervals of time which we perceive directly as they pass, belonging in a way to the 'present,' and longer intervals of time where we judge that so much time has elapsed since something happened. You may be able to judge how long it has been since you began to read this section, or how long ago it was that you came into the room, without your having been aware continuously in either case that time was passing. To make a judgment of elapsed time, you have to recall specific memories.

Let us consider the simplest case. How do we know that time passes at all? What is there about our present experience which makes it part of the stream of consciousness, anchored on the one side in the past and on the other side in the future? Do we have some kind of a time sense which, acting by itself, tells us of the passage of time? Psychologists agree that the answer to this last question is pretty obviously *no.* Time cannot be appreciated directly, nakedly, as such; it can only be known through some process which goes on in time. For the physicist such a process may be the motion of a pendulum or the rotation of the earth. For the psychologist the processes which give us our impression of time are those which underlie the perception of what William James called "the specious present." We seem to sit perched on a sort of saddleback of time with a certain length of its own. The present, as we experience it, is a very small bit of duration between the past and the future, the bit which can be spanned in any one instant. A phrase of a melody is somehow a unitary thing, spread out in time and yet sensed in one instant. By trying to hold the notes of the melody or the ticks of a watch clearly in mind, it is possible to estimate how long is this directly perceived duration. Normally it is not more than one or two seconds. Certain observers have claimed that it may stretch out to eight or even twelve seconds. On what does this durable present depend?

(1) First, we should note that each experience we have persists for a very brief time. Cut off an experience suddenly by removing its stimulus and it seems to glow for a moment like the tail of a comet. It is as if the processes underlying consciousness have a certain inertia which they have to expend before they can return to quiescence. Our consciousness is somehow like the scene from the back of a moving train. Objects flash into view and then gradually fade into the distance. Sometimes this persistence is called *memory* or, more particularly, the *primary memory image,* but in general it seems better to speak simply of the *persistence of consciousness.*

(2) The flow of experience must be marked off by distinct events. Something must flash by. If what we experienced in one moment were just exactly like what we experienced the moment before, we should not be able to distinguish them, to know that the one was new, the other hanging on from the moment before. It would be as if our train were moving in a dense fog, or even in inky blackness. There would be nothing to tell us that we were moving, that time was passing. An event which marks off time is necessarily a change. Something is present now which a moment before was not there, or something is gone

now and our experience of it is fading away.

Once more we see how important *change* is to perception. As a matter of fact, the perception of time depends so fundamentally upon the perception of change that in many specific cases they amount to the same thing.

(3) Many of the changes which are fundamental to the perception of time are internal. The important background of events which furnishes the framework of time consists of subtle experiences from the body, the rhythms of pulse and breathing, occasionally the peristaltic movement of digestion, the flow of memories and images before the mind's eye. Insomnia would be no trial at all were it not for the insistent flow of these internal experiences which assail us when sleep will not come. They form the ground against which the events of the external world appear as clear figures.

Experience is a continuing, unbroken process. The experience of each moment belongs with that of the moment before. One flows smoothly and without interruption into the next. At the same time experience is constantly changing. Against a uniform background of internal pulsations and muscular strain, constant light or steady noise, one change after another erupts into our field of attention. Each momentary event appears, persists for a moment and then fades away. Fitted between other events fore and aft, it belongs to the present; it is neither imagined nor recalled.

The *present* includes everything of which we are aware just now. Some of these experiences, which have persisted, really represent the recent past. And yet they do not seem old, for they have not yet passed the threshold into the past. We experience them as being here *now* because we cannot clearly label them as belonging either to the future or to the past. To sense time fully, therefore, requires that we be able to *discriminate* between experiences that belong to the present and those that belong to the past.

It would be a mistake to think of the durable present as a problem peculiar to man's conscious experience. There are aspects of the behavior of animals which raise much the same problem. We shall have more to say later about certain time-telling rhythms which occur in animal activities. In addition to these rhythms, the simplest, free-swimming organisms possess a very elementary kind of memory, a memory in the sense that the animal 'keeps in mind' what happens from one moment to the next. The best example is the collection of bacteria in a ring about an oxygen bubble. They are exhibiting what Jennings called *trial behavior*. Imagine a bacterium swimming about in a body of water which is short of oxygen. It comes to the favored zone near the oxygen and passes readily from the poorer area into the better one. Later it starts to cross the boundary in the opposite direction. Once it touches the unfavored area, its forward motion stops and it turns back into the better area. The bacterium has made, in its simplest form, a kind of successive comparison. It is just this kind of reaction to change which is the essential first step in the perception of the passing of time.

This is the place to interrupt the argument with a brief remark. It must now be clear that the psychological problem of *the present* is very different from the philosophical one. Psychologically, the present is a part of a substantial continuing process, whether it is regarded as our experience or as some activity in our brain. The psychological present is the segment of this process which, at any moment, can influence what we do. It is a good solid chunk of time even if it lasts only a second or two. Philosophically, on the other hand, the present is but an infinitely small particle of time which has no duration. It is only the boundary between the future and the past, like the edge of a sharp shadow through which events pass. There is no movement, no flow, no existence.

TEMPORAL PATTERNS

Time not only passes; it is also patterned or structured. It is divided and subdivided by a sequence of events which follow in varied order. Let us see what happens as the rate of these events changes. Imagine that you are listening to a series of short sounds or watching a flashing light. At a high rate of speed the sounds or flashes merge into each other so that the sensation which results is smooth and continuous. Slow down the rate of interruption and a point is reached at which the tone begins to waver or roughen, the light to flicker. This critical rate may be called the *threshold of discontinuity* (or the threshold of continuity, depending upon whether you are speeding up or slowing down). The threshold will be somewhat different for light and for sound or for widely different conditions of stimulation. As a rough estimate, however, it can be said that sounds must be separated by at least one-twentieth of a second if they are to be heard as two, or that a light must flash less than twenty times per second if it is to appear to flicker.

A series of clicks or flashes at a rate slower than the threshold of discontinuity will seem nevertheless to fill up the time as it passes. We see simply a flickering light, hear a 'beating' tone or a rough noise. There is no perceptible pause between the ticks of a watch or the explosions of an idling automobile engine. The sounds or flashes are bound together into a firm series.

Let the time between sounds become long enough, however, and we begin to hear pauses. When more than one-half second comes between two clicks, we hear a click-pause-click, in which the pause has a sensible duration. Longer and longer intervals will seem to last quite a while up to the point where the beginning of the interval has slipped out of mind and can be recalled only from memory. At this point, judgment of duration depends no longer on a perception but rather on all the memories which fill up the gap between the starting point and the end.

Short Intervals

The accuracy with which short intervals of time can be estimated has been the subject of a great many experiments. It has been found that intervals of less than a second are commonly overestimated, and intervals of more than a second tend to be underestimated. Between the two lies an *indifference point,* an interval which is judged correctly since it is neither over- nor underestimated.

Our estimates of time are much affected by the way the interval is filled. If two clicks mark off the period of silence, the interval is called *unfilled.* On the other hand, a series of five or ten clicks might be presented in which the first and last clicks would define the interval to be judged. This would be a *filled* interval. Filled intervals are perceived as longer than unfilled intervals of the same objective length.

More disturbing to the judgment of time

than the number of events filling an interval is the *meaning of the material* for the listener. The duration of a word, for instance, is judged to be shorter than a noise which actually lasts the same time, and meaningful sentences seem to be shorter than an equivalent series of nonsense syllables. Other factors which increase the interest of the listener in what is going on have much the same effect. On the other hand, an interval with a striking beginning and end will be perceived as longer than one with indifferent boundaries. Either the sharp intense stimuli call particular attention to the passing of time, or they add a short bit of duration on either end of the interval.

Rhythm

Rhythms are patterns in time which are marked off by regular beats with varying emphasis. Simple rhythms have every second, third or fourth beat accented. But the accent alone is only part of the pattern. Subjectively the important thing is the way the beats are grouped. Thus, the count of *one,* two, three is different in grouping from a count of one, two, *three,* or one, *two,* three; and in poetry iambic meter differs from trochaic meter, depending upon the place of the stress in the foot. Rhythm depends, then, on two basic factors, *grouping* of beats into measures or feet and the *accenting* of one or more of the beats in each measure. Rhythms become more complicated when (1) the time intervals between beats are no longer equal and regular and (2) when more than one level of accentuation is introduced, giving rise to subgroups within the measure.

In the absence of any accentuation in the objective rhythms, the person listening will nearly always supply his own. Try to listen to a series of absolutely uniform clicks and you will find yourself involuntarily grouping them into twos, threes, fours, or even groups of six or eight beats. The commonest subjective groupings are of two or four beats; if a larger group of six or eight beats is heard, it is almost sure to be subdivided into two sets of three or two sets of four.

For the perception of rhythm the rate at which the beats follow each other must be neither too slow nor too fast. The possible range is from about two-thirds beats per second up to 8 beats per second. The most pleasing rates usually fall between 70 and 90 beats per minute or roughly 1.2 to 1.5 beats per second.

Rhythm plays a great part, of course, in artistic expression. All the basic forms of music, dancing and poetry are rhythmic. Curiously enough, a comparable form of art which makes important use of visual rhythms has never developed. Perhaps this is a result of technical difficulties in producing rhythmic visual patterns; more probably it reflects rather a fundamental difference between the sense modalities. Rhythm appeals to the ear and to the sense of bodily movement, the *kinesthetic* sense. These are the senses which offer us sharply defined events against a continuing background. Visual events are not nearly so abrupt and discrete as those of hearing; visual objects are, after all, substantial and do not suddenly appear and disappear. Sounds, on the other hand, start and stop under circumstances where the seen object remains steadily in view. Furthermore, sound, or silence, furnishes us with a continuous background whether we care to listen or not. Vision can be shut off by our own fiat; we shut our eyes or turn our heads away. Kinesthesis resembles hearing in these particulars. Perhaps it is not so strange that rhythm belongs peculiarly to sounds and to bodily movement.

ORIENTATION IN TIME

Our ability to tell time, to wake at a particular hour, to judge periods several hours in length without recourse to a timepiece, presents quite a different problem from the one we have just been discussing. This ability has been tested in an experiment in which a subject spent nearly four days in complete isolation in a soundproof room. The subject was provided with a bed, supplies of food and water, paper, pencil and a telephone with which he could communicate with the experimenter at will. At irregular intervals the subject reported what time he thought it was then. Between reports he ate meals, made notes, slept and amused himself as well as he could under such restricted conditions. Within the first day the subject's personal 'clock' had gained more than four hours. Then it began to lose and at the end of the experiment his guess about the time was less than forty minutes in error, closer to the correct time than it had been since the start of the experiment.

How this man was able to maintain his orientation in time will be better understood if we digress for a moment to see what is known of some of the important time-telling rhythms in animal behavior. The longest, and yet highly precise, rhythms are those connected with the migration of birds and fishes. Year after year we see the ducks and geese flying north in the spring and south again in the autumn. Each flock sets off on its flight at almost precisely the same date each year. Bird lovers are accustomed to finding individual species of warblers arriving each spring within a few days of a customary date. How are these migrations controlled? Our best guess at the present time is that the length of the day is the principal factor. Temperature and food supply appear to be secondary factors. Changes in the total light are known to produce fivefold to tenfold changes in the size of the pituitary gland, which in turn secretes more or less of several hormones. These control many other organs of the body. Nature apparently uses this mechanism to start many species of birds north to their breeding grounds in the spring.

Many other long-term rhythms are known in other animals. Arctic animals such as the weasel, hare and fox change the color of their coats with the season. Certain marine worms swarm with the full moon. Army ants alternate between a nomadic and sedentary life. In all these cases we find evidence of the same thing, *environmental control of a particular physiological mechanism.* The animal is sensitized so that he can tell time from nature's clock.

By far the most general rhythm in animal behavior is the diurnal one, the daily pattern of sleep and activity. Animals vary, of course, as their peak activity comes during the day or night. But their hunting and eating, their hiding and sleep, even their sex life follow a daily cycle that is governed by the sun. Offhand it would look as if this diurnal rhythm, like the longer ones, is controlled by light, temperature, sound or some other environmental stimulus. In some measure this is true. Female rats, for instance, always come into heat at night. If the lighting cycle is changed so that it is dark during the day and light at night, the rat's estrus peak comes in the dark during the day. Its occurrence is obviously controlled by the cycle of light and dark. But there is this very important difference. A blind rat, or one kept continuously in the light, shows little or no disturbance of the normal four-day estrus cycle. In other words, the light acts only to synchronize the already rigidly established rhythm within the animal with the changes in the environment.

There is evidence to indicate that the diurnal rhythm generally is something of this kind. Normally sleep and activity are synchronized with the environment, but in the absence of environmental changes the rhythm will maintain itself with considerable precision. A group of rats were placed in a room with a 28-hour 'day'; lighting, watering and feeding were all geared to the longer day. It might have been thought that they would adapt to this new day, but apparently they did not, for in each 28-hour cycle they showed a peak of activity just 24 hours after the time they had been previously fed. In these diurnal and estrus rhythms, then, we are dealing with a *self-maintaining physiological rhythm.*

The behavior of men does not show such neat control as the behavior of rats. Remnants of both the types of mechanisms which we have discussed above probably exist. It is not hard to believe that the restlessness of spring fever has its roots in surplus hormones brought forth at that season of the year. Physiologically rhythms such as estrus are quite clear-cut. Diurnal rhythms are harder to discover because they are so strongly reinforced by social conventions as to cast doubt on their underlying physiological nature. Travelers report, for instance, that Eskimo life north of the Arctic Circle continues around the clock during the month-long summer day. Nevertheless, we do get clues from our bodies when we make temporal judgments. Four psychologists had their alarm clocks set at odd hours between 12:15 and 4:45 A.M. When awakened, they guessed the hour. They discovered that depth of sleep was one of their most obvious clues, followed closely by the dark brown taste of indigestion and the necessity to urinate. These clues do not belong to the basic diurnal rhythm, and a more clever experiment will be required to settle whether our sleeping once a day is a social convention or sound physiology.

Two other important mechanisms can be recognized in our time telling. The first of them is the conditioning, often unconscious, of particular behavior to some clue in the environment. Some of the best examples can be found in individuals who wake up in the morning "like clockwork." A careful examination nearly always shows that there is some particular happening to which each of these people responds. For some people the clue is the sunlight, for others it is the sounds of traffic or the arrival of the milkman or the early departure of a neighbor for work. Similar conditioning establishes our hunger at mealtimes or our drowsiness in the late evening. Daily habits of long standing apparently can go quite far in regulating our basic bodily mechanisms. These habits represent a sort of involuntary keeping of time. Intentional estimates of time would be well anchored by this habitual framework.

In addition to this subtle sort of conditioning, it is possible for us to make quite explicit use of memories in gauging the amount of time which has passed. If you think of how long it has been since you arrived home, you are able to recall that you went to your room and washed up for supper, that you talked briefly to your roommate, that you read a letter waiting for you when you arrived, that you have now glanced over certain features of the evening paper. Some memories may afford you quite exact estimates, such as the known time of your accustomed walk from school to home. In other memories the clue may be the sheer number and clarity of them which crowd into your mind. A morning in a new and strange place seems very long in retrospect because of the many novel experiences it contained, or, again, your estimate may be influenced by the restlessness and boredom which you recall or by the absence of memories of moments when time was heavy on your hands. Whatever may be the whole pattern of these explicit memories, it is evident that they form a most substantial clue against which we all can check our personal clocks.

To sum up, we can say that orientation in time depends on four factors: (1) externally controlled physiological rhythms, (2) self-controlled physiological rhythms, (3) habitual acts conditioned to environmental cues, and (4) the pattern of memories which belong to the interval being judged. From all these factors we build up a framework of time in which our present actions are set. External events and our own actions have special meanings for us as they fit into this framework. Thus we come finally to have a kind of 'time perspective' pointed both toward the past and toward the future.

REFERENCES

1. Boring, E. G. *The physical dimensions of consciousness.* New York: Appleton-Century, 1933. Chap. 5.

   A fairly modern view of mind-and-body. This chapter deals with the perception of time.

2. Boring, E. G. *Sensation and perception in the history of experimental psychology.* New York: Appleton-Century, 1942.

   Describes the historical setting of the more important current problems in perception, and in vision and hearing as well.

3. Carr, H. A. *An introduction to space perception.* New York: Longmans, Green, 1935.

   A simple, and not too complete, summary of the conventional material on space perception.

4. Harrower, M. *The psychologist at work.* New York: Harper, 1937. Chaps. 2 and 3.

   A popular account of how a Gestalt psychologist deals with a few of the facts of experience and their relation to behavior.

5. James, W. *Psychology: briefer course.* New York: Holt, 1892. Chaps. 17, 20 and 21.

   James' discussion of space and time and of the stream of consciousness; it has been modified by many new facts, but the breadth of his account is still without peer.

6. Köhler, W. *Gestalt psychology.* (2nd ed.) New York: Liveright, 1947. Chaps. 4, 5 and 6.

   Three chapters on Gestalt principles applied to some problems of perception. Still the best introduction to this school.

7. Koffka, K. *The principles of Gestalt psychology.* New York: Harcourt, Brace, 1935. Chaps. 3, 4, 5 and 6.

   Contains a comprehensive account of perception written from the Gestalt point of view. Difficult and erudite.

8. Woodworth, R. S. *Experimental psychology.* New York: Holt, 1938. Chaps. 24 and 25.

   Chapters on form, color, space and attention. Factual and readable, the best single advanced text on experimental psychology.

CHAPTER 11

Sensation and Psychological Measurement

THE chief business of the living organism is adaptation to its ever-changing environment. The protozoan, swimming along near the muddy floor of a pond, turns aside from the sharp cold of a fresh current and moves toward a safer region. Man's problems and man's responses may be more complicated than the protozoan's, yet man, crossing the street in traffic, dodging taxicabs in the five-o'clock rush hour, solves similar problems of avoidance in similar ways. Both cases involve perception: the protozoan perceives cold and the man perceives the oncoming rush of steel and glass which is the taxicab. All organisms, from protozoan to man, preserve themselves in a careless universe by a knowledge of the external world which comes to them through their sensory mechanisms.

The preceding chapter has dealt with problems of perception. In perception the organism does all it can to get the best possible information about the external world. A piece of coal in the sunshine may reflect more light than a piece of notepaper in the shade; yet we see the coal as black and the paper as white. The constancy phenomenon has come into play here; it helps us to recognize these and other objects in a way which has most meaning for us. So too the organism gets the third visual dimension of space; it sees that a mountain or a trolley car has not only height and width but also solidity. As it 'interprets' the data from its two eyes, so also the organism 'interprets' the data from its two ears, not merely hearing a sound—the horn of the taxicab—but knowing also the direction from which it came. In short, in one way or another the organism musters all its resources to the end that it may get the most valuable information about its environment; and this process we call *perception.*

Sensation Is the Core of Perception

The way from the external world to the brain is via the sense organs, and these remarkable organs, responding to light, sound, heat, cold, pressure, touch, etc., are the windows through which we look out at the world about us. The sense organs start the messages along the nerves, the highways to the brain. When these messages merge at the higher centers of the nervous system, when they organize themselves and modify one another through interactions and associations, we call the re-

This chapter was prepared by S. Smith Stevens of Harvard University.

sult perception. But the bare messages themselves, isolated and apart from their mutual influences, we call sensations.

We get at sensations by analysis, by paying attention to certain aspects of our perceptions. It is much like the artist painting his landscape. Where the casual observer sees a valley partly shadowed by a rocky hill, the artist sees a patch of purple jutting into a field of green and speckled by reddish brown dots. By selective attention he analyzes the organized scene into patches of color and he translates these sensations into pigments on canvas.

The student of sensation goes farther. He learns to attend not only to color as such but also to its several modes of variation, to its redness and whiteness and grayness. And the object of his analysis is an understanding of the behavior of sensory processes: How do sensations arise? what causes them to change? how many aspects of them can be separately distinguished and how can the aspects be measured? what takes place in the sense organ and in the sensory nerves? and how do these events depend upon the physical, chemical or mechanical happenings in the world outside? The answers to these questions are the laws of sensation, laws that are based upon careful experimental measurements.

STIMULUS AND ATTRIBUTES

In order to understand the laws of sensation we must first know what is meant by a stimulus and by attributes of sensation such as quality and intensity.

Stimulus

A stimulus is any change in external energy that activates a sense organ and its receptors. It is a stimulus only when it stimulates. Light is not a stimulus to a totally blind person. The radio waves that fill the air are not a direct stimulus to any organism that we know of. Many phenomena of nature affect no sense organs, and these phenomena come to our attention only indirectly by way of their effects or by way of the elaborate inferences of science. The important phenomena that can be classed as stimuli are mechanical, thermal, acoustic, chemical and photic.

Man himself reacts to many kinds of *mechanical* stimulation. He has the tactual sense of his skin, by which he appreciates the presence, size and shape of the objects with which he comes in contact. He can feel pain, which warns him of violent or dangerous contact. He perceives his own posture by means of the proprioceptive organs that lie in his muscles and joints. By their use and by vision he maintains his erect position. He perceives certain contractions of his stomach and calls them hunger. He perceives dryness in his mouth and throat and calls it thirst. These instances are samples of the wide variety of mechanical events which can act as stimuli in man.

Thermal stimulation is also effective for man. He must keep the temperature of his body constant. If it varies a little he may be ill; if it varies much he may die. Although his body is equipped with a remarkable system for automatic thermostatic control, he needs also to help out by conscious adaptive behavior. The thermal sense tells him when to put on heavier or lighter clothes, when to start the electric fan, when to turn on the radiator.

Acoustic stimulation affects most animals that live in the air and some that live in water. Hearing, which shares with vision the important function of giving information about distant stimuli, is a very important and highly developed sense. Persons suddenly made deaf, and deprived of speech and music, seem to suffer even more from their deficiency than the blind. These people say that they live in a "dead world." Sound, more than anything else, signifies that the world is alive and moving.

Taste and smell are *chemical* senses, the direct descendants of the chemical sense of fishes. Taste is a liquid sense; it is stimulated only by substances in solution. Smell is an air sense; it is activated by small particles of substance diffused in the air. Although a highly developed sense, smell is little used by man, who, with his erect posture, keeps his nose away from the ground where most of the smells lie. The dog, nose to ground, finds how extremely informative olfactory stimuli can be.

Vision is the *photic* sense, and light is man's most important stimulus, even though the other senses may, in the blind, become remarkably effective substitutes for vision. Whereas the lower animals sense only the intensity of light, man and some of the higher vertebrates can discriminate its wave length as well; that is to say, they can see hues as well as blacks, grays and whites. Probably this sensitivity to difference in the wave length of light is one of man's most recent sensory acquisitions, for the development of color vision is still incomplete in that an appreciable portion of the population is color blind. Most animals are also color blind, responding to differences in the energy, but not differences in the wave length, of light.

Attributes of Sensation

Since there are many ways in which a sensation can change, an observer, experiencing a sensation, describes it completely only when he has specified its value with respect to every possible dimension of change. These possible dimensions constitute the attributes of sensation.

Suppose a congenitally blind man were suddenly given perfect vision and shown a red square. This single experience would not teach him anything about the attributes of visual sensation, but we could soon show him what some of them are. First, we could change the square in *quality* by altering its hue toward orange or purple or gray, telling the man that this sort of change is a change in the qualitative attribute of color. Then we could change the square in size to teach him about the attribute of *extension*. To change the time of its exposure would be to exhibit *duration* to him. Some psychologists think that hues also have an attribute of *intensity*, which they call *brightness*. A difficulty arises here, however, because *brightness* is *whiteness*, and white is a color quality. At any rate all the other sensations have an intensitive attribute. Tones can be loud, smells and tastes strong, pressures and pains intense.

It is conventional to classify the sensory attributes under four main heads: *quality*, *intensity*, *extension* and *duration*. There can be, however, many more than four sensory attributes, for there are just as many attributes as there are possible modes of variation of sensation. In his course in psychology the college student often discovers attributes that are new to him, for most people do not know, until they are taught, that colors vary in three dimensions in a system that is represented by a solid figure and that tones change in volume and density as well as in pitch and loudness. Perhaps there are some sensory attributes which the psychologist himself has not yet discovered.

The problem of attributes comes up for animals as well as persons. For instance, size is an attribute of visual experiences. Can a rat perceive *size?* Yes, because he can learn to choose, for a reward, the larger of two circles. Can a rat perceive *shape* as such, independently of all the other spatial properties of visual stimuli? Probably not. Figure 98 shows the stimuli of an experiment which was arranged to test the capacity of human and animal subjects to perceive triangularity as such. The subject was first trained to choose the triangle and avoid the square in the standard pair of stimuli, *S.* He was then tested to see whether he would choose the triangle instead of the other figure in each of the other seven pairs of stimuli, *A* to *G.* If he chose the triangle in preference to the square in *S* because it was a triangle, he should choose the triangle instead of the circle in *A* and the inverted triangle in *B;* he should choose the triangle instead of the rotated square, without regard to the rotation of the triangle, in *C* to *F;* and he should prefer the dark triangle to the dark square in *G.* Since each pair of figures is equated in total area and thus in total brightness, and since the triangle was shown as often on the right as on the left, it can be argued that shape—not brightness, angular position or size—must have been the basis for the original discrimination in *S.* The general problem has proved, however, too hard for the rat. A chimpanzee almost succeeded in it, and a child did succeed. Thus it is apparent that a human being is able to analyze a perception more specifically into its attributes than a rat or even a chimpanzee.

It is important to realize that a person has to learn about particular attributes before he can describe experience in terms of them. People learn readily enough to distinguish between size and brightness, but most animals do not. Color-blind persons do not easily discover the defects in their color sense because they are not especially trained to analyze their color experiences. Instead they are told that the grass

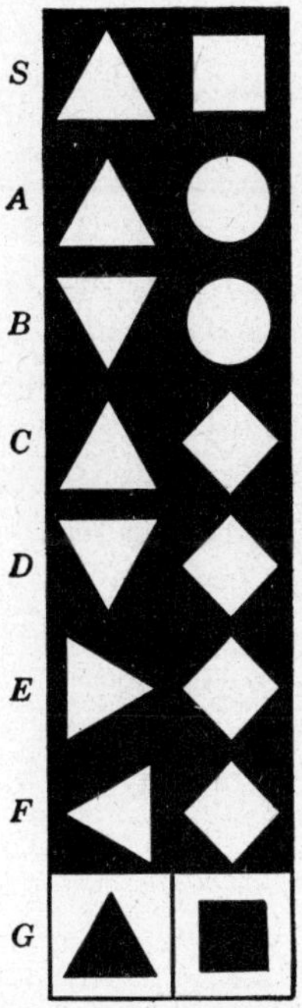

FIGURE 98. DISCRIMINATION OF SHAPE

The subject was trained to choose the triangle in pair *S.* Then the experiment was arranged to discover whether he would choose, without further training, the triangle in each of the pairs *A* to *G.* The stimuli were large, and were presented with the triangle as often at the right as at the left. A child learned to discriminate 'pure triangularity' in this way; a chimpanzee almost, but not quite, succeeded; a rat failed. [From L. W. Gellerman, *J. genet. Psychol.,* 1933, **42,** 14.]

is green and that the rose is red, although these two objects may be to them the same color. And faced with the task of making an impossible color analysis, they avoid giving attention to color attributes, and rely, when they can, upon their knowledge of the nature of objects. No roses, they remind themselves, are green, and grass is never red.

Quality

All the senses but hearing seem to be based upon a few *unique qualities,* which may unite in fusions to give other secondary qualities.

In *vision* the seven unique qualities are red, yellow, green, blue, white, gray and black. All other colors occur as blends of these unique colors. (See pp. 270–274.) In *smell* the unique qualities are fragrant, ethereal, spicy, resinous, burned and putrid, and a huge number of intermediates that fit in among these six. (See p. 356.) In *taste* the unique qualities are sweet, saline, sour and bitter, and for these, too, there are intermediates. (See p. 353.) In *somesthesis,* the body sense, the unique qualities are pressure, pain, warmth and cold. There are also a great many complex patterns of these four qualities, like hunger, dizziness and itch. (See p. 360.) *Hearing* is the one sense that cannot be reduced to a few unique qualities. The tones form a continuous series of qualities from the lowest pitch to the highest. Instead of a mere four or seven unique qualities we have in hearing all the separate pitches the ear can hear, a thousand or more.

Why do we experience different qualities? Why is a sight so different in quality from a sound? How can the brain tell a smell from a pat on the hand? Actually, there is almost no satisfactory physiological theory of sensory quality. All we know about quality is that the fibers for each of the five senses lead to a particular part of the cerebral cortex. It seems probable that of the four unique qualities of the sense of touch each has its special nerve fibers; that, in hearing, although a given tone excites many fibers, its quality may be dependent upon the excitation of one particular fiber more than the others. In vision it seems likely that there are only three kinds of nerve fibers in the optic nerve, and that the six or seven unique colors are not differentiated physiologically from the others until the excitation has reached the brain. There the mystery is complete. All we can say is that, when an organism is making a qualitative discrimination, it is distinguishing between the excitation of different systems of nerve fibers.

Quality indicates *what* neural system is functioning, which fibers are excited. Intensity, extension and duration merely tell *how* the system is functioning. That is why quality seems to be more fundamental than the other attributes, why we talk about the loudness of a pitch but not the pitch of a loudness, about the duration of a red but not the redness of a duration.

Intensity

Usually the intensity of a sensation increases when the energy of its stimulus is increased. A paperweight makes more noise if it drops from the desk to the floor than if it drops only a few inches. On the other hand, intensity of sensation also varies with the sensitivity of the sense organ. In hearing, for instance, sensitivity is greatest in the middle of the musical scale. A tone in this region, therefore, requires less energy than a low tone in order to sound equally loud.

Both vision and hearing are senses tuned to respond to certain limited ranges of a continuous stimulus. The electromagnetic waves, some of which we call light, extend through a long range (see Fig. 114, p. 275); yet the retina responds to only a limited range of these wave lengths. The long infrared waves and the short ultraviolet waves are invisible under most circumstances. For visible light the retina is least sensitive at the two extremes of the spectrum and most sensitive in the middle. (See Fig. 126, p. 291.) Similarly the ear responds to only a limited range of tonal frequencies, being completely deaf to very low and very high frequencies and most sensitive to the middle frequencies of the musical range. (See Fig. 154, p. 324.) Thus it is plain that, if we wish to predict the intensity of a sensation, we must know about the stimulus, its frequency and its energy, and we must know about sensitivity as well. The sensitivity of the organism to a given stimulus is just as important as the energy of the stimulus.

PSYCHOPHYSICS

The obvious fact about sensation is that it arises from an interaction. Some form of energy impinges upon a sensitive receptor in a living organism, and the organism reacts. The organism sees, hears, smells, tastes, feels. These reactions are psychological processes, set in motion by physical events. When we study sensation, therefore, what we discover is the relation between those two aspects of the universe commonly called the *mental* and the *physical.* We learn how experience depends upon stimulation. We learn what it takes by way of a cause to set off a response in a perceiving organism.

Psychophysics was christened by G. T. Fechner, a physicist and philosopher, who in 1860 gave us a treatise on a new science of the "relation between mind and matter"—meaning the relation between sensation and the stimulus that causes it. Fechner's basic notion was simple. He believed that, if he could measure both the strength of a stimulus and the magnitude of the sensation it arouses, he would have a formula relating physics and psychology. He asked, for example, how great is the loudness we experience when we listen to a sound wave of a given energy. Or how bright, subjectively, is a light of so many candle-power?

These are complicated questions, as later chapters will show. We no longer give them the same answers that Fechner gave, for psychophysics has moved ahead, and new methods of psychophysical investigation have been evolved. These methods are used nowadays to answer practical, everyday questions as well as to settle theoretical problems. They are essential to engineers and designers as well as to psychologists. All attempts to adapt machines and gadgets to the sensory capacities of human beings raise problems in psychophysics which can be solved by its methods.

The story of the telephone is a case in point. The earliest instruments were unreliable devices. You spoke your message and the listener asked, "What did you say?" You shouted into the mouthpiece and he still did not understand. Trial-and-error on the part of inventors brought improved clarity, but the last word in high-fidelity transmission was impossible until the psychophysics of hearing had been explored. In one of the world's largest research laboratories careful studies were made of the behavior of the ear: its sensitivity to different frequencies, its response to sounds of varying intensity, its ability to hear tones masked by noise. These researches established the performance requirements of the telephone: how it should transmit the sounds of speech in order for them to be correctly perceived. Knowing what they were aiming at, the designers could then proceed.

Psychophysical Problems and Methods

The procedures used in psychophysical studies are as varied as ingenious researchers confronted by complex problems can make them. There are two useful ways, however, of classifying them: (1) by the type of judgment or reaction made by the subject in the experiment; (2) by the method of presenting, controlling and measuring the stimulus. Thus the problem has two facets: the psychological and the physical. There are several ways of getting at the psychological experience of the subject—ways of having him respond—and there are many procedures for manipulating the physical energies and forces to which he is exposed. In general, our choice of procedures is guided by the nature of the problem we set ourselves, but we often find it impossible to follow what might be the ideal method. We cannot, for example, change the intensity of a smell by known physical amounts in the way we can alter the intensity of a light. Many problems in psychophysics must wait on further developments in the other sciences.

It is the business of psychophysics to ask questions about the behavior of man and animals. And since the character of a science is revealed by the kind of questions it poses—and by the way it tracks down the answers—we do well to list the types of questions asked and answered by psychophysical procedures. Of course these are technical, scientific questions, designed to reveal the laws and principles of behavior. They are the kinds of questions that involve measurement and experimentation guarded by careful controls. Broken down into their principal categories, we find that these questions raise seven kinds of psychophysical problems.

(1) *Absolute thresholds.* What is the smallest stimulus that will set off a response on the part of an organism?

> *Example.* How faint is the faintest light a man can see? (*Answer.* Five to seven quanta of light energy falling on the retina may produce a visual response. A quantum is the smallest package of light energy possible in nature.)

(2) *Differential thresholds.* What is the smallest *change* in a stimulus that can be detected?

> *Example.* How many ounces must be added to a pound in order to make it feel heavier? (*Answer.* About half an ounce.)

(3) *Equality.* What values must two stimuli have in order to produce equality in a given attribute?

> *Example.* What intensity of red light appears as bright as a given intensity of green light? (*Answer.* The red light must have about eight times the physical intensity of the green light.)

(4) *Order.* Given a set of stimuli, what is their order of progression from least to greatest with respect to some attribute or quality?

> *Example.* What is the relative merit of the music of these composers: Bach, Beethoven, Chopin, Grieg, Tschaikovsky, Wagner? (*Answer.* By 308 members of four leading symphony orchestras the music of these composers was preferred in the order: Beethoven, Wagner, Bach, Tschaikovsky, Chopin and Grieg.)

(5) *Equality of intervals.* When is the apparent difference between two experiences the same as the difference between two other experiences? Or, as a special

case, when does one sensation appear to be equidistant between two other sensations?

Example. What note on the piano has a pitch that sounds equidistant between middle C and the c four octaves above it? (*Answer.* Not the c at the second octave above middle C, as you might suppose, but the note g above this c.)

(6) *Equality of ratios.* When is the apparent ratio between two experiences the same as the apparent ratio between two other experiences? Or what stimuli produce sensations having a given ratio with respect to each other?

Example. How many ounces *feel* half as heavy as a pound? (*Answer.* About eleven ounces. Eight ounces feel much less than half as heavy as a pound.)

(7) *Stimulus rating.* How accurately can a person name the correct physical value of a stimulus which he can sense but cannot measure directly?

Examples. Several of them, mostly unanswered questions: How accurately can aviators estimate their height in feet above the ground? How well can policemen estimate the speed of passing cars? How precisely can a farmer estimate the area of a field? In trying to answer these questions the experimenter would usually be interested, not only in the accuracy of the estimate itself but also in the factors which tend to increase or decrease the accuracy. Some of these factors would come under the heading of what we commonly call illusions.

To each of the types of problems listed above we can apply a variety of psychophysical procedures. In other words, we can present the stimuli in a variety of ways and we can ask the subject to indicate his response in several manners. These methods and their many variants have important uses in psychology in all its branches. Some of them permit the detailed scrutiny of the function of the sense organs themselves. Some of them enable us to measure sensation and tell how one sensory experience compares with another. Others have more practical uses. They make it possible to grade commodities like leather and perfumes and wines in terms of psychological scales set up by experienced judges. They even provide the basis of techniques that are used in the polling of public opinion and in the assessment of consumer attitudes.

SCALES OF MEASUREMENT

Measurement is the backbone of the scientific method. Primitive peoples usually speak of "a lot of" this or "a little of" that. Scientists, trying to get away from being primitive, like to pin numbers on things. They are not content with the mere statement that something is hot or cold. Instead, they ask what its temperature is in terms of degrees on a scale. Not many centuries ago there were no scales of temperature and no way of making hot and cold a quantitative matter. Methods of measuring temperature had to be devised. Someone in the middle of the seventeenth century had to invent a thermometer.

Psychology uses many of the scales employed in the other sciences, and it also invents scales of its own with which to measure in psychological dimensions. We have scales for measuring attitudes, intelligence, learning, sensation, etc. Some of the scales are rather crude affairs; some show considerable refinement. The accuracy and usefulness of any scale depend, of course, upon the care and ingenuity of its creator, but they also depend upon other things, particularly upon which of the four basic kinds of scale is being used. These four categories of scales are called by the names (1) *nominal scale,* (2) *ordinal scale,* (3) *interval scale* and (4) *ratio scale.*

(1) The *nominal scale* is the most primitive of the four. In fact it is not, in the ordinary sense, a scale of measurement at all. But for the sake of completeness we must include it here, because it is what we achieve when we pin numbers on objects or on classes of objects in order to keep track of them. For example, a coach numbers the football players on his team, or a manufacturer uses a model number to stand for a class of automobiles. There is actually more to this simple-minded procedure than meets the eye, for if the coach could not tell his players apart in the first place, he could not give each player a different number. And it is only because the automobile maker thinks all of a certain group of cars are equal in some respect that he gives them all the same model number.

We see, therefore, that the nominal scale is not entirely trivial. It has great practical importance, and, what is of more interest to us, its creation really depends upon our ability to determine (*a*) that something is present (so that we can give it a number) and (*b*) what other things are equal to it (so that we can give them the same number). In other words, we have to be able to answer the psychophysical problem of equality—problem 3 in our list above.

(2) The *ordinal scale* is more interesting. It is the kind of scale we can set up whenever we can determine the rank order of a set of items. Thus the composers listed on page 256 are arranged on an ordinal scale of merit, from greatest to least, in the opinion of other musicians. A scale of rank order cannot be set up unless we can solve problem 4 above: the determination of the direction of a difference.

On the ordinal scale of musical merit we find that Beethoven is better than Wagner, who is better than Bach. But this scale does not tell us how much better Beethoven is than Wagner, nor whether the difference between these two is the same as the difference between Wagner and Bach. In other words, the ordinal scale is not a quantitative scale in the layman's sense of the term quantitative. It is nevertheless a very useful device, as is shown by the fact that many such scales are in daily use. They are used to rate applicants for jobs, to scale personality traits, to measure intelligence and to grade examination papers. (See Fig. 99 for ordinal scales.)

When the instructor gives you A, B, C or D on a term paper he is using an ordinal scale. Of course he may give a numerical instead of a letter grade, but that does not change the situation. When you get 90 and your friend gets 70, it means that your paper is somewhat better than his (from the instructor's point of view), but you cannot say how much better it is. This is true simply because there is no way of knowing whether the *units* on the instructor's grading scale are equal from unit to unit. Is the difference between 70 and 80 the same as the difference between 80 and 90? Since neither you nor the instructor can answer that question, we are forced to conclude that he grades on an ordinal scale.

Actually, if you were to count up all the scales described in books on psychology, you would find that most of them are or-

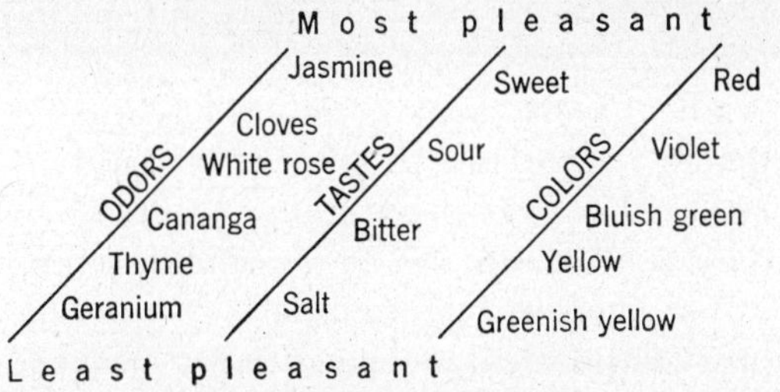

FIGURE 99. SOME ORDINAL SCALES OF PLEASANTNESS-UNPLEASANTNESS

Odors: samples from a list of 14 olfactory stimuli ranked by 8 observers using the method of paired comparisons (each stimulus compared with each other stimulus).

Tastes: average rank order obtained from 7 to 10 observers who rated each taste on a three-point scale. The concentrations used were 20 times the threshold concentration (the least concentration detectable as different from plain water). At other concentrations the rank order may be different. For example, at 10 times the threshold concentration salt is preferred to bitter.

Colors: 18 squares of colored paper were ranked by 1279 college students using the method of paired comparisons. Many factors and causes may alter a person's preference for colors.

[Data from J. G. Beebe-Center, *Pleasantness and unpleasantness,* Van Nostrand, 1932.]

dinal scales. It is far easier to arrange things in rank order than it is to devise scales for measuring them in terms of equal units. But rank ordering is not always easy. How, for example, would you scale the following traits in order of their importance for success in business: perseverence, courage, honesty, initiative, optimism, friendliness, intelligence, loyalty?

(3) The *interval scale* is one on which the units are equal but on which the zero point is arbitrarily chosen. The ordinary Fahrenheit temperature scale is a good example. The units (degrees) are equal, but the zero point is just an arbitrary temperature chosen by the German physicist, Fahrenheit, that of a freezing mixture of ice and salt. The centigrade scale is another example of an interval scale, and it has a different zero point, the temperature of ice water without salt (Fig. 100). On both these scales we know that the units are equal because we set up the units by marking off equal distances on a column of mercury or alcohol, which expands with increasing temperature. Then each rise of one degree in temperature lengthens the

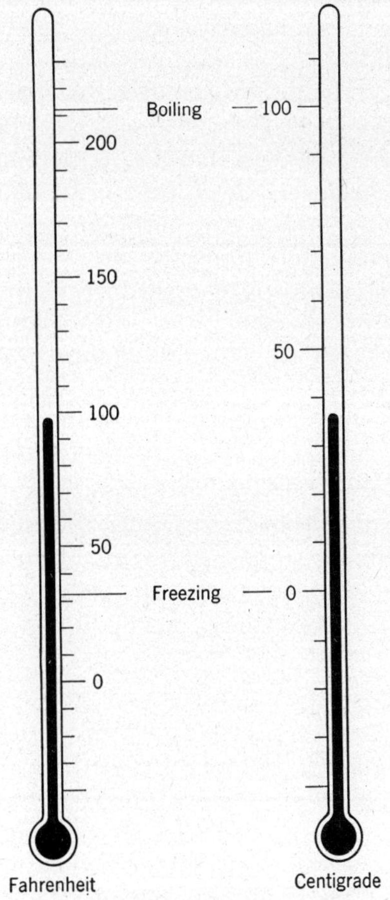

FIGURE 100. INTERVAL SCALES

On each scale the units are of equal size, but the Fahrenheit units are five-ninths as large as the centigrade units. Each scale has a different zero point, and neither zero point on the scale represents a 'true' or 'absolute' zero in temperature.

column by the same amount. By this procedure we solve for temperature scales the problem of equality of intervals, the same kind of problem we listed on page 256 as psychophysical problem 5.

When equal intervals can be determined for sensation, intelligence or some other psychological variable, scales having equal units can be established. The intelligence tester makes the units on his scale as equal as possible by adjusting (*a*) the difficulty of the items on his test and (*b*) the numerical credit given the testee for passing a given item. He then concludes that the units are equal if a large group of children, chosen at random, make scores that distribute themselves according to the normal curve (p. 262). His conclusion is correct, of course, only provided the intelligence of the children is really normally distributed—something the psychologist can *assume* but not prove in advance. Nevertheless, by proceeding on this assumption of a normal distribution, we get highly useful scales for measuring human traits and abilities, scales having reasonably equal units but whose zero points are generally arbitrary. An uncritical critic might make the rash claim that his competitor has no intelligence whatever, but he would speak loosely, for no one knows what zero intelligence is.

(4) True zero points are possible only on *ratio scales*. And in order to set up a ratio scale we must be able to determine not only equal intervals but equal ratios as well. Scales of length, weight and electrical resistance are examples of ratio scales. In fact so are most of the other scales used in physics. We can demonstrate that two inches is half of four inches and that four inches is half of eight inches. If we knew nothing about these ratios we should not know where to put the zero point on the scale, and *vice versa*.

The *stimuli* used in psychophysical experiments are nearly always measured on ratio scales. The *sensations* produced by these stimuli can also be measured on ratio scales whenever we can solve the psychophysical problem of sensed ratios (problem 6, p. 257). For example, if we can find out what weights feel half as heavy as what other weights, we can set up a ratio scale of perceived weight, as distinct from the physical weight which we measure in pounds and ounces. With the aid of the psychological scale of weight, we might then be able to tell the grocer how to package his dried beans so that a package of one size will feel fifty per cent heavier, say, than the next smaller size.

Figure 101 shows a ratio scale of perceived weight. This scale was obtained by the simple procedure of having a group of subjects select from among a graded series of weights the one that felt half as heavy as a given standard. Standards weighing different amounts were used, of course, and the complete data were employed to construct the curve in Fig. 101. The dotted lines illustrate the basis on which the curve was drawn; a weight of 100 grams gives a psychological impression which we say arbitrarily corresponds to one psychological unit or, to name the unit, one *veg* (from an old Anglo Saxon word meaning "to lift"). Then 0.5 psychological unit must correspond to the physical weight that feels half as heavy, since 0.5 is half of 1.0. But our experiment tells us that 72 grams feel half as heavy as 100 grams. Therefore our graph must pass through the cross and also through the circled point on the plot—the point indicated by the dotted lines connecting the value of 0.5 veg on the vertical scale with 72 grams on the horizontal scale.

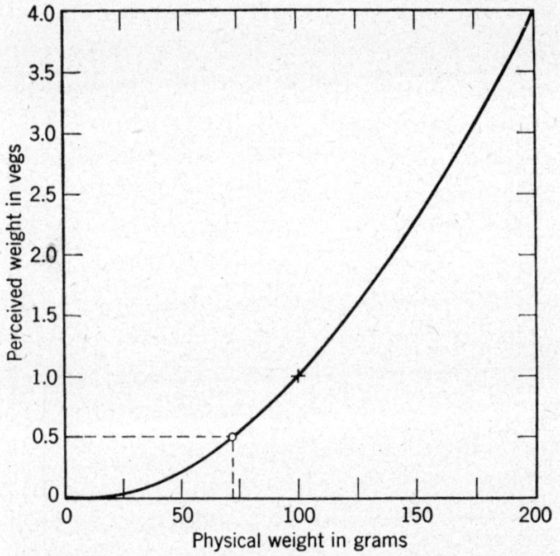

FIGURE 101. PSYCHOLOGICAL RATIO SCALE

Relates perceived weight in vegs to physical weight in grams. A *veg* is defined arbitrarily as the value of the subjective impression obtained by lifting a weight of 100 grams. By experiment it is determined that 72 grams feel half as heavy as 100 grams. Therefore half a veg corresponds to 72 grams. The curve shows that perceived weight increases much more rapidly than physical weight. [Data from R. S. Harper and S. S. Stevens, *Amer. J. Psychol.*, 1948, **61**.]

By extending this logic we obtain other points on the curve, and eventually we map out the entire graph relating perceived weight and physical weight.

STATISTICS AND MEASUREMENT

None of the seven basic problems of psychophysics can be solved without the use of statistics. The reason for this is obvious. The behavior of living organisms is variable. Seldom does their behavior repeat itself exactly from moment to moment. Nor does the behavior of one individual always duplicate that of another. For this reason the answers to psychological questions are nearly always statistical answers. They are usually given in terms of averages and variabilities—the elementary but important concepts in what has lately become a highly developed branch of mathematics.

Central Tendency

The common everyday notion of an average—so familiar to baseball fans—is usually one of three measures of *central tendency*. The statistician's name for the average is the *mean*. And two other measures of central tendency are the *median* and the *mode*. We shall define these measures with the aid of an illustration.

Suppose we show a group of ten subjects a horizontal line twenty-four inches long and ask them to estimate its length. The ten estimates might give us the following distribution of guesses: 17, 18, 20, 20, 20, 22, 22, 24, 27, 30. What, then, is the mean or average estimate? In order to obtain the mean we add up all the individual estimates (scores) and divide by the number of scores. This gives twenty-two inches as the mean estimate of the group of ten subjects. We conclude that on the average they underestimated the length of the line.

We might also ask another question about these estimates: What value divides the scores into two groups such that the estimates of half the subjects are equal to or lower than this value and half are equal to or higher than this value? The answer gives us the *median* of the distribution. In our example the median would be the value midway between the scores for the fifth subject, who guessed 20, and the sixth subject, who guessed 22. The median then is 21 inches. Fifty per cent of the guesses lie above this point and 50 per cent lie below.

The *mode* is simply the value in the distribution that occurs with greatest frequency. Since 20 inches was guessed more often than any other value, we see at once that the mode is 20 inches.

Which of these three measures of central tendency should we use? The answer depends upon what we want to know, the kind of question we ask. Generally speaking, the mean is the most useful measure in that the line tends to be underestimated, but they also show that the judgments above the mean are spread out further than those below. In other words, the distribution tails off more gradually at the right than at the left. If we observed 1000 cases instead of 10, we should get rid of all the small irregularities in the curve, but these other two features might remain

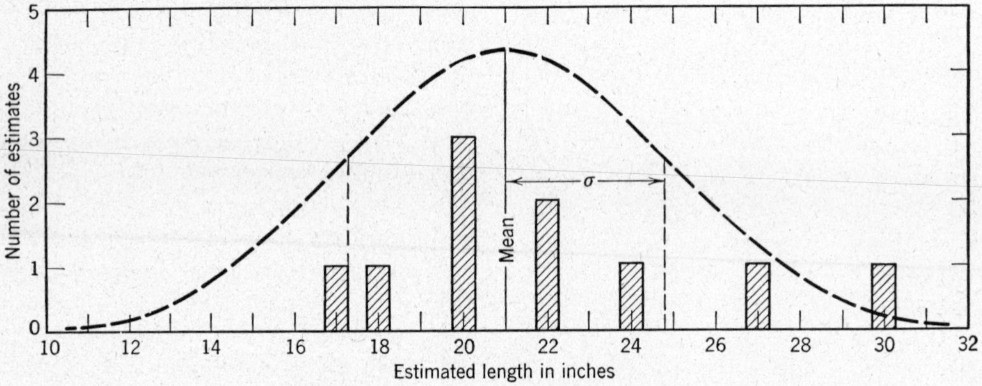

FIGURE 102. DISTRIBUTIONS OF DATA

The heights of the vertical bars show how many times each value on the horizontal scale was given as the estimated length of a line. The dotted curve shows the shape of a *normal distribution* (see text). The distance indicated by σ is the *standard deviation* of the distribution.

the sense that it is the most stable. If we were to enlist another 10 subjects for our experiment and get 10 more guesses, the mean of the second group would probably not be very different from that of the first—not so different, at any rate, as the median of the second group compared with the median of the first. And the mode would be the least stable of all. This fickleness on the part of the mode is unfortunate, because the mode is extremely simple to determine. Apparently what comes easiest in statistics is often not worth very much.

The data for 10 subjects, plotted as vertical bars in Fig. 102, show a roughly bell-shaped distribution: the judgments tend to cluster near the mean. They indicate as the facts of the case, provided we still use this scale of inches for measuring them. More often than not we get underestimations, yet the overestimations, when they do occur, show larger departures from the average of the group.

The dotted curve of Fig. 102 is the so-called curve of *normal distribution.* Observed data very often approximate it when the deviations from the mean are due to a multitude of chance factors and when the total number of cases is large. When the data do not approximate the normal curve, the scientist often changes the scale of his distribution, stretching it at one end and pushing it together at the other, so as to force the curve to be more nearly normal.

He does that because he wishes to treat his data under the conventional rules of statistics, many of which have been worked out in their simplest forms only for the normal curve.

It is clear that when data can be properly represented by the normal curve, their mean, median and mode all have the same value, for the normal distribution is symmetrical about its single mode. (On normal distribution, see also pp. 418 f.)

Variability

Measures of variability tell us how widely the data scatter about their mean. The important measures of variability are the *range,* the *standard deviation* and the *probable error.*

The *range* is simply the difference between the highest and the lowest score. As with the mode, we come by it easily but it tells us relatively little. The range of guesses for the length of the line in our experiment is $30 - 17 = 13$ inches. Common sense tells us that another group of ten subjects would probably not scatter its guesses over precisely this same range. So what is needed is a more stable measure of variability.

The *standard deviation* gives us this greater stability and is the most important measure of variability in the whole field of statistics. In technical language the standard deviation, designated by the Greek letter sigma (σ), is defined as the square root of the mean of the sum of the squares of the deviations from the mean. What this boils down to is simply that, in order to compute σ, we first find the mean, then we subtract the value of the mean from each score in turn. We then square each of the results, add them all up, divide by the number of scores and finally take the square root.

Apply this formula to the ten estimates of the length of the line, and you will find that the standard deviation of the distribution equals 3.8 inches. In Fig. 102 the upper and lower standard deviations on either side of the mean are indicated by vertical dotted lines.

It is interesting to note that the area lying under the normal curve and between the upper and lower standard deviations is equal to about two-thirds of the total area. If we were to draw verticals to points on either side of the mean so that just half the area lay between them, we should have to pick points nearer the mean. Those points, with half the area below the curve lying between them, are the values defining the *probable error* (P.E.). In numerical terms it turns out that the probable error is equal to 0.6745σ. The probable error gets its name from this fact: If the scores that scatter about the mean are regarded as errors, the probability is 50–50 that a particular error will lie inside the limits set by the probable error.

THRESHOLDS

All living organisms exhibit the phenomena known as *thresholds.* Some stimuli affect them; others do not. Some lights are too faint to be seen, some sounds too faint to be heard. But, as the intensity of a light or a sound is increased, there comes a point at which it is seen or heard. At any instant, it appears, this point at which a stimulus just crosses the threshold must be fixed, definite and precise. But, unfortunately, at two different instants the threshold point is not the same. The organism's properties do not stay put. Instead, its sensitivity bobs up and down from moment to moment. Consequently, when we want to determine the threshold we have to make repeated measurements and we have to apply statistical procedures to the resulting data. For this reason it is commonly said that *the threshold is a statistical concept.*

When we examined the seven basic problems of psychophysics, we saw that there are two kinds of threshold, *absolute* thresholds and *relative* or *differential* thresholds. The absolute threshold is the value of a stimulus which is (on the average) just noticeable or just detectable. The differential threshold is that difference between two stimuli which is (on the average) just noticeable. The measurement of both types of threshold has long been an important problem in psychology, and for their measurement elaborate procedures and precise statistical treatments have been devised. All these methods have one aim in common: They try to draw stable conclusions from measurements on variable organisms. These conclusions are important to science, and they are often of great practical importance as well. Some people earn their living measuring other people's thresholds.

Suppose, for example, a man is applying for a job as a radio operator. Obviously he must have normal hearing. That means that his absolute threshold for sound must not be significantly above normal. Since speech is the most important kind of sound he must hear, we might say that he must have a normal absolute threshold for speech.

Standardized threshold tests for speech were developed during the recent war as an aid in the rehabilitation of aural casualties. Carefully chosen words were recorded on phonograph records, and by means of special electrical circuits these words could be reproduced at the listener's ear in graded steps of intensity. The problem then is (1) to determine the faintest intensity at which the listener can hear the speech and (2) to compare this intensity with that at which a normal listener hears the words. How this is done can be illustrated with the aid of Fig. 103. We shall assume that our listener has a fairly large hearing loss, sufficient to cause his friends to raise their voices.

First let us consider the threshold of the normal listener. We find, of course, that at a given faint intensity he hears some of the words and not others, because his sensitivity varies. If we raise the intensity slightly, he hears a larger percentage of the words. Finally, if we make the speech loud enough, he hears all the words. If, therefore, we plot the percentage of the words he hears at each level of intensity, we obtain the curve in Fig. 103. This is usually a long S-shaped curve. It approximates, in fact, the *ogive* form of the normal distribution curve, the form which shows us, not the number of cases for each value of the stimulus, but the number of cases *up to and including* each value of the stimulus. It is a cumulative curve. It starts at zero per cent for the stimulus that is always ineffective and reaches 100 per cent at the stimulus that is always effective.

Having plotted the percentage of words which the listener hears at successive intensity levels, we are ready to decide what value we shall call the threshold for speech. Both common sense and convention tell us that the threshold ought to be defined as the intensity corresponding to the 50 per cent point on the curve. This is the speech intensity that will be heard correctly half the time. If we regard the listener's responses to the words as comprising a frequency distribution, this 50 per cent point is the *median* of the distribution.

For the hard-of-hearing listener we carry

out precisely the same procedure. We plot a curve showing how his correct responses depend upon intensity and we pay attention to the 50 per cent point. Then, since we measure hearing loss relative to the normal threshold, we simply take the spread between the two 50 per cent points as the quantitative measure of hearing loss. In the example before us this loss is 45 decibels, a large enough loss to call for a hearing aid. (For a fuller account of the intelligibility of speech, see pp. 345–349.)

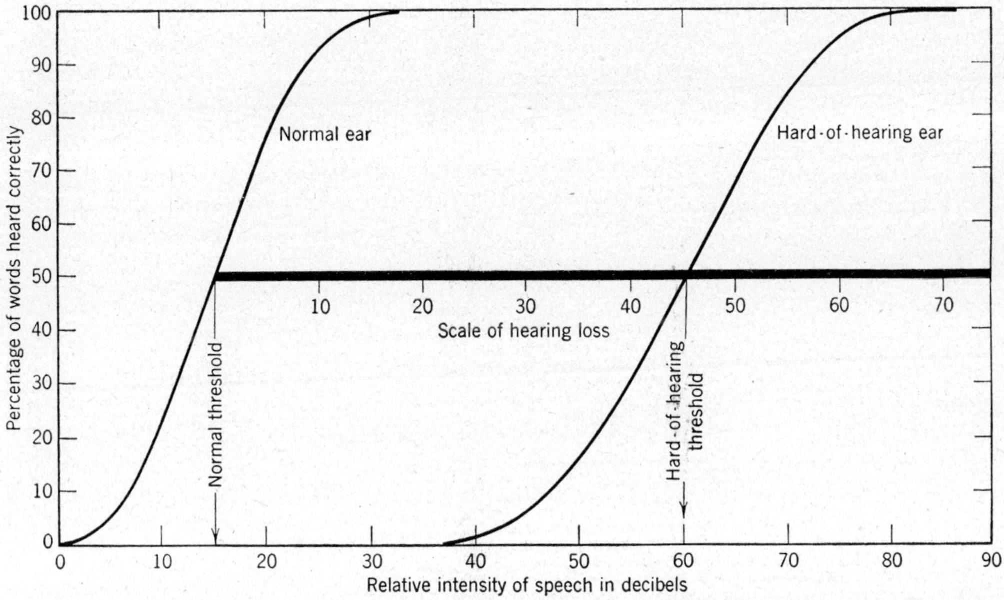

FIGURE 103. PSYCHOMETRIC FUNCTIONS FOR ABSOLUTE THRESHOLDS

The two curves (psychometric functions) show how the percentage of words heard correctly increases as the intensity level of the speech (in decibels) is raised. The intensity at which half the words are heard correctly is defined as the absolute threshold. Amount of hearing loss is the difference between the threshold of the patient and the threshold of a normal ear.

The S-shaped curves in Fig. 103 are known as *psychometric functions.* Curves of this sort are obtained whenever we present carefully graded stimuli and record the frequencies with which a subject responds to them. The curves in Fig. 103 measure absolute thresholds, but similar functions are obtained when we measure relative thresholds by the same method.

Thus we can present pairs of stimuli graded as to the *difference* between them and ask the subject to respond by saying whether the second stimulus in each pair is *greater* or *less* than the first. We should then obtain two psychometric functions (one for judgments *greater,* one for judgments *less*). The two functions would cross each other at their 50 per cent points. This crossing would usually fall near the value corresponding to *no* physical difference between the stimuli. On these two functions we should then have to decide the value of the differential threshold, obviously *not* the 50 per cent point. Here convention tells us we should choose the value of the physical difference which gives judgments of *greater* (or of *less*) 75 per cent of the time. This is reasonable enough if you think about it. The 75 per cent point

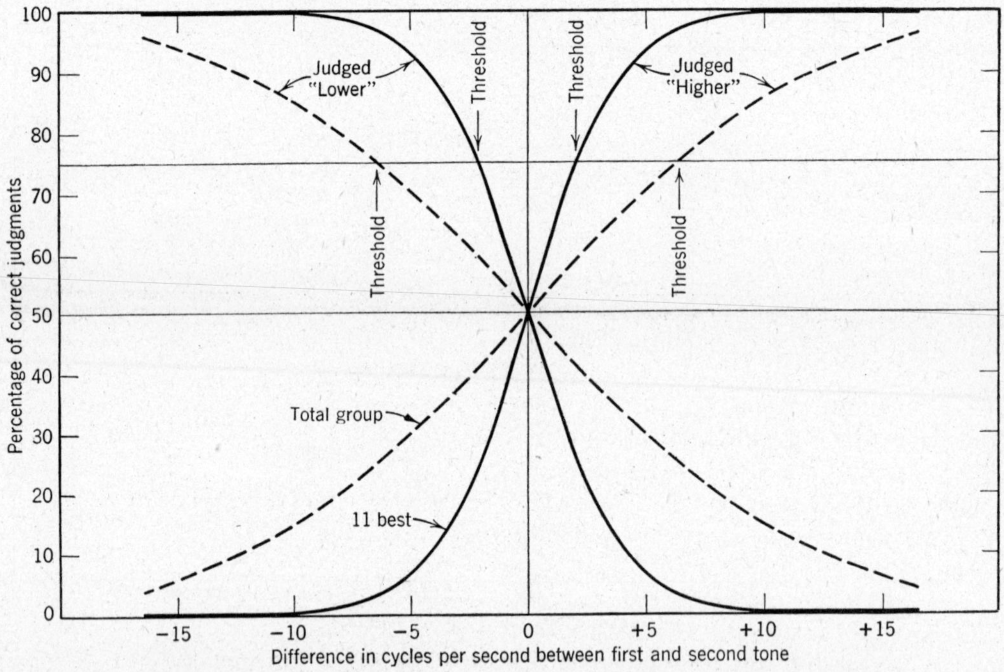

FIGURE 104. PSYCHOMETRIC FUNCTIONS FOR DIFFERENTIAL THRESHOLDS

Psychometric functions show how the correctness of pitch judgments depends upon the size of the stimulus difference. The dotted curves represent the composite scores made by 95 high school students who took the Seashore Test for Musical Talent. The solid curves are for the group of 11 students who scored highest on the test. The curves for the judgments *higher* and *lower* cross at the 50 per cent point, which coincides with zero difference between the two tones presented as stimuli. Thus, when there was no difference to be heard, the judgments followed the chance expectancy of 50–50.

is the midpoint of the distribution of judgments falling on *one side* of equality.

Figure 104 shows how all this works out in a practical situation. A group of 95 high school students was given one of the Seashore Tests designed to gauge musical ability. This test calls for the discrimination of small differences in pitch. Pairs of tones are sounded, and the listener tries to tell whether the second tone of each pair is higher or lower than the first tone. The percentages of correct judgments may then be tabulated and plotted as in Fig. 104. There we see plots for the average of the group of 95 students and plots for the average of the 11 best students. These 11 listeners are clearly better at discriminating differences in pitch than the group as a whole. If we measure pitch discrimination as the difference in frequency (cycles of the tonal stimulus per second) correctly noticed 75 per cent of the time, we find that the group as a whole has an average differential threshold equal to 7 cycles per second. For the 11 best listeners the average is only 2 cycles per second. On the average these 11 people could tell the difference between a tone of 1000 cycles and a tone of 1002 cycles—which is very good discrimination indeed.

Pitch discrimination as good as this is a necessary asset to a musician. But a word of caution is in order here. Although good pitch discrimination is necessary, the fact of having it does not make a person a musician. Other important talents are called for in addition. Pitch discrimination is to the musician what visual acuity is to the artist. It is what is called a *necessary* but not a *sufficient* condition for success.

THE WEBER FRACTION

There is another important aspect of the problem of differential thresholds that we must consider. It is important because it is a law of relativity in psychology. This law says that in order for it to be perceived the increase that must be made in a stimulus depends upon the amount that is already there. If to two lighted candles in a room a third is added, there is a greater increase in the sensed illumination than there would be if a twenty-first candle were added to twenty. The additional light has more effect when added to a lesser illumination. A cough counts for more in church than in the subway. In other words, the differential threshold for intensity gets larger as the intensity gets greater.

It is usual to measure relative sensitivity by taking the ratio of the differential threshold, which we may call ΔI, to the total intensity at which the threshold was obtained, which we may call I. This ratio $\Delta I/I$ is called the Weber ratio or the *Weber fraction,* because a century ago the physiologist, E. H. Weber, thought that it remained constant at different intensities. Modern research has corrected his view. Figure 105 shows the typical form of the *Weber function,* that is, the way $\Delta I/I$ changes with I. Although Weber held that such a function would be a horizontal straight line, actually the Weber function

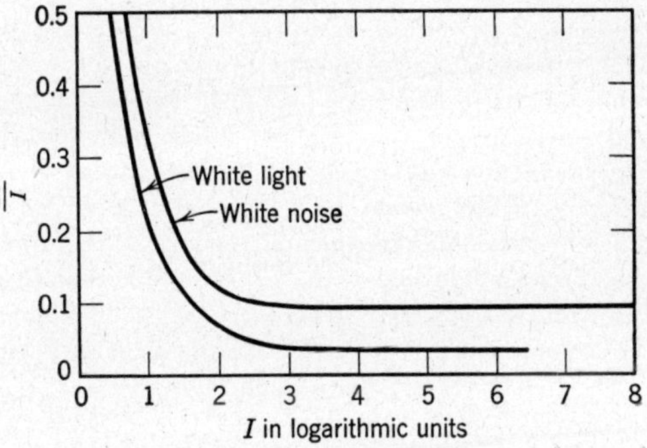

FIGURE 105. TYPICAL WEBER FUNCTIONS FOR VISION AND HEARING

The curves show the relation between the Weber fraction $\Delta I/I$, and the intensity of the stimulus, I. Log $I = 0$ = absolute threshold. On the intensity scale each unit represents a tenfold increase in energy. White noise is a purely random mixture of all frequencies. It sounds like a sustained *Sh-h-h*. It is called *white* because, like white light, it is composed of all the perceptible frequencies acting simultaneously. [Data from G. A. Miller, *J. acoust. Soc. Amer.,* 1947, **19,** 609–619.] The measurements for white light were made with a small patch of light (visual angle = 28 minutes of arc) falling on the retinal fovea.

is, as the figure shows, a curve. The value of the Weber fraction first decreases rapidly as the intensity increases and then more slowly until it reaches a minimal value. Thereafter, it may remain constant, or occasionally it may again increase slightly.

In terms of the Weber fractions, it is possible to compare one sense with another with respect to differential sensitivity. Since the fraction varies within a single sense, we must choose for each sense some one representative value, and it is obvious that the minimal fractions best lend themselves to comparison, since each minimal fraction shows the maximal sensitivity of which that sense is capable. In Table XVI

TABLE XVI

MINIMAL WEBER FRACTIONS

For all cases below, except tones and smells, the Weber fraction has a minimal value in the middle range of intensities. The minimal values for tone and smell are for the maximal intensities after the Weber function has leveled off. Although each of the different values would be somewhat altered by a different choice of experimental conditions, the difference between 1/77 and 1/5 is so very great that there can be no doubt about the general fact that different sensory mechanisms differ significantly in sensitivity.

	Weber Ratio	*Weber Fraction*
Deep pressure, from skin and subcutaneous tissue, at about 400 grams	0.013	1/77
Visual brightness, at about 1000 photons	0.016	1/62
Lifted weights, at about 300 grams	0.019	1/53
Tone, for 1000 cycles per second, at about 100 db above the absolute threshold	0.088	1/11
Smell, for rubber, at about 200 olfacties	0.104	1/10
Cutaneous pressure, on an isolated spot, at about 5 grams per mm	0.136	1/7
Taste, for saline solution, at about 3 moles per liter concentration	0.200	1/5

these minimal values are listed for seven well-established cases. It is true that these figures apply only to particular experimental conditions; nevertheless, the general relation of the senses is clear. Tonal sensitivity is less than visual. The skin is not so sensitive to a difference in pressure as the muscles to a difference of lifted weight.

Despite the fact that for a given sense the Weber fraction is only approximately constant, we must not lose sight of the fact that the Weber function is a general statement that *relativity* is approximated in the world of sensory intensities. The principle of relativity signifies that a little thing means more to another little thing than it does to a big thing. A dollar means more in poverty than it does in wealth, whereas an error of an inch in the length of the equator matters less than an error of an inch in the fit of a shoe. Just so the Weber function means that differences that seem large at small intensities become quite unnoticeable at large intensities.

REFERENCES

1. Bartley, S. H. *Vision.* New York: Van Nostrand, 1941. Chap. 2.

A discussion of the principal facts of brightness discrimination with emphasis on the underlying physiological processes.

2. Boring, E. G. *The physical dimensions of consciousness.* New York: Appleton-Century, 1933. Chaps. 2, 3 and 6.

A systematic discussion of the sensory attributes of intensity and quality in terms of a physical theory of mind.

3. Boring, E. G. *Sensation and perception in the history of experimental psychology.* New York: Appleton-Century, 1942. Chap. 1.

Chapter 1 summarizes the work and thought on sensation and perception during the last three centuries.

4. Guilford, J. P. *Psychometric methods.* New York: McGraw-Hill, 1936. Chaps. 2 to 6.

A comprehensive treatment of the classical psychophysical methods and their statistical bases.

5. Stevens, S. S., and Davis, H. *Hearing: its psychology and physiology.* New York: Wiley, 1938. Chaps. 2 to 5.

A systematic analysis of the facts of auditory sensation with respect to pitch, loudness and the other tonal attributes.

6. Troland, L. T. *The principles of psychophysiology.* New York: Van Nostrand, 1930. Vol. 2, especially sections 53, 54 and 61.

A systematic account of the psychophysical facts of all the senses with especial emphasis on vision.

CHAPTER 12

Color

WHAT the eye sees is color—greens, oranges, pinks, grays, whites. The location of the seen colors in space and the patterns that make up the perceived visual field are problems of visual space perception with which the next chapter deals—the how and why of shape and size, of flat and solid, of near and far. This chapter is about the visual qualities, the relationships and laws of colors.

CHARACTERISTICS OF COLORS

We begin with the appearance of colors, what can be said about color without reference to its stimuli or to the conditions of its arousal.

Color Names

An attempt to catalogue all the various color qualities at first appears impossible. When we think of the many lavenders, pinks, purples, reds, oranges, yellows, browns, tans, greens, blues, grays, blacks and whites of our everyday experience, the accepted estimates of 100,000 to 300,000 discriminatively different colors does not seem too high. Colors were first named by reference to particular objects, and many such terms are still retained in our everyday speech, for instance, orange, violet, olive, straw. Others have lost their object reference and now are simply color names, as purple, scarlet, sepia, maroon, crimson, azure, taupe. In addition, it has been the custom for a long time to invent color names, particularly for clothing, and such names have changed with the styles of the time. In the sixteenth century, for instance, French women wore colors called *rat color, widow's joy, envenomed monkey* and *chimney sweep*. The eighteenth century produced *rash tears, Paris mud, stifled sigh* in France and *red-hot bullets* and *smoke of the Camp of St. Roche* in England. Only yesterday (1930) they could be matched with *folly, lucky stone, elephant's breath* and in 1946 with *sun love, town blond* and *cocoblush* or *Virginia turf, radar blue* and *avenue gray*. Obviously, such fantastic names have no value for scientific purposes, though the textile industry has systematized them for sales promotion.

The most comprehensive dictionary of color gives over seven thousand samples of

This chapter was prepared by Forrest L. Dimmick of the U. S. Naval Medical Research Laboratory at New London.

The opinions or assertions contained in this chapter are the private ones of the collaborator and the editors and are not to be construed as official or reflecting the views of the Navy Department or the Naval Service at large.

colors but finds only about half that many color names, some of them repetitions and others obsolete. An attempt has been made by the National Bureau of Standards and the Inter-Society Color Council to standardize and simplify color names. They have found that the long list of color names commonly used can be reduced to twelve applied singly (blue) or in combination (bluish green) with certain modifiers (light blue-green). (See Table XVII.)

TABLE XVII

COLOR NAMES

The diagram shows how a few color names and modifiers can be combined to represent a large range of colors in the Inter-Society Color Council and the National Bureau of Standards system of color names. The five rows give alternative names for five different greens.

GREEN

Greenish White	Very Pale Green	Very Light Green	Very Brilliant Green	
Light Greenish Gray	Pale Green	Light Green	Brilliant Green	
Medium Greenish Gray	Weak Green	Moderate Green	Strong Green	Vivid Green
Dark Greenish Gray	Dusky Green	Dark Green	Deep Green	
Greenish Black	Very Dusky Green	Very Dark Green	Very Deep Green	

Unique Colors

It is not necessary to have a separate name for every color, because colors can be grouped according to their resemblances to a few outstanding or *unique* colors. A unique color is a color that is describable in terms of itself alone, that is to say, it must be displayed or demonstrated. There are seven such unique colors, namely, Red, Yellow, Green, Blue, White, Gray and Black. No one of the unique colors looks like or implies the existence of any other unique color, but all *non-unique* colors can be referred to two or more of the unique colors because they resemble the unique colors. Thus *non-unique* colors fall into *series* of gradations from one unique color to another. For example, *purple* refers to a group of colors that look both reddish and bluish. There are bluish reds (purples), blue-reds and reddish blues (violets). Some investigators use the terms *purplish red, reddish purple, purple* and *bluish purple,* as well as *red-violet, violet* and *blue-violet.* Any color in the group can be described by giving its relative redness and blueness. Careful experimental observations have established the fact that the *seven unique qualities* mentioned above *are necessary and sufficient for precise description of all visible colors.*

The Color Equation

The fact that every color can be described precisely by stating its likenesses to the several unique colors can be expressed in the equation:

$$\text{Color} = (\text{Red or Green}) + (\text{Yellow or Blue}) + (\text{White or Black}) + \text{Gray}$$

or, more simply,

$$C = (R,\ G) + (Y,\ B) + (Wh,\ Bk) + Gy$$

The equation pairs six unique colors, expressing the fact that there are no red-green, no blue-yellow and, as a matter of fact, no black-white colors. (The intermediate colors, from black to white, are mix tures of black or white with the gray color in various proportions.) This fact is the basis of the *complementarism* of colors, a relationship which, as we shall see, appears in several other ways. There are no colors which look reddish green or bluish yellow, although there are reddish yellows, bluish greens and reddish blues (Fig. 106). That is why the equation for color reduces to four terms instead of seven.

Unique colors. There are seven of them, *R* (red), *Y* (yellow), *G* (green), *B* (blue), *Wh* (white), *Bk* (black) and *Gy* (gray). They are unique because they are the points of orientation for all the other colors and no one resembles any other one. They are also *simplex.*

Duplex colors. They lie on the color series connecting any two unique colors. There are eighteen such series:

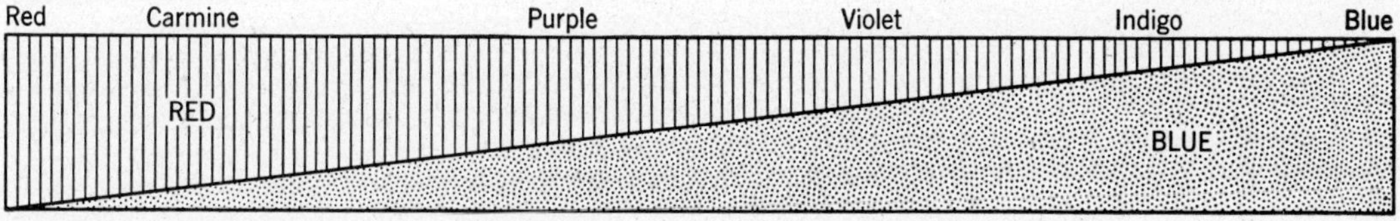

FIGURE 106. DUPLEX SERIES OF COLORS

The second point about the color equation is that it shows how many different ways colors can vary in their relations to one another. The *unique* colors are simple and points of reference, for all the other colors are designated by reference to them. Then there are *duplex* colors, like the carmines, purples, violets and indigos of Fig. 106, which form a series between unique red and unique blue. Unique red is an end point of five such duplex series, red-blue, red-yellow, red-white, red-gray and red-black. For duplex colors two of the four terms in the color formula are equal to zero and disappear, and the other two terms characterize the color. When there are three terms used in the color equation the color is *triplex,* like a light purple (red + blue + white) or a grayish orange (red + yellow + gray). The great majority of colors are, however, *quadruplex,* like a light pastel jade (green + blue + white + gray).

We shall do well to summarize these relationships.

1. *R-Y*	7. *G-Wh*	13. *R-Gy*
2. *Y-G*	8. *B-Wh*	14. *Y-Gy*
3. *G-B*	9. *R-Bk*	15. *G-Gy*
4. *B-R*	10. *Y-Bk*	16. *B-Gy*
5. *R-Wh*	11. *G-Bk*	17. *Wh-Gy*
6. *Y-Wh*	12. *B-Bk*	18. *Bk-Gy*

In these groups what are sometimes called 'good hues' appear in series 1–4. The bright colors are in series 5–8, the dark colors in series 9–12, the poorly saturated or grayish colors in series 13–16 and the achromatic colors (the whites, grays and blacks) in series 17 and 18. These series are the lines in Figs. 107, 108, 109 and 110.

Triplex colors. A great many colors have only one term in the color equation missing, being related to the other three unique colors. Such colors lie in the triangular spaces of Figs. 107, 108, 109 and 110. There are twelve such triangles:

1. *R-Y-Wh*	4. *Y-G-Wh*	7. *G-B-Wh*
2. *R-Y-Bk*	5. *Y-G-Bk*	8. *G-B-Bk*
3. *R-Y-Gy*	6. *Y-G-Gy*	9. *G-B-Gy*

10. *B-R-Wh* 14. *Y-Gy-Wh* 18. *Y-Gy-Bk*
11. *B-R-Bk* 15. *G-Gy-Wh* 19. *G-Gy-Bk*
12. *B-R-Gy* 16. *B-Gy-Wh* 20. *B-Gy-Bk*
13. *R-Gy-Wh* 17. *R-Gy-Bk*

See the triplex series from orange to white in Fig. 111.

Quadruplex colors. They represent the great majority of colors which have to have positive specification in respect of all four terms of the color formula. There are eight such combinations:

1. *R-Y-Wh-Gy* 5. *G-B-Wh-Gy*
2. *R-Y-Bk-Gy* 6. *G-B-Bk-Gy*
3. *Y-G-Wh-Gy* 7. *B-R-Wh-Gy*
4. *Y-G-Bk-Gy* 8. *B-R-Bk-Gy*

The Color Pyramid

The facts expressed in the color formula can be represented in a spatial schema. If we put the unique colors at points and the various qualitative series on straight lines, the framework of our structure builds itself. For a start let us take the four points and four series representing red, yellow, green and blue. The resulting shape is a square with each one of the four colors at a corner (Fig. 107). If we had taken blue, white, yellow and black, or red, white, green and black, similar squares would have resulted (Figs. 108, 109). Gray goes in the middle of each of these squares because of the complementariness of the remaining three pairs. You cannot go from red to green, from yellow to blue, or from white to black without passing through gray.

To bring these three squares together, as we must, since we have in all only *six* corner points, we can set white and black

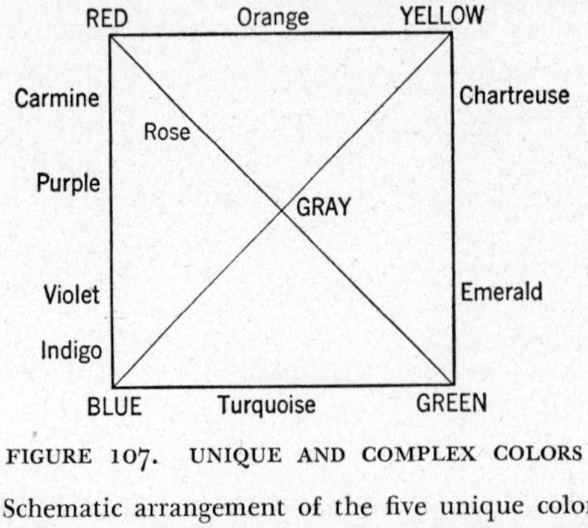

FIGURE 107. UNIQUE AND COMPLEX COLORS

Schematic arrangement of the five unique colors, red, yellow, green, blue and gray, showing examples of duplex colors lying along the straight lines connecting the uniques. Triplex colors lie within the four triangular spaces.

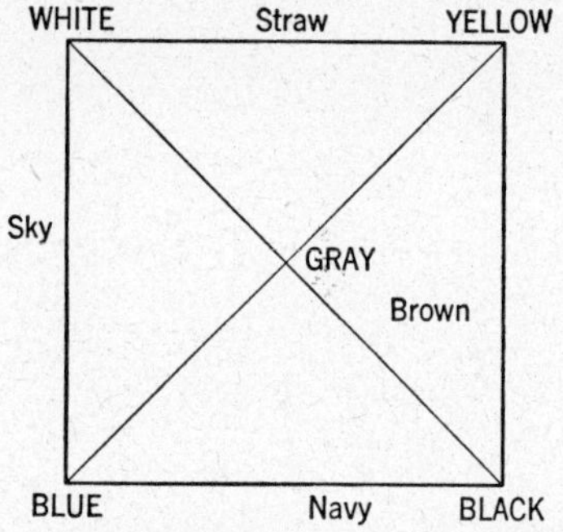

FIGURE 108. UNIQUE AND COMPLEX COLORS

Schematic arrangement of the five unique colors, white, gray, black, yellow and blue, with duplex colors along the lines, and triplex colors in between.

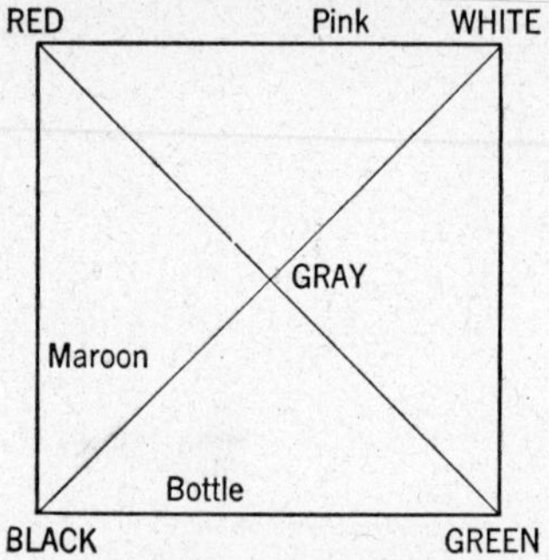

FIGURE 109. UNIQUE AND COMPLEX COLORS

Schematic arrangement of the five unique colors, white, gray, black, red and green, with duplex colors along the lines, and triplex colors in between.

respectively above and below the middle of the red-yellow-green-blue square and connect them with its corners. The identical grays at the middle of each square coincide in the middle of the solid figure which results. This figure is a double square pyramid or octahedron. Gray, as we have said, stands at one end of series that run to *all* the other unique colors. Its place, obviously, is at the center of the system. (See Fig. 110.)

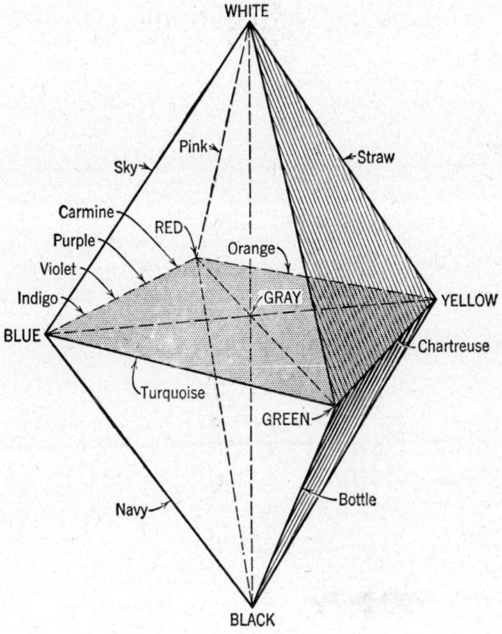

FIGURE 110. COLOR PYRAMID

The duplex colors lie on the eighteen lines of the pyramid, the lines which form the edges, and the six lines which radiate from gray. Figure 112 is one of the eight tetrahedrons which make up the color pyramid. This tetrahedron has four unique colors at its four corners, six series of duplex colors along its six edges, four sets of triplex colors in its four triangular faces and all the red-yellow-white-gray quadruplex colors inside its volume. Salmon and pink (see Fig. 111) would lie near the top of the front face (Fig. 112).

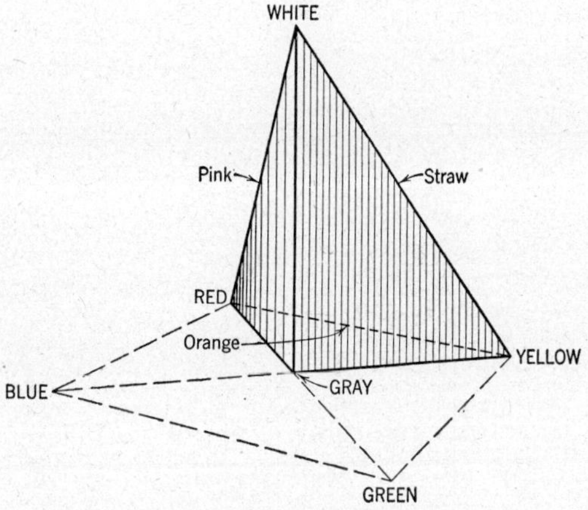

FIGURE 112. TETRAHEDRON FROM COLOR PYRAMID

One of the eight tetrahedrons in the color pyramid. All the colors in this tetrahedron may be specified by the equation Red + Yellow + White + Gray = *C*.

The color pyramid and its color equation represent every known or hypothetically

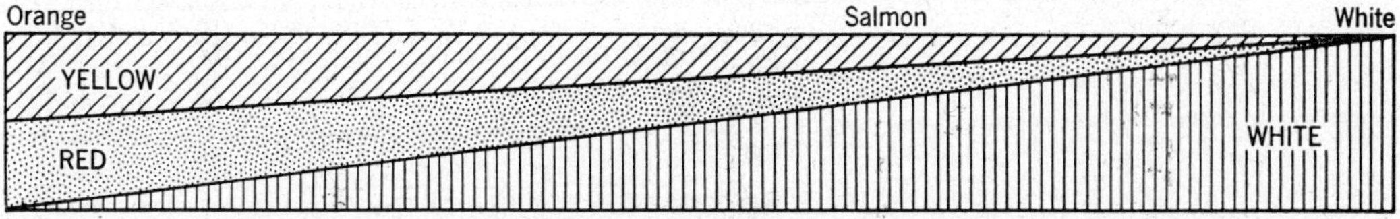

FIGURE 111. TRIPLEX SERIES OF COLORS WITH WHITE CONTENT VARIED

The diagram shows an orange getting whiter. The proportion of yellow to red remains the same, but the proportion of white to orange (yellow-and-red) increases.

visible color quality. The only other ways in which visual appearance can be altered are by putting qualities from the pyramid into a spatial pattern or by making them change in time or by both together or by presenting simultaneously one color to one eye and a different color to the other eye. In the last case we sometimes see luster.

Chromatic and Achromatic Colors

This is the newer view of the classification of colors. The older and more conventional view separates white, gray and black from the rainbow colors, labeling the former *achromatic* or 'uncolored' colors and the latter *chromatic* or 'colored' colors.

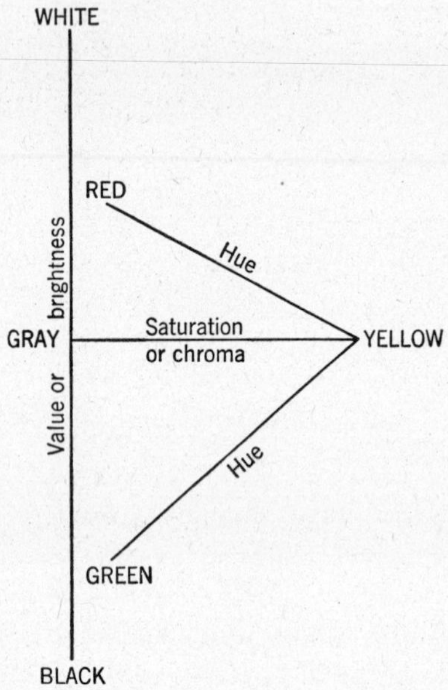

FIGURE 113. DIMENSIONS OF THE COLOR FIGURE SHOWING HUE, SATURATION AND BRIGHTNESS

Hue, saturation and *brightness* are the conventional terms which are used to characterize the attributes of colors. Again we have here simply a different set of terms, not any new facts. (See Fig. 113.)

Brightness (sometimes called *lightness, tint* or *value*) refers to variations along the achromatic scale, black-to-gray-to-white. Since other colors also show gradations toward white and toward black, a chromatic color may also vary in brightness.

Saturation is represented most simply by a series of gradations from one of the chromatic colors, like red, to one of the achromatic colors, like gray. In the conventional terminology, the series representing change of saturation would be all the radial lines that could be drawn from gray to the colors on the outside of the color square of Fig. 107. The newer view puts gray at the middle of the color pyramid. All radial lines that go from it to any color in the surface of the pyramid are series which show increasing richness of the chromatic or achromatic color toward which the line leads and diminishing grayness. This view really makes the pyramid into a double hedgehog, with saturation lines sticking out from gray toward the other colors in all directions.

Hue, in the older system, refers specifically to the several 'chromatic' colors—red, yellow, green, blue and their intermediates.

THE STIMULUS TO COLOR

It is not enough to know the number of color qualities and their relations to one another. We must know also how the colors are produced, the nature of their physical stimuli.

Nature of the Stimulus

The stimulus to color is light. When electric charges are moving through space at a uniform rate, they release radiant energy in the form of oscillations in intensity of the electromagnetic field whenever their uniform motion is altered. This radiant energy is light. Its visible aspects are related to three important characteristics of these electromagnetic oscillations. (See Fig. 114.)

The most fundamental characteristic is the distance from pulse to pulse of the vibration, the *wave length* of light. Such wave lengths cover a wide range, from those measured in units of 10-trillionths of an inch to those many miles long. Light waves are among the shorter ones, lying between 16- and 32-millionths of an inch or, in the more usual notation, between 400 and 800 millimicrons (millionths of a millimeter, abbreviated mμ). A particular beam of light may consist of a set of waves that are all of a single length (homogeneous), of several wave lengths (heterogeneous) or of all wave lengths between the visible limits (heterogeneous).

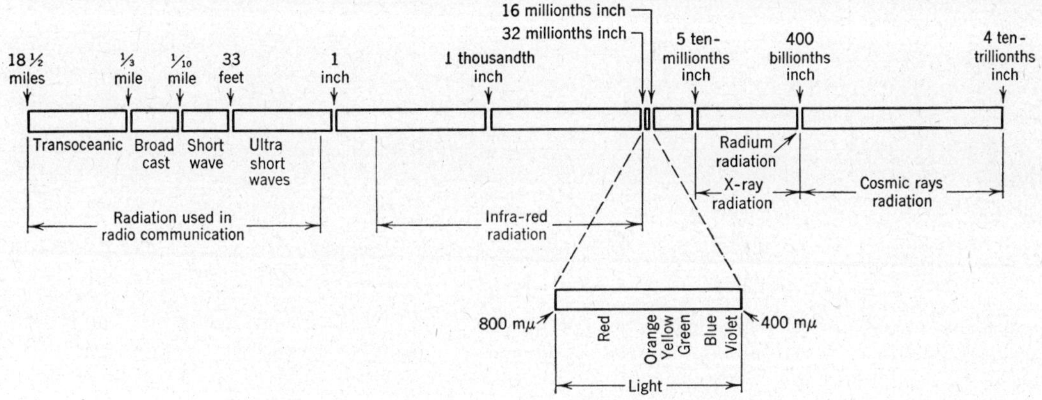

FIGURE 114. THE RANGE OF ELECTROMAGNETIC RADIATIONS

The range is so wide that this diagram had to be plotted on a logarithmic scale in order to place it on this page. Note the small portion of the spectrum in which visible light is radiated.

It was in 1666 that Isaac Newton discovered that a beam of heterogeneous light ('white' light) upon passing through a triangular glass prism is dispersed or spread out into a wide band so that every wave length falls in a different place. Thus the heterogeneous light is broken up into its homogeneous components. What you see, of course, is the spectrum, a brilliant band of colors shining out in the dark in which you are working. Newton called this apparition in the dark a *spectrum* because of its specterlike appearance. It is from the spectrum that the wave lengths of light are determined. You never *see* wave lengths directly. They have to be computed from physical measurements.

In addition to wave length and homogeneity, radiant energy varies also in amount or *intensity*. The intensity of the color stimulus is always proportional to the rate at which energy comes from a given surface. You measure amount of radiant energy to measure the intensity of the stimulus.

The physical stimulus may vary, then, (1) in *wave length,* (2) in *homogeneity* (number of wave lengths combined) and (3) in *intensity* of luminous energy. We must examine the dependence of the various characteristics of color upon these physical properties of the stimulus.

Dependence of Color on Its Stimulus

There is a fairly simple and consistent correlation between wave length and the first half of the color equation, that is, red, yellow, green and blue (the chromatic colors, the hues). The long waves of the spectrum beginning at 700 millimicrons are seen as red tinged with yellow. As we go from that point toward the shorter wave lengths, colors become more yellow wave length. At the red end there is no change of color toward yellow until you get below 635 millimicrons. The colors there get less black, less gray, more red, but not yellower. Between that point and 450 millimicrons the difference in wave length necessary to get a noticeable change in color varies around 2 millimicrons. (See Fig. 116.) Differential sensitivity is greatest near yellow and blue and least near

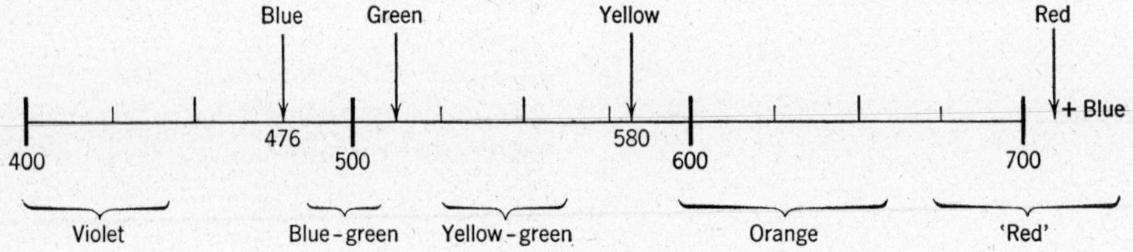

FIGURE 115. RELATION OF HUE TO WAVE LENGTH

Wave lengths of spectral light indicated in millimicrons. Duplex colors shown below the line. Four unique colors shown at arrows above the line. Unique red is nonspectral. Spectral red is duplex (yellowish).

and less red, passing through the red-yellow series until unique yellow is reached at about 580 millimicrons. Between that point and green at 510 millimicrons lie the greenish yellows and yellow-greens. Between 510 and 476 millimicrons is the series from green to blue. Shorter wave lengths, from 476 millimicrons to the end of the visible spectrum at about 435 millimicrons, give reddish blues or violets. (See Fig. 115.) Purples and bluish reds have no simple spectral correlate but must be obtained by mixtures of the wave lengths from both ends of the spectrum. Unique red itself requires a complex physical stimulus, since the longest wave length visible is distinctly yellowish. We can get unique red by mixing a little spectral blue with the yellowish spectral red.

Changes in color through the spectrum are not uniform for equal steps of physical green. Below 450 millimicrons the only change in color is toward black.

This relationship holds for the middle intensive range of radiant energy, but for high energies all the colors become whitish and for low energies blackish.

The whiteness or blackness of a color depends in a general way upon the amount of visible radiant energy, upon what is called the total *luminance.* An illuminated spot will appear lighter or darker, whiter or blacker, as the intensity of the luminance increases or decreases. Whether the spot actually *looks* white or gray or black depends, however, upon the luminance of the surrounding field. A spot of intermediate luminance may look white on a black field, black on a white field. The ratio of the spot's luminance to the average luminance of the entire field is the determining condition.

For example, a spot radiating 0.2 unit of energy (or, exactly, 0.2 lambert per square centimeter) set in a field which radiates an average of 1 unit will look gray. A spot which radiates 1 unit in the same field will look white. Radiation less than 0.03 unit will look black. If, now, the luminance of the whole field is raised to 10 units, it will require 2 units to look middle gray, whereas the 0.2 unit of the preceding example will now look black.

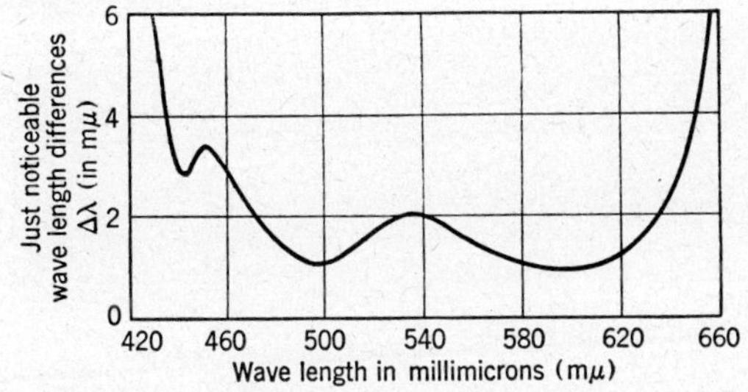

FIGURE 116. DISCRIMINATION OF HUE AS A FUNCTION OF WAVE LENGTH

Typical hue discrimination curve for a normal observer using a 2-degree stimulus. The ordinate gives the just noticeable difference in hue at every wave length throughout the spectrum.

The whiteness or blackness of a spectral color depends upon the same ratios of luminance as those of the white-gray-black series. With a white surrounding field, emitting a luminance of 1 unit, a spot of any homogeneous spectral wave length (for instance, 520 millimicrons which looks green) of 0.2 units of energy will look neither blackish nor whitish but will have a brightness of gray. If we increase the energy of the 520 millimicrons to 0.5 unit, the color will appear whitish green (light green); if we reduce it to 0.1 unit it will look blackish green (dark green). These appearances, however, also depend on the laws of color constancy and may be altered in accordance with them (pp. 234–237).

Purity and Saturation

We saw that light can be broken up by dispersion into many different wave lengths and that each wave length gives a specific color. When light consists entirely of a single wave length it is said to be 'spectrally pure.' For the physicist 'white' light means that the luminous energy is distributed at random among all wave lengths. It is maximally heterogeneous. Its *purity* is zero. Between the two extremes of complete homogeneity and maximal heterogeneity are all gradations of spectral purity. When spectral purity of a light stimulus changes alone with no change in its luminance relative to the field which surrounds it, the color changes principally in grayness. Grayness tends to diminish and saturation to increase as purity increases. That is why spectral lights are so impressive; the colors tend to be better saturated than the colors from mixed lights which objects reflect.

Sensation versus Stimulus

There are three important ways in which the stimulus to color can change: (1) in wave length, (2) in energy and (3) in purity. The preceding sections indicate the more obvious ways in which color is affected by changes in these three dimensions of its stimulus. Change wave length, and you get change in the red-yellow-green-blue dimension of color quality. Change energy, and you get change in the black-gray-white dimension of color quality. Change purity and you get change in the grayness of the color quality. That is very simple, but, alas, the truth is more complex! All three of these kinds of color change can be made to occur, under certain specific conditions, by changing any one of these three dimensions of the stimulus. Here are the complexities.

Change of color in the red-yellow-green-blue chromatic series occurs when wave length changes, when energy changes (with diminished energy all colors converge on red and green, with increased energy on yellow and blue) and when the heterogeneity of the light changes (see the laws of color mixture in the next section).

Change of color in the black-gray-white achromatic dimension occurs when energy changes, when the wave length of homogeneous light changes (pure 'yellow' light is brightest, pure 'blue' light darkest) and when heterogeneity changes (adding more lights together to get greater heterogeneity makes the color whiter).

Change of color in grayness occurs when purity changes, when energy changes (very dark and very light colors have little gray in them; they are near to unique black or unique white) and when wave length changes (for instance, the two ends of the spectrum, being very black have but little gray in them).

There is an important lesson to be learned here. *You do not see the stimulus.* You see the colors which the stimulus (operating under the laws of perception) creates. It is not true that in seeing hues you are seeing wave lengths. If you see a green, it is most likely a complex mixture of wave lengths, and there are many different mixtures that will make you see the same green. If you see a white, you are not seeing an amount of energy. You may be seeing great energy for a single wave length, but more likely you are seeing many wave lengths of which the whiteness depends in part on color constancy and the looks of the field around the white. If you see a gray you need not be seeing maximal heterogeneity of light, for the gray may come from all the visible wave lengths mixed together at low energy with a bright field around them, or from a mere two wave lengths mixed in the right proportions.

Physics depends on observation as much as psychology, but its observations are different. Usually they are the visual observations of scales on instruments. You can 'see' a wave length by reading a scale on a spectrometer. You can 'see' light energy by reading an illuminometer. And wave lengths themselves are not colored, even if they do stimulate the retina to see colors.

COLOR MIXTURE

A great deal happens to light before it becomes a proximal stimulus to act upon the retina and produce color. 'White' light from the sun is a heterogeneous mixture of all the visible wave lengths, as well as the invisible infrared and ultraviolet beyond the spectrum. It falls upon green foliage and a great deal of the energy of every wave length is absorbed. The darker the foliage, the greater the absorption. The rest of the light is reflected, but not in the random balanced mixture that makes 'white' light. Light from the green-yellow region of the spectrum predominates, although some red and some blue are also reflected. The laws of the mixture of color stimuli tell that the reflected combination is what makes the foliage look yellowish green. Most 'colored' objects reflect all the wave lengths, but in combinations that give the objects their specific colors. The color of an object is the result of what it reflects and does not absorb.

The color of a transparent object depends on what it transmits and does not absorb. Red goggles transmit mostly the 'red' end of the spectrum, absorbing the 'blue' end.

Laws of Mixture

Three laws govern the mixture of color stimuli. The first two were laid down by Isaac Newton in 1704. The third is not yet quite a century old. They apply to what is called *additive color mixture,* the addition of the wave lengths of one stimulus to the wave lengths of another to make a total wave length pattern for the mixture. You have additive mixture when you have two colored lights and can shine them superposed on the same spot on a white screen. Or for additive mixture you can use the device of Fig. 117, where light from one stimulus is reflected from a half-silvered mirror at forty-five degrees, while light from another stimulus is transmitted directly through the mirror, so that you get both sets of light added together along the same common path. Here are the laws of additive mixture.

Law I. For every color stimulus there is another color stimulus which, when mixed with it in the right proportions, will cancel it. The wave lengths of both stimuli will be present in the mixed stimulus and the total energies of the two will be summated. The mixture will be the color of the stronger or, if the two are equally strong, the mixture will be gray.

This is the law of complementaries. It agrees with the color equation. No colors can be found that resemble both members of a complementary pair, both red and green, both blue and yellow, both black and white. Complementariness, however, does not always work out quite so simply.

The mixture of black and white gives a perfect cancellation, leaving, of course, gray. Mixture of unique blue with unique yellow gives gray. The mixture of red and green lights on the other hand gives a gray so yellowish as not properly to be called gray. It is more usual to say that the complementary of unique red is bluish green, and the complementary of unique green a bluish red or purple.

Law II. Color stimuli which are not complementary, when mixed, give resultant colors that resemble all the components to the same degree that each one is present in the mixture. This principle is most obvious in the combination of pairs of hues such as red and yellow to give orange, blue and green to give bluish green or greenish blue, etc., and it holds equally well for the addition of black, gray or white to any mixture.

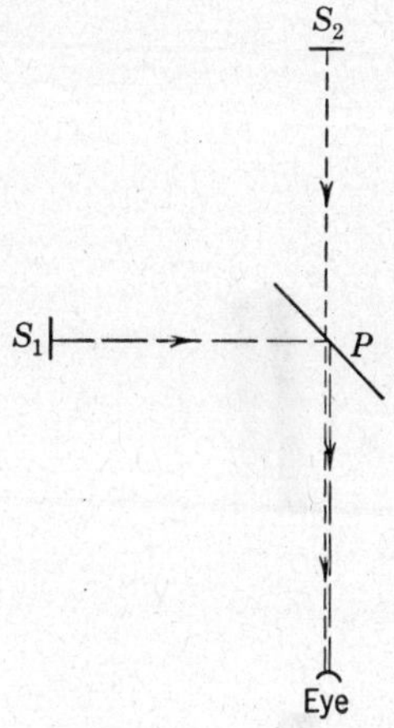

FIGURE 117. SCHEME FOR EXPERIMENTATION ON THE MIXTURE OF COLORS

The glass plate *P* reflects the light rays from S_1 into the observer's eye; the rays from S_2 pass directly through the glass and enter the eye in the same direction.

The stability of the colors obtained by the mixture of stimuli is guaranteed by the third law.

Law III. A mixture of mixtures that match will match either of the original mixtures (provided the light conditions remain constant). The law guarantees that colors can be dealt with as visual resultants on the basis of their resemblances or matches without reference to the physical composition of their stimuli. Thus another wording of the law is: Colors combine no matter how they are composed. You cannot tell the composition of a color by looking at it, of course, but that fact does not matter—so the law says. If you have a red and a bluish green which mix to make gray, you can substitute for the red any other red that looks like it to the eye, no matter of what spectral lights it is composed, and the new red will cancel the bluish green just as well as the old. You can make colors gray by mixing gray with them, although gray can be made of all the wave lengths, of any two complementary wave lengths or in hundreds of other ways. You have only to be sure that, when you substitute one gray for another, the grays match. You may need to keep the illumination constant, but that is because grays and other colors differently composed change color differently when illumination shifts from daylight to the depths of night vision.

While certain exceptions occur, the laws of color mixture are so well established that the important technology of colorimetry is based upon them.

Methods of Mixture

There are three important scientific devices for mixing color stimuli. The first two are additive, the third subtractive.

(1) Two beams of light may be combined so that they act as a single effective stimulus. Such a mixture produces a physical resultant which is the sum of the physical components. The method already mentioned (p. 279 and Fig. 117) may be used. The simplest way to do it, however, is to project two beams of light upon the same area of a nonselective, diffusely reflecting surface, for example, matte white (Fig. 118). Another way is to bring the two beams together by means of prisms so that their

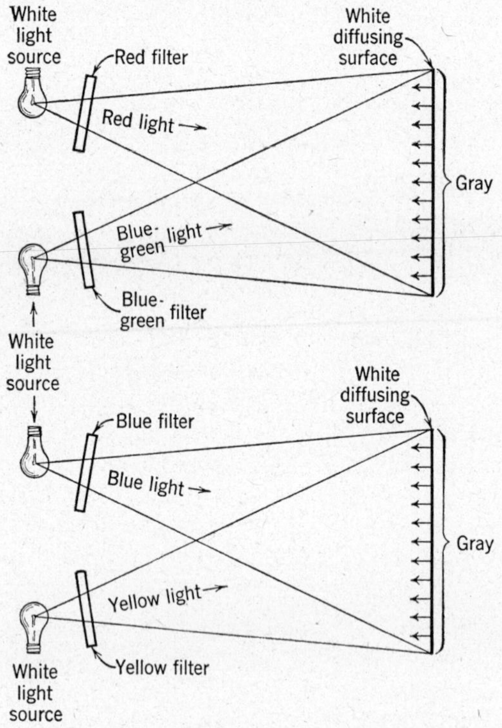

FIGURE 118. COLOR MIXTURE: THE FIRST LAW

sources are viewed directly as in the same place.

(2) Light from two areas may be rapidly alternated so that the two components are continuously effective over the whole area. The usual device of this sort is a rotating disk made up of two or more sectors. At four thousand revolutions per minute the component sectors fuse and summate proportionately, giving a single uniform color.

This is a convenient method to use because of its simplicity. The method is limited, however, because its summation is proportional, not absolute, that is to say, the color of each sector is effectively spread over the whole disk, thus reducing the stimulus effect per unit of area and making the mixture grayer. For instance, if you want to mix the red of a red paper with the yellow of a yellow paper, you can view both papers simultaneously in the same place by the use of prisms, and you get an orange that has in it the energy of all the red and all the yellow. But, if you put the two papers on a rotating disk, you have to make the disk half red and half yellow, and you get altogether from the disk only half as much energy as you would from mixing a whole red disk with a whole yellow disk. The result is that colors made by rotation of components are duller and grayer than they would be by simple addition.

(3) When a beam of light is passed through two or more transparent colored filters in succession, we have what is known as *subtractive color mixture.* The results are quite different from those of additive color mixture. In fact, the subtractive procedure should not properly be called color mixture, although it is a way of getting new colors from the combinations of others.

Two or more filters in combination will transmit only those wave lengths common to both or all. For example, if a filter that transmits only short waves below 550 millimicrons is placed over one that transmits only the long waves above 550 millimicrons, no light will pass the combination, and it is without meaning to talk about the color of the combination. It is not only complementary filters that cancel each other. A red filter may cancel a blue because the two filters transmit no common wave lengths. On the other hand, a yellow and a blue filter that are complementary may give a green, even though the yellow and blue are complementary. Why? The two filters overlap in transmission. The yellow filter lets through wave lengths from the red, yellow and green regions. The color looks yellow because the stimulus has more yellow than red and green and because the red and green tend to cancel and make a gray which mixes with the yellow. The blue filter lets through green, blue and violet light, and looks blue because blue predominates. *Together* the filters let through only the green light which is all that is common to both of them. So yellow and blue, which would give gray by additive mixture, in this case give green by subtractive mixture. The yellow filter subtracts the blue and violet, and the blue filter subtracts the red and yellow. Only green is left.

(4) In the mixture of color pigments, all the foregoing factors may be involved. Pigments consist of fine particles which modify the light falling upon them by selective reflection, by selective transmission, by both at once, and by refraction. All these effects are modified by the medium in which the pigments are suspended. In addition, one size or type of pigment particle has effects on another size or type that cannot be anticipated from the mere color of either. Therefore, although a particular yellow pigment and a particular blue pigment may result in a green, other pigments, visually identical to the original yellow and blue, may mix to give red or, perhaps, gray. In all cases the laws of color mixture are operative, but other factors control the selection of available wave lengths. For instance, to change the color of a certain yellowish red pigment toward bluish red, it may even be necessary to add white pigment, not blue.

Colorimetry

Within the last twenty years optical instruments have been so developed that a relatively simple operation can obtain a precise quantitative physical measurement

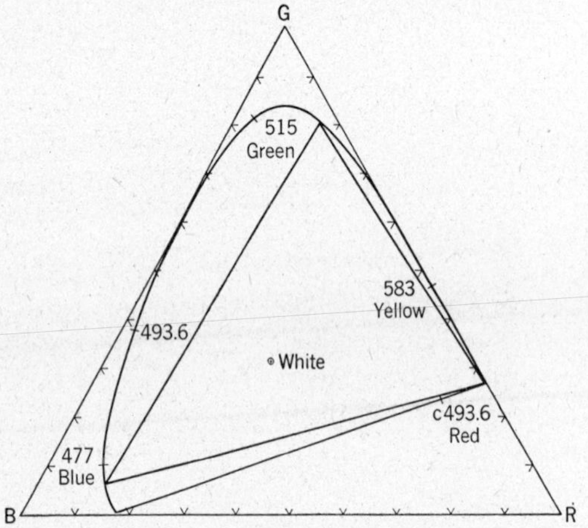

FIGURE 119. THREE-COLOR MIXTURE TRIANGLE

Curved line shows spectrum; small triangle, mixtures from three spectral colors; large triangle, three primaries whose mixture would give all the spectral colors; c493.6 (red) is nonspectral and complementary to 493.6 (bluish green).

of the spectral components of any light source, transmitting medium or reflecting surface. Given a spectral distribution curve for some color, it is not, however, easy to say from the curve just what the appearance of the color would be. Colorimetry puts the three laws of color mixture to work so that any spectral distribution can be translated easily into a statement of what color the distribution would give. (See Fig. 119.)

Since every component wave length in a spectral distribution combines with all the rest under one or the other of the first two laws of color mixture, and since under Law III any resultant is equivalent psychologically to any other resultant which it matches, it is possible to equate the color of any spectral distribution to a much simpler combination of wave lengths. For practical purposes three wave lengths have been found to answer most of the needs of such a reference system. Obviously the wave lengths must be carefully chosen and must be such that their normal colors will include unique red, yellow, green and blue. There are many possibilities, all of which will work out satisfactorily. The set must include a wave length near each end of the

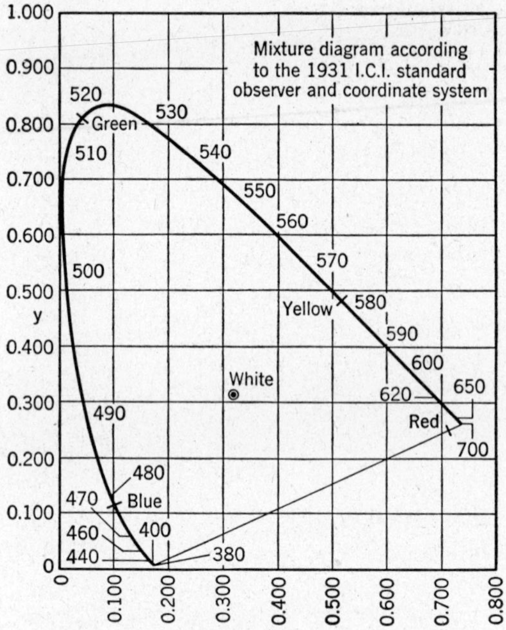

FIGURE 120. STANDARD TRICHROMATIC COLOR COORDINATES

The figure shows the spectral colors plotted on the standard ICI (International Congress on Illumination) coordinates. This plot permits specification of all unique or duplex colors. The yellow in this diagram can be specified by $x = 0.512$, $y = 0.488$.

spectrum and one near the middle. The international standard that has been adopted specifies wave lengths 700, 546.1 and 435.8 millimicrons, which give, respectively, a slightly yellowish red, a yellow green and a reddish blue.

Data have been obtained which standardize the amounts of these three stimuli ($R + G + B$) that will match every one of the monochromatic spectral stimuli. These quantities are known as the *tri-stimulus values* of a color. All colors having the same tri-stimulus values, no matter what the physical composition of their stimuli may be, will look the same. That is Law III of color mixture.

A still simpler form of representation has been made by taking the proportions of the tri-stimulus values, for R, G and B, respectively, that is, $R/(R + G + B)$, $G/(R + G + B)$, $B/(R + G + B)$. Any two of these proportions determine the third and thus specify the spectral equivalent of a stimulus, but not its black-white component. The *trichromatic coordinates* can be plotted on a two-dimensional diagram (Fig. 120). Trichromatic colorimetry which has a wide field of applications is based upon this system of representation.

COLOR PHENOMENA

We come now to a consideration of the more general psychological phenomena of the occurrence of color in human experience—the laws of adaptation, contrast and indirect vision, and the facts of color blindness and night vision.

Adaptation

When color stimulation is continued, the color changes, at first rapidly and then more slowly, tending toward gray. A bright light retains its extreme brightness for only a brief time. The sun on snow gives a blinding glare when we first go out of a more dimly lighted building, but the glare soon moderates. Similarly, the blackness of the dark does not last. The darkened theater is hopelessly black when we first enter, but when we have been there a half hour, the blind behavior of a new arrival seems ludicrous. The same thing happens to all the other colors. The yellowness of artificial illumination, as it is first turned on, soon disappears.

The phenomenon we are describing is known as *sensory adaptation* and is effective for all visual qualities with one exception, the ever-constant gray. The law of color adaptation may be stated as follows: *With continued duration all colors tend toward gray.* Blacks and whites, as well as reds, oranges, yellows, greens, blues and purples, get grayer when the stimulation for them continues on the same part of the retina.

FIGURE 121. SENSORY ADAPTATION

Steadily fixate the line between the two fields. Notice how the black lightens and the white darkens.

Sensory adaptation can be observed and described most accurately if you fixate steadily a small patch of color or a particolored field, to give a basis for comparison. Hang up side by side a sheet of white cardboard and a sheet of black cardboard, and stare fixedly at some point on their line of junction. (See Fig. 121.) Almost at once, clouds of gray begin to form over the two fields, lightening the black and darkening the white. The clouding increases as fixation continues until both halves of the field approach gray. You could get the whole particolored field a uniform gray if you could but keep your eyes still. Instead you find that you keep twitching them, losing fixation and then regaining it.

Afterimages

The effects of any visual stimulation persist after its removal, and the longer

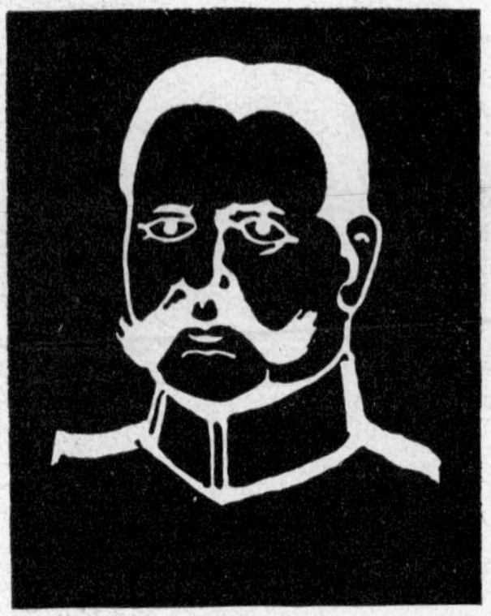

FIGURE 122. NEGATIVE AFTERIMAGE

Fixate steadily, for about a minute, one of the eyes in this negative portrait. Then shift the fixation quickly to a blank sheet of white paper. You will see a negative afterimage of this negative, that is to say, a positive. [After A. Noll (1926).]

the original stimulation, the greater and more persistent are the after-effects. The glare of the sun on the snow will be modified to some extent according to the illumination of the house from which we have just come. The theater is darker when we enter from a bright day than when the day outside is dull and overcast. When colored glasses have been worn for a time and then removed, everything takes on a color complementary to the color of the glasses. If, after you have stared at the particolored card for a time, someone covers it with a uniform screen, the screen appears blackish where the card was white and whitish where the card was black. (See Fig. 121.) The effects are even more striking if other colors are substituted for black and white. If the color fixated is red, the after-effect will be green; if blue, yellow; and vice versa. Thus white follows black and black, white; red follows green and green, red; yellow follows blue and blue, yellow. This phenomenon is known as the *negative afterimage.* The complementary relationship of the opposing color pairs of the color equation appears again. (See Fig. 122.)

The facts of adaptation and negative afterimage show that we are dealing with a single process. Adaptation to one color means sensitization to its complementary. That is what you are seeing when you try to fixate the line between the black and white fields of Fig. 121. As your eyes twitch, the image of a narrow edge of white field falls upon the black-adapted, white-sensitized part of the retina, and the white looks even whiter than it did at first. So with the black, when the eyes twitch the other way.

The after-effects of continued color stimulation are not, however, limited to this complementary or negative afterimage. There is also a *positive afterimage,* so called because its color resembles the original color although somewhat grayer. A color experience does not cease immediately when the color stimulus is removed, but persists for a measurable time and may, after disappearing, reappear again. It is the reappearance that is the positive afterimage. Sometimes the inevitable lag of every sensation after its stimulus has ceased may be prolonged without an interval into the positive afterimage. Positive afterimages, especially when they occur after long adaptation to the dark and short exposure to a brilliant stimulus can be very vivid, showing detail and reproducing all the colors. The circle of light produced by the revolving pinwheel in a display of fireworks is mostly positive afterimage.

Contrast

The quality of a color varies with its background. If a red which is unique when it occupies the entire visual field is restricted in size and surrounded by blue, it becomes yellowish. If the surrounding color is changed to yellow, the red turns bluish. As we have seen, white in the background may give an appearance of black, and vice versa. A green background makes the red redder, and conversely. The only background color that does not alter the original quality is gray. For this reason, when we wish to examine a color accurately, we always place it upon a gray background. Similarly we can study the effect of a background best by placing a gray strip or patch upon it. The gray becomes tinged with color complementary to the background. This effect of background upon a color is a third instance of the complementariness of colors. (See Fig. 123.)

We may state the general *law of contrast* as follows: *Every color in the visual field affects and is affected by every other color.*

Several secondary laws made specific the nature and degree of the effect. (1) The quality of the induced color is always that of the complementary of the inducing color. (2) The induction increases with a decrease of gray in the inducing color. (3) The induction is greatest when there are no sharp outlines between the background and the induction field. (4) The induction is greatest at the margins near the inducing field. (5) The induction is greatest when the background and the induction field are in the same plane. (6) The inducing effect of red, yellow, blue and green is greater when there is no white or black contrast.

Everyday experience affords many examples of color induction. Gray stripes on a green material will appear a purplish red. A bright light in the visual field makes everything else dark. This is one

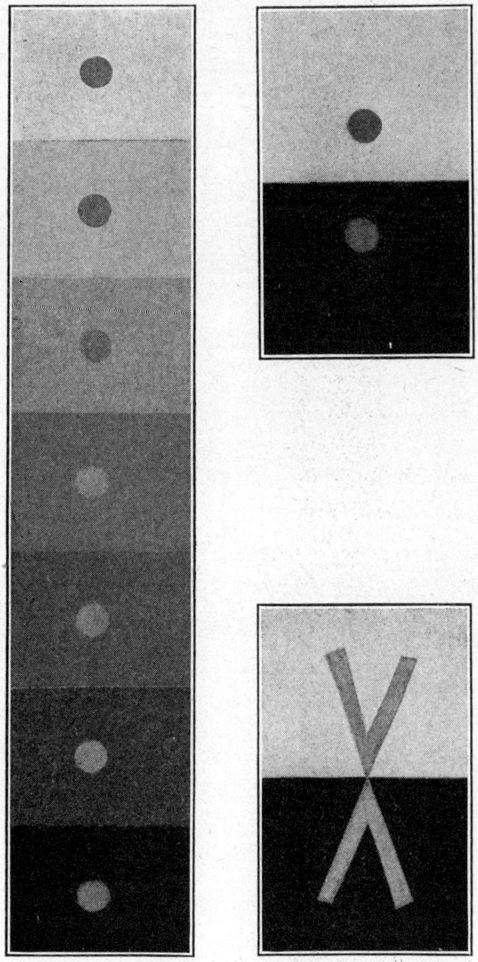

FIGURE 123. SIMULTANEOUS INDUCTION OF CONTRAST

A white background induces an increment of black in a small area of gray placed upon it, and vice versa. The gray dots and figures are all identical but appear dark on the light background and light on the dark background.

reason why the lights of an oncoming car 'blind' you. They cover everything else with a black that blots out contours. A student of art soon learns that he can color some objects by painting only the surrounding objects. A sailboat against a blue sky will be tinted with yellow. Color contrast contributes to everything we see and must be taken into account when we wish to specify or control the color of an object.

A manufacturer once tried to make a green and gray gingham. When he wove the gray threads among the green, he had a green *and pink* gingham. Undoubtely the gingham fulfilled the conditions of the secondary laws of contrast. There must have been little gray in the green. The gray and green threads must have been equally white or equally black. The checks of the gingham must have been small, must have appeared to be in the same plane and without contours.

Shadows, when black-white equality is secured, are especially subject to red-yellow-green-or-blue contrast effects, because a shadow lies exactly in the plane of the surface on which it is projected and has no prominent contours. If you stand under a red neon light you will notice that your shadow is green.

A piece of gray paper on a field of red paper looks greener if the whole field is covered with thin white tissue paper. Why? Because the tissue paper cuts out perceived contours and puts the red and the gray in the same plane, as if the gray were a shadow. The tissue works against contrast because it decreases the relative intensity of the red, making it grayer, but the laws of contour and of plane are more important and make up for the disadvantage of the grayer red.

Indirect Vision

The quality of a color varies with its position in the visual field. If, as we fixate steadily on a point straight ahead, a color stimulus that is not too intensive enters the visual field from the side and approaches the fixation point, the color undergoes a series of changes. In the extreme periphery it appears gray, light or dark according to its whiteness or blackness. A little farther in, a blueness or yellowness may appear, but not until the stimulus has reached a position near the center of the field is it reddish or greenish. If the entire visual field of each eye is explored in this manner, there will be found a fairly restricted zone in the center of the field of vision where all color qualities can be seen. Surrounding this area lies a second zone in which no redness or greenness is visible but where blueness and yellowness can be seen. In the extreme periphery all color experience is restricted to blacks, grays and whites except with very intensive stimuli. In this spatial distribution the colors have appeared again in their complementary pairs. (See Fig. 124.)

Thus a dark purple disk, being moved from the outside of the field to the center, will appear first black, then blue, then purple. A light orange disk will appear first white or light gray, then yellow, then orange.

The boundaries of the color zones in the field of vision are not rigidly fixed. The more effective the stimulus, the farther from the center can the color be seen. The zones are larger for a spot of spectral light than for a patch of colored paper, because the spectral light is less gray. The zones are larger for large stimuli than for small. You might think that you could see your own color zones by looking with one eye at

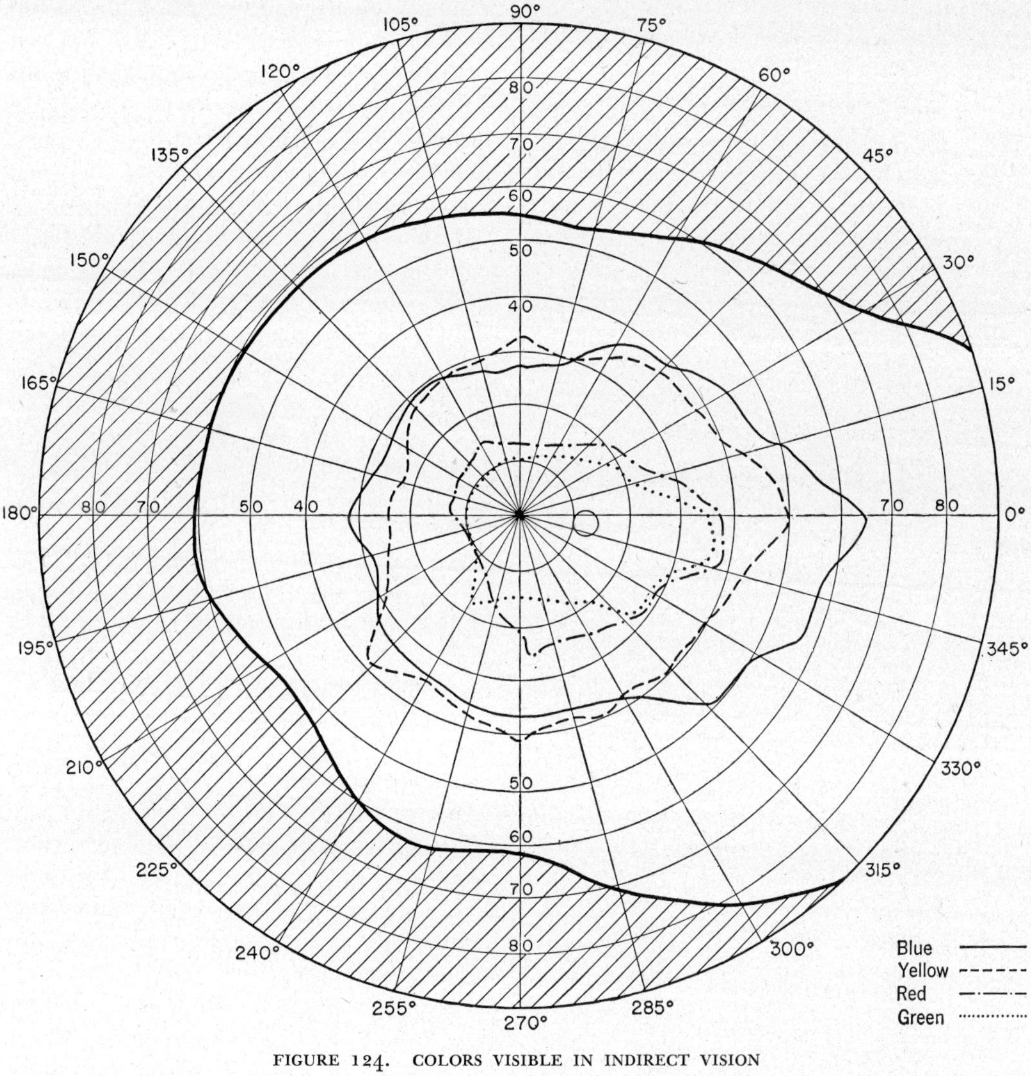

FIGURE 124. COLORS VISIBLE IN INDIRECT VISION

Chart shows the portion of the visual field of the right eye within which each of the unique colors can be seen when the stimulus is a small patch of homogeneous light. At these intensities red and green are limited to an area of approximately 20 degrees about the fixation point, whereas yellow and blue can be seen out to 40 or 50 degrees in the vertical and 50 to 60 in the horizontal meridian.

a large sheet of purple paper which fills your entire field of vision. You cannot. The large color stimulus is so effective that it causes you to see the purple all the way to the limits of your field of vision.

In the course of exploration of the visual field of a single eye with a small stimulus we find an area of some size where the stimulus completely disappears. Known as the *blind spot,* it occurs because the eye's retina is practically blind where the optic nerve enters it. You do not see your own blind spot in ordinary vision. For one thing, the blind spots in the two eyes do not coincide, so nothing is missing in two-eyed vision. Still you cannot see your blind spot for one eye when you close the other. That is because in perception you fill in the field with whatever the surroundings would make you think belonged there. As we have seen before, perception tries to keep objects constant. In a neutral field, however, with only a fixation point and one other object present, the existence of the blind spot can be readily demonstrated. (See Fig. 125.)

FIGURE 125. BLIND SPOT

Close your left eye, hold the book at a distance of about 14 inches in front of you, and fixate the dot with the right eye. If you see the face at the right, move the book a little nearer or farther away. When the right distance is found the face will disappear and the page will appear blank.

Color Blindness

A certain deviation of color vision appears as a special peculiarity. About four per cent of the population, nearly all males, never experience the color qualities red and green. They see only five unique colors, blue, yellow, black, white and gray. All redness or greenness of normal vision appears to them gray, just as they do outside the central zone of the field of vision. They do not need a color pyramid to diagram the colors visible to them. They see only what appears in the color square for yellow-white-blue-black with gray in the center. (See Fig. 108, p. 272.)

Many curious instances of this deficiency have been reported. Attention was first called to the defect by Huddart in 1777, but the truth of his assertions was discounted. In his memoirs Sir John Dalton, a noted chemist of the late eighteenth century, gives an excellent account of the difficulties into which his own peculiarities of vision had led him. His description of them gives us a good idea of how the world of colors looks to a color-blind person.

Dalton wrote: "My observations began with the *solar spectrum,* or coloured image of the sun, exhibited in a dark room by means of a glass prism. . . . I see only *two* or at most *three* distinctions. These I should call *yellow* and *blue;* or *yellow, blue,* and *purple.* My yellow comprehends the *red, orange, yellow,* and *green* of others; and my *blue* and *purple* coincide with theirs. That part of the image which others call red, appears to me little more than a shade, or defect of light; after that the orange, yellow, and green seem *one* colour, which descends pretty uniformly from an intense to a rare yellow, making what I should call different shades of yellow. The difference between the green part and the blue part is very striking to my eye: they seem to be strongly contrasted. . . . All crimsons appear to me to consist chiefly of dark blue; but many of them seem to have a strong tinge of dark brown. I have seen specimens of *crimson, claret,* and *mud,* which were very nearly alike. Crimson has a *grave* appearance, being the reverse of every shewy and splendid colour. Woolen yarn dyed crimson or dark blue is the same to me. *Pink* seems to be composed of nine parts of light blue, and one of red, or some colour which has no other effect than to make the light blue appear dull and faded a little. . . . My idea of red I obtain from *vermilion, minium, sealing wax, wafers, a soldier's uniform,* etc. These seem to have no blue whatever in them. . . . Blood appears to me red; but it differs much from the articles mentioned above. It is much more dull, and to me is not unlike that colour called *bottle-green.* Stockings spotted with blood or with dirt would scarcely be distinguishable. . . . I take my standard idea [of green] from grass. This appears to me very little different from red. . . . Green and orange have much affinity also. . . . Green woolen cloth, such as used to cover tables, appears to me a dull, dark, brownish red colour. . . . When this kind of cloth loses its colour, as other people say, and turns yellow, then it appears to me a pleasant green." *

In the same class with Dalton's experience is the inability of color-blind persons to distinguish ripe red cherries from the foliage of the tree upon which they hang, and red flags of a golf course from green turf. We must not, however, confuse a lack of accuracy in color naming with the true lack of red-and-green color experience.

Upon careful examination color blindness has been found to be not a simple all-or-none phenomenon. There are varying degrees and kinds of deficiency in color vision. A few, no more than one hundred cases, have been reported in which the only colors seen are black, gray and white. For them color vision is reduced to something like the extreme peripheral vision of a normal observer. Most color deficiencies, however, involve only red and green.

A further complication is that red-green color blindness is of two different types. Most color-blind persons see gray in place of both red and green with the relative brightnesses of the spectral colors unchanged. Such persons have been called *deuteranopes.* A few color-deficient persons have color vision further complicated by a shift of relative brightness away from the long wave lengths toward the short wave lengths, so that in place of red they see black and in place of green they see a whitish gray. Such persons have been called *protanopes.* The names are derived from the fact that protanopic vision is supposed to be more primitive than deuteranopic, just as all red-green color blindness is supposed to be a more primitive—evolutionarily older—kind of vision than normal vision.

Between deficiencies in which all sensitivity to green and red is lacking and cases of normal sensitivity, lie many degrees of color weakness. It appears, moreover, from recent measurements that red-green deficiency is accompanied by a loss in blue-yellow sensitivity. The color blind suffer an overall loss. They do not compensate for the loss of one pair of complementaries by increased sensitivity for another pair.

In spite of their deficiency, color-blind persons name colors correctly more often than not. There is sufficient difference between other colors and the dull dark yellow which they see for red, or the light yellowish gray that green appears to be, for them correctly to identify objects designated by those color names. It is undoubtedly for this reason that color deficiency is so recent a discovery. In our complex civiliza-

* John Dalton. Extraordinary Facts relating to the Vision of Colours: with observations. Read Oct. 31st, 1794. *Memoirs of the Literary and Philosophical Society of Manchester,* 1798, **5**, Part 1, pp. 31–35.

tion of today, color discrimination has increased in importance so that color deficiency is a disadvantage, often a menace, in numerous occupations (for instance, at sea or in transportation where colored signals are used). Hence many tests have been devised for its detection. Identification of color samples or matching and sorting can be used to bring out color anomalies. Accuracy of results depends on the care with which the color samples are prepared. In an early test devised by Holmgren, the subjects were asked to find among a variety of skeins of yarn samples similar to three standards. From the errors exhibited, a color-blind subject should be detected, were it not for the fact that many such people learned to correct their errors and so appeared to pass the test. Matching tests, with carefully graded series of color chips, work better and can be used to measure the degree of the defect.

In many ways the most interesting type of test is one in which patterns are made up of two colors which appear identical to a color-blind person but are quite different to normal vision, such as orange and yellow-green or blue-green and lavender. A number is outlined in dots of one color on a background of the other color. The color-blind subject is unable to make out such a concealed pattern. Still other tests present small areas of filtered light for recognition and diagnose color deficiency on the basis of confusions of 'white' light with 'green,' or 'yellow' with 'red,' or 'red' with 'green.' With properly chosen filters this test can be very accurate.

Night Vision

Vision in the ordinary ranges of daylight from fairly faint twilight up to the brightest blaze of the sun is called *daylight vision* or *photopic vision*. Nearly all the facts described thus far in this chapter are facts of daylight vision. Vision from the point where twilight falls down to what you see in the country on a moonless night when the clouds obscure some of the stars (you do not see objects unless you have been some time in the dark) is *night vision* or *scotopic vision*. In twilight, daylight vision and night vision overlap; both function together. The next section shows that we believe that there are in the retina two kinds of receptors for these two kinds of vision: cones for daylight seeing, rods for night seeing. That theory gives us still another set of names for the same difference: *cone vision* and *rod vision*.

What happens when the energy of the general illumination is gradually diminished from a level necessary for good daylight vision to the level at which night vision is working alone? You can see the answer for yourself if you watch the light fade on a variegated field of color samples. You can make the observation during a couple of hours at twilight or you can hurry the process up by arranging very gradually to shut the door of a room which will be pitch dark when the door is completely closed. At first, as the light fails, the colors remain the same in respect of the red-yellow-green-blue series, though they become somewhat blacker and grayer. Then at a particular point the reds begin to darken considerably and the greens and blues to lighten. This change is called the *Purkinje phenomenon,* after the physiologist who discovered it in 1825. Red finally turns to black while green and blue become a silvery light gray. Thus in complete night vision all colors reduce to shades of black, gray and white. As adaptation goes on, the blacks disappear, leaving only grays and whites, which have the bluish cast that is taken for granted as a characteristic of moonlight. Thus in motion pictures, almost any scene can be converted into 'moonlight' simply by dyeing the whole film blue without reducing the intensity of the illumination.

We can, therefore, in this continuous process, distinguish two stages. In the Purkinje phenomenon daylight and night vision act together. We can still see reds, yellows, greens, blues and violets, but the reds are very dark, and the blues and violets very light. In complete night vision the reds have become black, the blues and violets light bluish gray, and the yellow-greens bluish white. After long-continued night vision, most of the blacks disappear under adaptation, since there is nothing darker than a lightless region for the night eye to see as black. (See Fig. 126.)

Full sensitivity of night vision is not attained at once, if illumination suddenly drops to a low level. It develops gradually at a decreasing rate over a period of half an hour to an hour. In that time your ability to discriminate small intensities of light increases by at least ten thousand times. Thus *dark adaptation* means not only that the blacks have become gray, but also that sensitivity has increased enormously. In the Second World War the psychology of night vision became suddenly important, because all at once there was need for men to see in the dark. In peacetime the way to see in the dark is to turn on the light. In war you dare not—not if you are a night fighter or a naval lookout or an infantry patrol on duty at night. Such men stayed in the dark half an hour before they went on night duty so that their night vision might be maximally sensitive after thorough dark adaptation. Or else before duty they wore red goggles, the kind of red goggles that let through only the very long wave lengths. In this way they kept the rods in their retinas sensitive, because red light does not affect the rods or cause them to become desensitized. (That is why red looks black in rod vision.)

A third characteristic of night vision is that objects become more difficult to see when they are looked at directly. That is because the very center of the retina is blind at night; there are no rods there.

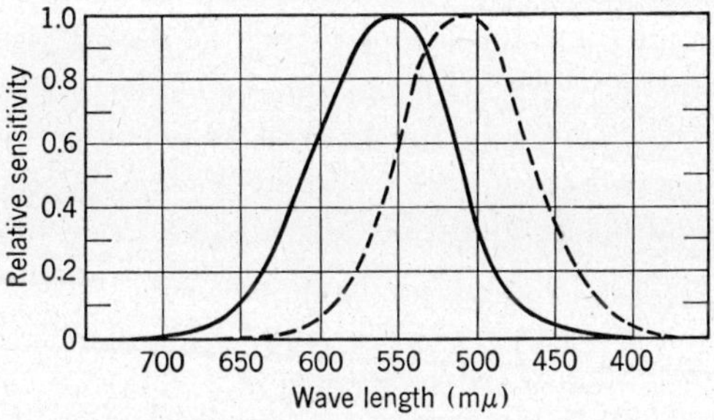

FIGURE 126. SENSITIVITY CURVES FOR DAYLIGHT AND NIGHT VISION

The solid curve is the sensitivity curve for daylight vision, and the dashed curve is for night vision. The curves show relative sensitivity, and hence brightness, in different parts of the spectrum when the light at all wave lengths is of equal energy. In daylight vision hues are seen at the various wave lengths. In night vision only grays of different whitenesses are seen.

You can demonstrate this fact by setting in a dark room a source of light which is completely covered except for two pinholes a few centimeters apart. Try to fixate, from a distance of three or four yards, one of the pinholes. The light which is fixated will disappear while the other shows up fairly clearly. A shift of fixation from one pinhole to the other will make the hole at which you look invisible and the hole at which you do not look directly visible. With fixation elsewhere in the field, both points are visible. Small weak stimuli cannot be seen at all in the center of the field of vision where, in good light, details are seen best. The region in the center of the retina is called the *fovea.* One of the characteristics of night vision is *foveal blindness.*

In summary we may note that night vision differs from daylight vision in four ways. (1) All color qualities, except black, gray and white, disappear. (2) The grays and whites that remain are slightly tinged with blue. (3) The whitest colors at night occur for color stimuli which at normal intensities give yellow-green. (4) The fovea, at the center of the field of vision and the spot which is most competent in daylight, is blind at night.

PHYSIOLOGY OF COLOR VISION

The eye is a simple form of photographic camera consisting essentially of a dark chamber with a *lens* at the front and a sensitive film (retina) at the back. (See Fig. 127.) In front of the lens is a diaphragm (pupil) and a shutter (eyelid). The dark box is approximately spherical and is kept in shape by the liquid with which it is filled. The lens is a relatively thick transparent capsule filled with a liquid whose refractive power is different from that of the liquid in the dark chamber. The focus of the lens is altered by the *ciliary muscle,* a circular muscle attached to its edge, which stretches and flattens it or allows it to bulge, according to the distance of the object viewed. The precise nature of the sensitive membrane, the *retina,* which lies at the back of the dark chamber has been studied by physiologists and psychologists who are interested in the functioning of the eye.

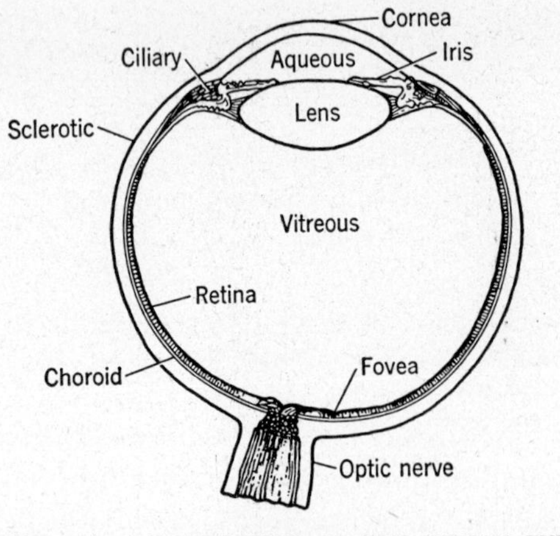

FIGURE 127. CROSS-SECTION OF THE HUMAN EYE

This figure represents a cross-section of the right eye, as viewed from above. [After L. T. Troland, *The principles of psychophysiology,* 1930, II, p. 98; by permission of D. Van Nostrand Company.]

Microscopic examination of the retina shows that it is made up primarily of nerve cells and their special endings. The latter are of two types. One, the *rod,* is cylindrical in form and ends in a nerve fiber with a cell body somewhat removed from the base of the rod. The other, the *cone,* is shorter and thicker and somewhat conical in shape, and the nerve-cell body is incorporated in its base. The nerve fibers, which thus have their origins in the rods and cones, end within the retina in synaptic connections to another set of nerve cells, the *bipolar cells,* which in turn connect with a third group of *ganglion cells* with long fibers which join to form the optic nerve and run back to the nuclei in the brain and thence to the cortex. (See Fig. 128.)

The latest microscopic examinations show the neural connections at the retina to be very complex. A single cone is connected to several bipolar cells and by way of them to as many as half a dozen ganglion cells whose fibers form the optic nerve. Some bipolar cells are connected to both rods and cones and all of them run to two

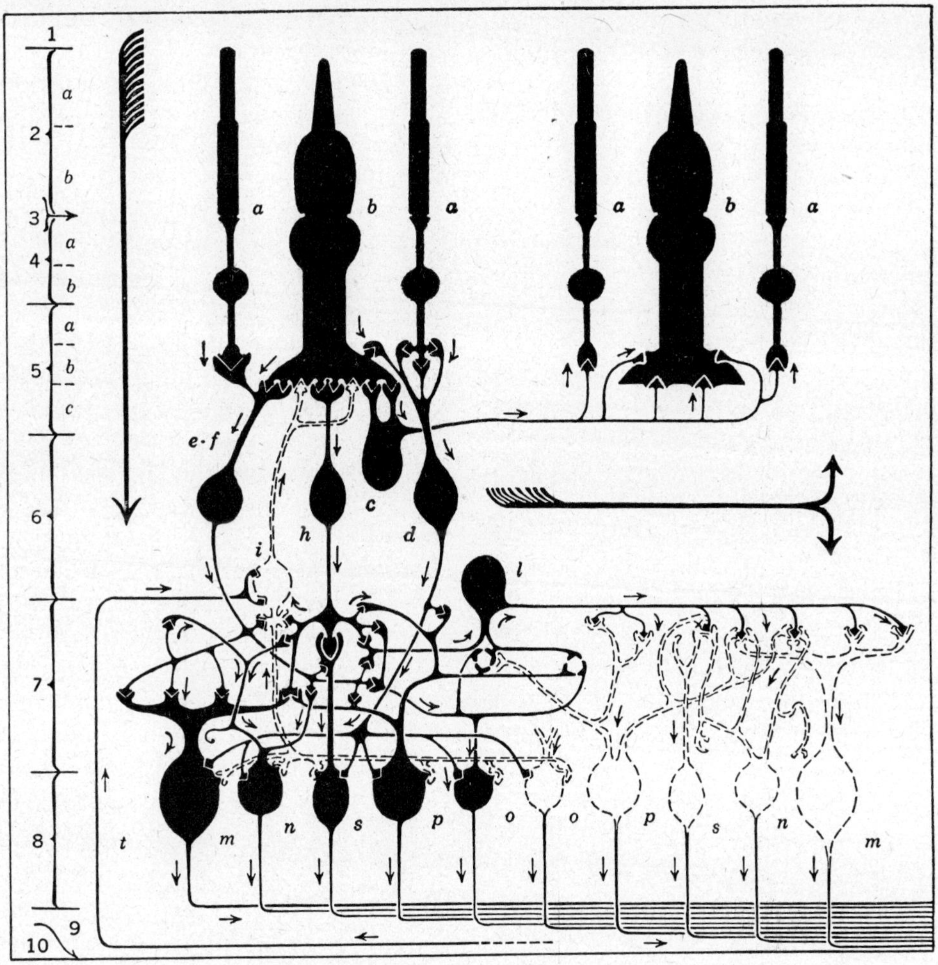

FIGURE 128. CROSS-SECTION OF THE RETINA

The numbers on the left indicate different layers of the retina. The arrows indicate the direction in which the nerve impulse travels. The rods (*a*) and cones (*b*) transmit their excitations through the various kinds of bipolar cells (*d, e, f, h, i*), sometimes across the retina through horizontal cells (*c, l*), to the ganglion cells (*m, n, s, p, o*), and on through the optic nerve (layers 9, 10) to the optic nuclei and the visual cortex. [From S. L. Polyak, *The retina,* Chicago: University of Chicago Press, 1941.]

or more ganglion cells. In addition there are horizontal cells that connect one cone with another and with near-by rods, and others that make horizontal connections among the bipolar and ganglion cells. Finally, there are several different types of connections between the various cells. It is believed that all this complication is significant in the functioning of the retina, not just a matter of accident. After all, in many phenomena the retina is known to act as a whole and not in isolated parts. We can, for example, see purple at the periphery of the retina provided the same kind of stimulation affects all the remainder of the retina.

Active sensory nerves have been found to exhibit electrical phenomena in the form of changes in electrical potential which give rise to *action currents.* In recent experiments action currents have been recorded from retinal elements in response to light stimuli. From them it appears that some retinal elements—rods or cones or both—respond to all ranges of light stimuli. Other retinal elements, however, respond to only limited light-wave ranges. Response to blue has been definitely isolated and possibly the responses to green and to red.

Since the cells which give rise to the optic fibers lie in the innermost layer of the retina, the fibers, in order to leave the eye, must pass back through the retina. All the fibers come together as they leave the eye, producing a gap in the retina. At the corresponding area in the field of vision there is but little sensitivity, and that is the region which is called the *blind spot.* Since the optic nerve leaves the eye about three millimeters to the nasal side of the center of the eye, the blind spot lies to the temporal or outer side of the field of vision of each eye.

The diameter of the retinal blind spot is about two millimeters. Such an area on the retina subtends an angle of about six degrees in the visual field.

Duplexity of Retinal Function

An adequate account of the way a sense organ functions consists in a careful correlation of the physiological and physical facts, on the one hand, with the parallel psychological data, on the other. Usually not all the necessary facts in both fields are available, and the psychologist must attempt to put together the available facts in such a way as to bridge the gaps in knowledge. Some of the resulting psychophysiological correlations are quite firmly established. Others are tentative. One of the best-established correlations is the principle that the retinal rods are the organs of night vision and the retinal cones the organs of daylight vision. Let us summarize the facts by which this correlation is established.

Vision is of two kinds. (1) First there is full color vision as represented by the color equation. (*a*) Such vision is maximal at the center of the field of vision in the region surrounding the point of fixation. (*b*) It diminishes in regions away from the central zone, losing first the red-green member of the equation and then the yellow-blue member in regions that approach the periphery. (*c*) Color vision requires the relatively greater stimulus energy of daylight vision. If the energy of the stimulus falls below a certain level, color vision disappears.

(2) Second, there is vision that consists (*a*) only of black, gray and white (modified by bluishness). (*b*) Such vision is completely lacking in the center of the field of vision and improves progressively toward the periphery. (*c*) It requires a relatively low level of stimulus intensity, the maximum being slightly above the minimum level for color vision. In some cases, therefore, the two visions overlap, and we can then observe that various stimuli do not have the same effectiveness in both kinds of vision. (*d*) Red stimuli have no effect in low-level vision, whereas green and blue are relatively more effective than they are in color vision. Moreover, (*e*) low-level vision is not turned on immediately as color vision is turned off, but requires a considerable time to appear, during which dark adaptation takes place.

Now, on the physiological side, we have found, first, that the retina contains two distinctive types of nerve endings, and, second, that these two endings have significant distributions over the surface of the retina. Cones are closely packed in the fovea of the retina and thin out toward the periphery. Rods are completely absent from the fovea and increase in number, both absolutely and relative to the number of cones, toward the periphery.

Putting these two sets of facts together gives us what can be called the *duplexity theory,* the generalization that the cones are the organs of daylight or color vision and that the rods are the organs of night vision.

Further physiological facts are known about the rods, facts which fit in with psychological facts and tend to confirm the duplexity theory. A substance known as *visual purple* is found around the ends of the rods. Its chemical formula has been determined and many of its properties recorded. It is a highly unstable compound, related to vitamin A. It quickly decomposes in the presence of light and recombines in darkness, when the proper substances are present. The ideal conditions for the formation of visual purple occur in the retina in total darkness, where its increase will continue for a considerable period of time. We can conclude, therefore, that the visual purple of the retina acts as a sensitizer for the rods. In its absence they fail to respond. After a large accumulation of it has been built up, the sensitivity of the rods is ten thousand times that of the cones in daylight. The rate of the accumulation of visual purple within the natural conditions of the retina in darkness parallels the progress of dark adaptation. Since the visual purple absorbs yellow and green light, it responds more vigorously to those wave lengths. Correspondingly, yellow-green wave lengths are seen in night vision as whiter than other wave lengths, whereas red wave lengths give no white at all and are seen as very dark or as black. Such a psychophysiological correlation affords an acceptable theory of night vision in terms of rod function.

By elimination, then, color vision is ascribed to the cones of the retina, but physiological facts concerning their functioning are insufficient to afford a detailed correlation. It has been supposed that various cones may contain differently selective photochemicals, but no such substances have been isolated from the retinal tissue. Another hypothesis supposes that the various connecting cells respond differently to give qualitative differences in color. We have noted that one investigation has found that the electrical discharges from various retinal elements indicate that some elements respond to all light waves whereas others are more selective. This finding may mean that the early theorists were right in ascribing the differentiations among colors to the retina, but there is other evidence that the nerve impulses are not completely differentiated until they reach the brain. An acceptable psychophysiological theory of color vision still waits upon future discovery.

REFERENCES

1. Bartley, S. H. *Vision.* New York: Van Nostrand, 1941.

   The psychophysics and psychophysiology of most of the phenomena of visual sensation and perception except the correlates of wave length.

2. Graham, C. H. Vision: some neural correlations. In C. Murchison (Ed.), *A handbook of general experimental psychology.* Worcester, Mass.: Clark University Press, 1934. Chap. 15.

A technical handbook account of the neural mechanisms involved in visual perception.

3. Hecht, S. Vision: the nature of the photoreceptor process. In C. Murchison (Ed.), *A handbook of general experimental psychology.* Worcester, Mass.: Clark University Press, 1934. Chap. 14.

A rather technical presentation of the physiological data which form the basis for theories of the neural reception of light.

4. Ladd-Franklin, C. *Colour and colour theories.* New York: Harcourt, Brace, 1929.

Reprints of a score of the author's more important papers on color theory and the argument which supports her genetic theory of color.

5. Parsons, J. H. *An introduction to the study of colour vision.* (2nd ed.) Cambridge, England: Cambridge University Press, 1924.

The most complete handbook which reports the basic investigations on color up to 1924, but now out of date.

6. Troland, L. T. Vision: visual phenomena and their stimulus correlations. In C. Murchison (Ed.), *A handbook of general experimental psychology.* Worcester, Mass.: Clark University Press, 1934. Chap. 13.

An excellent and precise summary of the psychophysical relation of visual phenomena to visual stimulation.

7. Troland, L. T. *The principles of psychophysiology.* New York: Van Nostrand, 1930. Vol. II, Chap. 14.

A full discussion of the psychophysical relations of visual phenomena to visual stimulation, somewhat more complete than the preceding item.

CHAPTER 13

Visual Space Perception

THE human organism lives in three-dimensional space, orients itself in it, reacts to stimulus objects in it and is fully aware of it in all its tridimensionality. It has equipment for perceiving space, equipment with which heredity provides it—eyes with retinas on which a two-dimensional image of the visual field can be focused, eyes which can do the focusing, which can converge more or less toward each other, which, being separate, get dissimilar views of the world, which move in the head, thus changing the visual field. It has a head to hold the eyes and to move them around. It has also mobile arms and hands to explore the immediate universe and to respond within this universe to visual stimulation, as well as a mobile body to explore the more remote world and to make more responses to stimulation. This equipment the organism uses during its early lifetime to build up its knowledge and awareness of tridimensional space, to learn how to react with discrimination to objects in a three-way visual field. The retinas could not do this job alone. They depend on movements of the eyes to make images clear and to gauge distance, and on movements of the body and limbs to give spatial meaning to the core of the visual perception, a core which in itself consists only of a bidimensional pattern of colors. We have already seen how a man can learn to react properly in a three-dimensional world after he has become accustomed to wearing special glasses which turn his retinal images upside down and right for left (p. 242). That experiment showed how definitely the 'visual' perception of space depends on motor reactions to make it meaningful. For instance, a visually perceived object is localized in space when you know where to reach for it. If you reach up to get something off the floor simply because you think the floor is above you (as you may if you have just put on these special glasses), you must learn something before you know your 'visual' space.

The most surprising fact about visual space perception is that, with bidimensional retinas, we see tridimensional space. How do we do this? Where does the third dimension come from? At the retina the organism has surrendered one of the three dimensions of space, for only up-down and right-left are directly represented in the

This chapter was prepared by Forrest L. Dimmick of the U. S. Naval Medical Research Laboratory at New London.

The opinions or assertions contained in this chapter are the private ones of the collaborator and the editors and are not to be construed as official or reflecting the views of the Navy Department or the Naval Service at large.

retinal image. Yet in visual perception it has got back again the lost dimension. It sees solid objects in tridimensional space. How it has contrived to do that is the topic of the first section of this chapter.

VISUAL PERCEPTION OF THE THIRD DIMENSION

You can think of the perceiving organism as instantly knowing how to build up its picture of the stimulus world from *clues* which the senses furnish it. The organism is an instantaneous detective in these perceptual matters. It does not reason its perceptions out and sometimes it makes 'errors.' A standard habitual error we call an illusion. Nevertheless the organism does well with its clues. It has to have some basis for discriminative reaction and for accurate knowledge, and psychology's business is to determine the character of these clues upon which the organism acts.

The stimulation clues for up-down and right-left perception lie, obviously, in the stimulation pattern itself. The clues to adequate knowledge of the third dimension are less direct. Some of them come from eye movements and some from the disparity of images in the two eyes, due to their spatial separation; but the simplest are the clues implicit in the pattern of the projected retinal image, the clues to depth and solidity that you can see with one eye or in a photograph.

Implicit Clues

There are half a dozen of these implicit clues to tridimensionality which merit special mention.

(1) *Interposition.* If one object partially obscures another, it is perceived as nearer. The instantaneous operation of this clue, acting by itself, is evident in simple line drawings like the one in Fig. 129. Its effectiveness is increased when the images represent familiar objects.

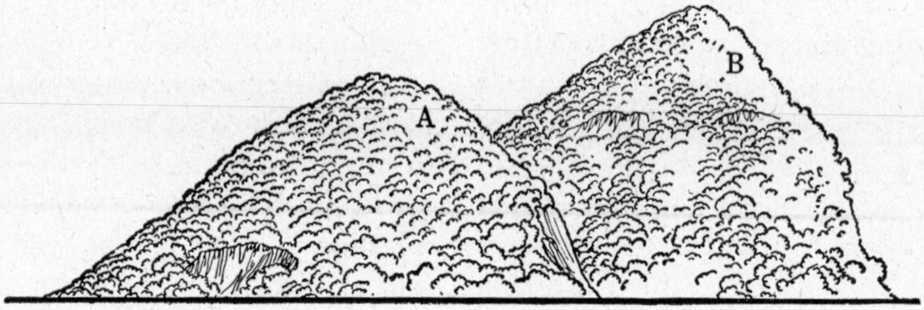

FIGURE 129. INTERPOSITION

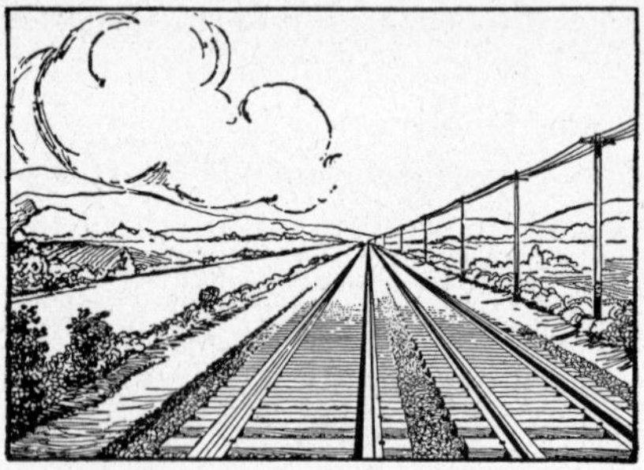

FIGURE 130. LINEAR PERSPECTIVE

(2) *Size and linear perspective.* The larger representation of an object appears nearer than a small one. Linear perspective consists in grading the sizes of a number of objects to represent their varying distances (Fig. 130). When objects do not

follow this implicit indication of distance, distortions of size or of distance result.

(3) *Aerial perspective.* Objects with sharp outlines are perceived as nearer than those that are indistinct or hazy. In actual scenes, objects vary in perceived distance as the changing clarity of the atmosphere alters their sharpness of outline (Fig. 131). On the stage, depth is increased by interposing layers of netting.

(4) *Light and shade.* Light is taken implicitly as coming from above. Thus highlights on convex surfaces are near the top, shadows below. Concave areas show the reverse. In a photograph with strong modeling the protuberances and indentations can be reversed by inverting the photograph (Fig. 132).

(5) *Movement.* Far objects appear to move in the same direction as the observer when he moves; near objects move in the opposite direction. As you ride in a train, the far hills move with you; the near fence posts snap backwards, so what moves with you is far. That is the clue.

(6) *Fixation.* Fixated objects tend to appear nearer than objects not fixated, but other implicit clues, like perspective, often conflict with the clue from fixation. It is thought that fixation is a clue because aerial perspective is. The fixated object is clear, other objects are blurred.

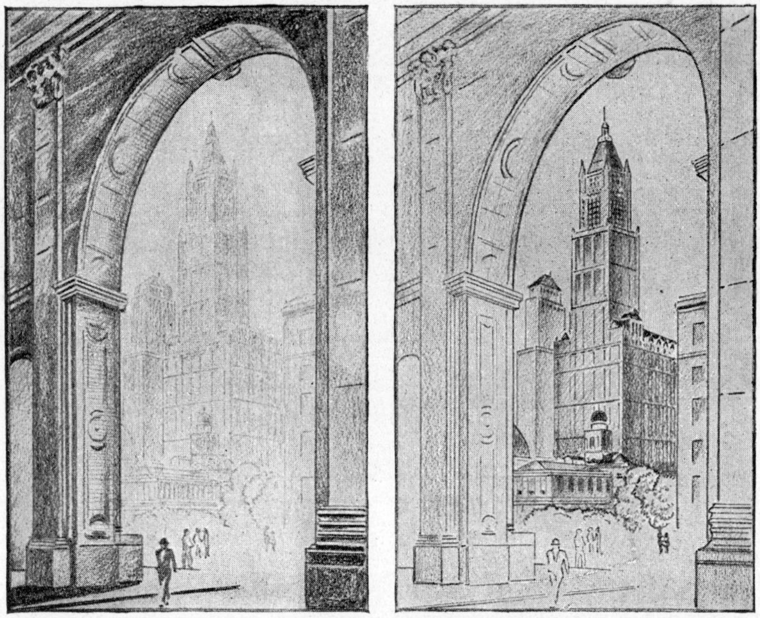

FIGURE 131. AERIAL PERSPECTIVE

These clues are deeply ingrained in perceptions, having long histories in the experience of an organism. They are sufficient of themselves to give an adequate apprehension of nearness or farness of objects, or to lead to proper responses to the distances of objects. Solidity, as perceived in pictorial art, is dependent upon the manipulation of such clues. The clues are so fully adequate that most persons have no difficulty in seeing moving pictures in three dimensions, though the presentation is only shadows on a flat surface. Moving pictures have much more depth than still pictures because they move. The relative movement of objects in the picture gives it great depth, which can be achieved in

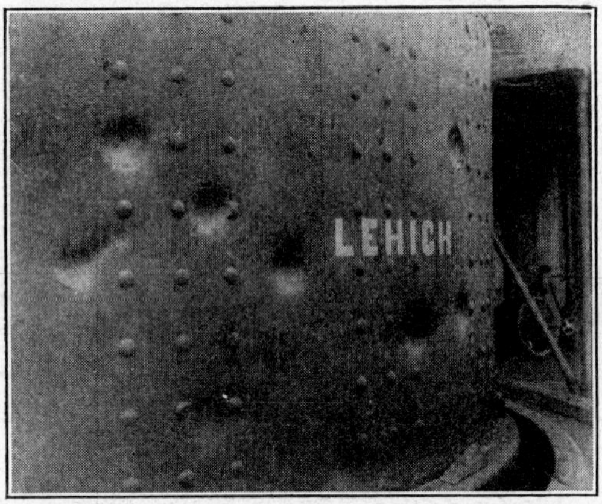

FIGURE 132. INFLUENCE OF LIGHT AND SHADE

The dents in the monitor's turret appear as dents if the light seems to come from above, and turn into bulges if this page is turned upside down, provided the light still seems to come from above. If the light can be imagined as streaming up from below, the dents turn into bulges without inverting the page. [Reprinted by permission of C. H. Stoelting, Chicago.]

still scenes by moving the movie camera while taking the picture.

Motor Context

Accurate vision involves constant motor adjustment of the eyes to the distances of the stimulating objects. Though only a single visual field is seen, the two eyes must be aimed coordinately in the right direction. This adjustment requires a pattern of muscular contractions and tensions characteristic of every distance. It is generally believed that these contractions and tensions give rise to proprioceptive clues to the distance of a fixated object. The clues could come from the convergence of the two eyes upon the object—convergence—or from the focusing of a single eye upon the object—accommodation.

Convergence. When the two eyes look at a distant object, their lines of vision are parallel and the muscles that move them are relatively relaxed. When the object moves in nearer than fifty to sixty feet in front of the observer, his eyes must be pulled out of their parallel position so that the lines of vision converge and intersect. A new pattern of muscular pulls is required, which may provide a proprioceptive clue for the perception of that distance. Certainly the clue is there. The only doubt is whether the observer actually has the proprioception to make the clue available to him. He is not directly conscious by somesthetic sensation of the convergence of his eyes, but not all proprioception is somesthesis. Some is effective without becoming conscious. (See Fig. 133.)

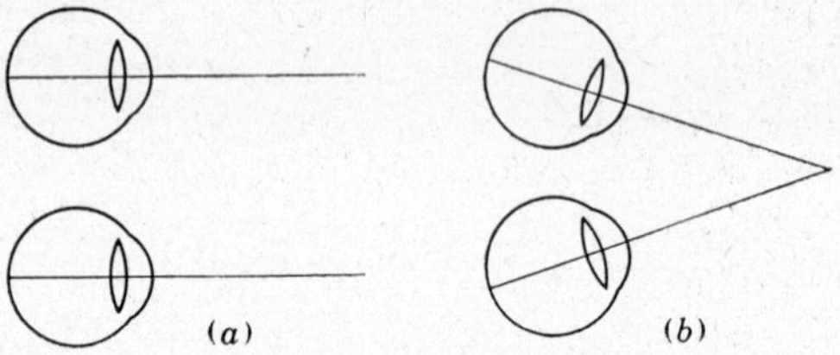

FIGURE 133. LINES OF SIGHT

In (*a*) the lines of sight are directed toward the horizon. In (*b*) they are converged upon a near object.

Accommodation. In fixating an object the lens in each eye must accommodate its focus to produce a clear image of the object on the retina, and this movement, if it gives rise to proprioception, would furnish a further clue to distance. (See Fig. 134.)

Normally accommodation and convergence work together to produce sharp images on the corresponding parts of the two retinas. When they do not cooperate, vision is impaired but can be restored by correcting either factor. If, for a given distance, the eyes converge too near for the correct focus, or focus too near for the correct convergence, the insertion of lenses to correct the focus or prisms to bend the lines of vision to the proper angle will correct the visual defect.

Accommodation appears to contribute less than convergence to the perception of distance. When convergence is partially removed by closing one eye, it becomes difficult to judge accurately, by accommodation alone, the distances of near objects and impossible for objects more than six feet away. One-eyed people must depend upon the implicit clues to a much larger degree than those with two eyes and are greatly handicapped when these clues are lacking. For this reason, monocular vision is not considered adequate for airplane pilots, and even pilots with binocular vision must be carefully tested for ability to judge distance accurately when the only available clues are accommodation and convergence.

As we have already noted, it is characteristic of an organism that its motor responses become stereotyped with repetition and that an habitual action gives meaning to the object or situation which touched it off. Accommodation and convergence are no exceptions to this rule. Most of the time our eyes aim and focus themselves automatically, making our perception of distance immediate and implicit. The first responses that make the perception a meaningful whole are these focusings and convergences. After them come the other reactions to complete the sense. I want my pen. Vaguely I see it lying on the desk in front of me. At once and automatically my eyes fixate it, focus on it, converge on it. Then I verify my perception of location, for I reach out and take it, my hand finding the pen at once. All that seems so easy and natural, and yet it is part of the learned structure of perception. If I had newly put on those special reversing spectacles, the perception would start off in the familiar way, but presently my hand would be groping vainly for the pen because the visual clues set off the wrong reaching behavior.

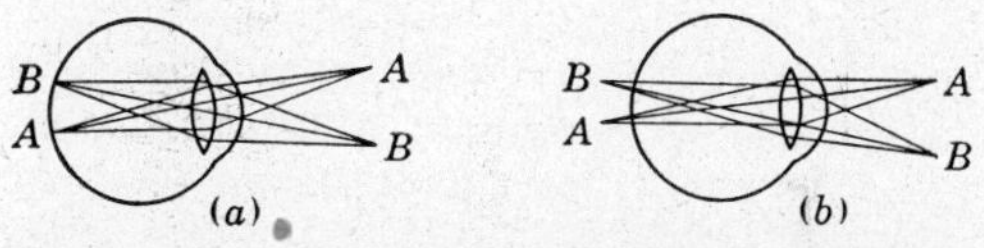

FIGURE 134. THE ACCOMMODATION OF THE EYE

In (*a*), with the lens more convex, the images are in focus on the retina. In (*b*) the focus lies behind the retina so that the images intercepted by the retina are out of focus.

Retinal Disparity

The fact that the eyes are set some $2\frac{1}{2}$ inches apart means that the two retinal pictures of an object are never identical. Only the point fixated and a few others will be projected upon identical points on the retinas. Everywhere else the two eyes, viewing the scene from different positions at different angles, get somewhat different views. This difference in the geometry of seeing is called *binocular parallax,* and the resultant difference in the two retinal images is called *retinal disparity.* Most of the pattern that falls on your retinas at any one time you 'ought' to see doubled, because corresponding lines in the pattern do not fall on corresponding lines in your retinas. But you do not. These doubled images do not remain distinct and disparate for perception. Instead, they integrate into, and are perceived as, solid or tridimensional. Within limits the greater disparity gives the greater depth or solidity. Here, if ever, you have a case of the effective operation of unconscious clues. The disparity can be of two kinds. (See Fig. 135.) If you look at a tree, *X*, in the middle of a grove, a nearer tree, *N*, will have disparity in one direction, but a far tree, *F*, will have the disparity reversed. The clues to distance depend on which eye sees which image. You yourself are, however, wholly unconscious of what it is that you see with one eye and what with the other. (You can figure it out by closing one eye and seeing what is left in the scene, and then trying out the other eye, but that is an elaborate inference, not the inference of immediate automatic perception.) Yet the clues work, even if you are not immediately aware of them. They enable your brain, without your knowing how it works, to 'decide' what is near and what far, and to build up space perception in accordance with what actually exists in the stimulus world outside. That is how two bidimensional retinas, working together, can between them get back the third dimension which they seemed to have lost.

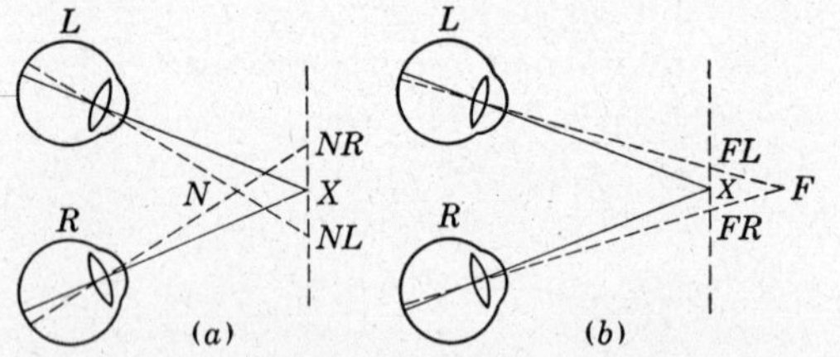

FIGURE 135. DOUBLE IMAGES

In (*a*) the double images of *N*, a point nearer than the point of fixation, *X*, are seen at *NR* and *NL*. In (*b*) the double images of *F*, a point farther away than X, are seen at *FR* and *FL*.

Stereoscopy

While the best depth perception is obtained by the cooperation of all three of the factors we have just discussed, the two proprioceptive factors can be eliminated and an excellently deep and solid perception obtained merely from two flat disparate pictures, presented each to its appropriate eye. This is accomplished by a device known as a *stereoscope*. Two photographs (stereograms) are taken at a certain distance apart and are then presented so that the right eye sees only the right picture and the left eye only the left picture. The two views are then integrated by the brain into a single perception that is solid or tridimensional.

Figure 136 shows how a hollow truncated cone looks to each eye when the cone is held near the face and binocular parallax is great. If these two drawings, each of a pair of images, are used as a stereogram in a stereoscope, you see down into a hollow cone for the disparity shown at the left of the figure, and you see a convex

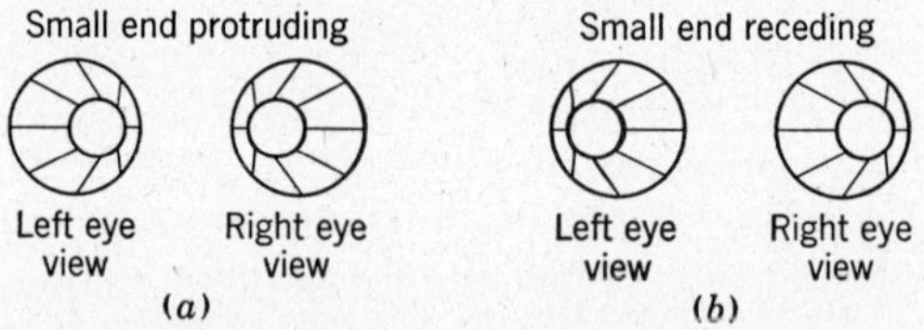

FIGURE 136. TRUNCATED CONE AS SEEN BY EACH EYE SEPARATELY

The small circles represent the small end of a hollow truncated cone, the large circles the large end, the straight lines the sides. In (*a*) are shown the views for each eye when the small end of the cone is near the observer; in (*b*) the views for the two eyes when the large end of the cone is near the observer. The retinal disparity for (*b*) would be the reverse of that for (*a*). It is also proper to regard (*a*) and (*b*) as two pairs of stereograms which, being reversed, would give opposite depths in perception.

cone tapered toward you for the disparity at the right. Figure 137 shows how binocular parallax gives retinal disparity. The two eyes look at the cube *A*, and the left eye sees the image *B* while the right eye sees the image *C*. The dotted lines show

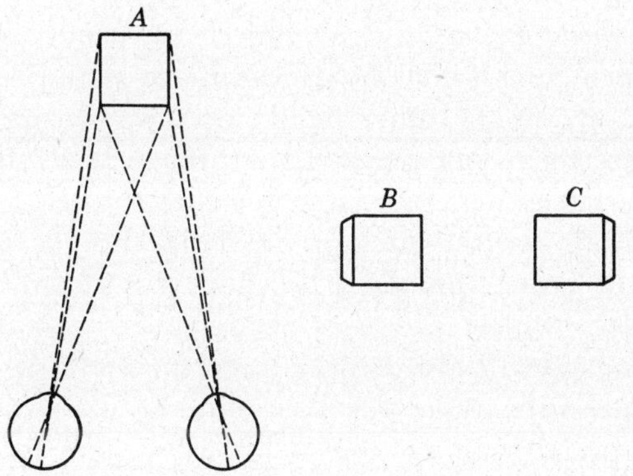

FIGURE 137. BINOCULAR PARALLAX AND RETINAL DISPARITY

A shows how binocular parallex gives to each eye a different image of a cube. *B* and *C* show what the images in the two eyes are like. [From E. G. Boring (Ed.), *Psychology for the armed services,* Infantry Journal, 1945, p. 41.]

why the views that the two eyes get are different.

If desired, solidity can be exaggerated in stereoscopic vision. You will perceive an exaggerated depth if the two photographs are taken at a distance apart which is greater than the distance between the two eyes (2½ inches). Separating the cameras which make the pictures by more than 2½ inches exaggerates the binocular parallax, and thus the retinal disparity, and thus the perceived depth. In fact this method can be used to reveal small differences in the distances of objects which are both miles away. It is then called *telestereoscopy.* In war, to find out which airplanes are flat dummies and which are solid and real, camoufleurs in airplanes at great altitudes take telestereoscopic pictures of the ground in order to distinguish the heights of camouflaged objects on the ground.

The *stereoscope,* by means of which the stereograms are observed, uses either a pair of lenses (as in Fig. 138) or a pair of mirrors to bend the lines of vision of the two eyes so that the two stereograms can be shown individually to the proper eyes while they are converged normally at a point some convenient distance in front. Naturally, if the stereograms are reversed so that the left eye sees what was the right picture, and vice versa, a *pseudoscopic* effect will be produced; near things look far away and far things near, providing the implicit clues are not too dominant. If they are, the result is usually confused or flat. By reversing the stereograms, you can make the outside of a teacup look like an inside, you can make a tennis ball look like a cup, you may even make the face of

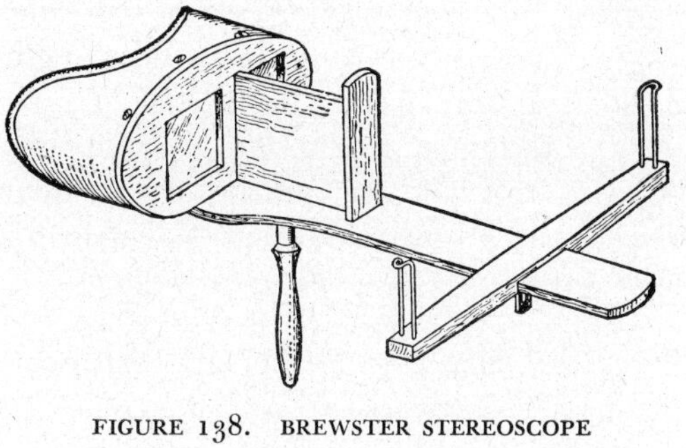

FIGURE 138. BREWSTER STEREOSCOPE

The double stereogram goes in the card holder. Each eye sees but one drawing or photograph. The lenses allow the eyes to converge so that the two images combine.

a plaster bust look like a death mask, but you cannot turn a human mobile face concave. There the implicit clues are too strong for pseudoscopy to work.

You can get this same reversal of the third dimension by looking at objects through a system of lenses called a *pseudoscope,* which reverses the images to the two eyes.

VISUAL PERCEPTION OF SIZE

The most obvious determinant of visually perceived size is, of course, the size of the retinal image, which stands in a fixed relation to the size and distance of the object. It is customary to state this relation in terms of visual angle. (See Fig. 91, p. 232.) To maintain a constant visual angle, and thus constant size of retinal image, the size (width, diameter) of objects must vary directly as the distance of the objects from the eye. With an object of constant size, the size of the visual angle varies inversely as the distance of the object. Thus, from a knowledge of the physical size of an object and of its distance from the eye, we can calculate the approximate size of the image which it produces on the retina; and, on the basis of this rule, we can predict how large the object ought to look at any given distance if its size were determined solely by visual angle. That is the rule for perceived size that Euclid, the geometrician, laid down in his *Optics* over two thousand years ago.

Perceived Size and Perceived Distance

Euclid was, however, wrong, as we already know from the facts of object constancy (p. 231). Under ordinary conditions the perception of size deviates from Euclid's law. A negative afterimage, for instance, since it subtends a constant visual angle, has constant retinal size and should therefore, under Euclid's law, remain constant in perceived size; nevertheless it appears to get larger with each increase in the distance at which the afterimage is projected. Its size is determined not by the visual angle and retinal image, but by the perceived distance of the projected surface. Conversely, if we look at two objects of the same physical size, but at different distances, the nearer object, with the bigger retinal image, looks no larger than the farther object. This is the principle of *size constancy,* a case of object constancy, a principle which holds within wide limits.

If, on the other hand, we view two objects with one eye looking through holes in a screen, cut in such a way that the conditions for the perception of distance have all been eliminated, we find that the object which produces the smaller retinal image will also appear to be smaller. Apparently, then, the constancy of size is a special case of the relationship between perceived size and perceived distance. Automatically the organism makes an adjustment of the perceived size which allows for the changes in perceived distance. The screen with the holes in it is the *reduction screen.* (See p. 235.) Here it reduces the sensory core of the perception to the retinal image, eliminating all the clues to distance by which retinally determined size might be corrected by the brain.

Nor does the principle of size constancy hold at all distances. It fails for small objects—such as a coin—when held within a few centimeters of the eye and for large objects at great distances. A man talking to you and five feet away is not five times as tall as the man twenty-five feet away, for size constancy holds approximately; but the man way down the street or across the valley may be a tiny little creature. A familiar object will, other things being equal, remain constant in size over a greater range of distances than an unfamiliar object. In general, then, you expect constancy of size for a middle range of distances. Within that range familiarity with the object increases constancy.

Perceived Size and Surrounding Objects

The relationship between size and distance is one of many instances in which the specific perception of things is determined by their situations. If an object appears at a great distance, as in a perspective draw-

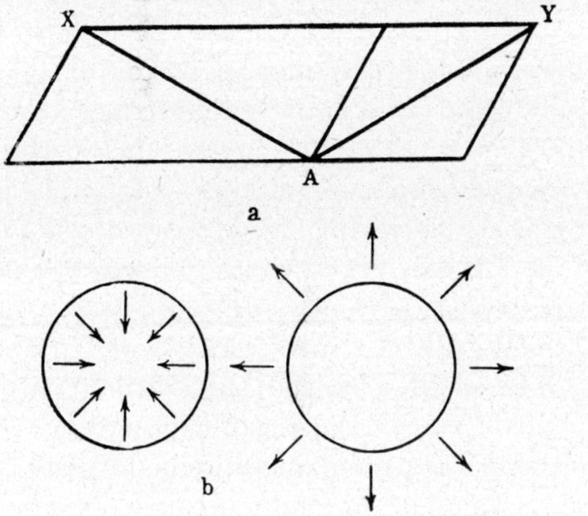

FIGURE 139. INFLUENCE OF LINEAR FIGURE TAKEN AS A WHOLE UPON THE SIZE OF ONE OF ITS PARTS

ing (see Fig. 130, p. 298), its size corresponds approximately to that distance.

The principle holds also for bidimensional situations. The line *AX* in Fig. 139*a* appears longer than the line *AY;* the former is apprehended as the diagonal of a larger, and the latter as the diagonal of a smaller parallelogram. Similarly, in Fig. 139*b* the difference in size between the two circles must be referred to the influence of the included and excluded lines. In the familiar arrowhead illusion (Fig. 140*a*) the line *c* appears longer than *d* because it is a part of the larger area suggested by the direction of the arrowheads. Similarly, in Fig. 140*b* it is almost impossible to see the distance between the outer limits of circles *A* and *B* as equal to the distance between the right extreme of *B* and the left extreme of *C*. The perception of the circles as objects constrains us to perceive the dis-

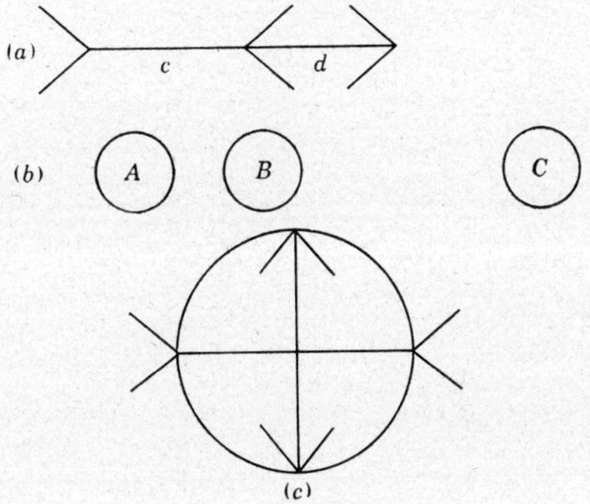

FIGURE 140. EFFECT OF A TOTAL FIGURE UPON AN ISOLATED LINEAR DISTANCE

In (*a*) the distance *c* equals the distance *d*. In (*b*) the right side of B is equidistant from the left side of *A* and the left side of *C*. In (*c*) there is a true circle which looks flattened.

tance as between circle and circle rather than as between point and point. In Fig. 141 the lower object looks shorter than the upper object, possibly because of a contrast between the short upper line of the lower figure and the long lower line of the upper figure, possibly because of a perspective effect induced by the convergence of the straight lines at the two extremes.

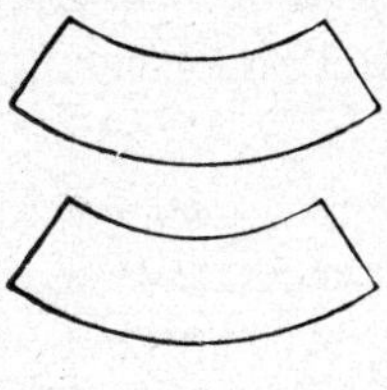

FIGURE 141. SPATIAL CONTRAST

The lower figure looks shorter and stumpier.

Within limits even such factors as whiteness may function as determinants of size. If two equal squares, one black and one white, are placed side by side against a gray ground, the white will usually appear larger than the black. Differences in hue may also have an effect on apparent size. To most people a red object will appear slightly larger, and nearer, than an equally bright blue object, and in some pathological cases such differences become pronounced. The apparent distance of color is sometimes used by artists in obtaining depth in their pictures.

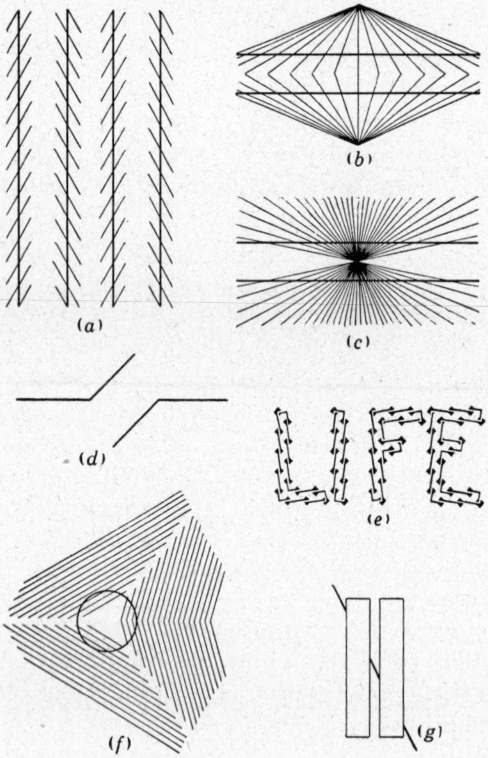

FIGURE 142. ANGLE ILLUSIONS

Distortion of straight lines and parallels by surrounding objects.

Apparent shape and direction of lines are similarly modified by surrounding objects that set up implicit perceptual attitudes. Because of the tendency to perceive all objects as tridimensional, lines in a drawing that cross each other at oblique angles are taken implicitly to represent right angles extending into space. For example, a vertical line with several oblique cross-lines is perceived as if set at an angle to the frontal plane like a telegraph pole with cross-arms. Similarly, all acute angles tend to be overestimated and all obtuse angles tend to be underestimated, making them approach right angles. Even in drawings to which perspective perception does not apply, distortion in direction of the lines takes place. Many of the so-called visual illusions are of this sort. Some of them are shown in Fig. 142. (See also Fig. 1, p. 6.)

Visual Acuity

The smallest object that can be seen depends upon several variables. A white spot on a black ground in sunlight can just be seen when it subtends an angle of about 10 to 12 seconds of arc; a black spot on a white ground in diffuse daylight requires an angle of 25 to 36 seconds. Similar values have been determined for the smallest perceptible degree of separation between two objects, a determination which depends upon a number of different factors. The sidewise displacement of two vertical lines, placed end to end, may be perceived when the ends are displaced by an amount equivalent to a visual angle of only 2 seconds.

The separation between points in space must, however, be larger in order to be perceived. In a well-lighted room two black dots can just be seen as two when they are separated by an angle of 60 seconds. In abnormally high or abnormally low illuminations the angle must be increased, as it must also if lines are substituted for the dots and the separation is apprehended as a gap in an otherwise complete figure.

The threshold of 60 seconds or 1 minute of arc for the just noticeable separation has been accepted by the oculist as the standard *visual acuity* for normal vision. If the eye can see a letter the distance between whose parts (for example, the horizontal bars of the test letter E) subtends an angle of 60 seconds, it is in that respect considered normal. If, on the other hand, the angle subtended by the parts of the letter must be, say, 120 seconds before the letter can be distinctly seen, visual acuity is said to be one-half normal. The test letters are, of course, always shown under good illumination.

VISUAL PERCEPTION OF MOVEMENT

When we look fixedly at the minute hand of a watch we see no movement; but if, after a brief interval, we look at the watch once more, we observe the hand in a new position. We perceive a change in position but not a continuous change. When we see an athlete doing a standing broad jump, on the contrary, we see him—as we saw the hand of the watch—first in one place, then later at another place; but, in addition, we see him moving or changing his position from one place to another. It is the perception of this continuous change in position of an object that is called the perception of movement.

General Conditions for Perceived Movement

Usually the visual perception of movement depends upon the displacement on the retina of an image of the moving object. There are exceptions. Movement in the near-far dimension may occur, as when the approach of an object is indicated by an increase in its brightness (lights of an approaching automobile), in its distinctness (ship coming toward you through the fog) or in its size (an approaching object). Watch a streetcar as it comes along toward you through an empty street from too far away for the law of size constancy to apply. It gets bigger and bigger, by little jumps, and you see this increase in size as a movement of approach.

All seen movement is, of course, relative. It occurs with respect to some frame of reference. So the clouds scurry across the face of the moon; or, if the larger object becomes the frame of reference for the smaller—and that is quite usual—the moon scurries behind the clouds (as was stated on p. 239). When the movement is a simple displacement, the initial position of the object may be the frame of reference. That is what happens when a spot of light is seen to move in the dark. With continuous movement of an object, its background and the surrounding objects become important and ordinarily furnish the frame of reference.

Frequently you have to include yourself in the system of relations which determines seen movement. You sit in the train in the station watching the other train, and all at once you feel yourself begin to move backward, because the other train, not yours, has started to move forward. You rise from the ground in an airplane, and suddenly you are not rising; instead you see the ground falling away below you. There are no simple rules that say which part of the system will be the frame of reference and which the moving object, but it is clear that the system can include the perceiving organism and that the visual perception of movement is not dependent solely on visual factors. If the other train makes you see that you and your own train are moving, then you both *see* your train moving and *feel* yourself moving.

Other complications arise because the eyes tend to fixate a moving object when it is the center of attention. The consequence is that the image of the object does not move across the retina because the eyes move with the object. Instead the image of the stationary background moves on the retina, looking blurred. It is really quite remarkable how well the neural coordinations take care of fixation when the head moves. You can watch a bird on a limb and move your body and head as you will, and your eyes remain fixed on the bird. Moving your head does not spoil your fixation for a moment. You do not have again to adjust your eyes after you have moved your head. The same innervation that moves the head moves the eyes compensatorily, so that they stay still with respect to the bird. When the bird flies off, you can still watch him, your eyes moving and converging to keep fixation, and, if you move your head then, compensation stays just as good.

There are really two different ways in which movement across the field of vision is perceived. (1) The bird flies across the field. Your eyes follow him. Other objects look blurred. The bird has been seen to move. (2) The bird flies across the field. Your eyes remain fixed on the distant tree. The tree and most of the objects in sight are clear. The bird is blurred, because your eyes did not follow him; nevertheless you saw him move. (3) The bird sits on the fence. You move your eyes along the top of the fence. Everything is blurred (except when your eyes stop momentarily). Nothing seems to move. Your eyes are moving, but you do not think about that.

How the brain puts these clues together in perceiving movement is not clear, but put them together it does. Here there are really five items that can change position in relation to each other: (1) the object of attention, (2) the visual frame of reference for the object, (3) your eyes, (4) your head and (5) your body. Proprioception, a great deal of it unconscious, tells your brain what your eyes, head and body are doing. If you are fixating an object—and almost certainly you are—your brain has already arranged to have your body and head movements compensated by your eye movements. The retinal sensations tell you what the retinal image of the object is doing in relation to the retinal image of the other things that make up the frame of reference. Any wise man could figure out what the object is doing with respect to any frame of reference, if he had all these clues. The brain has the clues, solves the problem and puts the answer into perception. The wonder is that it does the job so immediately and accurately, and does it without setting up any consciousness of the process by which it works.

Afterimages of Movement

If you look fixedly for fifteen or twenty seconds at a slowly rotating white disk upon which has been drawn a heavy black spiral line, the disk will seem to contract or expand, depending upon the direction of rotation of the spiral. If you then turn your eyes away and fixate a person's face, the face too will appear to expand or shrink depending upon the direction of rotation of the spiral. Similarly if you look steadily for a minute at a waterfall or at a flowing stream, and then glance away at the landscape, the latter will appear to flow in the opposite direction. If you are riding on the rear platform of a train which suddenly stops, you notice that the formerly shrinking and receding objects appear to broaden or come nearer. In short, under certain conditions a movement produces an after-effect which manifests itself as a movement in the opposite direction. The velocity of the afterimage of movement corresponds roughly, but by no means exactly, to the relative velocity of the moving object.

We see here that perceived movement exists in experience in its own right. It does not consist necessarily in the displacement of an object, for some of these movements move without getting anywhere. The rotating spiral keeps expanding, and yet is not found to have become bigger. You watch the waterfall and then look at the rocks. They are seen to keep moving up and up and up, and yet they never get away from where they were. There must be a physiological label for movement which the brain puts on to that part of a perception which is not the frame of reference.

Perceived Movement with a Moving Stimulus

A stimulus must travel a minimal distance before movement is perceived, a distance depending in part on the rate at which the stimulus travels. It depends also upon other conditions, such as the part of the visual field involved. Three things may be noted about the distance traveled by a stimulus before perception of movement occurs.

(1) The distance is always larger than the extent of the involuntary tremors of the eye that occur whenever we try to keep our eyes still.

(2) Except in the center of the visual field, the distance is always smaller than the threshold for the perception of the separation of two points. Thus movements in the periphery of the visual field may be perceived distinctly when objects are indistinct.

(3) Nevertheless, the magnitude of the threshold for movement varies with visual acuity, although in the periphery of the visual field the decrease in sensitivity to movement is not so great as the decrease in visual acuity. Thus at the center of the field the two thresholds are approximately the same, but at a distance of 20 degrees from the center the threshold for acuity is four times as large as that for movement. When you look directly at a moving automobile, for example, you can see the automobile as distinctly as you can see its movement. When you look out of the corner of your eyes, on the contrary, though you do not get either perception so clearly as you could in direct vision, still you can see the movement of the automobile even *before* you can see the automobile itself. That is another fact that convinces us that movement is a special kind of perception with its own 'label,' which is different from the 'label' of the object perceived.

What are the limiting rates of stimulation that will arouse the perception of movement? In vision, under optimal conditions and at a distance of 2 meters, an object must move about 0.2 centimeter per second before it is perceived as moving. When the rate becomes about 150 centimeters per second, the perception for the same distance will appear as a flicker or a blur. The minute hand of a watch would have to move five or six times faster than it does to be seen as moving.

In everyday experience the rate of 150 centimeters per second seems slow, for it is only about 3 miles per hour. If, however, while you were looking at the ground 2 yards away through a pipe a foot long and one inch in inside diameter, a mouse runing at the rate of 3 miles per hour passed through the restricted field of your vision, the mouse would be seen as a blur; it would be neither a mouse nor a moving object.

The remoteness of a moving object decreases the perceived rate of its movement. At a distance of a few yards an automobile traveling at 60 miles per hour will appear to be moving rapidly, but at a distance of a few miles only slowly. A ship on the horizon is not perceived as moving at all. The decrease in rate is not, however, proportional to the distance and hence not proportional to the rate of the movement of the object's image on the retina. The tendency for objects to maintain their size with increasing distance tends to keep constant the apparent rate as distance increases. Movement on the retina seems faster in perception when the moving object is perceived as distant, than if its distance were not perceived. If one backs away from a revolving barber's sign, both the perceived size of the sign and its rate of movement remain approximately unchanged. If perceived size stayed constant with changing distance and perceived movement altered with the rate of movement on the retina, we should have strange contradictions in perception.

Perceived Movement with Stationary Stimuli

Since stationary stimuli may appear to move (afterimages, autokinetic movement) and since normally the perception of movement results from displacement of the stimulus with respect to a frame of reference, there would seem to be no fundamental necessity for the stimulus itself to be moving. Discrete displacement under proper conditions might be enough to win the movement 'label' for the perception. The fact is that series of discontinuous stimuli will produce the perception of movement, provided the illumination, the distances and the rate of succession are within the proper limits.

Just this happens in what is termed *stroboscopic* or *apparent movement,* of which there are many examples in everyday experience. The simplest situation is at railroad crossings where two lights, placed side by side, light up alternately when a train is near. With continued fixation the light seems to move back and forth from one position to the other. Everyone is familiar with the motion seen in electric signs before theaters, stores, hotels and on billboards. There, of course, no actual movement is present. The lights are turned on and off in proper sequence and with proper timing.

The commonest example of all is the movies themselves. In the cinema a series of still photographs is projected on the screen, every photograph representing a slightly different position of a moving object. When the series is projected on the screen in the proper order and at the proper rate (usually twenty-four per second), normal movement is perceived. The quality of the movement changes with the rate of projection. If this rate is too slow, we see a succession of static pictures. If the rate is then increased, the movement becomes first a flicker, then normal movement, and finally, when too fast, jerky and blurry. At great speed of projection all movement disappears, and we see only a filmy surface.

A situation for the perception of apparent movement with two successive stationary stimuli at different places is shown in Fig. 143. If a vertical line *A* is shown, removed, and then, after an interval of 0.06 second, a horizontal line *B* is shown, the vertical line will be seen to rotate clockwise from the 12 o'clock to the 3 o'clock position, as in *C* of the figure. Should the interval between exposures of the lines be shortened to about 0.02 second, the two lines would appear simultaneously and form a right angle. If, on the other hand, the interval between the exposures were lengthened to 0.20 second, the two lines would appear successively with no movement perceived at all.

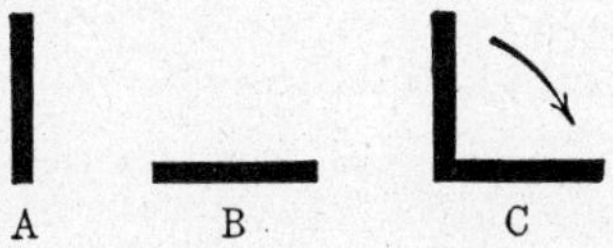

FIGURE 143. STIMULI FOR APPARENT MOVEMENT

When *A* is succeeded by *B* and the time intervals are correct, you see the stroboscopic or apparent movement as indicated in *C*. The line moves down through the angle.

Exposing the two lines a short distance apart always produces a better perception of movement than exposing them farther apart. The motion-picture cartoonist, recognizing this fact, makes sure that the difference between his successive drawings is slight. The less the displacement between successive drawings, the more lifelike and complete the movements of the figures.

Exposing each stimulus briefly gives an impression of swifter movement, whereas lengthening the exposure time slows down the movement and makes it jerky. Similarly, small stimuli tend to produce smooth movement, and large ones jerky movement. We reject the front seats in the movies to avoid jerkiness and flicker.

Apparent movement with discretely displaced stimuli is often perceived as actually 'better' and smoother than the movement of an object which is really moving. In one experiment two rectangles were projected, one above the other, at the left of a screen. Then one rectangle was made to move rapidly across the screen to a position at the right, while the other disappeared at the left and reappeared at the right without having moved through the intervening space. There was no fundamental difference between these two perceptions of the real movement and apparent movement, except that the real movement was described as a little more 'jerky' and less uniform than the apparent movement. That makes sense. All the brain needs to perceive movement is discrete displacement at the correct rate. It can be embarrassed by a surplus of clues.

Just as implicit clues add the meaning of depth to a flat picture, so the grayish flash that trails a moving object or that appears in the field of apparent movement can add the 'label' of movement to a stationary object in a picture. A blur in the form of a few indistinct lines behind the wheels of a car in an advertisement gives it

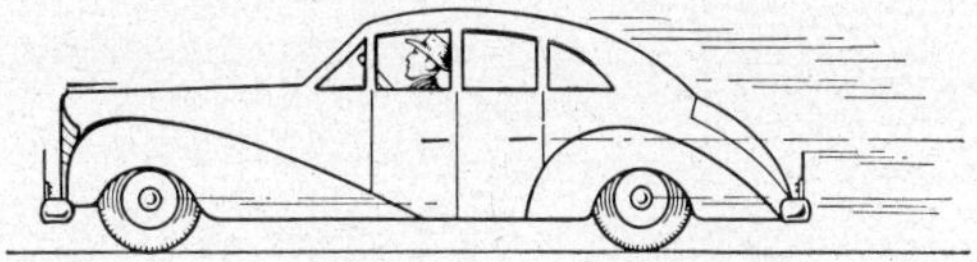

FIGURE 144. USE OF LINES TO GIVE THE IMPRESSION OF MOVEMENT TO OBJECTS

a dash as if it might move into the left column (Fig. 144). Modern illustrations furnish many more examples of the use of this clue.

REFERENCES

1. Boring, E. G. *Sensation and perception in the history of experimental psychology*. New York: Appleton-Century, 1942. Chaps. 8, 9 and 15.

The history of research and ideas in the fields of visual sensation and perception from the seventeenth century down to about 1930.

2. Carr, H. A. An introduction to space perception. New York: Longmans, Green, 1935. Chaps. 3, 6, 7, 8, 9 and 10.

A clear and readable handbook of the psychology of space perception (mostly visual) before the researches of Gestalt psychologists had affected the field.

3. Ellis, W. D. *A source book of Gestalt psychology*. New York: Harcourt, Brace, 1938. Sections, 11, 12, 13 and 14.

Translation of papers written by the leaders of the school of Gestalt psychology, with a dozen papers on topics of visual perception.

4. Vernon, M. D. *Visual perception*. Cambridge, England: Cambridge University Press, 1937. Chap. 11.

An excellent textbook on visual space perception, which includes the contributions of Gestalt psychology.

5. Woodworth, R. S. *Experimental psychology*. New York: Holt, 1938. Chaps. 22, 23, 25, 26 and 28.

Excellent up-to-date handbook chapters on the visual perception of color, form and the third dimension.

CHAPTER 14

Hearing

FOR the most part, with the eye we see what things are, and with the ear we hear what happens. Sight is primarily concerned with objects; hearing with events.

For man to hear, the most important events are the sounds of speech. It is doubtful whether any single achievement more sharply separates man from the apes than spoken, and heard, speech. It is the basis of our culture, the loom within which we weave and fashion our civilization. Two men talking to each other form the simplest element of society.

Only a little less important, of course, are the other events about which our ears tell us. We know when people come and go, when a car is approaching, when the clock strikes, or the telephone rings, when the baby is hungry or wet, when people about us are writing or coughing or asleep. While we may be looking with our eyes at some single object, we hear the flux of sounds which conveys to us news of the many events that happen around us.

The loss of hearing is in many ways more disturbing than the loss of sight. Many people fear blindness more than deafness. In a sense they are right, because the blind man is more critically dependent upon another person than the deaf man. It has been found, however, that the deaf adjust themselves to their loss more poorly. They feel cut off from other people and become resentful when they cannot take part in the give and take of conversation. Their feelings and interests grow more and more shut-in. Paranoid symptoms may appear in them. Complete loss of hearing warps the loser's personality and social adjustment far more seriously than it disrupts his ability to deal with his physical environment.

The ear, the instrument with which we hear, accomplishes a remarkable task. It is more sensitive than the element of any practical microphone. It can respond to a pressure as small as one three-millionth of a gram. This sensitivity is so great that the keenest ear can almost hear the random fluctuations produced when the individual molecules of the air strike the eardrum. When a person is listening to the weakest sounds, the movement of the eardrum is so small as to defy imagination, less than the billionth part of an inch.

At the same time, the ear can respond to pressures ten million times greater, although it must be said that such sound pressures are uncomfortable and result in temporary deafness. How a system having such extreme sensitivity can continue to respond so well over this enormous range of intensities is not well known, nor do we understand fully how the ear protects it-

This chapter was prepared by Edwin B. Newman of Harvard University.

self against damage while listening to the loudest sounds.

Apart from its job of relaying the slight energy of sounds to the brain, the ear also aids in distinguishing one kind of sound from another. We shall see later something about how this takes place. It is enough to note here that the ear has two functions, first, to receive sounds and convert them into nervous messages and, second, to respond in a different way to different sounds so that analysis and discrimination among sounds is possible.

STIMULUS FOR HEARING

To understand how it is that we hear, we have first to learn a little about the physics of sound.

Sound Waves

The immediate stimulus for hearing is normally a rapidly fluctuating pressure on the eardrum. This alternate rise and fall of pressure is the result of sound waves which are transmitted through the air (or through solid objects such as walls or windows) from some source of sound. Sound waves behave in much the same way as other forms of wave motion. Once the wave motion is started, it travels at a constant speed, depending upon the density and elasticity of the medium. In air the speed is about eleven hundred feet per second. A sound wave bends when it passes a corner or when it goes through air which is not all equally dense. In a closed room, sound waves are reflected very well (often more than ninety per cent of them) from all the walls and hard surfaces. If sound travels away from a point in the open, the amplitude ('height') of the wave is halved each time the distance is doubled. In all these ways, sound waves are like light waves or waves in water.

In other respects sound waves are different. Waves on the surface of water consist of a movement which is mostly up and down, at right angles to the path the wave is taking. Sound waves involve movement forward and back, in line with the direction of their travel. Each bit of air is pushed forward by the pressure from behind and moves back as it passes on this pressure to the air ahead. Also sound waves, unlike light waves, are commonly distorted in certain ways as they pass through the air. Generally, the sound on arrival at the ear has about the same wave form it had when it left the source. But if it is of very high intensity (a 'shock wave'), such as the sound of an explosion, it changes its shape in its hurry to leave the place from which it started. Furthermore, high-frequency waves fall off in energy more rapidly than low-frequency waves when they have to travel distance of a quarter mile or more. As we shall see later, we are able to make use of our familiarity with such distortions in judging the distance of a source of sound from the listener.

Sound is produced when an object is set into vibration. A single sharp sound arises when an object is struck. The drip of water, the banging of a door, the tick of a clock, the sound of a hammer or rifle are sounds of this sort. Each of them produces a single sound wave, or short train of waves at most, which is transmitted, pulse-like, to the ear. If there is a series of clicks or bangs which follow each other closely, yet in a random manner, the sound becomes continuous. The drip of water becomes the drumming of rain on the roof or the steady roar of the surf or the waterfall. The tap of one leaf on another becomes the rustle or rush of wind through the trees.

Air or steam in its disordered haste to escape from a pipe or jet produces an equally disordered train of waves which is heard as a hiss. All such sounds we call *random noise* (or *fluctuation noise*) because no two succeeding waves are the same; the amounts of pressure existing in successive moments is governed by chance. We may equally well speak of *white noise* because, as we shall see in a moment, noise can be broken up into many different frequencies much as white light can be broken up into a variety of spectral colors.

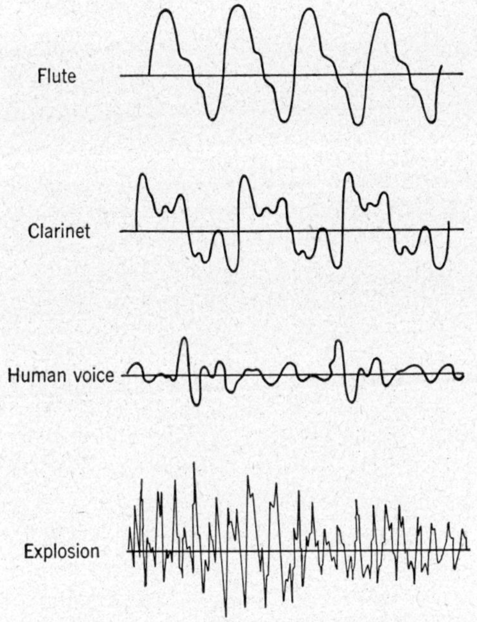

FIGURE 145. TYPICAL SOUND WAVES

The first three are periodic waves, repeated regularly. The last is highly irregular. [From D. C. Miller, *The science of musical sounds,* 1926; by permission of the Macmillan Company.]

So much for noise. Not all sounds are noisy. Instruments with strings, such as violins and pianos, are constructed in such a way that they produce smooth, simple sounds. Their strings, once touched, continue to vibrate at a regular rate. Each successive sound wave produced by the string is just like the wave which went before. The result is a musical tone. The column of air in an organ pipe acts in much the same way as the string. The air inside the pipe is like a coiled spring filling the pipe and attached at the closed end. Compressed slightly, then released, the column of air vibrates with a fixed period. Bells, bugles, bees, humming motors and the human voice all are sources of sound which produce trains of regular waves. We call the vibration of such objects *periodic.*

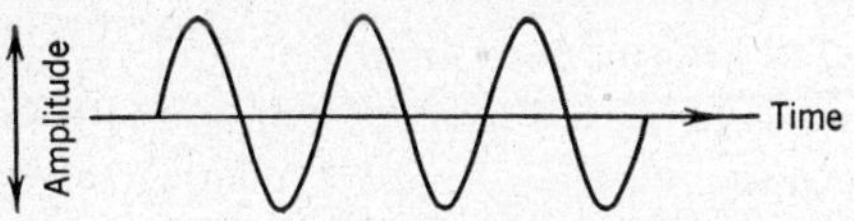

FIGURE 146. A SINE WAVE

Three complete cycles of a wave representing a pure tone.

In Fig. 145 are pictures of sound waves seen on the face of an oscilloscope. This is a device that traces the fluctuating pressure of the sound wave with a rising and falling finger of electrons which races across a screen. The first three patterns in the figure are of periodic waves; the last is the picture of a noise, a highly random sound which is dying away rapidly as it passes to the right.

A very few instruments produce what are called *pure tones,* dear to the heart of the experimental psychologist or physicist. Tuning forks, weakly blown pipes and, today, electronic oscillators coupled to suitable loudspeakers or earphones produce the pure tones with which these scientists work. In comparison with the notes of other instruments, pure tones sound thin and flat and have no interest for the musician.

They represent, however, the simplest possible wave motion, a sine wave, the form of which is shown in Fig. 146. This wave form can be represented by a simple mathematical expression, the sine function, familiar to students of trigonometry.

Simple Waves and Complex Waves

How can we start on the task of relating the many things that we hear to the large variety of physical sounds with their complex wave forms? What are the more important things to know about a sound wave? Just how may we describe it most effectively? We are faced here with the problem of *analysis* and must stop to become somewhat familiar with the methods of both *mathematical* and *physical* analysis of sound waves. Analysis provides the tools which we shall need to understand how we hear.

Fourier Analysis

In 1822, Fourier, a French physicist and mathematician, showed that it is possible to express any *periodic* wave form, such as the first three shown in Fig. 145, as the *sum* of a series of simple waves, each of which is a sine wave.

To illustrate how one complex wave is made up, we may look at the wave form shown in Fig. 147. A single complete period of the complex wave is shown at the lower right. It is roughly a square wave, such as that produced by some sirens. The Fourier analysis of this tone reveals five components, which are illustrated to the left. The relative frequency of each component is proportional to the numbers, I, III, V, VII and IX, to the left of each line, and you can check this frequency by counting the waves in any one period of the complex tone. To the right are shown the successive steps in the addition, starting with

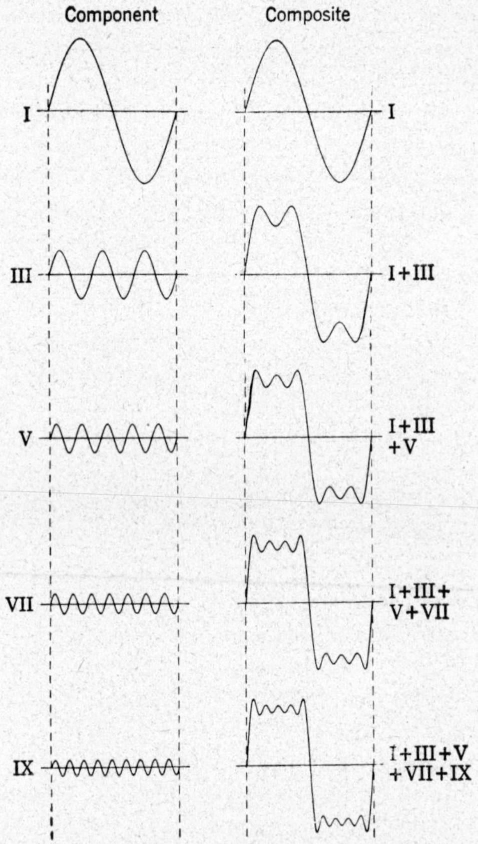

FIGURE 147. SIMPLE WAVES ADD UP TO A COMPLEX WAVE

The first five harmonic components of a single cycle of a 'square wave' are shown at left. Series at right show progressive change from a simple sine wave as each component is added. If enough additional odd harmonics were added, the 'square wave,' a rectangular form which is already apparent in the form at the lower right corner of the figure, would be even more closely approximated.

the wave of lowest frequency and then showing the composite wave as each additional component is added in. Examine carefully the composite waves and you can see how the wave form becomes more nearly square as this summing up goes on. The Fourier analysis is mathematical. It starts out with a basic or fundamental frequency which is the same as the frequency with which the complex wave repeats itself. To this fundamental are added sine waves of other higher frequencies. These added frequencies will always be some even multiple of the fundamental frequency. If the fundamental is n cycles per second, the harmonics will be $2n$, $3n$, $4n$, $5n$ or $6n$ cycles per second.

In the development of the physics of sound, the Fourier analysis is most important. It provides a mathematical expression which can be subjected to many further mathematical operations. These mathematical manipulations predict how sound waves will behave as they are transmitted in the air or are transformed into electrical waves and passed through electrical circuits. Without the Fourier analysis we should be at a loss in handling such theoretical problems. The Fourier analysis is very important for theory, but we should keep clearly in mind what it is, namely, a mathematical model which helps us to understand and predict the actions of periodic wave forms.

Analysis by Resonance

Physical methods of analysis, as distinguished from the mathematical, also start with the idea that a complex wave form is made up of a number of simple components. The physical analyzer has the job of responding separately to each of the possible component sine waves in order to discover which are present and which absent and to measure the amplitude (height) of those present. Most simply, this analysis is made with a series of *resonators,* one of which is tuned to each of the possible component frequencies in the complex wave. A resonator may be any device that has a natural vibration period of its own, such as a string or reed or pipe, and, in addition, is so sensitive to sound waves that it will be set into sympathetic vibration when series of waves strike it.

One such acoustic resonator, shown in Fig. 148, consists of a brass cylinder with an opening in the outer end to admit the sound and a small tip on the inner end for insertion into the ear. The length of the resonator can be adjusted by sliding the one part of the cylinder in or out of the other, like a telescope. The column of air in the cylinder reinforces by its own resonance one particular frequency as it passes through the resonator into the ear. With such a set of resonators it is possible to hear each of the component tones predicted by a Fourier analysis. If the tone is the square wave represented by the wave form of Fig. 147, resonators can be tuned to each of the five components and their frequencies and relative strengths can be estimated.

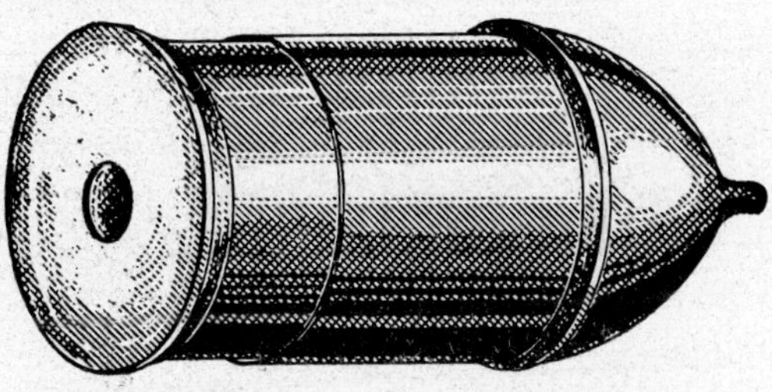

FIGURE 148. ACOUSTIC RESONATOR

The tip is placed in the ear and the length adjusted until the enclosed air vibrates in resonance with the component which is being analyzed out of the complex tone. [After R. Koenig (1872).]

The resonators can, however, do much more than the mathematical analysis. They are not limited to sounds whose component frequencies are in a simple arithmetic ratio to one another, which is the basic requirement of the Fourier series. Many large bells, for instance, give out component tones which are quite inharmonic, are not related by simple ratios.

The wave form produced by such a bell would never repeat itself exactly and it is therefore wholly unsuitable for a Fourier analysis. But by means of an acoustic resonator it is possible to discover just what these bell frequencies are.

Today we have the electronic wave analyzer, which is a far more accurate instrument than the acoustic resonator. The sound to be broken up is first picked up by a microphone and is then sent through many special circuits. Even then the action of the wave analyzer depends fundamentally upon a kind of resonance, but the resonance is electrical rather than acoustic. The advantages of the electronic analyzer are that the frequency may be determined easily by reading a single large dial and the strength of the component is measured on an accurate meter. With this analyzer it has been possible to find the components present in many kinds of sounds, particularly in many complex noises that previously were little understood. In fact, the physical composition of practically all sounds is now fairly well known, with the exception of a few extremely brief transient sounds.

Sine Waves

In describing a sine wave we have always to state its *frequency* (or wave length) and its *amplitude.* In acoustics frequency is stated in cycles per second (cps), the number of complete waves that pass a given point in a second. The amplitude is the size of the wave. In waves like those of Fig. 147 the amplitude is the height of the wave. There component III has a frequency three times the frequency of I and an amplitude somewhat less than half the amplitude of I.

In describing the relation of one wave to another, the *phase* relation of the two must be stated. In Fig. 147 the phase relation of III to I would be changed if III were shifted to the right a fraction of its wave length, but not if it were shifted one whole wave length. Two waves of the same frequency are said to be *in phase* when their crests (or troughs) coincide or to be *in opposite phase* when the crest of one comes with the trough of the other.

With these meanings in mind, we can now draw upon our knowledge of the results of the two methods of analysis of complex waves and formulate these conclusions.

(1) *Any complex stimulus to tone or noise may be described adequately as the combination of a number of components, each one a sine wave with its own frequency and amplitude.* In special cases it is necessary to say also what is the relative phase of the components or to tell how their amplitude rises and falls.

(2) So far as the acoustic and mechanical parts of the ear are concerned, *what happens to any complex sound is described fully by telling what happens to each of its sine wave components.* As we shall see later, *this rule no longer holds when we begin to deal with the action of the nervous system.*

(3) Sounds may be anything—an occasional pure tone, musical tones which have regularly spaced harmonic components (Fourier series), clangs and tone-like noises which have components of odd frequencies irregularly spaced and finally random and impulse-like noises in which the individual components can no longer be separated from one another. In this last case we speak of a *continuous* sound spectrum, meaning that all frequencies are present, although they will not all be equally strong (an analogy with the light spectrum). It

is clear that *the character or quality of a sound is determined by the number and distribution of the components which make it up.*

Harmonics

We think of a simple sine wave as being the stimulus for a pure tone, but actually exact sine waves are hard to create and, when they are formed in air by modern electrical means, they are almost certain to get distorted in transmission through any communication system, a telephone system or even the mechanism of the human ear itself.

If you pluck or strike a piano string, having pressed down the sustaining pedal, you get from it, not a pure sine wave, but a complex wave which is the sum of many waves having frequencies in the ratios of 1:2:3:4:5:6:7:8 and so on. If the string you plucked was the one for A of 110 cycles per second, you would have a complex wave of a frequency of 110 + 220 + 330 + 440 + 550 + 660 + 770 + 880 cycles per second, etc., that is, the notes A, a, e′, a′, d″, e″, g″, a″, etc. These notes, which tend to go together when an instrument produces the lowest one and which have these simple frequency ratios to one another, are called *harmonics* and are said to be in *harmonic relation* to one another. The lowest tone of a set of harmonics is called the *fundamental* and the rest the *upper harmonics.*

All notes of musical instruments are complex in different ways, according to which harmonics are emphasized in them—whether all the first ten, as in the plucked piano string, or the even harmonics, or the odd, or the high ones. The distinctive qualities of different musical instruments are due in part to the pattern of harmonics produced.

It is safe to say that no one has ever heard a loud pure tone. Unless the stimulus is very weak, even a pure sine wave is distorted by the transmission apparatus of the ear, so that for a pure sine wave outside we get inside a complex wave with all the components that the Fourier analysis gives for the distorted sine form.

SOUNDS: WHAT WE HEAR

Sound is, after all, what we hear. We have taken pains to understand the sources of sound, the sound waves, because, in the end, someone was going to hear the sound. Now we have to examine what is heard and relate it to the physical events outside the ear which preceded it. Our auditory experiences need to be arranged, and we have to find the common attributes, the dimensions, with respect to which these experiences may be ordered.

The simplest ordering of sounds is in terms of their quality. All sounds may be classified into *tones* and *noises.* Tones are smooth, blended, continuous; noises are rough, irregular, disorganized. There is, of course, no sharp line between the two. Many noises have a tonal character, and almost all musical instruments make noises that form a part of their normal tones. Noises may be *continuous* noises, like roars, rattles, squeaks and hisses, or they may be *explosive* noises, booms, thuds, bangs, clicks and pops.

Tones might be subdivided as they sound like a bowed string (violin), a plucked or struck string (piano), an open pipe (pipe organ), a reed instrument (clarinet), etc. Such a classification would be of little value, as it would serve to point out only what is obvious, that the ear can and does hear differences of this kind.

PITCH

For many centuries, certainly since the days of the early Greeks, men have recognized *pitch* as an attribute of tones. Pitch, and melody which in part depends on pitch, were used to further human enjoyment long before anyone understood how they come about. Indeed, it is sometimes disconcerting to realize how much men once achieved without the tremendous body of scientific knowledge on which we may draw today!

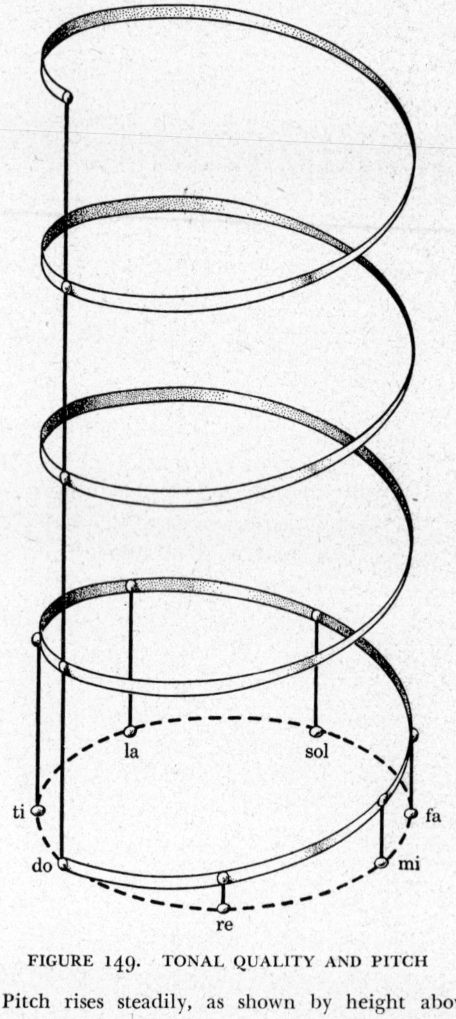

FIGURE 149. TONAL QUALITY AND PITCH

Pitch rises steadily, as shown by height above base. Tonal quality, as of a note on a musical scale, repeats itself through each octave and is shown around the circle.

Tones vary in pitch from *high* to *low*. Just why we use words describing space also to describe pitch is not clear, but the same pair of words is used in many different languages. A psychologist once put a loudspeaker behind a black curtain and then asked students seated in front of it where they heard a series of pure tones. They heard the higher pitches farther from the floor, the lower pitches nearer the floor. But the psychologist could find no explanation for this persistent impression.

Pitch is most characteristic of tones in the middle of the range, roughly within the musical scale. Some people would go so far as to say that pitch does not describe the extremely high notes. Such high tones, they say, are merely piercing, shrill, bright, etc. Nevertheless, a person who believed this would still put the notes in the same order from low to high, perhaps on the basis of brightness. Here arises a problem about the words we should use, and it is not important in understanding how the ear works. The important fact is that, whatever word is used, people who can hear the very high notes at all can tell them apart and put them in order.

A more difficult problem comes up because some pitches seem to be more closely related to one another than others. In particular, tones which are about an octave apart bear a very strong resemblance to each other. A person with little musical training will frequently make a mistake of a full octave in setting a pitch from memory, particularly if he is dealing with pure tones. It has been suggested that the proper way to represent pitch is not in a straight line, but rather in a spiral as shown in Fig. 149. The height above the base is the quality usually recognized by the psychologist as pitch. The notes within an octave, *do, re, mi, fa,* etc., would then be represented around the circle, and two notes an octave apart would come one over the other. Such a scheme is indeed useful, for it makes clear a set of relations among pitches which to the musician are all important.

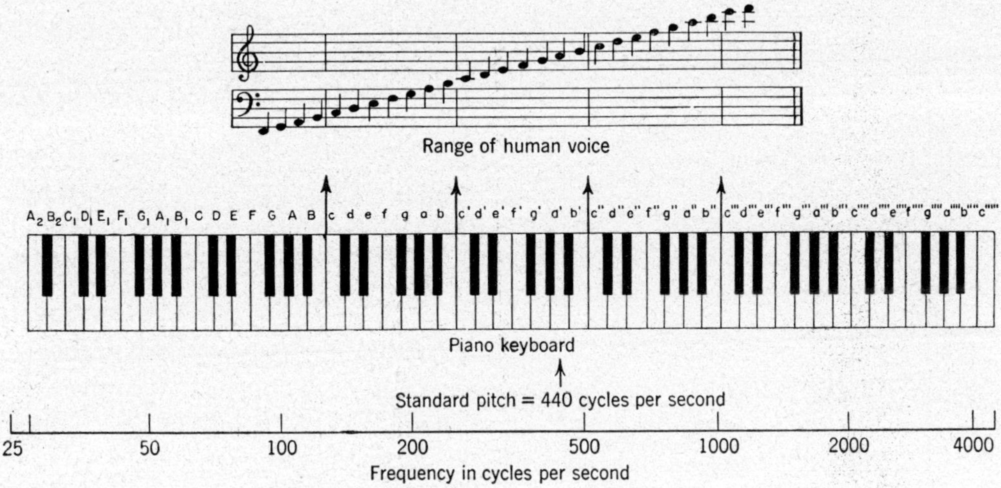

FIGURE 150. FREQUENCY OF MUSICAL TONES

The lowest scale shows frequency in cycles per second. Above this are shown the piano keys corresponding to each frequency, and the notes of the staff which are commonly sung. The musical scales are referred to standard orchestral pitch of a′ = 440 cycles per second.

Pitch and the Sound Wave

The pitch of a tone depends principally upon the *frequency* of the sound waves reaching the ear. High pitches are heard when the frequency is high; low pitches go with low frequencies. The frequencies of the notes on the piano keyboard are shown in Fig. 150, together with the notes that can be sung by the human voice. Naturally not all pianos are tuned to just these values, and some artists insist upon having instruments tuned a little higher or a little lower. Sometimes the terms pitch and frequency are used interchangeably. Engineers and physicists are particularly prone to this error, speaking of a 'pitch of 1000 cycles.' The reader should be careful not to make this mistake. Pitch is something we hear that is high or low; frequency is something measured physically by counting the number of waves per second.

Pitch Thresholds

The lowest pitch which can be heard is produced by a frequency of about 20 cycles per second, although a tone of this frequency must be quite intense to be audible. Still lower frequencies produce in the ear sensations which vary from intermittent pressure to a noisy flutter. At the opposite end of the scale, the highest frequency which can be heard is about 20,000 cycles per second. The exact threshold point depends again upon the tone's being sufficiently intense. There are plenty of sounds in the air, sounds produced by insects and by tiny objects, which, being above the upper limit, are never heard by human ears. Bats have been found to send out a series of short squeaks whose frequency is over 50,000 cycles per second. (See pp. 386–389.) By listening for the echoes, they are able while in flight to locate either obstacles or prey, much as a boat finds its way through a narrow channel in a fog by blowing its whistle. The greater sensitivity of some animals to these ultrasonic frequencies is almost certainly a result of the small size of the moving parts of their ears rather than to the possession of any special sense which man does not possess.

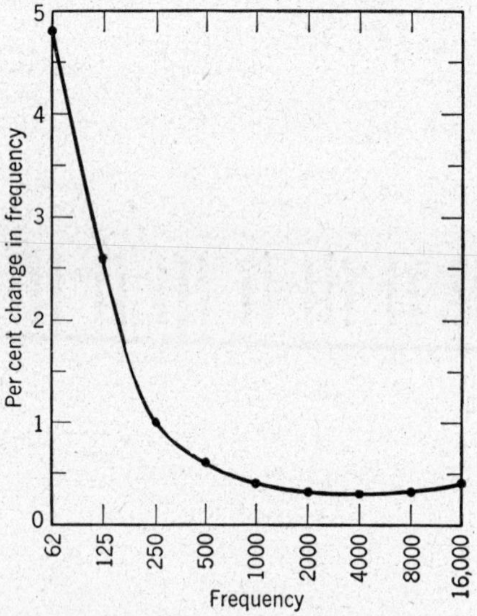

FIGURE 151. PITCH DISCRIMINATION

This figure shows the proportionate or per cent change in *frequency* necessary on the average to hear a change in *pitch*. Data are for tones 40 decibels above threshold. [From E. G. Shower and R. Biddulph, *J. acous. Soc. Amer.*, 1931, **3**, 284.]

Between 20 and 20,000 cycles per second there are about 1500 steps of pitch, each of which, under favorable conditions, is just as often as not distinguishable from the next one. They are threshold steps—differential thresholds. Their size is charted in Fig. 151. Notice that the measure of the differential threshold used in this figure is the *relative* amount of change in frequency. This is the way we should draw the figure if we expected something like Weber's law for frequency, and, indeed, *a constant proportion* appears to be necessary above 1000 cycles per second. Below that value quite the reverse holds, and the minimum change is marked off by a *constant number of cycles.* A rule of thumb is that a good listener can hear a difference between two tones 3 cycles per second apart up to 1000 cycles per second, and then a constant fractional difference of 0.3 per cent ($3/1000$) above 1000 cycles per second. Judged by any standard, this is truly remarkable discrimination.

The Scale of Pitch

These steps, that is to say, the series of notes which can just be distinguished from each other, give us one kind of unit in which to step off the scale of pitch. Are these the best units to employ? One other possibility would be to use frequency, but almost no one would listen to a series of tones 5 cycles per second apart, or 50 cycles per second apart, and say that they formed a series with equal steps. There are, on the other hand, many persons who would argue warmly that pitch is proportional to musical interval, such as the octave, the fifth and the third.

In its origin the diatonic scale, which is the basis of our music, used the octave as its unit or step. Then other intervals were added, the fifth and the fourth, then the third and sixth, until the octave had been divided up into the seven familiar, though unequally spaced, notes. The important fact about this musical scale is that the size of a given step depends on a *ratio* of the two frequencies. An octave, for instance, is always measured by doubling or halving the frequency. Thus if we start from 1000 cycles per second, an octave higher would be 2000 cycles per second, and the octaves lower would be 500 and 250 cycles per second.

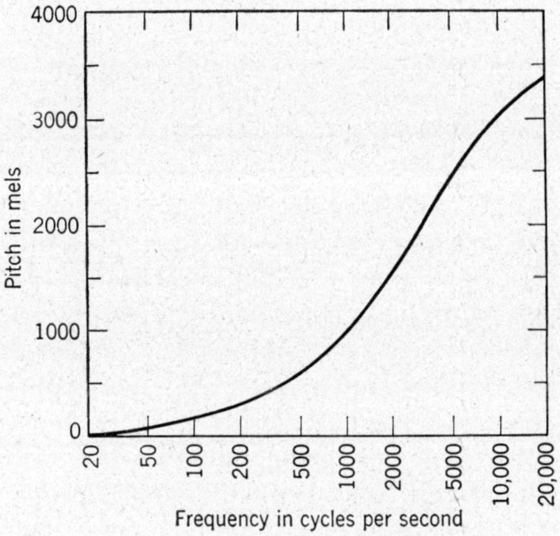

FIGURE 152. SCALE OF PITCH

The subjective magnitude of pitch is measured in mels. The curve shows how the number of mels increases as frequency increases. [From S. S. Stevens and J. Volkmann, *Amer. J. Psychol.*, 1940, **53**, 336.]

Recent experiments have shown that it is better to start out without knowing about ratios and frequencies, and simply to arrange a series of notes so that they sound to the ear equally far apart in pitch. The distance between any pair of notes in the series becomes a unit of pitch. One such scale is shown in Fig. 152 in which the unit has been called the *mel.* The figure shows just how the mels of pitch increase with cycles per second. Another way of showing the same thing is to distort the conventional piano keyboard so that each key is as wide as the number of mels it includes. The result, shown in Fig. 153, makes very clear how much the musical scale and the mel scale differ from each other.

LOUDNESS

An even more general characteristic of sounds than pitch is *loudness.* Both tones and noises can be called *loud* or *soft.* Loudness is easily recognized as the *intensitive* aspect of sound, the more-or-less, which corresponds to saturation in vision and the strength of a smell or taste.

For any single kind of a tone or noise, it is easy to say what is the physical change which makes a sound louder. Loudness depends simply on the amplitude of the sound wave. It is fairly difficult to say what will be the comparative loudness of two sounds of different frequency or of two noises. As we shall see (pp. 325 f.), we have to know much more than the relative amplitudes of the two waves.

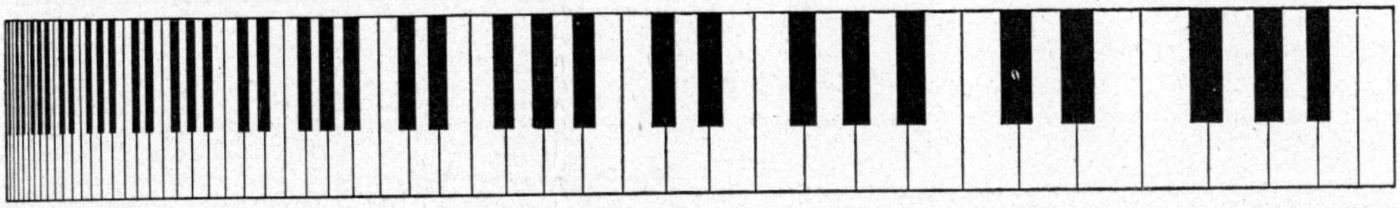

FIGURE 153. THE MEL KEYBOARD

The piano keyboard is distorted so that equal distance represents equal amounts of pitch rather than equal units on the musical scale. This shows why melodies are so much clearer when played in the treble than when played in the bass.

Loudness Thresholds

The softest sound, the weakest intensity which we ever hear, lies at the *absolute threshold* for hearing. If we measure the least sound pressure under an earphone at which a *tone* can be heard, we get results shown in the lower curve of Fig. 154. Notice how different are the amounts required

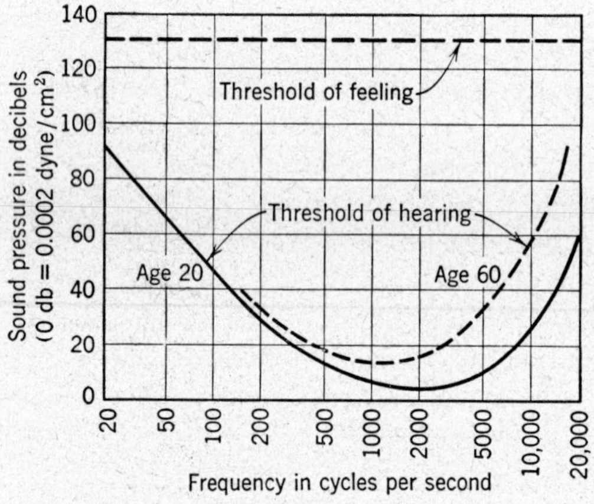

FIGURE 154. THRESHOLD OF HEARING

Lower solid curve shows the lowest sound pressure which can be heard by a practiced listener 20 to 30 years of age. Above this the dotted curve shows the threshold for an average listener of 60. The dashed line at the top shows initial threshold of feeling for both hard-of-hearing and normal subjects. All values are pressures under earphone at entrance to ear canal.

at different frequencies. A pressure 1000 times (60 decibels) greater is required at 60 cycles per second than at 2000 cycles per second. This curve shows what a person with good hearing can do when he is about 20 years old. As he grows older, the membranes in his ear stiffen and nerve fibers degenerate. The average sensitivity of a man of 60 is shown in the dotted curve. Note that he has lost completely his hearing for the very highest frequencies and that he has some loss in sensitivity through the middle range.

Just how loud sound can be before hearing is permanently injured cannot be specified with certainty. Moderately loud noise, if it lasts for a long time, will produce a measurable deafness. Instances are the deafness produced by long practice on a rifle range, flight in an open or uninsulated airplane or work in the pressroom of a large newspaper. More severe noises, noises that are actually painful, such as the rapid fire of anti-aircraft guns or the noise of the loudest sirens, will produce an almost complete deafness for high tones in a very short time. So far as laboratory experiments have gone, normal persons exposed to such very loud noises have always recovered—fortunately. The uncertainty arises from the fact that there are wide differences among people in the ease with which they suffer injury. Some people may perhaps incur not only temporary but also actually permanent losses from exposure to continued loud noise. Opinions on this point differ widely.

Before a level is reached which causes the most severe temporary losses, most laboratory subjects will object strenuously. As the sound grows louder it tickles, then can be felt as something jabbing at the ear. It is piercing and unpleasant, and finally painful. The level at which this takes place is shown in Fig. 154 as the *threshold of feeling*. Hard-of-hearing persons report the same experiences with the same levels of stimulation. Apparently the small hairs in the ear canal are being moved, and the drum stretched beyond its comfortable limit.

The Scale of Loudness

Just as for pitch, a scale must be constructed for loudness. The *physical* scale used to measure the amplitude of the sound wave is a logarithmic scale on which equal steps stand for equal ratios. The unit is the *decibel* (db), which represents a ratio of 1:1.13 between two pressures. In other words, a 13 per cent increase in pressure equals an increase of one decibel. Decibels are like compound interest, and successive decibel steps are given by $1.0 \times 1.13 \times 1.13$, not $1.00 + 0.13 + 0.13$. Decibels also have

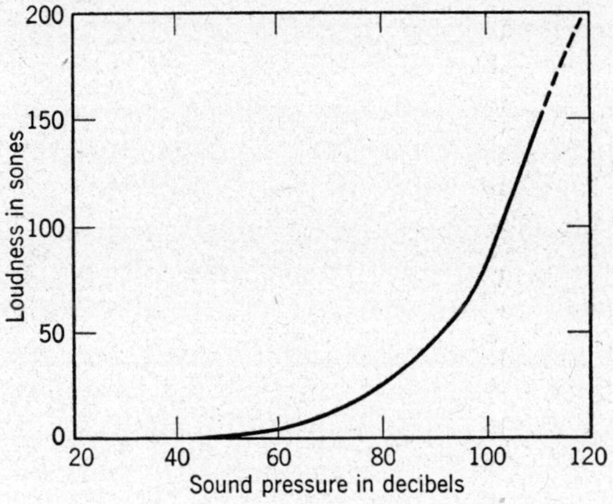

FIGURE 155. SCALE OF LOUDNESS

How loudness as judged subjectively grows as a function of sound pressure in decibels. Note that sound pressures below 40 decibels have almost no loudness, and only above 80 decibels does loudness grow rapidly.

to start from somewhere and be about something. Actually, decibels are just numbers, like 2 or 10. When we talk about sound pressure level, we arbitrarily use as a zero point 0.0002 dyne per square centimeter. Then 0-decibel sound pressure level equals 0.0002 dyne per square centimeter, 20-decibel equals 0.002 dyne, and 74-decibel equals 1 dyne per square centimeter.

This physical scale makes fairly good psychological sense, for the number of just noticeable differences of a sound above the threshold corresponds roughly with the number of decibels it is above its threshold. Difficulty occurs when we divide the whole range of sound intensities, for out of 120 decibels between the absolute threshold and the loudest sound commonly heard, the first 40 decibels just get up to an audible whisper and 80 decibels are only a good conversational level. To get a proper *psychological* scale it is necessary to resort to direct judgment. Suppose we begin with a certain faint sound and find a second sound that seems twice as loud; then we find a third sound that seems twice as loud as the second; and so on. From these results we can construct a scale of loudness like the one shown in Fig. 155. Loudness grows very slowly until a level of 60 decibels is reached, and then it goes up at an ever-increasing rate as far as the function has been measured.

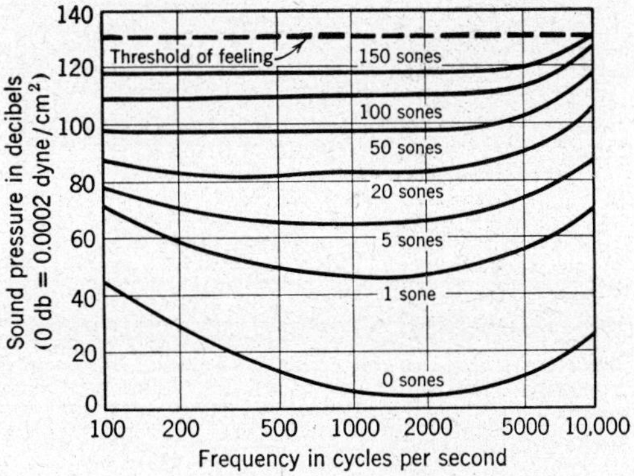

FIGURE 156. EQUAL-LOUDNESS CONTOURS

Tones corresponding to the points along each curve sound equally loud. Near each curve is given the loudness in sones. Zero sones equal the absolute threshold.

We noted earlier that, for a single tone, it is the amplitude of the sound wave which determines loudness. Now we must qualify that by saying that loudness depends also upon the frequency of the tone. First of all, we observe that the threshold for low tones and very high tones is much larger than the threshold for tones in the middle frequencies. That is clear in Fig. 154. At moderately high levels, well above threshold, loudness shows less variation with frequency. To show this, scientists construct an *equal-loudness contour* by adjusting a high tone to a low tone until one sounds just as loud as the other. Measuring the intensity of each tone makes it possible to draw the typical equal-loudness contours which are shown in Fig. 156. Since the distance in decibels from the one-sone to the fifty-sone contour is less at the low frequencies than at the high, it follows that loudness must grow more rapidly at low frequencies than at high.

INTERACTION OF STIMULI

Next we have to ask what happens when two or more tones sound together. How do they affect each other?

Beats and Combination Tones

To many a novice the skill of the piano tuner appears as something like magic, yet one of the devices he uses is so simple that only a little attention is required for anyone to hear it. This is the use of *beats* which occur whenever two tones sound together while differing only slightly in frequency. Beats sound like an alternate waxing and waning, a rhythmic wow-wow of the two almost fused tones. A keen ear can hear a very slow beat requiring as much as five or ten seconds to come and go. As beats become faster they sound like a pulsating tone, and then they lose their individual identity and become simply a roughness which is superimposed on the two now distinguishable tones.

A little consideration makes the origin of beats quite clear. Suppose two strings vibrate at slightly different rates, say, 500 and 501 cycles per second. If the strings are struck simultaneously both strings will move together, and the sound waves produced by each will *reinforce* each other. Now notice what will happen one-half second later; the one string will have completed 250 vibrations and the other 250½ vibrations. In other words, the strings will now be in opposite phases, one of them producing the peak of a pressure wave while the other produces a trough. Under these conditions the sound waves cancel each other, and a much weaker sound will be heard. Finally at the end of a full second, both will again be in phase.

Comparable is the phenomenon of *difference tones* which require more special circumstances if they are to be heard. When the two tones that are led to the ear are fairly strong, and have a frequency difference of about 50 cycles per second or more, one or more tones may be heard in addition to the primary pair. The most prominent of such tones is a *difference tone;* it has the pitch which belongs to the frequency equal to the difference in frequency of the primaries. Under good conditions, when the primaries are loud, a *summation tone,* whose pitch corresponds to the sum of the frequencies of the primary tones, can also be heard. Thus, for example, the tones 700 and 1200 cycles per second may produce a difference tone of 500 and a summation tone of 1900 cycles per second. If the primary tones contain strong upper harmonics, there may be other combination tones, although they usually are so faint as to escape notice.

Masking

Masking is the official name given to the familiar fact that one sound drowns out another. Interest in masking stems from the efforts of telephone engineers to improve service at those critical points where messages are lost in the background of noise. It is equally important in radio communication and in the choice of bells and alarms which must be heard under competition with other noise.

The facts about the masking of one pure tone by another are summed up in the curves of Fig. 157. The amount of masking is measured by how much *change* there

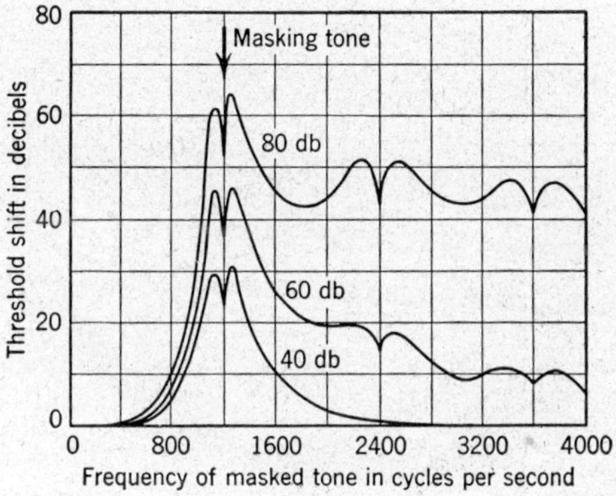

FIG. 157. AUDITORY MASKING

The curves show how much the threshold is raised at each frequency as a result of the masking by a 1200 cycles per second tone 40 decibels, 60 decibels, and 80 decibels above its threshold. [After R. L. Wegel and C. E. Lane, *Phys. Rev.*, 1924, **23**, 271.]

is in the absolute threshold for any given tone when it is masked by another. In this experiment, for instance, the threshold was first determined in a quiet room for many frequencies between 400 and 4000 cycles per second. Then a *masking* tone of 1200 cycles per second was turned on, and all the thresholds were found to have been raised by the amounts shown in the figure. The results for three levels of the masking tone are shown, with, obviously, the greater amount of masking when the masking tone is more intense. The curves also show one other important fact; the masking of high tones by a low tone is much greater than the masking of low tones by a higher one. The practical effect of this principle appears when some kinds of sound-deadening treatment give disappointing results in a room. The sound-absorbing material may remove the high frequencies quite well, but it usually has too little effect at medium and low frequencies. Yet it is just these low frequencies which do most of the masking.

If an engineer wishes to use the information about masking in finding out how well a given telephone or radio circuit will perform, he must know a good many technical details. In the final analysis the important thing is the ratio of the desired sound to the noise, the *signal-to-noise ratio;* which should be known for at least twenty bands of frequencies spaced equally along the *mel* scale.

HOW THE EAR WORKS

Up to this point we have been describing *what* the ear does; now we must see *how* the ear works. What kind of mechanism makes possible the discriminations of pitch and loudness? To answer this question, it will be necessary, first, to discover how the ear is constructed and, second, to explain what the various parts of the ear do in receiving a sound wave.

Unfortunately, the observation of the ear is made unusually difficult by its location buried in bones of the head. Anatomists have disagreed about the fine structure of the inner ear, either because they have damaged the ear while cutting the bone away or because the delicate tissues have disintegrated before preservatives could penetrate the bony shell. Only in very recent years has anyone seen the innermost parts of the ear actually working, and today the best observations leave much room for speculation and opinion.

In its basic design the ear is quite nicely adjusted for its job. It has three parts: first, the receiving part, a horn and funnel-shaped tube which collects the sound and leads it to the ear; second, the conducting part, a light drum-head diaphragm which is moved back and forth by the sound, transmitting this motion in turn through a set of rods to a small piston; and third, a hydraulic analyzer driven by this piston. Distributed to various parts of this analyzer are the nerve endings which start impulses up over the auditory nerve to the hearing centers in the central nervous system.

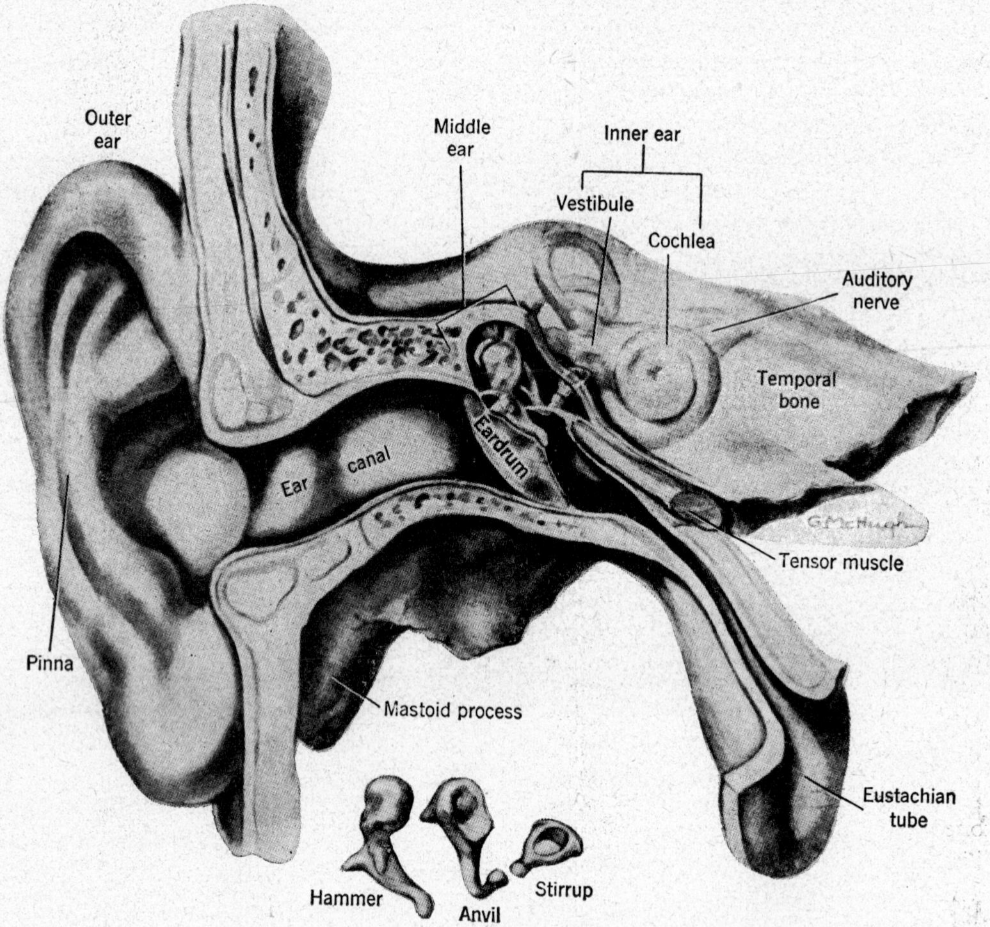

FIGURE 158. SECTION THROUGH THE EAR

This cross-section shows the principal parts of the outer, middle and inner ear, with the last buried within the skull. The inner ear has been rotated so it may be seen in better detail. The three ossicles, somewhat enlarged, are also shown separately at the bottom of the figure. [From G. McHugh, in S. L. Polyak, *The human ear,* Sonotone Corporation, 1946.]

A vertical cut through the head, made

in a suitable plane, would lay bare the hidden parts of the ear shown in Fig. 158. To the left is the receiving part, the *outer ear,* consisting of the pinna and the ear canal. The conducting part, the *middle ear,* consists of the cavity behind the ear drum and includes the tiny bones and muscles lying within that cavity. The analyzer is contained within the *inner ear,* which lies buried in the temporal bone in the floor of the case surrounding the brain. The important part of the inner ear for hearing is the snail-shaped *cochlea* which we shall examine in detail in just a moment.

The Outer Ear

In many animals the *outer ear* serves as an efficient collector of sound which increases substantially the intensity of the waves reaching the eardrum. Equally important to many animals is the fact that the pinna is often movable, a capacity which aids them in locating a source of sound. In some animals, such as the seal, the parts of the outer ear may be folded together to form a tight protective cover for the ear canal. Men get along without much help from their outer ears in any of these respects. Our pinnas help us slightly in locating high-pitched noises as being in front or in back. Moreover, our ear canals are effective horns for sound frequencies near 3000 cycles per second, amplifying the sound pressure six or eight times. But principally our outer ears are but vestiges of the more useful ears which our night-hunting arboreal ancestors once possessed.

Across the inner end of the auditory canal, and closing off the cavity of the middle ear, is the *eardrum,* a thin skinlike membrane pulled slightly inward at its center where it is attached to the hammer, the first of the bony links to the inner ear. The drum in area is a little larger than the end of a pencil. The drum itself is not under particular tension; the resistance it offers to movement by sound waves is a result of its inertia at high frequencies. The drum still works amazingly well when it is pierced; the loss in sensitivity can scarcely be measured. Even a small remnant of drum attached to the hammer bone of the middle ear permits some effective hearing.

The Middle Ear

The *middle ear* is a small air-filled cavity, lying within the temporal bone. Its location can be seen in Fig. 158. The front end of the cavity connects with the back of the nose through the *Eustachian tube,* and at the other end the middle ear broadens out into the sinuses of the mastoid bone. Its roof is a thin plate in the floor of the bony brain case.

The important parts lying within the middle ear are shown in Fig. 159. The three small bones or *ossicles,* known equally well by their English or Latin names, the hammer or *malleus,* the anvil or *incus* and the stirrup or *stapes,* form a bridge to carry sound from the eardrum to the cochlea. The hammer attaches firmly to the eardrum while the foot plate of the stirrup, in area roughly equal to a section of a pencil lead, is fitted into the *oval window,* one of two openings through the bone from the middle ear into the canals of the inner ear. The second opening, the *round window,* affords relief for the pressure produced in the inner ear as the stirrup moves in and out.

The action of the middle ear is to make the incoming sound wave most effective at one point in the inner ear, namely, at the oval window. The sensitive cells of the inner ear are immersed in fluid; their stimulation depends on movements of this

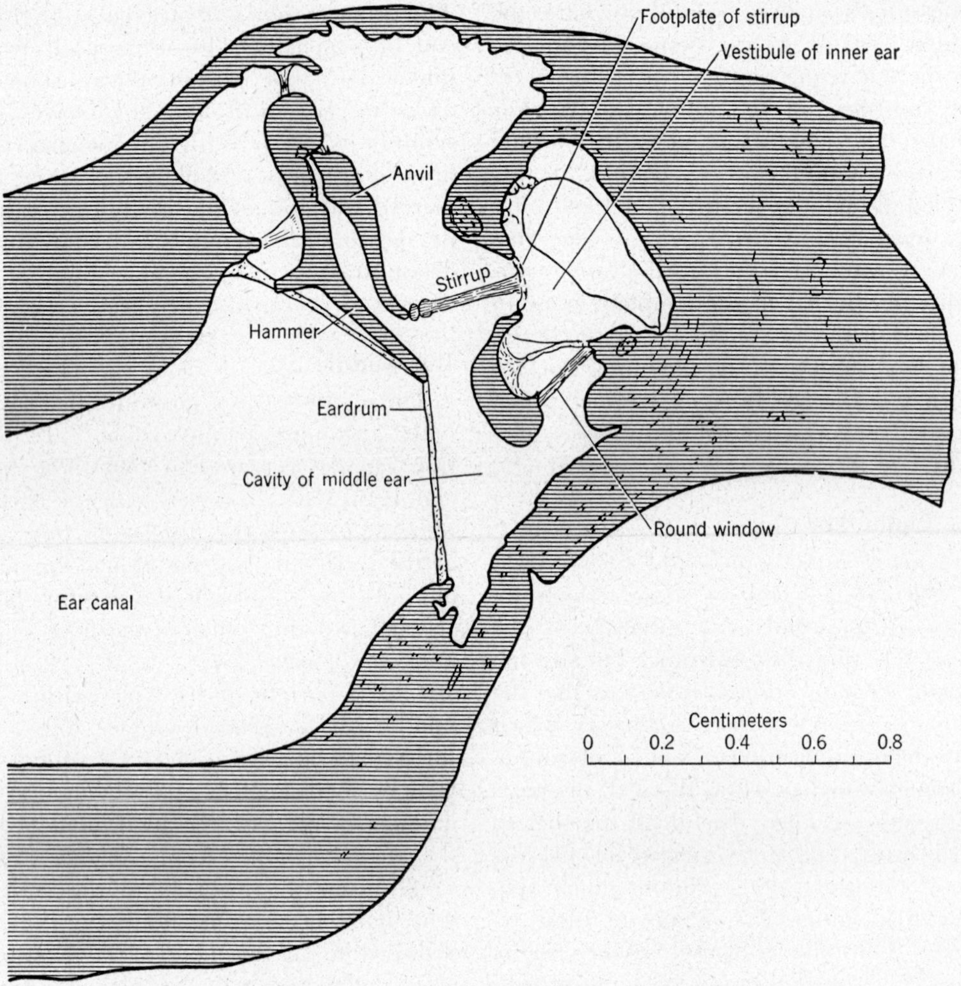

FIGURE 159. THE MIDDLE EAR AND THE OSSICLES

This cross-section has been constructed to show the relative size and spatial relations of the ossicles acting as a bridge to carry sound to the inner ear. [After A. Keith, in T. Wrightson, *An enquiry into the analytical mechanism of the internal ear,* Macmillan, 1918, p. 190.]

fluid. The sound waves consist of only small changes in pressure in the air, an easily compressible medium. Much more pressure is required to set the fluid in motion. This pressure is obtained by having all the relatively small air pressure over the large eardrum brought to bear on the small foot plate of the stirrup in contact with the fluid. Altogether, a mechanical advantage of about thirty to one is obtained by this device.

The Inner Ear

Immersed within the hard petrous portion of the temporal bone are the series of canals which contain the *inner ear.* They appear in shadowy outline in Fig. 158. The first chamber entered from the middle ear is the *vestibule,* one corner of which is shown in Fig. 159. Leading off to the back are the *semicircular canals* which serve an important function in our sense of bodily movement (pp. 374–377). To the front lies the snail-shaped *cochlea,* the important organ of hearing.

A cut through the center of the snail shell reveals the inside of the canals, as shown in Fig. 160. This reproduction is a considerable enlargement. The full width of the section shown is only about one-fourth inch. The human cochlea has three full turns; only two and one-half turns are shown here. Inspection shows that the cochlea is actually divided into three canals: a lower canal, called the *scala tympani,* an upper canal, called the *scala vestibuli,* and a small canal on the outer side, called the *cochlear duct.* The two larger canals are connected together at the very tip of the cochlea through an opening, the *helicotrema.* Feeding up through the very middle of the cochlea is the *auditory nerve.*

We can see the location of the actual

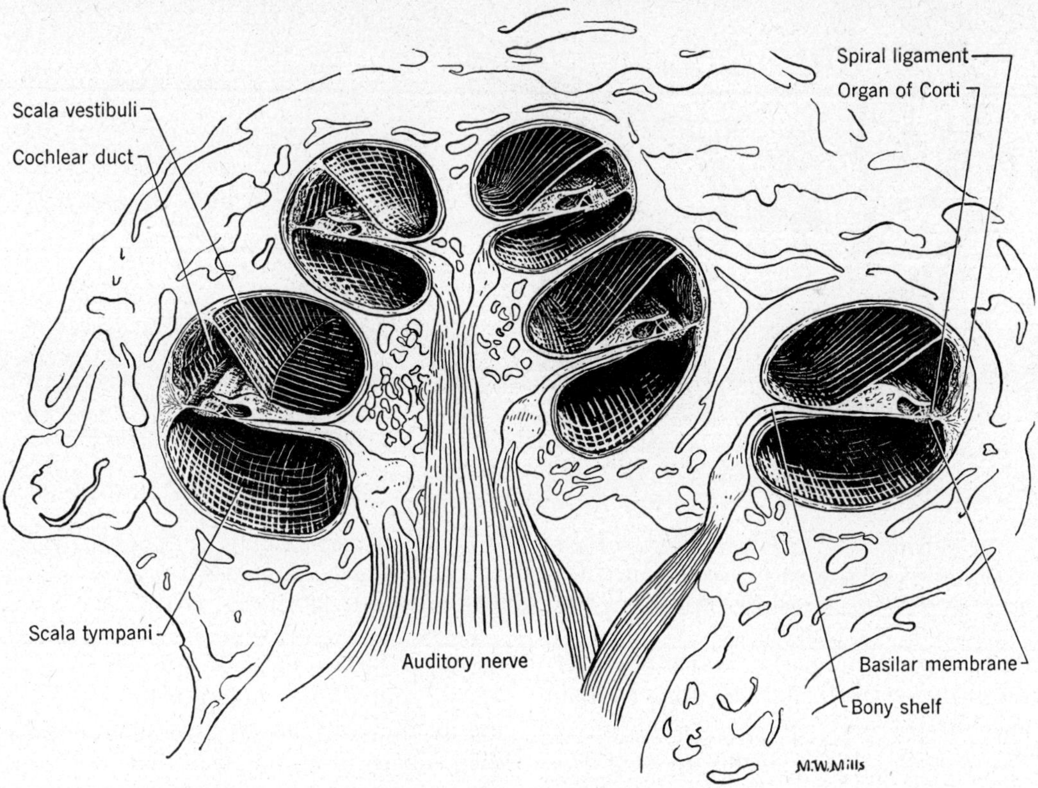

FIGURE 160. INSIDE OF THE COCHLEA

Section through the 'snail-shell,' the spiral cochlea. The scala vestibuli, the scala typani and the cochlear duct are spiral canals which can be seen to be receding and curving along with the basilar membrane, the organ of Corti, the spiral ligament and the bony shelf. (See Fig. 161.) The auditory nerve runs up the middle from below.

sense cells and the nerve endings more readily in the diagrammatic cross-section of Fig. 161. We can recognize here the larger features of the cochlea which appeared in the previous figure. In addition we can see organ of Corti are the nerve fibers from the *spiral ganglion,* the first way station on the path to the brain.

The organ of Corti itself consists, as Fig. 162 shows, of a framework which carries in

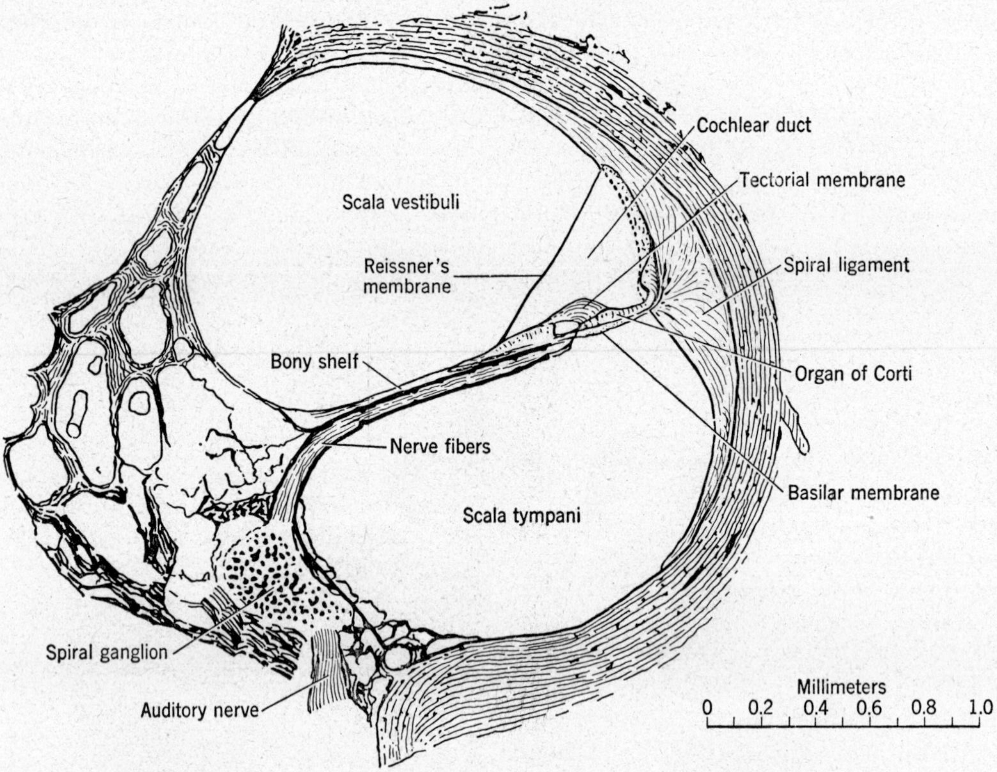

FIGURE 161. LOCATION OF THE BASILAR MEMBRANE AND ORGAN OF CORTI

The cochlear tube is divided into two parts by a partition consisting of the bony shelf, the basilar membrane and the spiral ligament. [After A. Keith, in T. Wrightson, *An enquiry into the analytical mechanism of the internal ear,* Macmillan. 1918, p. 192.]

that the partition, part of which is between the *scala vestibuli* and the *scala tympani* and part between the *scala tympani* and the *cochlear duct,* is made up of a *bony shelf* as inner part, the thick *spiral ligament* attached to the outer wall, and, suspended between them, the *basilar membrane* on which rests the *organ of Corti.* Passing out through the bony shelf to the its upper surface the *hair cells,* believed to be the source of stimulation for tiny endings of the nerve fibers. The hair cells get their name from the fact that each cell bears a series of fine hairlike projections on its upper surface, hairs which are embedded in the jellylike material of the *tectorial membrane.* The thin *Reissner's membrane* separates the two cochlear fluids, *perilymph* in the scala vestibuli and scala tympani and *endolymph* in the cochlear duct, but it has no important effect on the way the sense cells on the basilar membrane behave.

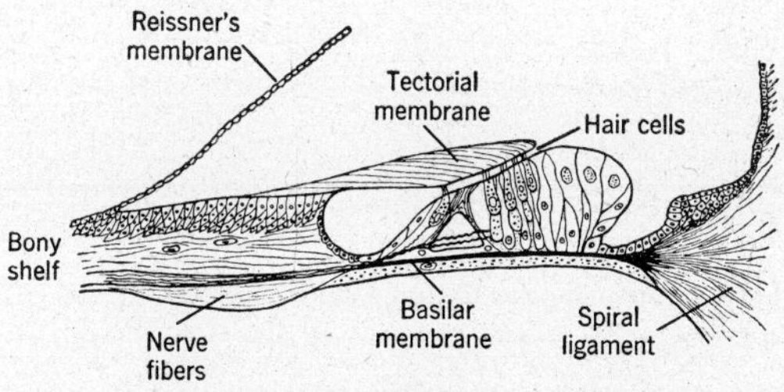

FIGURE 162. THE ORGAN OF CORTI

Much enlarged view of actual sensory cells. Note single inner row and multiple outer row of hair cells.

How the Cochlea Works

In explaining the action of the outer ear and of the middle ear, we have had to deal solely with physical principles, how sound waves in the air are turned into to-and-fro movements of the stirrup, which acts like a piston to pump back and forth the fluids of the cochlea. The crux of the problem of hearing comes when this physical movement in the cochlea has to be changed into the electrochemical message in the auditory nerve and, in particular, into a message which can be interpreted by the brain in terms of the psychological characteristics of pitch and loudness. Of course not all of this transformation from physical movement to psychological attribute need take place in the cochlea, but it must at least start there. Let us see first what happens in the cochlea to explain loudness. After that we may turn to the problem of pitch.

Since *loudness* is an intensitive attribute, we should expect to find some corresponding characteristic of the nervous response which can also be large or small, greater or less. On the other hand, the all-or-none response of each single nerve fiber does not permit a direct transformation from mechanical intensity into intensity in the individual fiber. Physiology tells us that the most common way intensity is represented in the nervous system is by transforming it into the frequency of response of any given fiber (p. 30). This probably happens in the ear as well as in other sense organs. When a weak sound reaches the threshold for a given fiber, it fires off only now and then; as the stimulus becomes more intense, the response of the fiber becomes more frequent until that fiber is working at top speed.

This cannot, however, be the sole explanation of loudness. There are two difficulties. First, the range of intensities over which the response of a single fiber can be graded in frequency is quite small, perhaps only as much as 30 to 1. The range of intensities over which the ear responds with distinguishable steps of loudness is very large, at least 10,000,000 to 1. The one can hardly be expected to take care of the other. The second difficulty complicates the first. At low frequencies, as we shall see in a moment, the nerve fibers are tripped off by the individual sound waves, so that the fibers tend to have the same frequency of response as the frequency of the sound wave.

Loudness must be explained, therefore, also in terms of the total number of active nerve fibers. At low intensities there are only a few fibers active, at high intensities a great many more. Loudness will depend both on how many fibers are working and on how often each one of them fires. It will be gauged ultimately by the total number of impulses in a large bundle of fibers. How is it that additional fibers go into action with increased intensity?

Probably two things happen. First of all, not all fibers have the same threshold. Quite different sound intensities are required to set off different fibers. Second, there are in the ear two mechanisms which may act much as do the rods and cones of the eye. They are the *inner* and *outer hair cells* which can be distinguished by a careful inspection of Fig. 162. The *inner hair cells* are much like the *cones* for they have each a single nerve fiber and require more vigorous stimulation of the ear to set them off. The *outer hair cells* are like the *rods,* connected in teams to each nerve fiber and so placed that the least movement will set them off. Third, as we shall see presently, the more intense sounds bring a larger proportion of the basilar membrane into action.

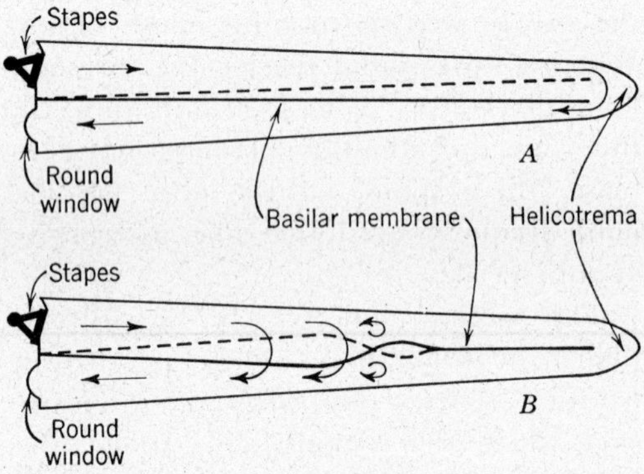

FIGURE 163. ACTION OF THE COCHLEA

Diagram represents cochlea unrolled, and indicates roughly how it responds differently to various frequencies. In *A,* slow movement of stapes depresses basilar membrane and pushes fluid through helicotrema. In *B,* fast movement of stapes depresses near end of basilar membrane up to limiting point where circular eddy marks end of stimulated area. [Adapted from G. Békésy, *Phys. Z.,* 1928, **29,** 793–810.]

To sum up, *loudness* depends on how many impulses arrive at some center in the brain. Just how many impulses there will be depends, in turn, upon how fast each single fiber is firing, upon the thresholds of each fiber, and whether all the fibers in one area have been called into action, upon the fiber's connection with the outer or inner hair cells and upon how wide a section of the basilar membrane is involved.

Pitch, in contrast with loudness, requires that the receptors make some discrimination in *kind.* Either there must be different types or varieties of the sense cells, as we suppose there are among the various skin senses, or else the location of the sense cell and the particular nerves to which it is connected is important, as in visual and tactual space. The first alternative is scarcely plausible, and the weight of evidence today favors the view that the receptors giving rise to the experience of a particular pitch have a particular location in the cochlea.

Let us look more closely at the cochlea. Imagine that the snail shell is unrolled so that it becomes a long socklike tube. Cut lengthwise it would look like Fig. 163. The tube is divided into an upper and lower half by the bony shelf and the basilar membrane. Only at the extreme tip of the tube do the two canals join (by way of the *helicotrema*). To the left, forcing liquid in and out of the upper canal, is the stirrup, driven by the sound wave. Closing the lower canal is the round window which can bulge into the middle ear as the stirrup pushes in at the top.

Now, if the stirrup is pushed *slowly* into the upper canal, fluid will flow up along the cochlea, through the helicotrema and down to the round window. At the same time the pressure will be slightly greater on the one side than on the other, and the basilar membrane will be bent down into the position shown by the solid line in *A* of Fig. 163. It will be depressed somewhat more *at the end away from the oval window* because *the basilar membrane grows wider toward the tip of the canal.* Pull the stirrup back and the reverse motion takes place with the basilar membrane in the position indicated by the dashed line.

Let the movement of the stirrup be more rapid, and there will no longer be time for the unhurried movement through the helicotrema. The pressure on the lower part of the basilar membrane will be greater, the membrane will be more distorted, while at a given point short of the upper end, something like an eddy develops and beyond this point little movement takes place. The cochlea acting in this manner is represented in *B* of Fig. 163. If the to-and-fro movement of the stirrup is still more rapid, the bulge of the basilar membrane will be confined to a very small area near the stirrup.

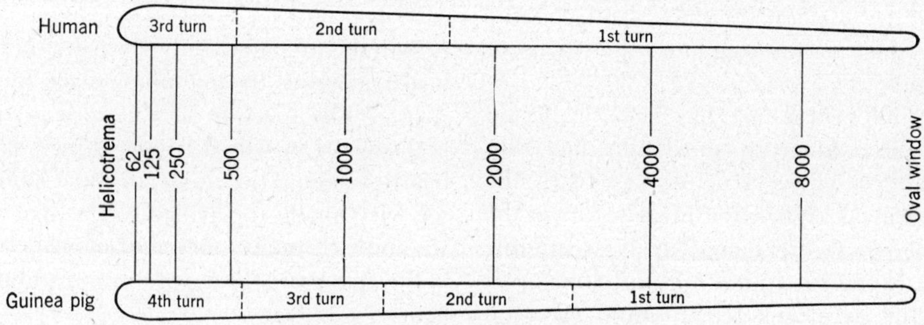

FIGURE 164. MAP OF BASILAR MEMBRANE

Narrow portion of membrane comes at base of cochlea. The maximum response to 1000 cycles per second comes at point indicated by line marked 1000. Experimental data obtained by drilling into cochlea of guinea pig. [From S. S. Stevens, H. Davis and M. H. Lurie, *J. gen. Psychol.,* 1935, 13, 312.]

It is one thing to know that different frequencies stimulate one part of the cochlea or another. It is a different matter to have a precise map and know that a given pitch is heard when a known point is stimulated. Such maps have been made by a number of different investigators, each using a different method. They agree about as well as we could expect on the basis of necessarily rough methods. Some of the maps have been made by relating deafness for particular tones in men, never a very precise affair, with postmortem examination of the cochlea. Other maps show how the conditioned responses of guinea pigs are upset by drilling holes in one part of the cochlea and destroying the underlying sense cells. Still other experiments make use of an electrical voltage generated when the hair cells are stimulated. One of these maps, of the guinea pig's ear, is shown in Fig. 164 together with the presumed parallel in the human ear. One interesting comparison appears. If the pitch scale of Fig. 152, page 323, which shows how pitch is related to frequency, is compared with this map of the cochlea, it turns out that *pitch is proportional to distances along the basilar membrane.*

The explanation of how the ear distinguishes *pitch* may be summed up in three points. *First,* while a large part of the basilar membrane may be deflected by any given sound wave, there is a point along the membrane where the deflection is maximum for a tone of a given frequency. *Second,* this maximum is near the base of the cochlea for high frequencies and is progressively farther from the stirrup and round window for lower frequencies. *Third,* the size of the area involved on either side of the maximum is probably proportional to the intensity of the sound wave, thus providing the additional factor needed to explain loudness and, at the same time, accounting for the facts of masking.

One important fact has been neglected in the account given above, the fact that nerve impulses are synchronized with the sound waves. When the impulses from the auditory nerve are picked up by a suitable device, they are found to reproduce precisely the frequency of the sound wave up to at least 2000 cycles per second. So exact is this synchronization that many sounds, even the human voice, can be recognized if the impulses are amplified and led to a loudspeaker.

Just what use the auditory centers in the brain make of these paced impulses is not fully known. They are certainly most important for the localization of sounds. They may contribute to the perception of rough and intermittent sounds. Furthermore, if the ear itself is not able to respond differentially to the very low frequencies, this mechanism could conceivably preserve the low frequencies and pass them on to some as yet undiscovered analyzer in the brain.

The means by which the auditory nerve can transmit a frequency as high as 2000 cycles per second when an individual fiber cannot respond more than 500 to 800 times a second is explained by the *volley principle,* in accordance with which all the available fibers are thought of as divided up into squads with each of the various squads firing in rotation. One squad of fibers fires on the first sound wave, another squad on the second, still another on the third, and then the first squad returns to fire again on the fourth or fifth wave. Many facts have been discovered which prove the correctness of the volley principle.

LOCALIZATION OF SOUNDS

Sounds are not only heard; they are heard coming from some place out in space. The space in which we hear things is the space in which we see things; having heard a sound we look at some point to see what made it. It is also the space that we know through touch and movement. It is the space in which we move around and act.

In one sense, therefore, there is no auditory space or visual space; there is a single perceived space about which we know through the joint and supplementary actions of several senses. Only a person who has been blind since birth would have an auditory space, uncontaminated by visual factors, but that is not the space that we wish to study. We are interested in normal space, everybody's space. The question is: How do we locate sounds in this space, what clues do we use, and what discriminations can we make?

Imagine that an experiment is performed with a person suspended somewhere in free space as suggested by the diagram of Fig. 165, so that sounds might come from any side of him. What will he be able to do with his ears?

First, he will almost never confuse any sound on the right with one on the left. He may sometimes report a sound located behind him when it is in front or overhead, or he will hear a sound to the right in front when it is actually to the right behind, but never will he confuse right with left.

Second, if his confusions are examined, it is found that both the actual and apparent positions lie at a constant angle from the median plane (the up-down-front-back plane, *F–U–B–D,* which separates his

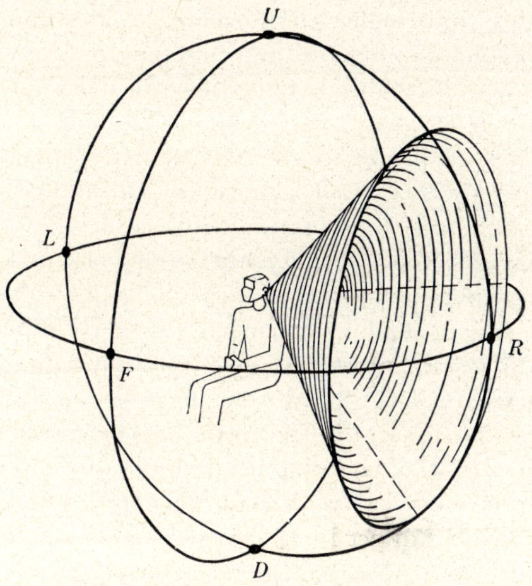

FIGURE 165. LOCALIZATION OF SOUND

The circles indicate possible positions of the sound source in the three principal planes of the head. Note especially the *cone* at one side. Any position on its surface may be confused with any other position on its surface.

right half from his left half) or, equally well, at a constant angle to his aural axis (the line, *R–L,* passing through his head from the right to the left ear). Thus, we may confuse front, back, up, down, up-front, up-back, etc., all of which lie in the median plane. We may confuse 45 degrees from the front toward the left, shown as *Z,* with 45 degrees from directly overhead toward the left in the vertical plane, shown as *Y.* The locus of a set of directions, which are confused with one another, is a double cone, formed about the aural axis with its apex at the very center of the head.

Third, if a sound stimulus is moved by a small amount, or given in two positions in close succession, the finest discrimination will be made in the horizontal plane directly in front of the listener, near the point *F,* and discrimination will become progressively poorer as the test is made in positions farther and farther to the side.

All these findings point very clearly to one conclusion, that localization depends upon the relative stimulation of the two ears, that is, upon *binaural clues.* These are not the only clues for the localization of sounds, but they are certainly the most important.

Binaural Clues

The binaural clues for localization may be of two kinds. Consider for a moment Fig. 166. Any sound from a point, *A,* in the median plane of the head will have reached the two ears by paths equal in all respects. On the other hand, a sound coming from a point to one side, such as *B,* will travel farther to reach the one ear than the other. The ear, of course, does not know how far the wave has traveled, but the brain may be able to recognize the *later* arrival of a given wave at the far ear. This clue is called *time difference.* At the same time, the nearer ear has a second advantage because it receives the sound directly, broadside, whereas the far ear is behind the head and in the *sound shadow* of the head. The two ears receive different intensities of sound on this account, and we speak of an *intensity difference* as the second clue.

Each of these clues should be examined somewhat more closely, for each is limited in its usefulness. Time differences will be produced when the stimulus is a sharp click. Nerve impulses will be set off, marking the arrival of the click at each ear and furnishing the auditory brain center with an adequate clue. The sudden starting or stopping of a tone or noise provokes an equally reliable neural event.

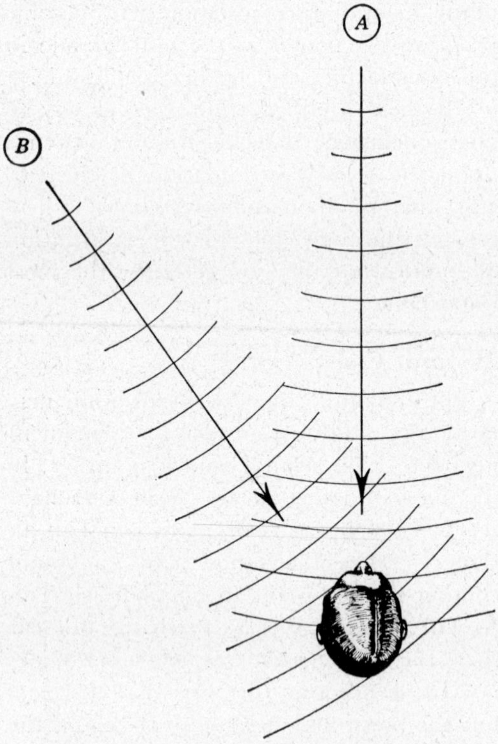

FIGURE 166. CLUES FOR SOUND LOCALIZATION

Sound waves coming from *A* in median plane affect both ears equally. Sound from *B* reaches left ear before right ear and is more intense because right ear is slightly 'shadowed.'

Tones, on the other hand, furnish adequate time clues only at low frequencies when the successive nerve impulses are slow enough to furnish distinguishable time intervals. The best localization is of tones 500 to 700 cycles per second. Very low frequencies have the disadvantage that the volley set off by one wave is ragged and scattered in starting, dulling the sharpness of localization. As the frequency becomes higher, on the other hand, a point is reached where the time difference between successive sound waves *at one ear* is twice the time difference *between the two ears.* At this point the ears fire alternately, and neither one is clearly first any longer. At this and higher frequencies, localization becomes ambiguous and may finally break down altogether. This difficulty starts for tones of about 800 cycles per second, located 90 degrees to the right or left. There are also classes of sounds for which there can never be significant time differences, notably tones of very high frequency and continuous noises.

Sound shadows are much less sharp than the shadows cast by light. We hear a person who faces away from us as he speaks, or the roar of surf before we come over the crest of a hill, but in both cases we hear them less well than when the sound comes in direct line. Measurements about the head show that only the very high frequencies can be substantially shut off by an object of the head's size—roughly frequencies above 3000 cycles per second. Thus there will be intensity differences for high-frequency tones and hisslike noises, and also for the high-frequency components of other, more complex sounds.

It is one thing to know what clues are available; it is another to know that they are used. The brain may not have 'learned' to use all the information that ears could provide. To test this point, experiments have been designed in which time differences or intensity differences have been created synthetically. If sound is led to the two ears by means of tubes, for instance, time differences can be created by lengthening and shortening the tubes with a trombone slide, and intensity differences by partially closing off one tube or the other. Electrical means would do the same thing more elegantly.

In such experiments, suitable time and intensity differences make the sound appear on one side or the other, just as we should

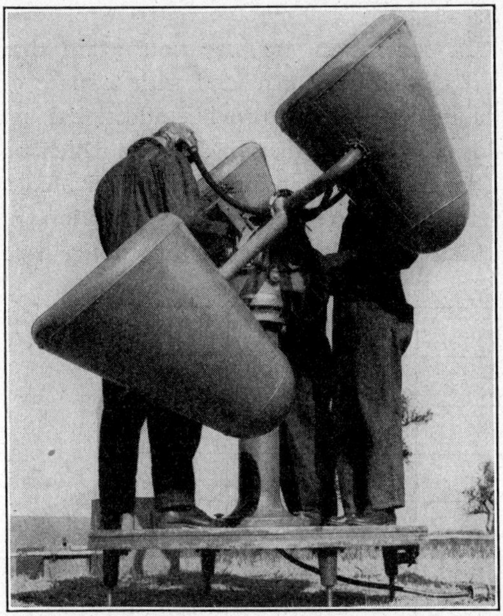

FIGURE 167. UNITED STATES ARMY SOUND LOCATOR

Tubes are led from a pair of horns to an observer's ears. One observer turns hand wheel controlling the horizontal traverse; the other observer tilts the horns in vertical elevation. [Courtesy of U. S. Army Signal Corps.]

expect from theory. On the other hand, what is heard is quite disappointing; for usually a phantom sound, starting at one ear, with an extreme difference in time or intensity, moves through the head or just back of the head to the other ear. Real, lively localizations far away from the listener do not often occur. It is apparent that each of these two factors, time and intensity, contributes to localization, but neither in itself gives the whole answer to the problem.

An instance of the use of a single binaural clue is the *sound locator* used by the Army for the location of airplanes. Figure 167 shows a model perfected in 1938. Using pairs of horns spaced well apart, the listener makes use of time clues to turn the horns until they point toward the sound. With this setting a sound image is heard located at the middle of the head. The locator is moderately successful in the hands of an experienced operator, but it suffers from the same difficulties as the synthetic experiments.

Secondary Clues

Three secondary factors are present in the natural activity of localization. In the first place, many sounds present double clues, both time *and* intensity. Thus in the sound of the voice there are starts and stops and low-frequency tones which give plenty of time clues, and there are also many high-frequency components which give intensity clues. Unless both sets of clues tell the same story, fuzziness and confusion result.

The second, and somewhat more spectacular, factor has to do with head or body movement. Just as it is important for a stable visual world that the shifting of the image on the retina should correspond closely with the movement of the head and eyes, so is it important for our heard space that *binaural clues change strictly in proportion to movements of the head.* It is this change of binaural clues with movement that gives us the out-there-in-space quality of sound localization. If the head is turned to the right, a sound that was previously straight in front of the listener shifts to the left of the head's axis. Or suppose that a sound is overhead and the head is tilted toward the right shoulder. Now the sound is heard to the head's left. In normal life we are continuously moving our heads and bodies and changing the binaural clues reaching our ears. In the synthetic experiment, where the clues fail to change with head movements, the phantom sound attaches itself to the head.

The third factor, which plays a subtle and changing role, is the effect on localization of our knowledge of sounds and our expectations about them. Sounds that are weaker than usual may be behind rather than in front of us. Sounds heard at a distance lose their high-frequency components, becoming more mellow. Sounds from another room or the other end of a large hall tend to roll as the echoes reinforce the original sound. Heard once, a sound may not be well localized; heard a dozen times, the listener will 'expect' a particular intensity, quality, degree of reverberation. As it departs from this expectation he hears the sound in a new place in space.

In conclusion, we may note again that our ears are not provided with a space of their own. They provide additional information about the same objects which we see with our eyes and touch with our hands. Usually ears tell about the direction in which something is happening, doing it so

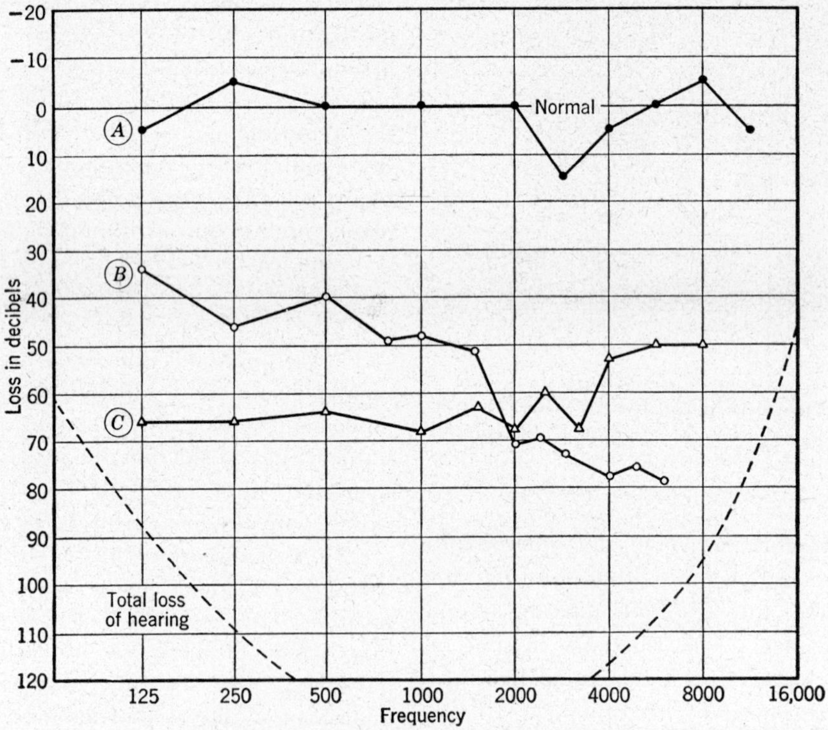

FIGURE 168. TYPICAL AUDIOGRAMS

Normal is the line at zero level near the top. Complete loss of hearing is shown by the dashed line near the bottom. (*A*) Typical normal ear. (*B*) Sloping loss, maximal in high frequencies. (*C*) Flat loss with all frequencies cut down nearly the same. (See also Fig. 169.)

quickly that the event is identified and confirmed by the eye before we can disentangle the contribution of each of the senses.

DEAFNESS

Normal hearing, like normal intelligence, is something which exists only in the averages of the statistician. All ears differ more or less from the average ear. Unlike intelligence, however, the ability to hear usually starts out quite near 'normal' in small children and declines through the natural processes of aging or, sometimes, through accident or disease.

A relatively small number of children are born deaf, perhaps one in six thousand. They are also mutes, that is, without speech, because without hearing they do not have the natural means of learning to speak words. A somewhat larger group of people lose their hearing entirely, often as a result of infection or the toxic effects of disease, less often through degeneration of the inner ear because of an obscure hereditary defect.

With no hearing the totally deaf person has to rely on visual or tactual means of communication. The easiest to learn is a sign language which is an elaborate system of manual gestures and finger spelling invented for the deaf. Better schools for the

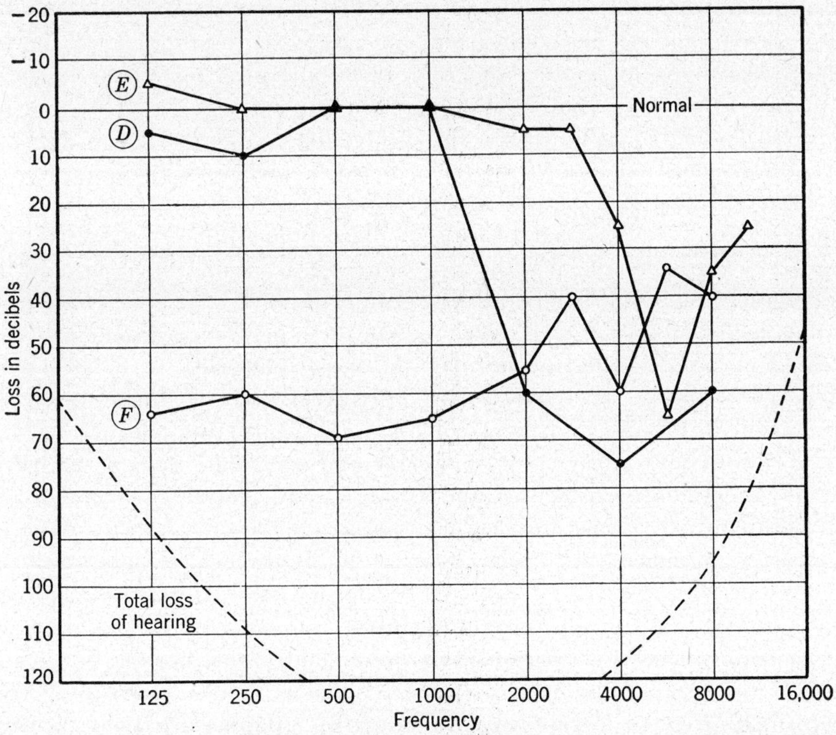

FIGURE 169. TYPICAL AUDIOGRAMS

(*D*) High frequency loss, with sudden drop between 1000 and 2000 cycles per second, frequently associated with exposure to damaging explosion. (*E*) High frequency loss with prominent 'notch.' (*F*) Rising curve with greater loss in low frequencies. (See also Fig. 168.)

deaf, however, insist on speech and lip-reading, more difficult skills to acquire, but skills that permit a far more normal adjustment of the deaf to ordinary life. The speech of persons who are totally deaf is generally intelligible, but it has a characteristic monotone quality and other peculiarities that are due to the lack of auditory control.

A far larger group than the totally deaf may be described as hard-of-hearing. Persons in this group have a measure of hearing, but their sensitivity is to a greater or less degree below normal. These are the people who may benefit from medical care or from the use of well-designed hearing aids. One in four over sixty-five years old falls into this group.

Loss of sensitivity for the hard-of-hearing is commonly shown by an *audiogram,* of which samples are shown in Figs. 168 and 169. This chart, which looks much like the curve of auditory sensitivity shown in Fig. 154, page 324, is actually an upside-down plot of the same function. 'Normal' hearing is represented by a straight line near the top of the audiogram. A person who can just hear the tone heard by the average listener is represented by points along the normal line. The curve *A* in Fig. 168 shows a typical audiogram with the ups and downs of a normal ear. Losses of sensitivity are then shown below this line in terms of the number of decibels by which a tone must be increased above the normal level in order to be heard.

Abnormal audiograms are grouped into three or four loosely defined classes. Curve *C* illustrates, for instance, a broad, 'flat' loss in which all frequencies are equally difficult to hear. Another common picture is shown in B where the loss gradually gets worse as frequencies from low to high are tested.

Not all audiograms are as smooth as these. Often there is a sudden drop in the audiogram, as shown in *D* of Fig. 169. This type of loss is common among soldiers whose ears have been injured by very close explosions. Some ears develop such losses without injury, as illustrated in *E* of Fig. 169. The loss often starts near 4000 cycles per second as a notch which widens and deepens. This notch was once called the "boilermakers' notch" because it was believed to be caused by the unusual noise of their work. Actually it can be found in any large group of people. The rarest type of audiogram is one shown as *F* in Fig. 169; it is down most at low frequencies and gradually rises toward the high end.

The cause of the deafness may be located in either the middle ear or the inner ear. If, for instance, scar tissue has grown over the eardrum, as a result of long-continued infection of the middle ear, or if the joints between the ossicles become fixed through otosclerosis, the resulting deafness we call *conduction deafness.* Sound is blocked before it reaches the inner ear, and the audiogram shows a large loss at all frequencies. On the other hand, if some acute infection, such as comes with scarlet fever or meningitis, strikes at the inner ear, the hair cells and the connecting nerve fibers may be destroyed over some part of the basilar membrane. The result is a 'perceptive,' or better, a *nerve deafness.* Particular frequencies are no longer heard. The resulting audiogram may show a sharp dip, most often at high frequencies but sometimes at the lower end or in the middle.

When a person has pure conduction deafness, sound can still be transmitted to the intact cochlea by means of *bone conduction.* The sound waves pass readily through the bones of the head and by compressing the walls of the labyrinth set the

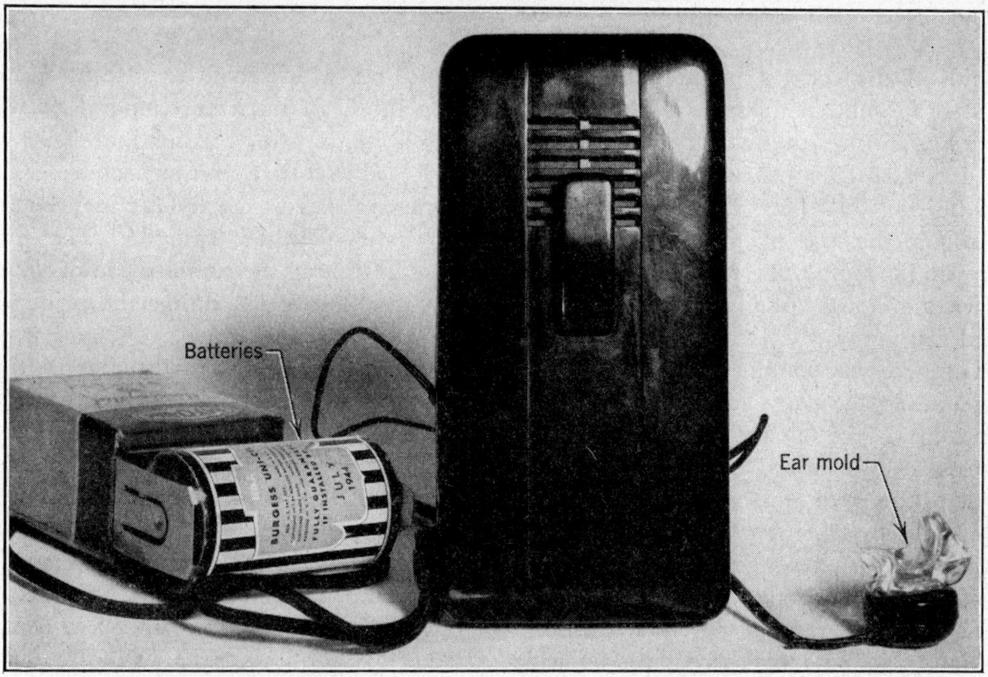

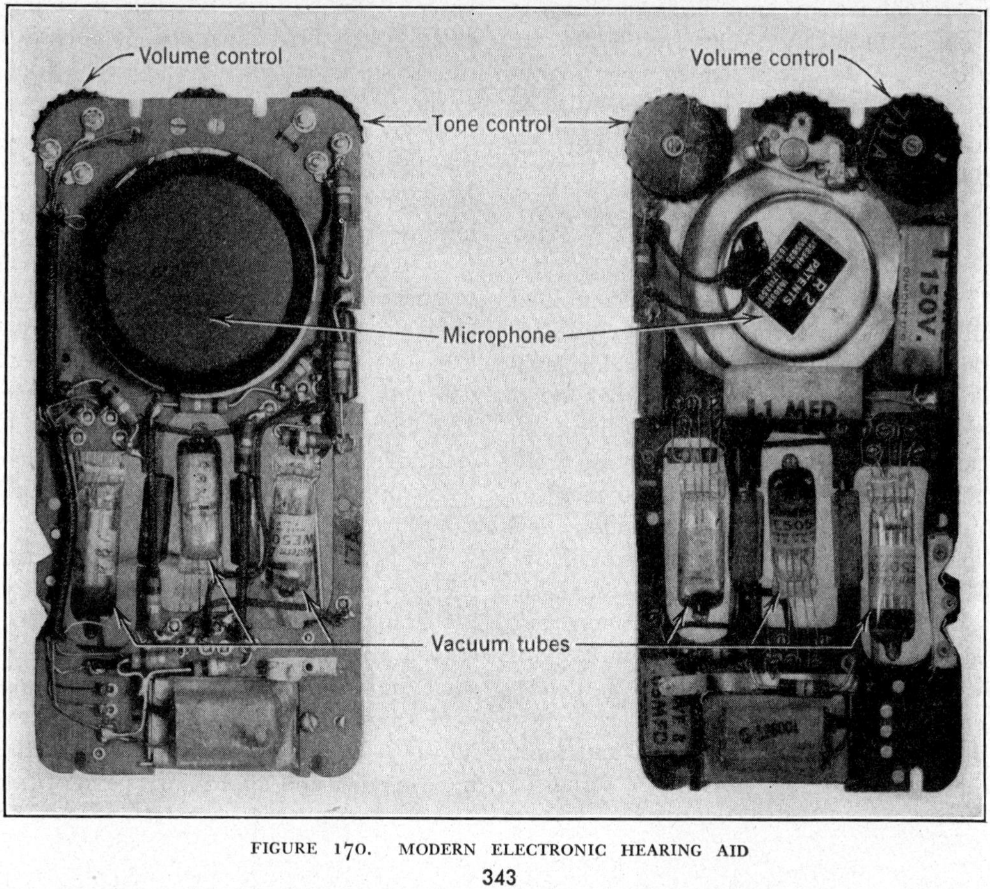

FIGURE 170. MODERN ELECTRONIC HEARING AID

fluids of the cochlea in motion. Anyone can hear bone-conducted sound by touching a vibrating tuning-fork to his teeth.

Tremendous improvements in the design of hearing aids have been made recently through the use of tiny vacuum tubes, shown in Fig. 170. Unfortunately these devices are still not so common as glasses, and too many people struggle along with an unnecessary handicap. The choice of a suitable hearing aid depends largely on the degree of hearing loss. Moderate losses are helped by almost any good aid. Purely conductive deafness can be overcome by the use of a bone conduction receiver which rests on the mastoid bone just back of the ear. Other forms of deafness merely require great enough amplification. To be sure, there must be wide-range, high-fidelity amplification, which it is not always easy to attain. Elaborate 'fitting,' widely advertised by some manufacturers, has recently been shown to be quite unnecessary provided high-fidelity hearing aids are available.

MUSIC

Sounds are not only useful. Combined and arranged to form music, they also afford us never-ending pleasure and relaxation. A few sounds are probably moderately pleasant by themselves, such as the tones of a fine violin or a rich and well-trained voice. But our real enjoyment of music springs from the movement, and color, and pattern of tones in combination.

Music starts, of course, with the basic discrimination of pitch and loudness, but it depends also on the more complex appreciation of *rhythm, melody* and *harmony*.

Rhythm is perhaps the oldest and most primitive feature of music. A series of sounds, in which some are accented, may form quite an intricate temporal pattern. In our music two, three or four beats are combined to form a unit or measure, which is then repeated. Each beat may be further subdivided or 'figured.' The principles governing the combination of sounds in a rhythm are not unlike the principles of grouping in vision (p. 222). For instance, two sounds close together in time form a strong 'pair.' A tempo has unique and compelling character as it is fast or slow. Rhythms distorted by syncopation have qualities distinct from rhythms with more even spacing.

Melody lies in the movement of a voice or instrument up and down the scale of pitch. The melodic line of a piece of music normally follows and adds to the underlying rhythmic pattern. But it is much more. In melodic patterns is found the richest source of feeling and expression in music.

Many elements of modern melody are highly stylized. We might use a scale consisting of five notes, or twelve, or perhaps twenty-four. Actually, in our culture, convention has chosen a scale with seven notes to an octave. A melody most often starts out with a note which establishes the tonality, that is to say, the key in which the melody is to be sung or played, and ends with a series of notes called a cadence which comes back to the keynote by a progression which provides 'resolution.'

The existence of these formal rules should not be stressed too much, however. Psychologically, a melody probably consists of a series of jumps or steps, some up, some down, some big, some small, some held for emphasis, others passed over lightly. Naive singers preserve carefully the direction and approximate size of these steps while they play havoc with the strict tonality of a melody. Moreover, melodies may easily be transposed not only by moving them up and down the scale but by cutting down all the intervals, producing 'micromelodies,' without upsetting the clear recognition of the original pattern.

Rhythm and melody are as old as music itself. *Harmony* is a relative newcomer. Harmony arises when two or more notes are sounded together. Certain combinations sound smooth and fused; others are harsh and rough. Combinations may also be rated rich or thin, sweet or discordant, or some nuance in between.

The element of harmony is the *interval,* a combination of two tones. Intervals are named by the number of notes on our scale which they include, such as the *second* for do-re, or fa-sol; the *third* for do-mi, or mi-sol; the *fourth* for do-fa, etc. The major intervals contain one more half tone than the corresponding minor intervals. For instance, do-mi is a major third, with two full tones, whereas mi-sol is a minor third with one full tone and one half tone.

Classical musical theory once ranked the intervals for their degree of fusion or consonance and gave a simple explanation of this order. The list, in order, together with the *ratio* of the two frequencies making up the interval, was as follows.

Interval	*Ratio*
Octave	1:2
Fifth	2:3
Fourth	3:4
Major third	4:5
Minor sixth	5:8
Minor third	5:6
Major sixth	3:5
Major second	8:9

The explanation given was based upon the small whole numbers which make up the preferred ratios; but such a theory can hardly be correct when we consider how an instrument is actually tuned off of these simple ratios to fit our arbitrary scale of equal temperament or when we discover how inexact is even a skilled musician when producing an interval.

Actual harmony is perhaps better illustrated by chords, combinations of three or more notes which form a set of consonant intervals. The major chord (like c-e-g-c′), for instance, consists of four notes whose frequencies stand in the ratios of 4:5:6:8. If you compare this chord with the table above, you will see that it contains the octave, fifth, fourth, major third, minor third and minor sixth.

A good explanation of consonance has not yet been given, but it will probably include some of the following factors: (1) the absence of disturbing *roughness* produced by beats lying in the range of 5 to 20 per second; (2) *richness* which arises when the notes in a chord are as close together as possible; (3) clear *tonality,* depending on the position of the tonic note in the chord; and (4) *balance* or proportion among the various notes.

Music is too rich a subject to be treated adequately here. It is also an elusive thing. Like other art, its perfection doubtless lies in a nice balance between simplicity and variety, between expected form and novelty. At its more elementary levels it has universal appeal, but fully developed it is appreciated by only the most sophisticated ear.

COMMUNICATION

We noted at the start of this chapter that men can live most easily together in a social group when they hear each other. Communication is as vital to a society as nervous activity is to an organism. It is the process by which an aggregation of men is changed into a functioning group. Moreover, the basic mode of communication is speech. Every normal man speaks, though only the more enlightened read and write.

The ready comprehension of spoken language is a truly remarkable feat. It requires the finest discrimination. A well-educated person will understand by ear alone perhaps ten thousand spoken words, each consisting of a short pattern of sound lasting less than one second. Furthermore, each of these words is a sturdy thing which keeps its identity in the face of marked changes. A word is understood when spoken by men or women or by people with the most varied accents and voice qualities. Even more remarkable are the distortions which speech undergoes in transmission over a radio or telephone circuit. Almost every conceivable characteristic of speech may be changed in some degree, and yet a large measure of intelligibility will remain. Finally, the ear is able to distinguish words and some measure of sense when presented against a background of several voices or of a steady noise. The sensory and perceptual achievement involved is almost without parallel elsewhere in man's experience.

Speech Sounds

The range of sound employed in understanding speech is limited not by the ability of the ear to hear but rather by the mechanics of the mouth and throat which produce the sounds. The lowest frequency to be found in speech is the fundamental of the vocal cords, about 125 cycles per second for men and 250 cycles per second for women. The highest useful frequencies are near 5000 cycles per second, just a bit more than five octaves higher. Thus the sounds of speech occupy just under a quarter of the total range of frequencies which can be heard at all.

The range of intensities is also relatively narrow. Between the softest sound and the loudest in any single sample of speech, there will be a range of only about 30 decibels. There will be a difference of perhaps an additional 40 decibels between a whisper and a shout, making a total of 70 decibels between the softest and loudest sounds in the human voice. But the whisper is still well above the softest sound that can be heard, and the shout well short of the loudest noise to be tolerated.

Many engineering calculations can be based on such facts about the overall properties of speech; but for a better understanding of how we make the many fine discriminations among words, we need to consider not the total spoken but rather the individual sounds out of which a language is built up.

Speech sounds, as we all know, can be divided first of all into vowels and consonants. Vowels are voiced sounds produced by the vocal cords with the help of the resonance of cavities in the throat and open mouth. Consonants, on the other hand, are those sounds which we make with some constriction of the passage through the throat and mouth. Roughly, the vowels are tones, and the consonants, noise.

The consonants can be divided in turn into voiced consonants, such as *b, g* or *z,* and unvoiced consonants of which *t, s* or *f* are examples. Or they may equally well be divided into the stops or plosive sounds, *p, b, t, d, k, g,* as opposed to the aspirate or fricative sounds, *h, ch, s, z, f, v.* A number of sounds which fall in between the clearly recognized vowels and consonants are called semivowels, sounds like *w, y, l, r, m* and *n.* For the final classification, the expert in phonetics points to the part of the mouth which is used. He speaks of dentals and labials, of front and back vowels. These distinctions, although real, are difficult for the layman to master.

A classification like this calls attention to several problems. For one thing our alphabet is fundamentally phonetic, and our spelling is supposed to reflect our speech. Written language does more, of course, than simply reflect speech sounds. The best written language would not necessarily be the one which gave the most accurate phonetic transcription. There is little doubt, however, that written English could be improved in its phonetic representation without losing its other usefulness.

Dividing speech sounds into these classes also helps to predict what sounds will be heard when listening is difficult. Vowels are by their very nature much louder than consonants, and, in turn, some consonants are much louder than others. Furthermore, the energy in a vowel sound is almost entirely in the frequencies below 2000 cycles per second whereas the characteristic components of a *th* or *f* lie above 3000 cycles per second. These facts are important in the design of telephone and radio circuits, for great care must be taken to preserve the weak consonants in the high range of frequencies.

Finally, a knowledge of speech sounds helps the teacher or speech pathologist to identify and correct wrong speech habits.

Sound Pattern in Speech

In order for the ear to distinguish the various vowels and consonants of speech, there must be differences among them which can be described in the more precise terms of the physical sound wave. A good account of these differences turns out, however, to be quite complex. Some of the sounds, such as *g* and *t* for instance, are really not unique sounds at all but are mostly ways of starting or stopping other sounds. None of the speech sounds consists of a simple pure tone. A few turn out to have a concentration of sound energy in a limited *band* of frequencies. These are sounds like *m* at the low end of the low end of the scale and *s, sh* and *f* at the high end. Most of the remaining speech sounds represent some complex *pattern* of frequencies.

In this connection *vowels* present perhaps the most interesting problem. How is it that they have a quality so much like a pitch (*oo* in *boot* seems low; *ee* in *beet* seems high) and yet they are not pitch alone, for the speaker's voice has its own pitch, separate from the vowel being spoken? The answer can be found by analysis of the vowel sound. The vowel is found to be a sound very rich in harmonics. Thus the fundamental frequency of a man's voice lies near 125 cycles per second, but various vowels, spoken at this pitch, will contain harmonics with frequencies all the way up to 2500 cycles per second. Furthermore, the distinguishing characteristic of each vowel is found to be the presence of harmonics in a particular frequency range. These characteristic regions are shown in Fig. 171. Some vowels, those in the upper part of the diagram, may have only a single region emphasized. Others, like *e* and *i,* always exhibit two regions of resonance.

The source of these characteristic patterns is to be found in the resonant cavities of the throat and mouth. In the first instances the entire mouth acts as a resonator to emphasize a single band of frequencies; in the latter instances, the back of the mouth and throat are cut off from the front of the mouth by the tongue and palate, forming two distinct cavities. Recently a machine has been invented which presents the characteristic regions of resonance as bars of light. A well-trained person can recognize at once in this 'visible speech' what vowel or consonant is being spoken and in this manner may listen with his eye to continuous speech.

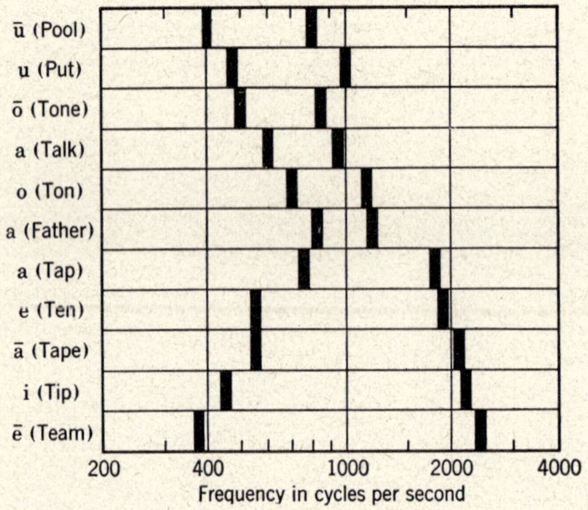

FIGURE 171. RESONANT FREQUENCIES OF VOWELS

Bars indicate regions in which strong harmonics are found when given vowels are spoken. Note especially wide separation of bars in lower part of figure. [From data of H. Fletcher, *Speech and hearing,* Van Nostrand, 1929, p. 58.]

The analysis of speech into sound elements is artificial in one important respect. The unit of speaking is really the syllable. The chest and diaphragm control the puff of air that forms the syllable unit. Within the syllable the rise and fall of sound, and its duration and relative stress, are fully as important as the exact quality of the vowel or consonant. This is evident when the actual vowels or consonants in speech are changed but the pattern is kept the same. Try reading aloud, for instance, this paragraph using one vowel throughout. See if most of the words are not understandable. (See eef meest eef thee weerds eere neet eendeersteendeeble.) Syllables are so important, in fact, that they are sometimes used as the phonetic unit, as in written Japanese.

Perception and Speech

The recognition of a pattern of harmonics as a vowel, or of a sequence of sounds as a word or syllable, requires the operation of mechanisms in the brain as well as in the ear. In contrast with the analytical functions of the ear, we are dealing here properly with auditory *perception.* The hearing of a word is much like the seeing of an object. Sound waves reaching the ear are broken up in the sense that they set off impulses in different parts of the ear. The excitation of each part is transmitted to some higher center where it is put together and interpreted. Just as in vision a person can see a hidden face in a puzzle picture (Fig. 78, p. 220), so also in hearing the fragments of a word or phrase are fitted together to form understandable speech.

The precise manner in which this integration is accomplished is something of a mystery. We shall have to be content here with the demonstration of how important auditory perception is rather than with its explanation. As with many abilities, the hearing and understanding of words are most evident when it is absent. Brain injuries, for instance, in certain parts of the temporal lobe produce disorders having to do with words. One of these is *aphasia* in which the patient loses his ability to form or speak words, although his vocal mechanism is intact. In *alexia* he sees but cannot get the sense of words that are read. In still other cases, words and sounds are heard but they have no meaning. These brain injuries appear to abolish the particular mental processes by which the sensory stuff furnished by our ears is collated and synthesized into words and language.

A rough measure of the *plus* furnished by perception comes from a study of speech which is chopped or distorted. In one set of studies whole bands or ranges of frequencies were completely removed from the speech of men and women. The intelligibility of the sound that remained was amazingly good. For instance, the removal of all frequencies *above* 1900 cycles per second left about 70 per cent of words intelligible, and the removal of all sound *below* 1900 cycles per second had the same result. The complete results are shown in Fig. 172. In other words, just half the component frequencies in speech are enough to give much *better* than half intelligibility.

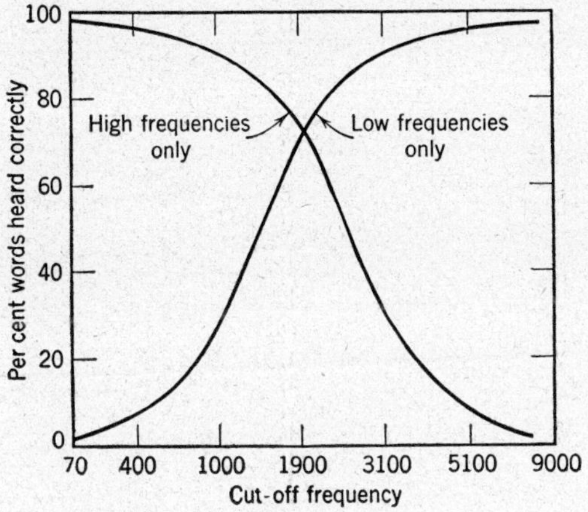

FIGURE 172. INTELLIGIBILITY OF FILTERED SPEECH

Curves showing number of words correctly understood when all frequencies above a given point are removed (leaving low frequencies only) or all frequencies below a given point are removed (leaving high frequencies only). [Derived from N. R. French and J. C. Steinberg, *J. acous. Soc. Amer.*, 1947, **19**, 90–119.]

Blanking out sections of the flow of speech with a masking noise, when done at moderate rates, has the same effect. Intelligibility is upset much less than we might expect. Conversation, blanked out for 50 per cent of the time (at a rate of 9 times a second), lost only 15 per cent of its words. The amount heard for other proportions of blanking can be seen in Fig. 173. To be sure, not everyone will understand such distorted or chopped speech equally well. Some people understand garbled speech without trouble, can listen successfully on a telephone with a bad connection; other people find this very hard. One person fits together, fills in, hears the words; the other does not.

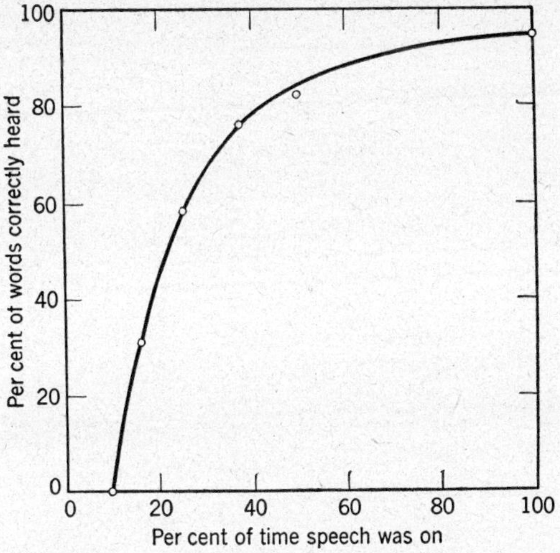

FIGURE 173. INTELLIGIBILITY OF CHOPPED SPEECH

Speech was turned on and off nine times per second. Quite short bursts of speech are enough to give good intelligibility. [G. A. Miller, *Psychol. Bull.*, 1947, **44**, 120.]

REFERENCES

1. Beatty, R. T. *Hearing in man and animals.* London: G. Bell, 1932.

Intended for the layman, but worth while for his readable account of hearing in general. It traces briefly the evolution of the ear and hearing.

2. Davis, H. *Hearing and deafness.* St. Louis: Mosby, 1947.

A recent account of the psychological aspects of deafness, written for the clinician and the intelligent layman.

3. Fletcher, H. *Speech and hearing.* New York: Van Nostrand, 1929.

A standard reference on the physical nature of speech sounds and the psychophysics of the ear that hears them.

4. Geotschius, P. *Theory and practice of tone-relations.* New York: G. Schirmer, 1917.

The rules and conventions followed by composers when writing music in our times.

5. Polyak, S. L. *The human ear in anatomical transparencies.* Elmsford, N. Y.: The Sonotone Corporation, 1946.

An anatomist's view which makes it easy to see the relation of the ear to the other parts of the head.

6. Stevens, S. S., and Davis, H. *Hearing, its psychology and physiology.* New York: Wiley, 1938.

A standard reference work on hearing, containing much that is new since the vacuum tube revolutionized our knowledge of audition. Stevens is a psychologist and Davis a physiologist.

7. Wood, A. *The physics of music.* Cleveland: Sherwood, 1944.

A delightful summary of what is known about musical instruments and how they work.

8. Wood, A. B. *A textbook of sound.* New York: Macmillan, 1941.

The physical characteristics of sound, including the mathematics used to describe it.

CHAPTER 15

Taste and Smell

THE sense of taste, by which we detect the flavor of sugar or salt, the sense of smell, by which we detect the aroma of coffee or the scent of perfumes, and the common chemical sense, by which we feel the sharpness of pepper and the irritation of chlorine gas, are known as the *chemical senses.* It is by them that we obtain not only information concerning the external chemical environment, but also information concerning the internal chemical environment of our own bodies.

Although adult persons of our culture are largely influenced in their choice of food by social custom and personal idiosyncrasy, it appears that, when given a choice, savages, young children and animals select food that satisfies their nutritional needs. (See pp. 119–121.) These preferences seem to depend in great measure on the chemical senses, particularly the sense of taste.

In lower animals smell probably plays an important role in sexual selection and mating. Some animals, like the musk deer or civet cat, apparently find their mates by means of the extremely strong odors arising from glands in the genital regions. In the white rat experiments show that, although the surgical removal of the sense of smell does not impair normal copulation, the level of sexual activity is reduced.

In man generally, olfaction is probably less important, yet its role is not altogether negligible; strong body odors may have a direct effect on the course of sexual excitement. It has been suggested that the use of perfumes to disguise personal odors is a late development, that the more primitive functions of perfumes may have been to heighten and fortify the natural body odors for sexual ends. Even today some of the finest perfumes derive their potency from the presence of the crude animal sexual odors like musk or civet.

Smell may also give warning of the presence of undesirable objects. We tend to avoid the foul putrid odors of decaying animal matter. The common chemical sense warns of irritating and noxious fumes. Yet these senses are not infallible indicators of the nature of our chemical environment. Poisonous elements in food which do not readily dissolve in the saliva may not be tasted, or, when tasted, they may not be particularly unpleasant. Certain war gases like mustard gas can do great harm in concentrations too weak to be detected, and lewisite can prove fatal without being smelled at all.

Each of the chemical senses has distinct sense organs located in particular parts of the nose or mouth, and each possesses certain distinctive characteristics. Yet in

This chapter was prepared by Carl Pfaffmann of Brown University.

everyday life they function together so intimately that most persons are unaware of their separate existence.

TASTE, SMELL AND THE COMMON CHEMICAL SENSE

The receptors for the sense of taste consist of spindle-shaped cells assembled in groups to form *taste buds.* They are located in papillae on the surface of the tongue and neighboring areas such as the epiglottis, the larynx and parts of the throat. (See Fig. 174.) Mild concentrations of salt, sugar, acid or quinine solutions elicit sensation qualities of saline, sweet, sour or bitter respectively, being effective only in those regions containing taste buds. Strong salt or acid may also elicit sting or pain from any region of the mouth cavity by stimulating the free nerve endings of the common chemical sense.

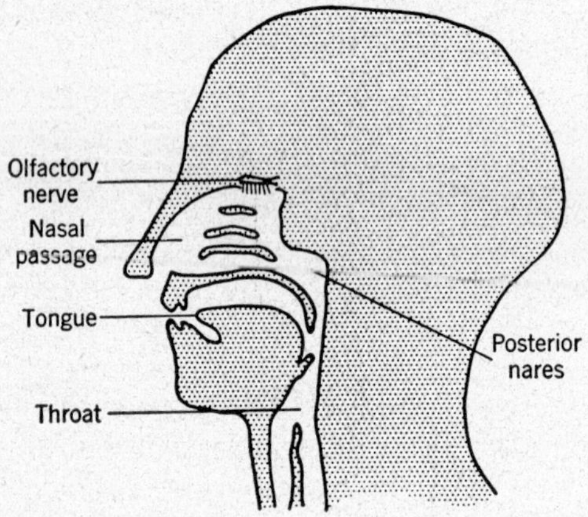

FIGURE 174. SCHEMATIC CROSS-SECTION OF THE HEAD

The olfactory receptors are located high in the nasal passage, the taste buds are primarily distributed over the tongue and the free nerve endings of the common chemical sense occur throughout the mucous membrane of both the nose and the mouth. [From C. Pfaffmann, Smell and taste, in T. G. Andrews (Ed.), *Methods of psychology,* Wiley, 1948, p. 268.]

The receptors for the sense of smell are threadlike cells embedded in a pigmented patch of the mucous membrane of the upper nasal passages. Odorous vapors may enter by way of the nostrils or from the mouth cavity by way of the posterior nares. (See Fig. 174.) The normal air currents of quiet breathing may not reach up to the olfactory cleft. Sniffing spreads the air currents more widely into the upper parts of the nasal passage, resulting in more effective olfactory stimulation. *Fruity, flowery, foul* and *burnt* are the names of typical olfactory qualities. They are not experienced when the nostrils are plugged so that the odorous vapors cannot enter the nasal cavity. In addition to stimulation of the olfactory receptors, many vapors stimulate the free nerve endings in the nasal passages. Substances like ammonia have, in addition to their typical aromatic odor, a painful or stinging quality which can be readily detected by persons who lack the sense of smell. Many odorous substances excite the sense of taste, and few are purely olfactory stimulants. Alcohol, for instance, has an ethereal odor, a sweet taste and a stinging quality. Its odor can be detected in the weakest concentration, its taste at a somewhat higher value, whereas its mild sting appears only in a still higher concentration. One might say that the sense of smell is more sensitive than the sense of taste, and taste more sensitive than the common chemical sense.

The mucous membrane of the mouth and nose is also endowed with cold, warm, touch and pressure sensitivity much like that occurring in the skin. These frequently add still other components to our normal perception of food, drink or other chemical stimuli.

Savor a mouthful of good cold Coca-Cola. What do you sense? It has an odor which probably belongs near the spicy group (that is smell), and a slightly bitter and very sweet quality (taste), and the sting of all carbonated drinks (touch), and cold (temperature sense) and the awareness of a liquid in the mouth (somesthesis).

TASTE

Primary Tastes

It is generally agreed that there are four primary taste qualities: saline, sour, bitter and sweet. Typical stimuli for these four are:

Saline	sodium chloride (common salt)
Sour	hydrochloric acid
Bitter	quinine
Sweet	cane sugar

In order to become a stimulus, a substance must be in solution or be soluble in the saliva which fills the pores of the taste buds. A large number of substances will elicit the pure sour, bitter or sweet tastes. There is, however, only one stimulus, sodium chloride (common salt), which calls out the pure saline taste. All other mineral salts have such complex tastes as salty-bitter, sour-salty-bitter, etc. These complex tastes can be compounded by appropriate mixtures of the four typical stimuli named above.

The surface of the tongue is not equally sensitive to each of the primary tastes. The tip is most sensitive to sweet, the sides to sour, the tip and sides to saline and the back to bitter. Consequently certain substances taste differently at the tip and at the back of the tongue. Epsom salts taste salty at the tip and bitter at the back; other substances are sweet at the tip and bitter at the back.

These findings suggest that a different type of taste receptor exists for each of the primary tastes, and that each type predominates in a different part of the tongue. Recent experiments in which the sensory nerve impulses in the single nerve fibers of the taste nerves were recorded by electrophysiological methods indicate that there are, in fact, these different kinds of taste receptors. In the cat, although all taste nerve fibers respond when acid is placed on the tongue, some of the fibers respond only to acid, whereas others respond to salt as well as to acid, and still others to quinine as well as to acid. This discovery suggests that, although there are different types of receptors, they may not correspond exactly to each of the four primary taste qualities. Similarly the retina is known to receive stimulation which is perceived as combinations of the seven unique colors, although it is usually supposed that there are only three different kinds of cones in the retina.

Sensitivity

Of the four tastes, the sensitivity for bitter is the keenest. Quinine can be detected in a solution of 0.00005 per cent. Sweet is next for such synthetic sweeteners as saccharine, although the sensitivity for sugar is not nearly so great. Sour and salty are next and in that order.

Not all persons are equally sensitive. The most dramatic examples are cases of 'taste blindness' for PTC (phenyl-thio-carbamide). For some persons the crystals of this substance are bitter, for others they are tasteless. This deficiency appears to be inherited as a Mendelian recessive character. Actually this deficiency is relative rather than complete, for nearly everyone can taste PTC in a sufficiently concentrated aqueous solution.

Taste sensitivity falls off with increasing age. Not only do children have a greater number of taste buds than adults, but their taste thresholds are lower than those of older people. The use of tobacco reduces taste sensitivity, but this effect appears to be temporary. Other drugs like cocain will reduce or abolish taste before the other senses of the tongue are desensitized.

Temperature of the taste solution has a definite effect on the intensity of taste. Extremely high or low temperatures usually lower taste sensitivity. The sugar in hot tea becomes more sweet as the tea cools. Such effects account in part for the way flavor changes with temperature. Those components of flavor which depend on smell are, on the other hand, usually enhanced by increased temperature, for more aroma is given off by warm substances.

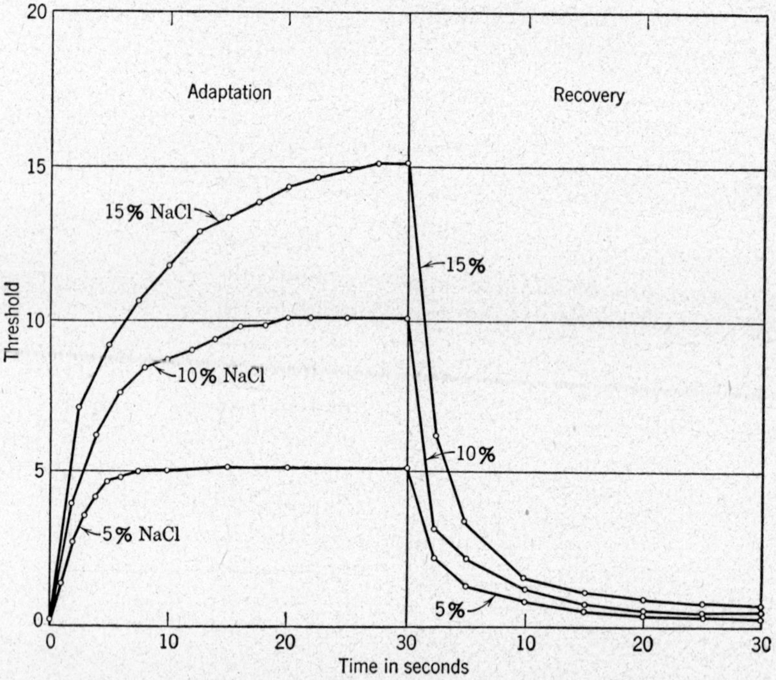

FIGURE 175. ADAPTATION AND RECOVERY CURVES FOR SODIUM CHLORIDE

The course of adaptation to three concentrations of sodium chloride, 15, 10 and 5 per cent, is shown for an adaptation period of 30 seconds and a recovery period of 30 seconds. Each curve indicates the threshold values at various intervals after adaptation or recovery had begun. The unadapted threshold is 0.24 per cent. [After H. Hahn (1934).]

Adaptation

Continuous exposure to a stimulus leads to sensory adaptation, the diminution or even the disappearance of the sensation along with a reduction in sensitivity. (See Fig. 175.) Sweet candies or drinks taste less sweet after several swallows.

Adaptation not only affects the taste undergoing adaption but may also enhance the sensitivity to other stimuli, a phenomenon sometimes called *successive contrast.* For instance, adaptation to salt lowers the threshold for sour, sweet and bitter. The sweet taste of water after sour pickle or sour lemonade is an example familiar to all.

they will take enough salt to keep themselves alive and in good health (Fig. 176). If the taste nerves to the tongue are cut by surgical intervention, however, the animal loses the ability to make this selection and soon dies.

This craving is accompanied by an increased sensitivity to salt. All rats will

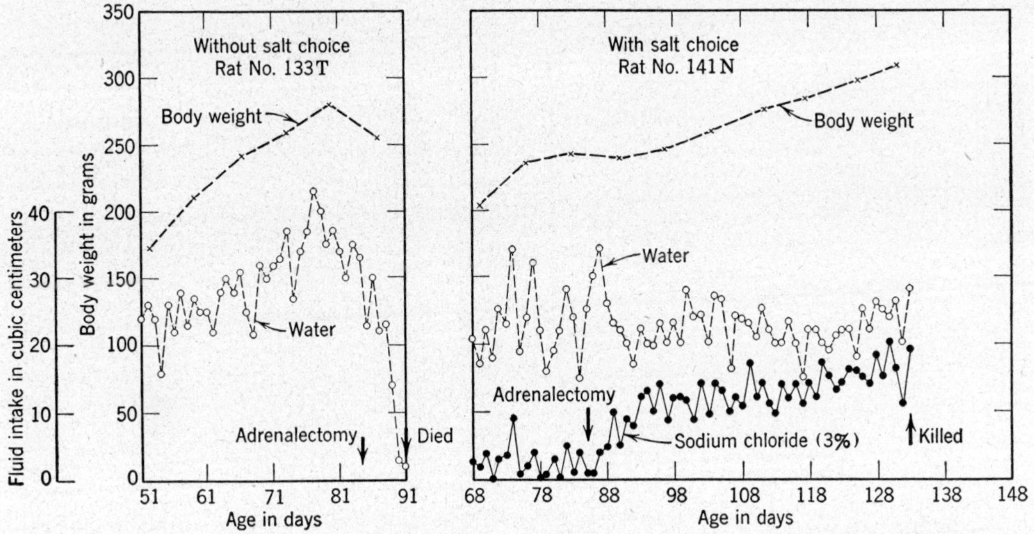

FIGURE 176. THE INCREASED SALT APPETITE AFTER REMOVAL OF THE ADRENAL GLAND

Rat 133 T had no access to salt and died a few days after removal of the adrenal gland (i.e., after adrenalectomy). Rat 141 N, which had access to 3 per cent sodium chloride solution, started taking more salt after being adrenalectomized and was still living seven weeks later. Arrows show when the adrenal glands were removed. [After C. P. Richter, *Harvey Lectures 1942–1943,* p. 66.]

Physiological Effects

Changes in taste may follow changes in the physiological condition of the organism. Diseases of the adrenal gland or removal of the same organ in animals profoundly upsets the salt balance in the tissues of the body. Large amounts of salt will be excreted and, unless the intake of salt is increased, the animal will die. Animals with this gland removed show a great craving for sodium chloride if they are given access to a salt solution. In fact,

show a preference for weak salt solution over plain water. Normal animals first show this preference at concentrations of 0.055 per cent. Animals with their adrenal glands removed first show a preference for salt at concentrations as low as 0.0037 per cent, a concentration too low to have any beneficial effects. Presumably there is a salt deficiency in all the tissues of the body, a deficiency which may sensitize the taste cells or make the animal more on the alert for salt.

That such a process can occur in human beings is suggested by a number of clinical reports. One of the most dramatic of these relates the case of a 3½-year-old boy with a disease of the adrenal gland. This boy kept himself alive for more than two years by eating salt by the handful. When this exaggerated salt intake was reduced by restriction to a regular hospital diet, he soon developed symptoms of salt deficiency and died.

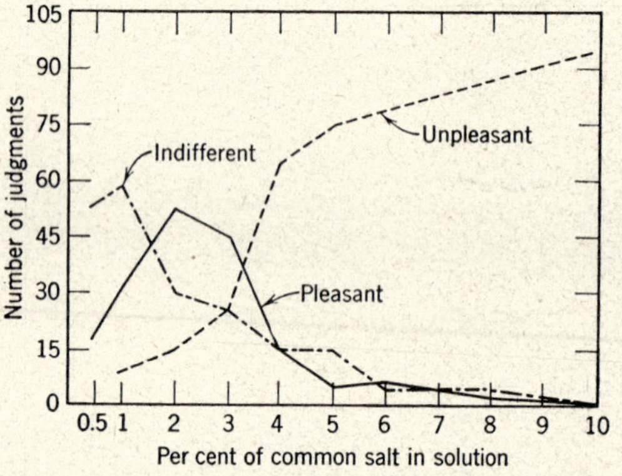

FIGURE 177. THE EFFECT OF STRENGTH OF SALT (SODIUM CHLORIDE) SOLUTION ON THE PLEASANTNESS OF TASTE

The total number of pleasant, unpleasant and indifferent judgments given by seven subjects in seven sittings are shown. [After R. Engel (1928).]

The four primary tastes are not all equally pleasant. Some, like quinine, are almost always unpleasant and even nauseating in all but the weakest concentrations; others, like sugar, are nearly always pleasant; still others, like salt or citric acid, tend to be pleasant in mild concentrations but unpleasant when strong. Figure 177 shows this relation for salt expressed quantitatively. In the weak concentrations the indifferent taste predominates. At 2 and 3 per cent, the taste is pleasant, but in stronger solutions the taste is mostly unpleasant. Although this relationship is typical for most of the persons tested, there may be individual differences. One subject, liking salt, usually reported the salt as pleasant in all but the most intense concentrations. How stable this preference for salt would remain on other occasions when his salt metabolism might have undergone some change is still an unanswered question. Physiological changes are not, of course, the sole determinants of the pleasantness or unpleasantness of taste. Many of the more sophisticated tastes may be pleasant only to the initiated, like black coffee, which is bitter but beloved by many. Many pleasantnesses have to be acquired before they can be appreciated. Some unpleasantnesses are acquired too. The gourmet does not accept a child's judgment as to what foods need sugar.

SMELL

Primary Odors

The fundamental odor qualities are less well established than the qualities of taste. For one thing there are many more odors, and the chemist is continually fabricating new compounds with new smells. One classification that is recommended by its relative simplicity and clarity is the one suggested by Hans Henning. He argued for six fundamental qualities as follows:

Fragrant	like the odor of violets
Ethereal	like the odor of oranges
Spicy	like the odor of cloves
Resinous	like the odor of balsam
Burnt	like the odor of tar
Putrid	like the odor of fecal matter

In general, putrid and burnt odors tend to be unpleasant; fragrant, ethereal, spicy and resinous are most often pleasant, although there are many exceptions. Some people like garlic (fragrant-burnt-putrid), some dislike wintergreen (fragrant-ethereal-resinous).

It is obvious that many of the smell names are the names of objects. *Fragrant* describes a quality like that produced by flowers. The real stimulus, of course, is not the flower but some property, as yet undetermined, of the molecules or molecular groups given off by evaporation of the essential oils in the flower. These particles ultimately reach and dissolve in the mucus which covers the olfactory sense cells. Odorous substances, for the most part, are organic substances, that is to say, they are compounds of carbon. A few of the inorganic chemical elements like chlorine and bromine are odorous. The constituent of the highly fragrant attar of roses, which is largely responsible for rose odor, has been identified as geraniol. Since substances responsible for the typical odors of many flowers and plants have been isolated, the perfume chemist can often describe his product in chemical terms. The essences from plants are, however, such complex mixtures that often the exact odor of the natural product can be duplicated only by adding a small amount of the natural essence to the synthetic odor. The chemical laws of olfactory stimulation are largely practical rules which at the present time cannot be unified by any simple or rational principle.

Sensitivity

The sense of smell is extraordinarily sensitive to odorous materials. Substances like natural or artificial musk, vanillin or the mercaptans can be detected in exceedingly small concentrations. Only 1/23,000,000th of a milligram of mercaptan per cubic centimeter of air is required for stimulation. The olfactometer is used for such measurements (Fig. 178).

Impairment of sensitivity, called *anosmia*, may be partial or complete, congenital or acquired, permanent or temporary. The frequent colds and catarrhal conditions of modern civilized life are frequently responsible for the temporary anosmia that we have all experienced from time to time. A kind of partial anosmia has been observed in which the sensitivity to certain odors differs markedly among a group of apparently normal individuals. For instance, in one group of persons, some were able to detect fragrance in a particular red verbena plant, but not in a pink one. The converse was true for other people. Only a few could detect fragrance in both. These effects appear to lie quite within the range of normal sensitivity. The same odor may

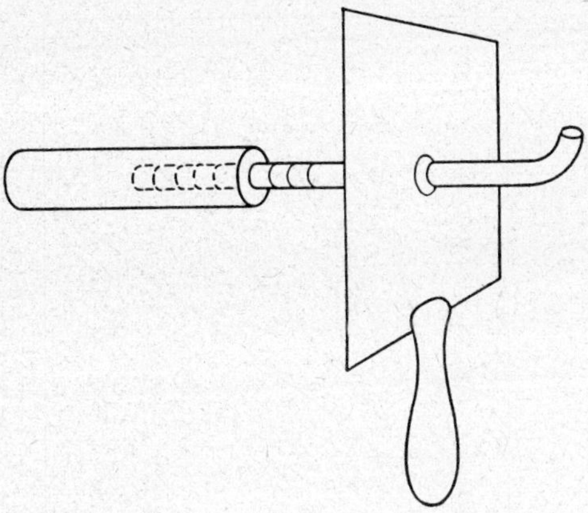

FIGURE 178. A SIMPLE OLFACTOMETER

The subject sniffs at the end of the bent-up tube. Over the other end of this smaller tube fits a larger stimulus tube made of an odoriferous substance, like India rubber. The amount that the stimulus tube projects beyond the outer tube measures the distance that the air, which the subjects sniffs, passes over the stimulus substance, and hence the intensity of the odor. The smaller tube is marked in stimulus units, called *olfacties*. [After H. Zwaardemaker (1888).]

even have different qualities in the right and left nostrils of the same person.

Adaptation

Sensitivity may be reduced as a result of fatigue or adaptation to the continued presence of an odorous stimulus. This phenomenon makes it possible for persons working in a foul atmosphere to endure the stench. Medical students in the dissecting rooms soon become adapted to the odors of the cadavers.

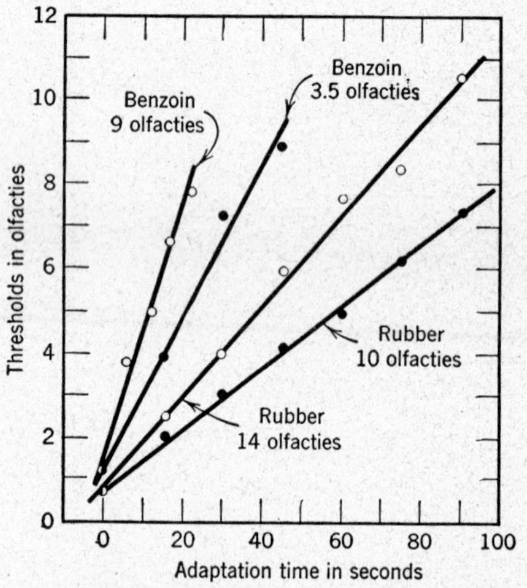

FIGURE 179. OLFACTORY ADAPTATION CURVES

Increasing adaptation is measured by the increase of the olfactory threshold (in olfacties). Adaptation is shown to be faster for benzoin than for rubber, and also with each substance it is faster for the more intense stimulus (as indicated in olfacties). [After H. Zwaardemaker (1895).]

The amount of adaptation depends on the nature and intensity of the adapting stimulus. Complete adaptation to camphor may occur in 5 to 7 minutes; to balsam in 3 to 4 minutes. The stronger the odor the faster the adaptation (Fig. 179). Complete adaptation to a weak stimulus is only partial adaptation to a strong one. It can be shown, for instance, that the use of camphor lotion for chapped lips elevates the threshold for camphor, and that chewing peppermint chewing gum elevates the threshold for peppermint.

During adaptation not only will the apparent intensity of the smell diminish, but sometimes the odor quality itself may change. Ionone, which at first resembles cedarwood in odor, becomes less intense and then changes to a quality like violet. This change in quality of the odor may sometimes be disastrous for cheap perfumes, which shift from a flowery odor toward putrid as the stimulation continues.

Adaptation may be selective. Sensitivity is then reduced most for the adapting stimulus, somewhat for other substances and not at all for still others. Adaptation to camphor reduces the sensitivity to cologne, cloves and ethereal oils. Adaptation to ammonium sulphide reduces the effectiveness of hydrogen sulphide and bromine, but not of etherial oils and coumarin.

Recovery after complete adaptation is relatively rapid, seldom requiring more than 5 minutes. The rate of recovery depends on the time of adaptation and the intensity of the stimulus. On the other hand, fatigue or the action of such drugs as anesthetic ether or gasoline may lead to a reduction in the sensitivity which lasts for hours.

Physiological Effects

Physiological changes may also influence the acuity of smell. In women, for example, an enhancement of sensitivity has been observed just prior to the onset of menstruation and during pregnancy. Changes in smell in relation to nutrition have not been studied systematically, but diminished thresholds are said to occur during prolonged fasts.

Odor Mixtures and Blends

Odors mix in two ways. In one way the odorous materials interact chemically to produce a third substance. That is not a true example of the mixture of stimuli, because a new stimulus is created. True odor *mixture* occurs when two or more odorous compounds, which do not react chemically, are combined. If the components are of unequal strength, the stronger predominates. If the two are equally balanced, a fusion or blend results. Selective adaptation to one of the components brings out the unadapted member of the pair.

In certain mixtures another effect, *compensation,* may occur. The effectiveness of each component is reduced by the presence of the other. Hence the resultant is weaker than either component alone. Compensation has been said to operate in the effectiveness of certain perfumes in overcoming body odors. This effect of compensation was used particularly a few centuries ago when bathing was not common.

REFERENCES

1. Crocker, E. C. *Flavor.* New York: McGraw-Hill, 1945.

The contribution of taste and smell to flavor is presented largely from the point of view of the food technologist.

2. Moncrieff, R. W. *The chemical senses.* New York: Wiley, 1946.

A more extensive work which includes a comprehensive treatment of the chemistry of taste and smell.

3. Parker, G. H. *Smell, taste and allied senses in vertebrates.* Philadelphia: Lippincott, 1922.

A clear, concise, general account of the chemical senses.

CHAPTER 16

Somesthesis

SOMESTHESIS, which means literally 'body feeling,' is the general name for all systems of sensitivity present in the skin and internal organs of the body. The classical view is that there are five senses: sight, hearing, smell, taste and 'feeling.' Aristotle had it that way, and current popular usage preserves the traditional list. However, from time to time other classifications have been made, some of them distinguishing more than a score of separate senses. Always, when the list has been expanded beyond five, the new senses have come out of 'feeling,' and whenever the list has dwindled the extra senses have gone back into feeling again. The reason for uncertainty appears to lie in the multiplicity of sense processes in the skin and internal organs. The skin, a complexly formed organ, contains nerve endings of several kinds. The endings are, moreover, variously embedded in the skin and can be stimulated in a variety of ways. Deeper lying tissues, such as muscles and organs of the viscera, are supplied with still differently housed nerve terminations. There are, however, similarities among the sensations coming from these different parts of the body, a fact which leads us to regard somesthesis as involving several systems of sensibility that essentially belong together. We shall consider first the types of sensibility present in the skin, then those found in internal bodily structures, the muscles, visceral organs and the nonauditory labyrinth of the inner ear.

CUTANEOUS SENSIBILITIES

The skin mediates at least four fundamental qualities of sensation—pressure, pain, cold and warmth—and is supplied with a variety of receptors.

The Skin and Its Receptors

From its external aspect the skin presents a highly variegated structure. In some parts of the body it has a relatively smooth appearance, it is deeply creased and furrowed in others; in some places it is stretched to the point of tautness, in others it is relatively mobile; in some regions it is thickened and tough, but in others thin and pliable; in some places it is hairless, but in others highly endowed with hairy appendages. Moreover, the nerve supply to the skin is highly variable. In some parts of the body, such as the lips and fingertips, there are abundant nerve terminations; in others, such as the middle of the back, nerve endings are sparsely distributed. If different skin regions show widely differing sensitivities, it should not be surprising. In fact, were it not for some

This chapter was prepared by Frank A. Geldard of the University of Virginia.

fundamental uniformities of subsurface structure, we might even regard the skin as a collection of quite separate organs.

Several successive layers comprise the skin, and it is conventional to mark off three major groupings of them: the *epidermis,* the *corium,* or true dermis, and *subcutaneous tissue* (Fig. 180). The epidermis, over most of the body surface tough and resistant to external influences, serves as a protective coat. It varies from a thin layer only a few cells thick at the lips to a relatively thick structure several millimeters deep in the callous ball of the foot. Fine nerve fibrils, 'free nerve endings,' penetrate the lower epidermal layers. The corium, subjacent to the epidermis, is continuous with it, the boundary between the two being generally irregular. The uppermost level of the corium consists of *papillae,* conical mounds of connective tissue projecting into the basal floor of the epidermis. It is the regular lineal arrangement of the papillae, giving form to the overlying epidermis, that provides the orderly lines of fingerprints and toeprints. As well as housing the smaller hair follicles, the ducts of sweat glands and the greater portion of the smaller blood vessels of the skin, the corium contains nerve fibers and, especially, the great majority of cutaneous nerve terminations. They exist in a multiplicity of forms and occur at varying depths. The legend of Fig. 180 provides an introduction to some of them. In the subcutaneous tissue, made up largely of fatty cells and loosely interwoven connective tissue fibers, which form a bond with underlying muscles and bones, are to be found the major blood vessels, the larger hair follicles, sweat glands and also a vast network of nerve fibers.

The nerve endings found at all levels of the skin are unquestionably the receptors for the various kinds of cutaneous sensations, though whether a particular type of end organ exclusively initiates a certain kind of sensation is by no means established with certainty. As we proceed we shall

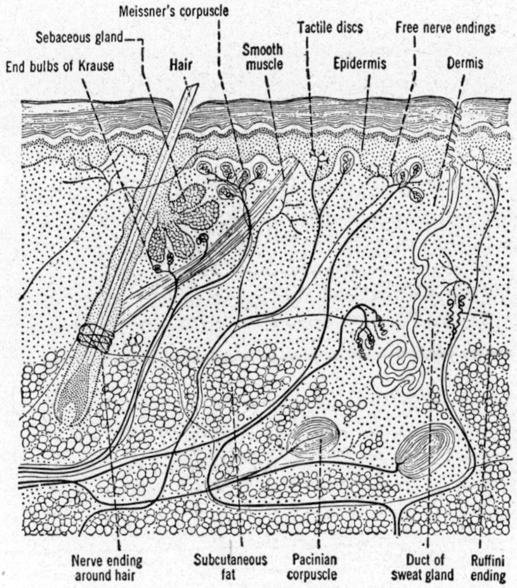

FIGURE 180. THE SKIN IN CROSS-SECTION

A composite drawing of the skin, showing the epidermis, the underlying dermis and, below the dermis, the subcutaneous tissue, with the stump of a hair and seven kinds of cutaneous nerve endings: (1) tactile discs within the epidermis, (2) free endings at the epidermis, (3) Meissner corpuscles beneath the epidermis, (4) Krause end bulbs in the dermis, (5) Ruffini endings in the dermis, (6) free endings about the hair follicle and (7) Pacinian corpuscles within the subcutaneous tissue. [Modified from H. H. Woolard, G. Weddell and J. A. Harpman, by E. Gardner, *Fundamentals of neurology,* Saunders, 1947, p. 111.]

examine briefly the evidence for the various proposed correlations between types of sensibility and kinds of nerve terminations.

Exploration of the Skin Surface

The first thing to be noted about the skin's sensitivity is that it is not uniformly distributed, even within relatively restricted areas. If a pencil point is moved gently across the back of the hand, sensations of touch or pressure are aroused at some places. At others cold sensations are likely to flash out, and at some point in the course of stimulation tickle or even itch may be aroused. Moreover, if the exploring stimulus is changed to a sharper or duller object, or if the mode of attack is varied to involve direct pressure into the skin, or if warmed or cooled metal points are substituted, a considerable range of sensations may result. This suggests that the skin's potentialities for sensations may be gauged by exploring sample areas in a systematic manner and by using a variety of stimuli. The possibilities are extensive, for the skin proves to be responsive not only to mechanical force exerted on it but also to electrical, thermal and chemical stimuli as well.

To make possible systematic exploration it is obviously necessary to use some sort of mapping technique. You can mark the skin off by using a rubber stamp which impresses on it a large grid, divided into many tiny squares, each one millimeter on a side. Then you study separately the sensitivity of each square millimeter; or, using a binocular microscope, you can study and map the cutaneous topography (furrows, hair stumps, sweat ducts, etc.) and localize your stimuli with respect to these signs.

PRESSURE SENSITIVITY

For the arousal of pressure sensations the conventional stimulus is a hair, human or animal, of suitable length, diameter and stiffness. Several hairs, each attached at right angles to a wooden holder, may be arranged to provide a graded pressure series. You place the end of the hair over the spot to be stimulated, then press the holder down to the point of bending the hair.

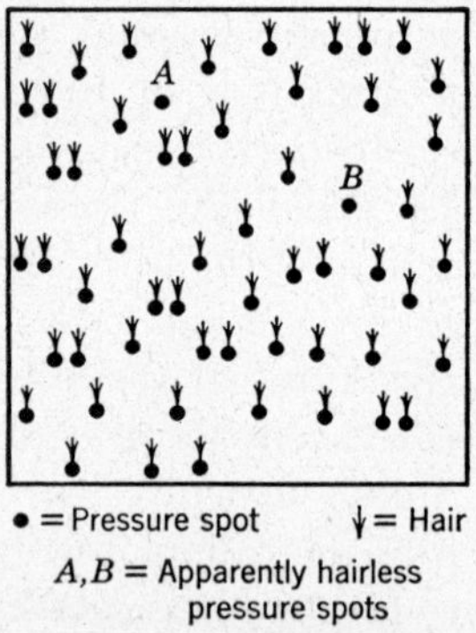

FIGURE 181. PRESSURE SPOTS AND HAIRS

Map from volar side of middle forearm. [After H. Strughold (1925).]

If a sample area on the under side of the forearm is explored point by point with a hair stimulus of moderate strength, the kind of map of pressure sensitivity shown in Fig. 181 results. The striking thing about the distribution of sensitive points is that it almost coincides with the distribution of hairs, which, in this region, are plentiful. Moreover, it is notable that the 'spots' of high sensitivity found in this man-

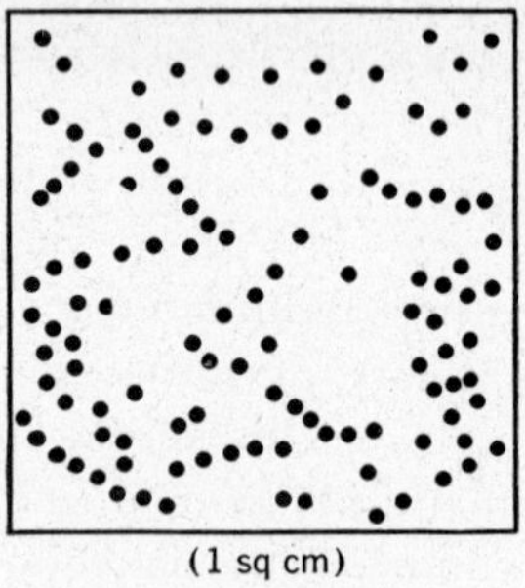

FIGURE 182. PRESSURE SPOTS ON HAIRLESS REGION OF SKIN

Map from web between thumb and index finger. [After A. Goldscheider (1885).]

ner are quite consistently located to the 'windward' of the hairs as they emerge obliquely from the epidermis, as if the receptors lay below the surface at the bases of the hairs. Nevertheless, a similar exploration, confined to a hairless region,

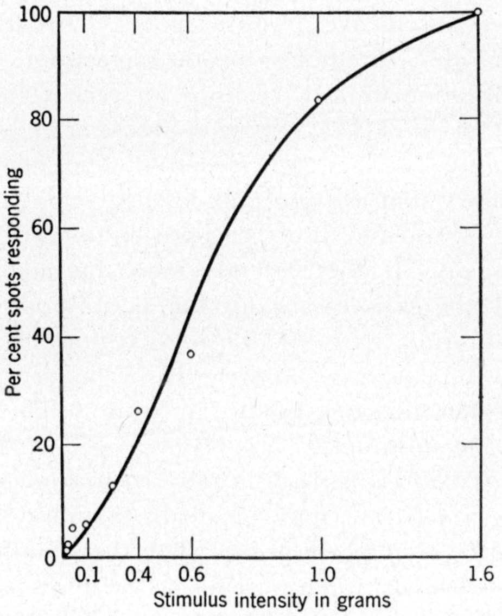

FIGURE 183. PRESSURE SENSITIVITY AS DETERMINED BY INTENSITY

Proportions of spots, in a one-centimeter area, responsive to hair stimuli of graduated intensity (grams). [From the data of J. P. Guilford and E. M. Lovewell, *J. gen. Psychol.*, 1936, **15**, 154.]

such as the web between the thumb and index finger, also yields a pattern of 'spots' of high sensitivity (Fig. 182). If pressure reception in the hairy regions of the skin is in some manner connected with end organs at hair follicles, this explanation will not serve for the hairless regions.

Something more about the way pressure sensitivity is distributed may be learned by repeating the exploration, in either of these areas, with stronger stimuli. If this is done, more 'spots' will appear and, if strong enough, there is no place where the stimulus hair may be set down without evoking a response. The relation between stimulus intensity and the percentage of 'spots' in a sample area one centimeter square is shown graphically in Fig. 183. It would appear that every point on the skin has the potentiality for arousing pressure sensations.

The effect of mechanical impact on the skin is not, of course, confined to a single point, however small the stimulus may be.

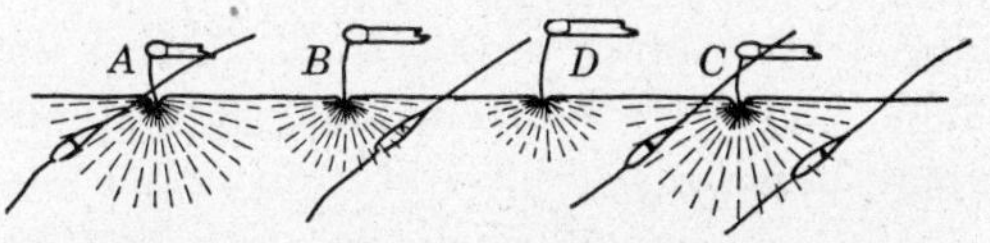

FIGURE 184. EFFECT OF STIMULI OF DIFFERENT INTENSITIES APPLIED TO DIFFERENT SPOTS OF THE SKIN

The stimuli are hairs which are pressed against the skin. The longer and finer the stimulus hair, the less the pressure. The diagonal lines are hairs protruding from hair follicles in the skin. [After K. M. Dallenbach (1935).]

The cutaneous tissues are highly elastic and transmit to considerable distances and in all directions disturbances created at a point on the surface. The greater the surface distortion, the farther into the skin and along its surface will the deformation be carried. Thus are set up tensions, which, occurring in the right places, may initiate nerve discharges. Figure 184 shows four possibilities of stimulation by hairs. Stimulus *B* in this case is most favorably located to affect end organs and thus arouse pressure sensations.

Experiments have shown that the stimulus can consist of an outward distortion of the surface, and the resulting sensation will be the same. An upward tug on a hair or on a thread glued to the skin surface may produce a pressure sensation indiscriminable from that brought about by a depression made by a stimulus hair. Herein lies another reason for supposing that the true stimulus for the pressure sensation is tension set up within the skin and not actual pressure on the skin.

Perception of Vibration

The skin is very sensitive to vibration and to differences in rates of vibration. It it possible to discriminate accurately between 420 and 425 cycles per second, when the two rates are vibration pressures produced by holding tuning forks against the skin. There has been some talk about there being a special 'vibration sense,' but recent experiments make it clear that vibration is perceived by way of the pressure receptors, that perceived vibration is *pressure in movement.*

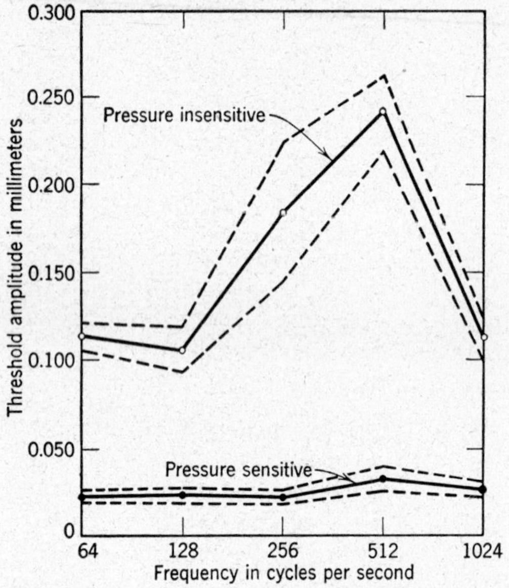

FIGURE 185. VIBRATORY THRESHOLDS FOR PRESSURE-SENSITIVE AND PRESSURE-INSENSITIVE REGIONS

Absolute thresholds for the 'whirring' feeling determined at five frequencies (64 to 1024 cycles per second) on a region especially sensitive to pressure and on another region especially insensitive to pressure. Sensitivity to vibration increases greatly with sensitivity to pressure. Dotted lines show variability of measurement. [After F. A. Geldard, *J. gen. Psychol.,* 1940, **22**, 286.]

The results of such an experiment are shown in Fig. 185. Two regions of the skin were selected, one containing ten very sensitive pressure 'spots,' and one with ten very insensitive pressure 'spots.' Then the absolute thresholds for the perception of vibration were determined for each region at each of five vibration frequencies (64 to 1024 cycles per second). The figure shows that the pressure-insensitive region is in all cases also the vibration-insensitive region. It does not take much movement of the skin to set up the perception of vibration. In the sensitive region 0.025 millimeter was enough. In the insensitive region the thresholds ran from 0.100 to 0.250 millimeter.

Tickle, sometimes introduced to students as a separate sense, is really a vibratory perception which occurs when the stimulus 'teeters' or when several nerve fibers are successively activated. It is not known certainly why some intense stimulation of this sort gives rise to reflex movements of escape or laughter.

Pressure Adaptation

Pressure sensitivity displays the phenomenon of adaptation. Continuous stimulation results in a fading and, eventually, in complete abolition of sensation. The time taken for the sensation created by a weight resting on the skin to disappear completely is directly proportional to the size of the weight and inversely proportional to the skin area contacted.

There is good evidence to believe that pressure adaptation has a simple mechanical basis. A weight placed on the skin surface continues to compress the underlying tissues and 'settle' into the skin for a surprisingly long time. In one experiment it was shown that pressure sensations remain only as long as the settling continues or until the rate of movement into the skin is reduced below the intensitive threshold. At that point adaptation is complete, for effective stimulation has ceased.

Aftersensations, which occur commonly in the realm of pressure sensitivity, represent a renewal of positive stimulation. Upon removal of the deforming stimulus the skin tissues tend to resume their normal positions. So long as restorative movements are occurring within the cutaneous tissues aftersensations will be aroused, actually in the absence of an external stimulus.

Localization of Pressures

The ability to localize pressure sensations varies greatly, depending on the bodily region involved. If an observer is blindfolded and is touched lightly on the fingertip, he will usually indicate the spot touched with an error under two millimeters in extent. At the tip of his tongue his error is almost too small to be measured. Touch him on the thigh or upper arm, however, and he is likely to miss by several centimeters. Localization is best in relatively mobile areas of the skin, in the hands, feet and mouth regions.

A different kind of capacity for localization is found in exploring the body surface with compass points to find the so-called *two-point threshold.* In each skin area there is some separation of two points which just gives rise to two discrete impressions; if the points are brought closer together and are simultaneously applied, they arouse a unitary impression. On the average the values of the two-point threshold shown in Table XVIII will be found to hold for the normal observer. In certain cases of brain tumor and other abnormalities of the central nervous system, the ability both to localize touches on the skin and to discriminate two simultaneously applied points becomes markedly impaired or is even absent, despite retention of bare pressure sensibility. Tests incorporating these two performances are, therefore, made a part of routine clinical examination of the nervous system.

TABLE XVIII

REPRESENTATIVE VALUES OF THE TWO-POINT THRESHOLD

	Millimeters
Tip of the tongue	1
Palmar side of the last phalanx of the finger	2
Red part of the lips	5
Palmar side of the second and dorsal side of the third phalanx of the finger	7
White of the lips, and metacarpus of the thumb	9
Cheek, and plantar side of the last phalanx of the great toe	11
Dorsal side of the first phalanx of the finger	16
Skin on the back part of cheek bone, and forehead	23
Back of the hand	31
Kneepan, and surrounding region	36
Forearm, lower leg	40
Back of foot, neck, chest	54
Middle of the back, and of the upper arm and leg	68

Receptors for Pressure

The receptor organs for pressure have not been identified with certainty. The common location of spots of highest pressure sensitivity to the 'windward' of hairs suggests that the receptors should lie at the hair follicles, which are known to be well supplied with sensory nerve terminations. These fibers twine so freely around the base of a hair that they have been called *basket endings.* Presumably they are pressure receptors. But what about hairless regions? Pressure sensitivity on the hairless palms is very high. The guess has been that *Meissner corpuscles,* sensory nerve endings situated in the papillae of the corium, are the receptors here. They are abundant in the palms of the hands and the soles of the feet, occurring in some profusion in the tips of the fingers and toes, and thus seem to have the proper distribution. However, the evidence is no more formidable than this. It may eventually turn out that other forms of specialized endings can also initiate pressure impulses.

PAIN SENSITIVITY

Pain, of all the cutaneous sensations, is aroused most generally over the skin surface. It is produced by several forms of stimuli: mechanical, chemical, thermal and electrical. If mechanical stimuli are used, they must either be applied with considerable force or they must be sharply pointed, sufficiently so to penetrate the epidermis or produce a deep depression in it. This deformation, of course, causes the prior arousal of pressure sensations, and with mechanical stimulation pain cannot be isolated from pressure. Many chemicals, when injected into the skin, elicit pain. The hydrogen ion is particularly powerful in this respect, the intensity of the pain being determined by the degree of acidity of the injected solution. Chemical stimuli cannot, however, be confined to a local area, and with their use it is difficult to determine the distribution of pain sensitivity and the exact mode of operation of the receptor.

The production of pain by extremes of temperature is familiar. As with mechanical stimuli, however, pain is not produced in isolation when warm or cold objects are used as stimulators. Pressure is a necessary accompaniment to warmth and cold. One recently devised technique, however, circumvents this difficulty. It consists in using radiant heat from the type of bulb used in a 'sun lamp' and focusing its rays sharply on the skin by means of a lens. Warmth is aroused by such a method, but it is not hard to distinguish the sharp, stabbing pattern of pain from the diffuse background of warmth. Concomitant pressure is entirely avoided. If the time of exposure is held constant and the intensity of the heat source is varied in small steps, it is possible to measure the pain threshold with some precision. For a group of 150 subjects of both sexes and of wide age range the absolute threshold proved to be constant at 0.21 gram-calories per second per square centimeter, with a variation of about 15 per cent.

Perhaps the best of the methods to arouse pure local pain and chart its distribution is to make use of electrical stimuli. A circuit may be arranged to permit a high potential discharge to the skin from an electrode held just above it. Such a 'sparking' method brings out the essentially punctate distribution of pain sensitivity. Not all local points on the skin respond with pain. Some spots give pressure, others cold, and some warmth. But pain is aroused from the largest number of points, and the distribution of its 'spots' appears to be quite haphazard.

Pain Adaptation

It is not immediately obvious that pain subsides with continued stimulation. A cut or bruise seems no less painful until 'something is done for it.' Cutaneous pain, however, does undergo adaptation. Press a needle into the skin with a steady, unvarying force and pain is aroused which gradually loses its intensity and eventually disappears altogether, leaving a sensation of pressure. Produce pain by radiant heat and, if stimulation remains steady, the pain will subside, leaving a residue of warmth. Similarly the pain accompanying extreme cold, such as is induced by dry ice held close to the skin, will fade out slowly leaving behind only cold. For a long time it was supposed that pain had no separate sensory existence but was simply the result of overstimulation of other senses. These facts of adaptation, however, taken together with the demonstration of 'spot' distribution, make it appear that pain constitutes a separate system of sensitivity with its own special receptors.

Pathways for Pain

The arousal of pain is notoriously slow. Touch a hot object or stub your toe and a noticeable interval passes before the pain is felt. Meanwhile there is appreciation, by way of pressure sensations, that the object has been contacted. The delay in the pain response suggests that it is carried by fibers of slow conduction rate. The weight of evidence is that pain is mediated chiefly by fibers of small diameter, and it is well known that the smaller the fiber the more slowly it conducts impulses. We should, therefore, expect reaction time to pain-producing stimuli to be relatively long, and it is. As much as a full second may elapse after the onset of the stimulus before pain is felt.

Not only is there evidence that pain involves a separate peripheral mechanism but it is known also that, in the course of conduction up the spinal cord, tracts differing from those responsible for pressure sensations are used for pain. Pain impulses ascend the spinal cord in the so-called anterolateral tract, a region through which impulses for pressure do not pass. In the disease known as syringomyelia, the central canal of the cord widens and interrupts these pain tracts. Consequently a loss of pain sensations (and usually of temperature) with full preservation of pressure sensitivity is brought about. The arrangement of the conduction paths also makes possible a surgical operation for persistent and unbearable pain. Cutting through the anterolateral tract at a suitable level abolishes pain sensitivity in the affected region but does not interfere with touch or pressure from the same area.

Pain Receptors

Since pain has been discovered to constitute a separate system there is naturally an effort to link it with a special type of nerve ending. The very general occurrence of pain in all regions leads one to attribute it to the operation of the most commonly found type of nerve termination, the free nerve ending. The most exquisitely painful regions of the body are the cornea of the eye and the inner reaches of the external auditory canal. Only free nerve endings can be found in these tissues. This sort of evidence cannot, however, be regarded as final. There must be receptors in the skin for pain, but we cannot yet be sure what they are.

TEMPERATURE SENSITIVITY

For the production of warm and cold sensations heated or cooled metal points will serve. The best temperature stimulators are arranged, usually by the aid of circulating water, to maintain constant a predetermined temperature.

Sensitivity to warmth and to cold, like sensitivity to pressure and pain, is distributed in 'spots' over the skin. Exploration with warmed or cooled metal points reveals 'spots' especially sensitive to cold, others readily responsive to warmth. As with pressure, however, the number of spots responding in a given limited region depends on the intensity of the stimulus. Let the point of the stimulator be maintained at a temperature just a little above that of the skin and only a few warm spots will be located; raise its temperature appreciably and the population will increase. A comparable rule holds for cold.

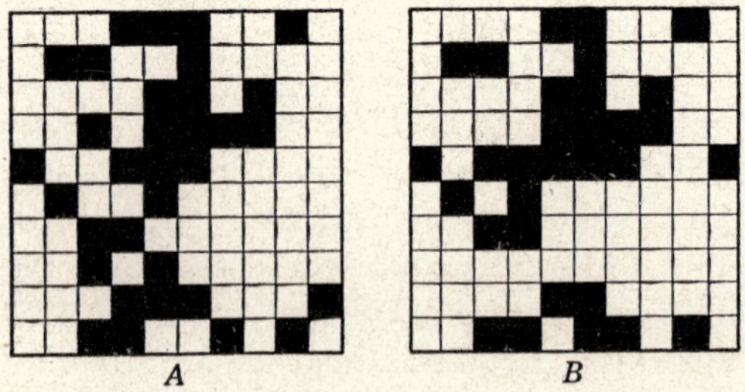

FIGURE 186. COLD SPOT PATTERNS

Successive mappings, *A* and *B*, 5 minutes apart, of a one square centimeter area on the forearm. In each exploration every square was stimulated once with a metal point, one millimeter in diameter, at a constant temperature of 17° C and at a constant pressure. Blackened squares indicate reports of cold. In *A*, 33 per cent of the millimeter squares responded with cold sensation; in *B*, 31 per cent. The two maps agree exceptionally well (88 per cent). [Unpublished data from F. A. Geldard.]

When careful measurement is undertaken, it is found that the sensitivity of the temperature spots varies from time to time, even from minute to minute. Figure 186 shows the same area mapped twice for the location of cold spots with the stimulus at 17° C and with an interval of 5 minutes between the mappings. The agreement is good (about 88 per cent) but not perfect, in spite of the fact that great care was taken to keep conditions the same. It is probable that the sensitivity of some of the spots has decreased in this short interval. On the other hand, it is possible to identify and mark especially sensitive temperature spots, finding that they respond with warmth or cold, as the case may be, whenever stimulated over a period of years.

Skin Temperature

At least a part of the apparent instability of warm and cold spots can be explained by reference to the temperature shifts within the skin itself. The cutaneous tissues are constantly undergoing thermal changes. Some of the changes result from heat radiation and the evaporation of moisture from the epidermis. The chief factor, however, is dilation and contraction of blood vessels in the corium and subcutaneous tissue. A vast number of influences can, by reflex nervous action, create changes in the size of cutaneous blood vessels. With dilation comes a larger blood flow and warming of surrounding tissues; with contraction there is a reduction of heat supply. Thus, with heat interchanges occurring at the site of nerve stimulation, it is not surprising that some of the less favorably disposed receptors are at times influenced, at others uninfluenced, by a small metal point set down on the skin surface.

The amount of heat delivered to or carried away from the skin by a thermal stimulator is not great. The epidermis is a good insulator. In experiments in which sensitive thermocouples have been embedded in the skin, it has been shown that a relatively large stimulus, 10° C above skin temperature and applied for 6 seconds, raised the local surface temperature only 5° C and the tissue 1 millimeter below the surface only 2° C. A large cold stimulus, 14° C below skin temperature, lowered surface and deep temperatures by corresponding amounts. The changes produced by a metal point of the size ordinarily used in exploration, particularly with momentary application, must represent only very small fractions of these values.

The net results of all the complex thermal adjustments being made unceasingly in the skin is that the body surface is normally held in quite stable heat equilibrium with its immediate environment. Over the clothed areas skin temperature remains at about 35° C, on the exposed hands and face it is about 33°, and under the tongue it is 37° (98.6° F). The temperature of the ear lobe, where blood flow is sluggish, may, however, be as low as 26° C.

Physiological Zero and Adaptation

The temperature to which a given skin region is thermally indifferent, that is to say, will respond with neither the sensation of cold nor of warm, is called its *physiological zero.* Thus plunging a hand into water at the temperature of its skin (33° C) normally produces neither a feeling of warm nor of cold. But let the hand previously be exposed to 40°, and the 33° water seems distinctly cold. Similarly, previous exposure to 20° will render the water at 33° decidedly warm. Physiological zero has shifted, in each instance, as a result of *adaptation.*

The phenomenon of thermal adaptation is familiar enough. Dive into a pool, and the cold may at first be breath-taking. Remain there, and the water may eventually be only pleasantly cool. Continued stimulation has lowered sensitivity and has brought physiological zero closer to the temperature of the stimulus. Complete thermal adaptation, reduction of the sensation of warm or cold to the zone of thermal indifference, occurs only within a restricted range of temperatures. For the hands the limits are, roughly, 17° C for cold and 40° C for warm. Temperatures below or above these points seem not to undergo complete adaptation but to continue to give rise to cold or warmth. The more extreme the temperature, the longer the time required for adaptation.

The fact that physiological zero can be moved by adaptation and the related fact that both warm and cold sensitivities are simultaneously affected are important because they suggest that either both kinds of temperature sensations are mediated by the same mechanism, behaving in two different ways, or the two systems of sensitivity, if they are separate, have certain operating characteristics in common.

Paradoxical Cold and 'Heat'

Two phenomena occurring in the realm of temperature sensitivity are remarkable and of considerable theoretical importance. One of them concerns the arousal, by a *warm* stimulus, of the sensation of *cold.* If a number of spots especially sensitive to cold are located, then are gone over with a very warm stimulus (43° C or higher), a certain number of them are likely to respond with their own proper sensation, cold. Since it seems paradoxical that a hot stimulus should arouse cold, this phenomenon has received the designation *paradoxical cold.* The theoretical significance of paradoxical cold lies in its support of the view that both cold and warm sensations involve their own specific receptors and nerve paths.

The other phenomenon has to do with a complex perception, usually called *heat.* The condition necessary for its arousal is the simultaneous stimulation, within a given area, of both the warm and the cold mechanisms. This can be accomplished by the use of the 'heat grill,' a device consisting of parallel metal or glass tubes on which the forearm or some other broad skin surface is rested. Cold water (about 15° C) runs through the even-numbered tubes; warm water (about 44° C) flows through the odd ones. There is nothing about either stimulus which would lead us to expect that the total pattern would be 'hot,' yet when the arm is placed on the grill the experience is uncomfortable and there is a strong tendency to pull it away. The experience is very similar to the feeling aroused by a large, hot object contacting the skin. There the receptor process is perhaps the same, warm spots giving their normal response, while cold spots are simultaneously and paradoxically aroused to action.

Receptors for Temperature

If uncertainty exists about the receptor organs responsible for pressure and pain, there is still more concerning those for warm and cold sensations. It has been seen that some facts point to a common mechanism for both kinds of thermal sensitivity while others seem to demand separate processes for the two.

A currently debated theory is that nerve endings in the walls of tiny blood vessels of the corium, the arterioles, mediate both warm and cold. When a warm stimulus is applied to the skin a local dilation of arterioles is produced, so this theory asserts that the nerve discharges created by relaxation of this smooth muscle tissue is the basis of the warm sensation. A cold stimulus causes the arterioles to contract, and this, it is said, sets up a pattern of discharge which eventuates in the cold sensation. The chief advantage of this *neurovascular theory* of temperature sensitivity is that it provides a ready interpretation of the facts of adaptation and shifting of the physiological zero. The unreliability of spot mapping would also be expected if nerve endings in the walls of the unstable blood vessels are responsible for temperature sensitivity.

The classic view is that two separate mechanisms are involved. Because they seem to lie at about the right depths in the cutaneous tissues to account for the time relations in thermal stimulation, it has been supposed that cold is mediated by *Krause end bulbs,* specialized nerve endings found in the upper portion of the corium, and that warm is cared for by *Ruffini cylinders,* sensory nerve terminations located considerably deeper in the corium and subcutaneous tissue. The quick arousal of cold and the relatively slow response of warm accord well with this guess.

We should suppose that a direct solution of the problem would be possible by mapping sensitivity in a given skin region, then excising the tissue and subjecting it for microscopical examination. Such experiments have been made a number of times, and the results have been, in general, disappointing. In one such attempt both warm and cold spots were carefully mapped and remapped. When the tissue was cut out and examined, not a single specialized nerve ending was found to be present; only free nerve endings appeared in the tissue sections. In general, the results are not such as to give any confidence in the conclusion that the receptors for warm and cold can be discovered in this simple and direct fashion.

KINESTHESIS

All the structures involved in bodily movements—muscles, their attached tendons and the articulations between bones —are well supplied with sensory nerves, and they originate patterns of sensation.

Kinesthesis ('feeling of motion') is the name given to these patterns. By its aid we are able, without the help of vision, to carry on complicated activities calling for considerable nicety of muscular adjustment or to judge accurately the positions of limbs.

The relative contribution made by sensations from muscles, tendons and joints that correct judgments of limb position are impossible. That muscle, by itself, has a sensory contribution to make is shown by the fact that movements of the tongue can be appreciated. Fine discrimination of tongue movements, however, is not possible kinesthetically, as may be amply demonstrated by noting, in a mirror, the discrepancy between what is seen and what

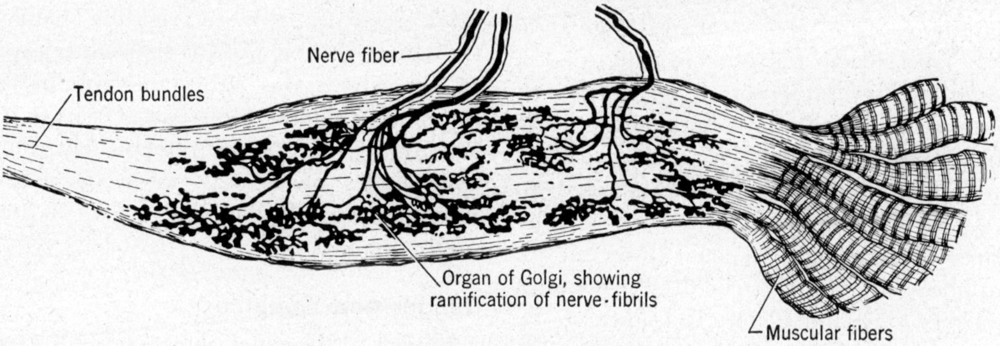

FIGURE 187. KINESTHETIC RECEPTORS IN TENDON

Freely branching sensory fibers with specialized terminations, the so-called Organ of Golgi, found in tendinous tissue. [From J. D. Lickley, *The nervous system,* Longmans, Green, 1931, p. 132.]

is not easy to assess by simply observing their 'feel' while making a limb movement. The patterns are massive and diffuse, and their exact localization is difficult. Abnormalities, however, provide a fairly conclusive answer. In certain rare nerve afflictions joint sensibility may be retained while sensations originating in muscles and their attachments, as well as those from the overlying skin, are abolished. In such cases the appreciation of posture and movement is very little affected, indicating that the joints play the major role in this capacity. Confirmation of this conclusion comes from pathological cases of the opposite variety. In a bone disease which destroys joint sensibility without disturbing the sensibility of muscles and tendons, it has been demonstrated is felt when the tongue is moved about the open mouth without touching the cheeks or lips. Sensations originating in tendinous tissue apparently make their chief contribution when heavy weights are supported or during extreme exertion. Then feelings of strain, even ache, appear.

Kinesthetic sensibility may be tested by mechanically moving a finger, toe or limb and measuring either the minimal observable rate of motion or the smallest angular displacement that can be detected. Surprisingly high sensitivity is found. The thresholds for the displacement of different joints vary between 0.2 and 0.7 degree. The lower value is for the shoulder. When measured by minimal rate of movement, again the shoulder proves to be the most sensitive joint,

Kinesthetic Receptors

The probable nerve endings for kinesthesis have been described fairly intimately. Whereas sensory nerves apparently do not terminate directly at the joint surfaces, large nerve endings known as *Pacinian corpuscles* are observed in the ligaments of joints and in the bone covering near joints. Free nerve endings are also found in these regions. Embedded in tendinous tissue are so-called *Golgi spindles,* specialized portions of the tendon containing several sensory nerve fibers each terminating in freely branching, club-shaped enlargements (Fig. 187). They seem admirably located and adapted to respond to changes of tension. The fleshy parts of nearly all skeletal muscles are supplied with special structures, a few millimeters long and definitely known to be sensory in function, called *muscle spindles.* These spindles are complex in their nerve supply, at least three different forms of terminations being found in them. Two types signal stretching, not contraction, of the muscle, whereas the third responds to varying states of tension. The muscle spindle would seem to be best adapted to providing information about cessation of muscle activity. Perhaps this is why recognition of posture and movement depends so much on the joints.

ORGANIC SENSIBILITY

As compared with the skin the deep-lying internal organs, even those of the alimentary canal, are very insensitive structures. Surgeons have long known that, in the absence of anesthetics, intestines may be cut, squeezed, scraped or even cauterized without so much as producing discomfort. Are visceral organs, then, normally anesthetic?

Experimentation provides a different answer. By means of stomach tubes and allied equipment it has been possible to establish the fact that the stomach and esophagus are sensitive to both warmth and cold. Internal distension of these organs, produced by inflating a balloon, may result in massive and vaguely localized feelings of pressure or, if the distension is rapid enough, pain. All visceral organs, indeed, seem capable of yielding pain if stretching of their walls is sufficiently rapid or extensive. Gas pains and cramps are common testimony to visceral sensitivity. Sensations from the deep organs have their own modes of arousal; large distending pressures are usually involved when pressure or pain is felt.

Hunger and Appetite

In view of the generally low level of sensitivity displayed by visceral organs, it may seem surprising that the unpleasant, gnawing pangs called hunger have their origin in local activity of one of them. Nevertheless the facts are clear. The hunger sensation has been definitely shown to come from strong contractions of the musculature of the stomach wall and thus to constitute a kinesthetic pattern. Figure 188 illustrates the recording of hunger pangs. A subject, habituated in advance to the presence of a balloon in his stomach and a rubber tube down his throat, presses a key whenever he feels the hunger pangs. His reports are seen to coincide with the occurrence of the strongest stomach contractions. While considerable activity of the stomach walls is going on between pangs, these movements are unknown to the subject through direct observation. Only the intense peaks of contraction, occurring every half minute or so, create sensations which get organized into a conscious somesthetic pattern.

A clear distinction must be made between the *hunger pangs,* which constitute a definite sensory experience, and *hunger-as-appetite,* which is the desire to eat and does not necessarily have any special sensory form. When you have the hunger pangs, you want to eat; that is true. On the other hand, you may also want to eat when you do not have the pangs, and then all the sensation you have is the kinesthesis of wanting to get hold of food when you see it. It is hunger-as-appetite that makes you eat desserts—all desserts, for the hunger contractions of the stomach and thus the hunger pangs are stopped by ingesting the food which precedes a dessert. If eating were entirely a matter of satisfying hunger, meals would become very brief affairs, but hunger-as-appetite carries on after the hunger pangs have lapsed. Even nonnutritive and indigestible substances—pieces of leather, bits of moss or clay—will temporarily allay these pangs. Hard swallowing or tightening the belt will do the same. Emotion is a very effective inhibitor of the hunger contractions and pangs. But appetite is the motivation that lasts when the pangs are gone. In modern civilization hunger pangs have become increasingly rare, but they are common enough in China and were too well known in Europe during and after the Second World War.

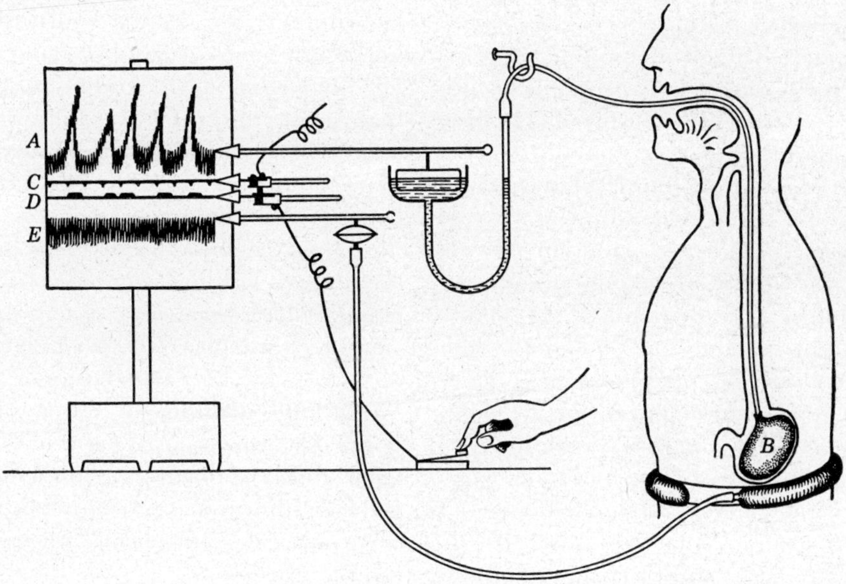

FIGURE 188. RECORDING OF HUNGER CONTRACTIONS

The subject records, by a magnetic marker on line *D,* the occurrence of hunger pangs, while the undulating record, *A,* shows the state of the muscular activity of his stomach. Time is marked off on line *C.* *E* is a breathing record, taken for control purposes. Note correspondences between *D* and *A.* [From W. B. Cannon, in *Handbook of general experimental psychology,* Clark University Press, 1934, p. 250.]

The psychologists use the word *hunger* both for the sensory pattern of the pangs and for the motive that makes animals eat when they have been deprived of food (pp.

115 f.). It is, therefore, important to remember this difference between *appetite* and *hunger pangs*.

Thirst

The chief source of thirst is not difficult to find. Direct observation tells us that thirst is primarily referred to the mouth and throat; a state of intense thirst consists in a very unpleasant dryness of the mouth cavity. Experiment confirms observation and demonstrates further that thirst arises whenever the mucous lining of the mouth and pharynx becomes dehydrated through a failure of the salivary glands to provide these tissues with a normal amount of moisture. Thirst may be induced by bodily changes quite remote from the mouth, as in the general drying out of tissues due to excessive perspiration or in the dehydrations of diabetes and certain kidney disorders. In such instances, however, it can be shown that there is also a reduction in salivary output and that the thirst is really of local, rather than of general, origin. Moreover, with full retention of body fluids, it is possible to create an intense thirst by subcutaneous injection of atropine, one of the first effects of which is greatly to interfere with output of saliva. Dryness of mouth tissues through salivary deficiency seems clearly to be the basis of the organic pattern we call thirst.

Thirst, this sensory perception of dryness of the mouth, normally acts as the first term in the stimulus-response pattern for satisfying the body's need for water. Thirst, like hunger, is a perception that acts as a motive.

EQUILIBRIUM

The cochlea is part of the labyrinth of the inner ear. It functions in hearing, as we have already seen (pp. 331–336; see Fig. 158, p. 328). The other divisions of the complexly formed labyrinth—the semicircular canals, the utricle and the saccule—are concerned with equilibrium of the body. (See Fig. 189.)

In the functioning of the nonauditory labyrinth we are dealing with a system of sensibility which, curiously enough, yields no direct sensations. Unlike the cochlear branch of the so-called auditory nerve, those branches supplying the remaining parts of the labyrinth do not have direct pathways to the cerebral cortex but, instead, make numerous connections at lower brain levels with outgoing fibers to striped muscles of the eyes, neck, limbs and trunk and also with fibers to smooth muscles of the viscera. The nonauditory labyrinth is thus the point of initiation of a vast array of proprioceptive reflexes, most of them concerned with the preservation of body equilibrium or with the making of new postural adjustments when equilibrium is upset.

There are, of course, consequences for sensation in all these changes, since kinesthetic, cutaneous and organic patterns are necessarily aroused by such widespread reactions. Unusual visual sensations sometimes attend labyrinthine stimulation also. Objects 'swim' in the visual field of a dizzy person because of a rapid involuntary jerking of his eyeballs, a response known as *nystagmus*. For the most part, however, labyrinthine stimulation sets up the unconscious proprioception that aids in maintaining equilibrium of the body.

The Semicircular Canals

Each labyrinth has three highly specialized branches called *semicircular ducts* or *canals*. The three lie at approximately right angles to each other, and each is sym-

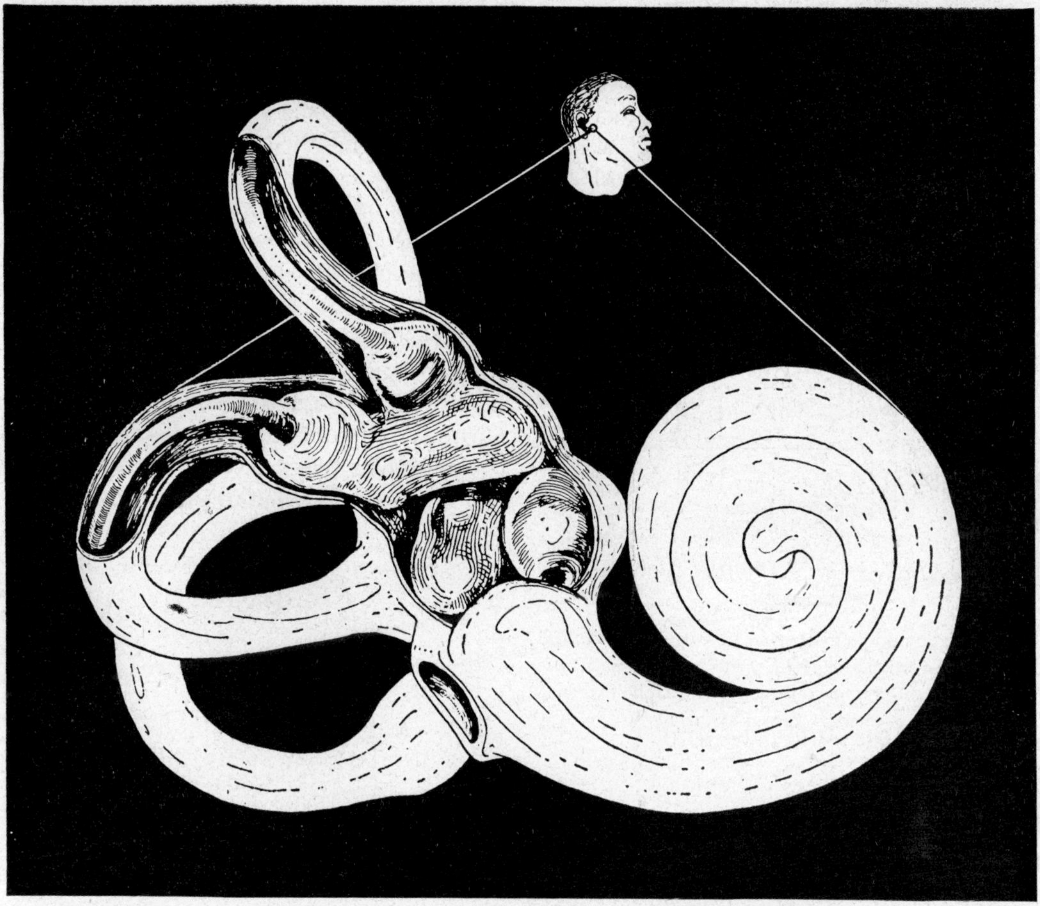

FIGURE 189. INNER EAR: SEMICIRCULAR CANALS AND COCHLEA

Three semicircular canals with outer bone cut away to show membranous labyrinth, including the utricle and the saccule. The cochlea is shown at the right. [Adapted from G. McHugh, in S. L. Polyak, *The human ear,* Sonotone Corporation, 1946.]

metrically paired in position with one on the opposite side of the head. Figure 190 shows the spatial relations among the six canals of the two ears. When the head is inclined slightly forward (about 25 degrees) the external canals are parallel with the ground, the anterior canals point forward at a 45-degree angle, and the posterior canals project backward at the same angle. It is clear that the arrangement of the canals in the head provides a three-dimensional coordinate system, and movement of the head will create, through lag, a flow of the watery fluid (endolymph) in one or more of the canals.

Each canal has a bulge near one end, an *ampulla,* within which are to be found specialized nerve endings, hair tufts called *cristae.* The hairs are embedded in a gelatinous mass, the *cupula* (Fig. 191), which extends across the ampulla and is bent over in one direction or the other, depending on the hydraulic pressure created by the flow of endolymph. It is this movement of the fluid, producing bending of the cupula and consequent distortion of the crista, that constitutes the immediate stimulus for the initiation of nerve impulses.

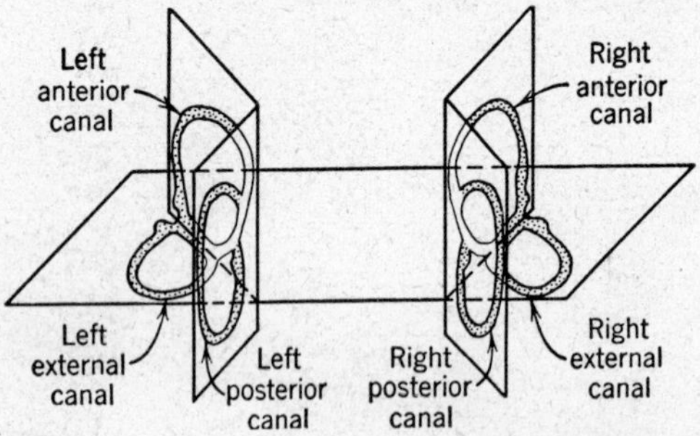

FIGURE 190. POSITIONS OF THE SEMICIRCULAR CANALS

The right and left sets of canals are paired: the left anterior with the right posterior, the right anterior with the left posterior and the right external with the left external. [From Wenzel.]

Since there is a certain amount of friction between the endolymph and the walls of the canals, it follows that, in any continuous movement of the canals, the endolymph will soon 'catch up'; then there will be no relative motion between the fluid and its containing walls and hence no stimulation. It is, therefore, only speeding up or slowing down of the canals, that is to say, positive or negative acceleration, that constitutes the stimulus for the hair cells of the crista.

This analysis of the action of the semicircular canals is borne out by a variety of experiments. Spin a blindfolded subject in a smoothly rotating chair, have him indicate his direction of motion by raising the appropriate hand, and the following events will ordinarily occur. First, as momentum is being gathered (positive acceleration), the subject will report the correct direction of rotation. Then, if speed is maintained constant (canals and endolymph moving together), he will drop his hand and indicate that he feels no motion at all. If brakes are then silently applied, quickly slowing him down (negative acceleration), he will raise his other hand. He feels himself to be rotating in the opposite direction (aftersensation). If, while traveling at high speed, he is stopped abruptly, there may be other reactions—compensatory movements of his arms, legs and head, all designed to prevent him from falling over. If, after rapid and uniform rotation to the left for a dozen revolutions, he is required to stand and hold his arms out forward, he will usually turn his head and arms to the left, his right arm will go up, his left down, and he may be in danger

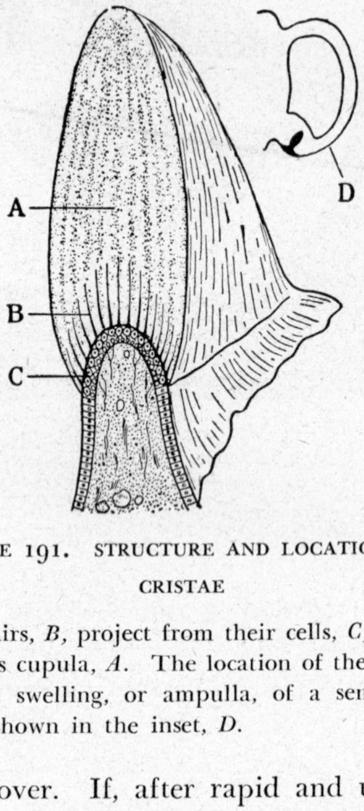

FIGURE 191. STRUCTURE AND LOCATION OF CRISTAE

The hairs, *B*, project from their cells, *C*, into the gelatinous cupula, *A*. The location of the crista in the basal swelling, or ampulla, of a semicircular canal is shown in the inset, *D*.

of falling backward and to the left. If his head position is then changed radically, he is sure to fall unless supported.

The amount of angular acceleration necessary to set the canals in operation is not great. You perceive rotation in the horizontal plane when your body is accelerated as little as one degree per second. There are also other ways of arousing your labyrinthine reflexes. Let the external auditory canal of your ear be syringed with water well above or below body temperature; compensatory movements of your head and nystagmic jerking of your eyeballs will result. The basic mechanism is the same as in rotary movements. Thermal changes in the endolymph create convection currents which affect the position of the cristae. The vestibular nerves, like all others, may also be stimulated electrically. If a direct current is passed transversely through your head, just back of your ears, your head will incline sharply to one side. In animals additional stimuli can be shown to be effective—heat applied locally to the exposed canals, mechanical pressure on the canals, better localized electrical stimulation and drugs applied near the cupula. Because in man the labyrinth is one of the most inaccessible of structures, the experimental possibilities are limited.

Receptors in the Sacs

The *utricle* and the *saccule,* the two structures continuous with each other and collectively called the *sacs* (Fig. 189), have nerve terminations of a different type, and they operate on a different principle. It is believed that the semicircular canals are stimulated only by motions involving changes of direction, whereas the sacs are continuously responsive to straight-line motions and to gravity. The sacs must have much to do with the maintenance of posture, though that they are not the sole determiners of this important function is attested to by the fact that many deaf-mutes who have degenerate vestibular apparatuses are able to get along quite well by substituting visual and kinesthetic clues.

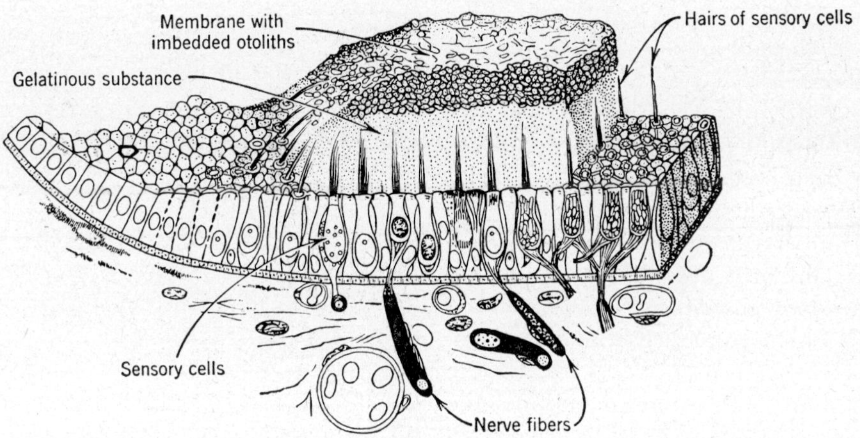

FIGURE 192. STRUCTURE OF THE MACULA

In three-dimensional cross-section. [After W. Kolmer (1926).]

The nerve endings of the sacs are contained in the *maculae* of these structures (Fig. 192). They consist of specialized hair terminations which have at their ends, embedded in a gelatinous mass, tiny crystals of calcium carbonate. It is believed that these crystals 'load' the hair cells and render them susceptible to stimulation by gravitational pull. Moreover, as the body speeds up or slows down, the inertia of the crystals causes the hair cells to bend in one direction or another, and the resulting tensions to initiate impulses in the attached nerve fibers.

Adaptation and Habituation

It has been noted, throughout the entire realm of somesthesis, that adaptation is a generally observed phenomenon. The non-auditory labyrinth provides no exception. In continuous oscillatory motion, which keeps the cristae constantly stimulated, sensitivity is reduced after a time. Both the perception of bodily movement and the nystagmic twitching of the eyes are reduced.

Adaptation should not, however, be confused with *habituation*. Many of the bodily reactions initiated by the labyrinth are subject to modification through central influences with the result that a man may learn to alter behavior in response to a given set of rotational and gravitational forces. Thus the ballet dancer, the whirling dervish and the acrobat, despite violent labyrinthine stimulation, make skillful muscular adjustments and achieve equilibrium through substitution of visual, tactual and kinesthetic clues for the usual proprioceptive ones from the labyrinth. Sailors do the same in acquiring 'sea legs.'

Nowhere is the importance of habituation greater than in learning to fly. The high speeds and maneuverability of modern aircraft place great demands on the ability of the flier to disregard many direct sensations and to learn to make his stick-and-rudder adjustments in accordance with his instrument board. In the beginning of a dive the pilot is very light and, at its end, extremely heavy. In evasive maneuvers his cristae and maculae prompt reactions which, if blindly carried out, would be disastrous. The pilot must learn to accept these new and unusual forces as normal to the flying situation and make suitable adjustments in terms of what he knows and what his instruments tell him. We have come a long way in aviation psychology since the days of the First World War when, because of the recognized importance of labyrinthine mechanisms in flying, it was the practice to select pilots for their high sensitivity to gravitational and rotational changes. It is important to the flier to have an intact labyrinth, but much more important that he be able to learn to resist many of the urges it creates.

REFERENCES

1. Boring, E. G. *Sensation and perception in the history of experimental psychology.* New York: Appleton-Century, 1942. Chaps. 13 and 14.

   Chapter 13 is an interesting and well-documented account of the development of ideas concerning the cutaneous sensibilities, and Chap. 14 performs a similar service for the internal sensibilities.

2. Cannon, W. B. Hunger and thirst. In C. Murchison (Ed.), *A handbook of general experimental psychology.* Worcester, Mass.: Clark University Press, 1934. Chap. 5.

   A brief but competent treatment of the theories and most decisive experiments on hunger and thirst.

3. Dusser de Barenne, J. G. The labyrinthine and postural mechanisms. In C. Murchison (Ed.), *A handbook of general experimental*

psychology. Worcester, Mass.: Clark University Press, 1934. Chap. 4.

A systematic discussion of the reflex mechanisms involved in the maintenance of equilibrium and posture, with an excellent bibliography to 1933.

4. Nafe, J. P. The pressure, pain and temperature senses. In C. Murchison (Ed.), *A handbook of general experimental psychology.* Worcester, Mass.: Clark University Press, 1934. Chap. 20.

The cutaneous sensibilities are treated in a systematic fashion, with particular emphasis on the problem of sensation-receptor correlations.

5. Ruch, T. C. Somatic sensation, and Neural basis of somatic sensation. *Howell's textbook of physiology.* (15th ed., J. F. Fulton, Ed.) Philadelphia: Saunders, 1946. Chaps. 16 and 17.

A clearly written and up-to-date account of the nervous mechanisms involved in cutaneous and internal sensations.

CHAPTER 17

Topographical Orientation

TO be successful in your daily business you must know where you are going, and your brain has few more important tasks than keeping you oriented in space. To know where you are going, you must know where you are now, and also know something of your immediate surroundings. This knowledge of special relationship with objects in your environment is called *topographical orientation.* A minimum of it is required when you move about by merely following a road, a trail or a leader. This type of locomotion is often called 'blind'; its opposite is the well-oriented behavior of a person who knows where he is and where he is heading. So basically true is this statement in its literal sense that the term *well oriented* has taken on the familiar connotation of competence to deal with social surroundings.

THE TOPOGRAPHICAL SCHEMA

Let us consider first the simplest type of topographical orientation, finding the way by following a path. It may be a footpath on a college campus, a city street, a numbered route on a highway or a blazed trail in a forest. At all times you need clues which tell you how to stay on the path; and usually they are obvious—the edge of the path or street, the undergrowth on both sides of the forest trail. If the path is well defined, it may be sufficient to follow your nose, provided it was pointed in the right direction to begin with; yet most paths have branches and crossings where some other procedure is required. Suppose that you are driving an automobile and seeking a certain numbered highway which you know leads to your destination. You may reach a crossroad which bears the correct route number; yet this clue is insufficient by itself. You must also know which way to turn. For example, U. S. Route 1 runs from Maine to Florida along the Atlantic coast; if you are driving east in Virginia and come to a highway marked "Route 1," you must decide whether to turn right (towards Miami) or left (towards Boston). Once this decision has been made correctly you need merely follow the signs.

Thus it is clear that even a simple path cannot be followed blindly without some idea of its spatial relationship to other objects. In practice the following of a marked path is supplemented by some sort of *mental map* or *schema* in which this path is perceived in spatial relationship to other paths and places. In familiar surroundings people are usually quite unaware that they are using such a schema, even though they can orient themselves correctly when placed in an unexpected part

This chapter was prepared by Donald R. Griffin of Cornell University.

of this familiar territory. They can recall the landmarks and other topographical clues in such a well-organized relationship to one another that each landmark can be related to any one of several others and serve for guidance along a variety of routes of travel.

Components of the Schema

Our mental map may include all sorts of memories of objects, once perceived as we moved about—visual memories of the appearance of buildings, trees or hills, bird's-eye views of buildings, pathways or streets and, in some cases, kinesthetic or auditory clues. The schema may also involve the realization that certain places or objects not immediately perceived lie in the same direction as other objects close at hand which we can perceive directly. We may think of the post office as beyond a seen window, or to our right, or over that hill yonder. Thus familiar places or parts of our own bodies become points of reference for other more distant objects or places. London lies in the same direction as the post office but beyond it; China is beyond the railroad station. If our schema has been much influenced by the use of maps, it will include the cardinal points of the compass.

Graphic Representation of the Schema

A map is, in fact, a graphic representation of such a schema, rendered more accurate by the techniques of surveying. The better oriented a person is, the more closely his schema is likely to resemble a map. For many people, however, geographical accuracy is not necessary or even important. A person who does all his traveling by street car may have a schema built around the street car lines. If asked to sketch the schema, he will simplify the street car routes, presumably smoothing curves into straight lines, and tending to show most turns as right angles. His customary stops are likely to be prominent, and other sections of the line may be telescoped or omitted altogether. Thus his schema will be quite distorted when compared with an accurate map, yet schemata of this kind fit the psychological needs of the person who travels over fixed routes. They are exemplified by the 'maps' inserted in railroad timetables, where the railroad route is usually made to appear straight with geography forced to conform to it. The motivation behind the drawing of railroad maps is partly a desire to make the route of the particular railroad appear short and direct, but the gross distortion of geographical fact also serves a real purpose for the traveler, for the railroad map conforms more closely to the topographical schema of the average traveler than the geographer's accurate maps. The traveler can turn this sort of schematic map into a mental schema more readily because it is already in the right form. The traveler is interested primarily in his starting point and destination. He has a secondary interest in the stations along the way and cares little or nothing about the twists and turns of the route. The railroad map and the mental map do not confuse him with geographical information which is of no immediate concern to him.

Not only are directions distorted in the topographical schemata of most people, but distances and the relative areas of various regions also reflect their importance to the individual rather than geographical reality. This is best illustrated by asking an adult person who has not for some years studied geography to draw a map of the United States. Almost invariably the area in which he lives will be

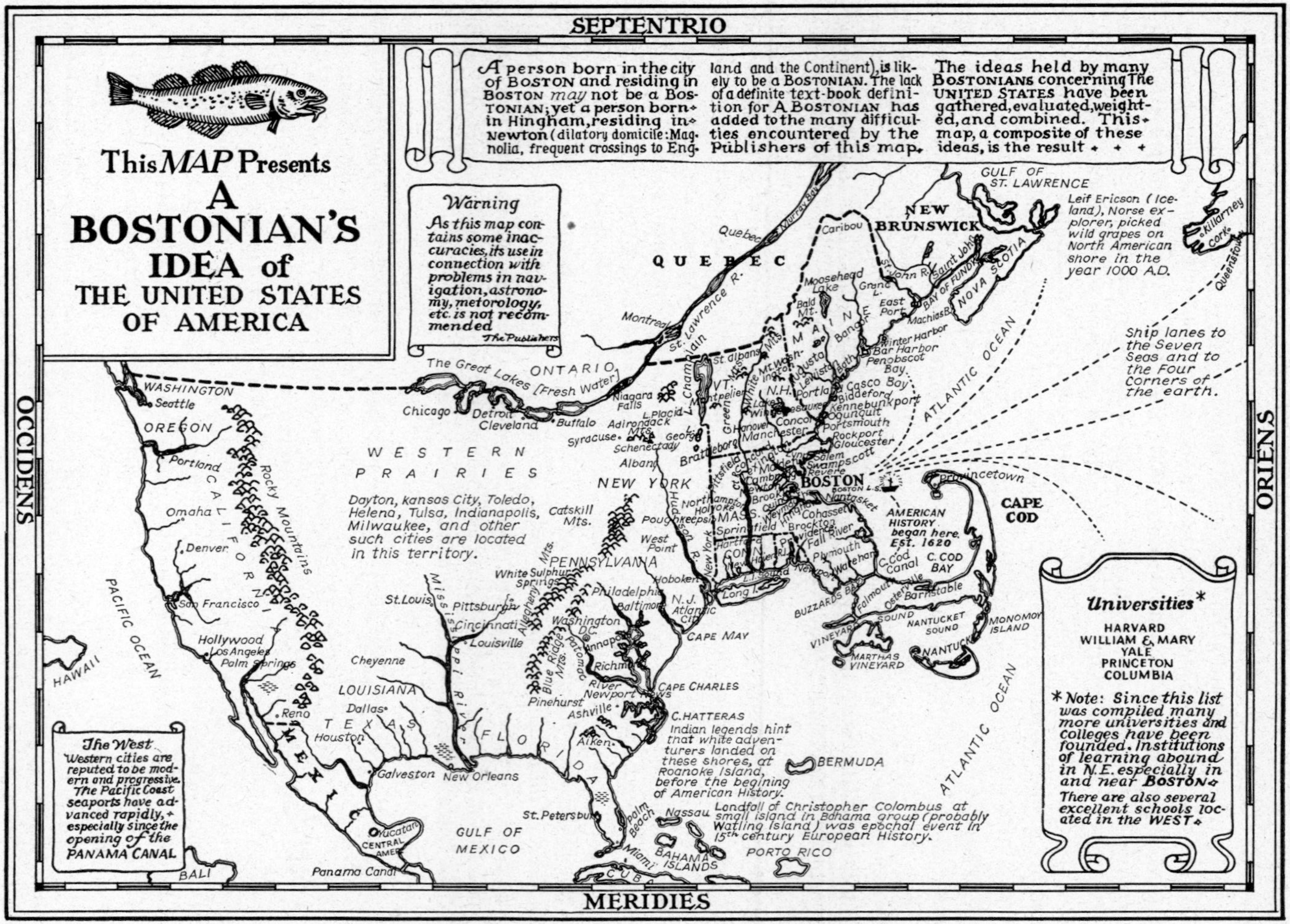

FIGURE 193. A BOSTONIAN'S IDEA OF THE UNITED STATES

[Adapted from D. K. Wallingford, *A Bostonian's idea of the United States of America,* 280 Madison Avenue, New York.]

drawn larger and in more detail than the rest of the country. A somewhat facetious map of this kind is shown in Fig. 193; it purports to show a typical New Englander's concept of the United States, and its distortions are but little greater than those characteristic of many persons' topographical schemata.

Extension of the Schema to New Territory

When a person goes to a strange place he takes with him parts of his old schema, which may, depending upon the circumstances, aid or hinder him 'in learning his way about'—in developing a new schema for the new locality or in extending the old one to include it. The old schema is an aid when it includes the points of the compass or other geographical relationships such as the bearings of shorelines, rivers and mountain ranges which remain pertinent when the old schema is extended to include the new area.

Often, however, the old schema does not fit because there were unnoticed turns in the road, and hence the extension is in error. Then part at least of the person's schema conflicts with the realities of his new environment. "When I was in Wilkinsburg, Pa.," a psychologist writes, "the trolleys for the eastern suburbs ran north through the town, but the east-bound trains ran south through the town. I arrived on the train and, of course, took the trolley going the wrong way to get to the west. My frame of reference was in conflict all that summer."

In learning a new schema, one may be led astray by the assumed directions of street or paths. If the assumption is wrong and the road, instead of being straight, runs at an angle or bends in its course, and if these deviations are not noticed, the topographical orientation becomes utterly confused. The Boston Common is surrounded by five streets which make approximately right angles with each other. Some of the streets are bowed inward enough to make this circumstance possible, but the stranger rarely notices the bends. Hence those who take the Common as a point of reference may often be ninety degrees out of reckoning.

What we call a 'sense of direction' is a skill at retaining orientation or expanding the topographical schema sufficiently to keep it up to date as we travel about. People vary greatly in this ability, which depends upon the rapid and accurate assimilation of new scenes into the schema. Like any type of learning, its perfection depends partly upon practice and partly upon motivation and attention. It is common experience that, in a strange city, we remain much better oriented if we find our own way about than if we cover the same ground in the company of a local inhabitant who leads the way. Active participation demands attention and facilitates learning (pp. 159–161).

Nonvisual Clues

We may use a topographical schema to find our way about even when the landmarks must be perceived through a different sensory modality from the one when they were first encountered. Often the landmarks are first learned as visual clues and later felt by means of other senses. A familiar instance of this is our ability to walk about in our own homes in the dark. We are likely to know, without conscious effort or counting, such topographical relationships as three steps from the bed and it is time to reach for the knob on the bedroom door, six more steps to the left brings us to the stairs, after four steps down we reach a landing and must turn right before continuing down ten more steps to the downstairs hall. (Perhaps the ten steps have to be counted, but the others usually can be perceived correctly without enumeration.) All this information gets organized into so coherent a topographical schema that a man can walk safely anywhere in his own house in pitch darkness even though he is nearly or quite asleep. In such case the mental schema was probably first erected on the basis of visual clues, but in the dark it gets transferred to substitute senses. We can recognize the round door knob, the hard hall floor and the mounting stairs by the somesthesis of hands or feet, the somesthesis of what it is like to take six steps. Hearing may also provide clues. The sounds of walking on a carpet and on a bare floor are different. We never have an auditory map, but we can have a kinesthetic one, the feel of how it is to cover the whole route; and we may have, not a verbal map, but a verbal guide by which we instruct ourselves how to go. In other words, the equipment of imagery that we use in other kinds of thinking is available for use in mental map making.

SENSORY BASIS OF ORIENTATION

Thus far we have outlined the mental processes involved in organizing into a mental schema certain sensory data which constitute topographical landmarks. Usually the schema is visual, the landmarks are carried as visual imagery. The real problem in building up a mental map is to select from a multitude of available visual impressions the few appropriate ones which can easily be remembered and serve as landmarks. There are, however, some situations where visual clues are lacking and successful orientation is nevertheless quite possible, and to such cases we may now turn our attention.

Orientation by the Blind

Consider the difficulties and dangers of traveling through a strange city when tightly blindfolded. At first thought such action seems impossible, and yet some blind people do it as a part of everyday life. Not all totally blind people can move freely about without the guidance of human friends or 'seeing-eye' dogs, but a few skilled and experienced members of that handicapped group can do so with astonishing precision. These blind men and women can walk about indoors without striking furniture or other obstacles, find doors, negotiate stairways and perform numerous other feats of orientation and obstacle avoidance which are quite beyond the ability of the newly blind and of sighted persons who are blindfolded.

A blind man who possessed this ability to a high degree has written: "Whether within a house or in the open air, whether walking or standing still, I can tell, although quite blind, when I am opposite an object and can perceive whether it be tall or short, slender or bulky. I can also detect whether it be a solitary object or a continuous fence, whether it be a closed fence or composed of open rails; and often whether it be a wooden fence, a brick or stone wall or a thickset hedge."

What sensory clues can enable a totally blind man to perceive such details when he is still at a distance of many feet from the objects which he is describing? Of the several explanations which have been advanced, two principal theories have generally been considered more plausible than a variety of other, semimystical explanations which postulate the development of a 'sixth sense' in the blind or their dependence on ill-defined 'waves in the ether' or even telepathy. The first of these two theories holds that the cutaneous senses of touch and temperature are developed to a keenness sufficient to enable the blind man to feel air currents as they are influenced by the proximity of obstacles. The face was believed to be the seat of this highly developed cutaneous sensitivity, and for this reason the term *facial vision* has been applied to the ability of the blind to perceive objects at a distance. Until very recently this theory of a facial cutaneous sensitivity was generally, though tentatively, accepted by most psychologists. It was supported by the reports of many gifted blind men that, when they approached obstacles, they felt cutaneous sensations on their faces, especially their foreheads.

Auditory Perception of Obstacles

The sense of hearing, however, has appealed to some psychologists as a more probable basis for the obstacle perception of the blind. Their opinions were based on experiments in which blind men lost much of their skill if their ears were covered. Since men can localize quite accurately the source of a sound, it seems possible that objects are detected at a distance by means of their effects on the total sound field perceived by the blind man. Many psychologists have believed, however, that a combination of cutaneous and auditory clues enables the blind to perceive obstacles at a distance.

Recent results have shown conclusively that the auditory theory is in the main correct. Blind men, as well as some blindfolded seeing persons who learned with practice to duplicate some of the feats of the blind, lost virtually all their ability when their ears were tightly stopped. This showed that cutaneous receptors by themselves were not sufficient for obstacle perception. The entire skin, furthermore, could be covered by heavy felt and similar materials without any impairment of the ability to detect obstacles before collision, provided that small openings were left over the ears. Thus the ears were shown to be both necessary and sufficient for the detection of obstacles. Finally, it was demonstrated that the ability could be retained when the judgment of proximity to an obstacle was based entirely on auditory clues transmitted by telephone.

In this crucial experiment one experimenter walked toward an obstruction carrying a microphone, while the subject—a blind man or someone else playing the blind man's role—sat in an isolated room listening with headphones to the sounds which the microphone picked up as it was carried toward the obstacle. The subject with headphones could detect the proximity of solid objects and signal to the carrier of the microphone when to stop within a few inches of the obstacle. To rule out any possible clues being given by the carrier of the microphone, another group of tests was conducted with the microphone carried not by a man but on a carriage moved by electric motor toward the obstacle and remotely controlled by the subject in another room. Both blind and sighted subjects could with practice bring the carriage close to the movable obstacle and stop it just before collision, even though at the start of a trial they did not know how far from the carriage the obstacle lay. Thus the entire operation of approaching the obstacle and stopping just before collision was accomplished with purely auditory clues.

It is not yet clear just what kinds of sound blind men use to detect obstacles, but we know that the ability is lost when there is no sound at all or when very loud distracting noises are present. Objects are apparently detected by noticing changes in the perceived quality of sounds, changes due to the presence of the obstacles. Street noises have a different sound when we are close to a building from their sound when we are walking past a vacant lot. Often the sounds are made by the blind man himself, consciously or unconsciously, to aid in the auditory perception of obstacles. There is the blind man's traditional tapping with his cane (as, for instance, the blind man Pew in *Treasure Island*), although he also uses his cane to feel out the ground immediately ahead. Or he makes sounds such as tapping, shuffling his feet, snapping his fingers or short sharp whistled or vocal sounds. In such instances blind men are apparently able to make use of the echoes of such sounds as clues to the proximity of solid objects.

The auditory clues must be very subtle indeed, since very few blind men are aware that it is hearing which warns them of obstacles. Yet that should not surprise us. A clue to be effective in perception does not have to be conscious in the sense that the organism which uses the clue knows that he has the clue or that he uses it. Unawareness of clues is rather the rule in well-established perceptions like the perceptions of spatial relations. Most proprioceptive clues are unconscious. We do not directly perceive excitation from the nonauditory labyrinth, although we perceive the effects in the perception of rotation, dizziness and the visual 'swimming' of nystagmus. Only by indirect means can we demonstrate that the retinal disparity, which comes about because of binocular parallax, provides the clues for the perception of depth and solidity. One clue used here involves the brain's 'knowing' what its owner never 'knows' in any full verbally expressive sense, that is to say, *which* eye perceives *which* disparate image. No man judging distance on the basis of the convergence or accommodation of his eyes knows that he uses these clues. The blind man in his 'facial vision' is thus not out of line with the psychology of perception. He presents simply a new, interesting case, which is somewhat surprising because facial vision is presumably learned and not necessarily learned in infancy.

Why do the blind think that facial vision is a cutaneous perception and not auditory? There may be, of course, some useful cutaneous clues for them, but the experiments have shown that such clues are neither necessary nor sufficient for the blind's perception of obstacles. Still, if there is some cutaneous experience and if the blind are constantly in fear of bumping into objects and have sometimes bumped into them, they may be especially aware of their cutaneous experience and may come to associate it with the auditorially conditioned facial vision.

Auditory Orientation by Bats

The use of sound for purposes of topographical orientation is also developed to a high degree of perfection in one group of lower animals, the bats. Bats are nocturnal flying mammals, mostly smaller in body than a mouse, and not only do they fly at night in thick woods but they are also very frequently found flying through the total darkness of underground caverns. Under these circumstances they are, nevertheless, able to negotiate tortuous passages without colliding with the irregular rocky walls or with each other. Furthermore, it was shown long ago that after being blinded bats can avoid obstacles as well as ever, even when the obstacles are wires as small as one millimeter in diameter. Just as cutaneous perception was once the most generally accepted explanation of the ability of blind men to find their way around, so the sensory basis of the bat's ability was long thought to depend on a highly developed sense of touch. And the parallel extends further; a few biologists felt that hearing was more important for the bats than touch, especially since bats lost much of their ability when their ears were stopped. The bat's flight, however, appeared to be quite silent, and for this reason the auditory theory was not widely accepted until it was shown recently that the animals were actually emitting sounds which were 'ultrasonic' in the sense that they were too high in frequency to be detected by human ears.

Although bats can make shrill cries which men have no difficulty in hearing, they also emit during flight special ultrasonic cries which have a frequency of 30,000 to 70,000 cycles per second, whereas the upper limit of human hearing is only about 20,000 cycles per second. The production of these ultrasonic cries is necessary if the bats are successfully to avoid obstacles. When a bat's ears are stopped, it becomes helpless and strikes whatever obstacles beset its path. In short, the bat's eyesight is so poor (at least in some species) that hearing has become for it the principal sensory avenue by which it perceives objects at a distance from its body.

Echolocation

More is known about the clues used by bats to detect obstacles than about the clues used by blind men. The bats apparently rely entirely on their own ultrasonic cries which, because of their short wave length, are propagated and reflected less diffusely than sounds in the audible range. The duration of a bat's cry is very short, usually 0.001 to 0.002 second. It is essentially a click, and the individual clicks are emitted as often as fifty times a second. Apparently the bat hears echoes of these pulses of high-frequency sound and detects obstacles by auditory localization of the source of the echo. The time elapsing between the original pulse and the return of the echo probably tells the bat its distance from the obstacle. The short duration permits the echo to be heard without interference from the original pulse even at close range. Figure 194 shows the waves in a single pulse of the bat's cry in true proportion to the animal's own size. Each curved line in this figure represents the crest of a sound pressure wave. The wave length of each sound wave is 5 to 10 millimeters, and the entire pulse is spread over a distance of only a foot or so.

There is an obvious parallel between the bat's method of locating obstacles and the newly developed sonar instruments. Sonar instruments send sound waves through the water and detect echoes from submarines, fish and other objects, including the bottom itself. In the last case the instrument becomes a sonic depth finder, an extremely useful aid to navigation. Thus bats, sonar instruments and blind men all seem to be employing the same fundamental process, the sending out of exploratory sounds and the detection of distant objects by means of echoes. In view of this similarity the term *echolocation* has been proposed to cover all such uses of echoes to aid in topographical orientation.

Strictly speaking, we cannot be certain *a priori* that a blind man always uses echo rather than unreflected sound. There are four possible ways in which objects could be localized by auditory means. (1) The object itself could be a source of sound, and as such it would be localized by any person with normal hearing. (2) There is nearly always a certain amount of random sound in any region, for absolute quiet is rare indeed. The presence of an object will affect the character of these random sounds, and they will also be reflected from it. A blind man could get clues in that manner. (3) An object can also indicate its presence by obstructing random sound or sound from other objects. Perceiving its sound shadow indicates something about the location of an object. (4) Finally, as we have seen, the blind man like the bat, frequently makes his own sound, the echoes of which, being localized, reveal the position of the object reflecting the echoes. There can be little doubt that echoes play an important role in the auditory perception of the position of silent objects, and we may accept the conclusion that blind men, as well as bats, use echolocation for their orientation in space.

The blind man's ability at echolocation, remarkable as it is, cannot, however, compare in refinement to the bat's. A blind man is expert if he can detect a lamp post six inches in diameter, but flying bats can dodge wires as small across as one millimeter. This three hundredfold difference in minimum perceptible size of a remote obstacle far exceeds the ratio in size between bats and men and likewise the difference in wave length of the sounds employed. It represents largely the difference in perceptual skill between an animal whose sensory world is largely auditory and a man who ordinarily relies primarily on vision and has learned only under stress of necessity to use his sense of hearing for topographical orientation. A congenitally

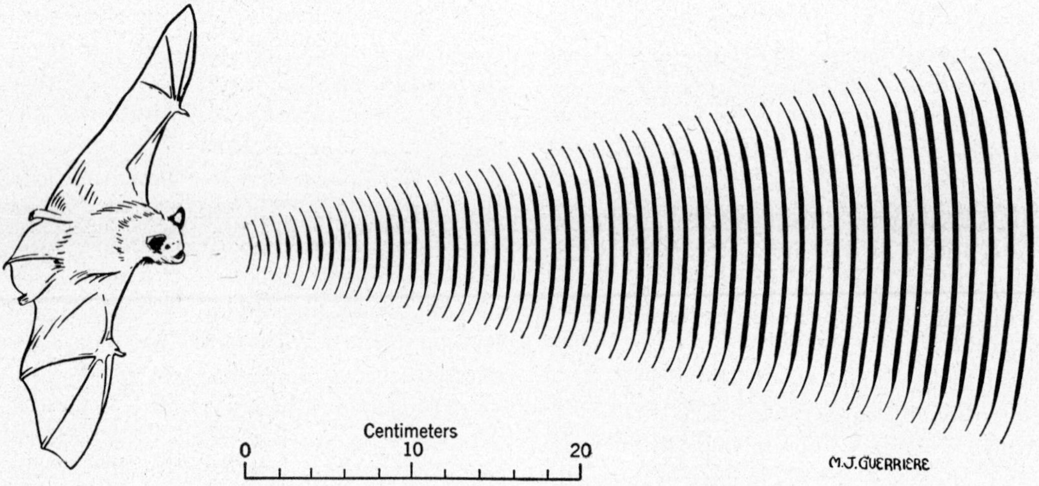

FIGURE 194. A FLYING BAT AND ITS ULTRASONIC CRY

The curved lines represent individual sound waves of a single pulse. Bats emit as many as 50 of these pulses per second and locate obstacles by hearing the echoes. The sound waves are represented here in true proportion to the size of the bat, and it is clear that the entire pulse occupies only a space of about a foot. This permits even objects at a short distance to be perceived without overlap of the original pulse and the returning echo.

blind man with special training from infancy on might be able to develop a skill at echolocation rivaling the bat's.

Other Problems of Animal Orientation

There are other infrahuman animals which keep themselves oriented under circumstances where a man would be quite unable to do so. In some of these cases we know the clues and the sense organs which are involved; in others we do not.

Animals such as dogs, cats, foxes and deer have the sense of smell far better developed than man. A hunting dog following the trail of a rabbit is analogous to the man following a marked path; here the edges of the path are fixed by the absence of rabbit scent. The direction in which to follow the trail presents a problem even to skilled dogs; they often start in the wrong direction and discover their error only after some distance, probably because of a decrease in the intensity of the scent.

Fish can detect food at distances of several feet through water, apparently because their chemical receptors are stimulated by molecules diffusing from the food material. Since fish can often turn quickly toward the food, they must perceive the direction from which the molecules are diffusing. Perhaps they do this on the basis of 'diffusion shadows' cast by their own bodies. If the food is to the fish's right, more molecules will strike the right side of its body than the left. Few details are known about the sensory basis of orientation or even the detection of food by other cold-blooded animals.

MIGRATION AND HOMING

Very remarkable is the ability of many animals to travel over long distances with a considerable degree of accuracy in their navigation. The annual flights of migratory birds are the most striking examples. Figure 195 shows the migration route of the golden plover, a bird which is little larger than a robin. It breeds on the shores of the Arctic Ocean and flies each year about eight thousand miles to a wintering range in South America. Furthermore, the route it follows during the southward autumn flight is quite different from its route returning in the spring. Other golden plovers migrate between Alaska and the Hawaiian Islands, and long overwater flights are regular occurrences with many other birds. In certain species the young birds apparently perform their first migration without the company of the older birds who might act as guides.

Long annual migrations are not confined to birds. Seals and whales migrate thousands of miles. Even some bats, dependent as they are on echolocation, manage to migrate at least five hundred miles between summer and winter quarters. Fish present us with equally baffling instances. Salmon spawn in fresh-water streams which are often tributaries of large rivers. Some species descend the rivers and swim many miles into the ocean, well away from the influence of the river water; yet in subsequent seasons they return to their own spawning grounds, not only finding the river as it flows into the sea but also selecting the correct tributary. Eels migrate in the opposite direction, spawning in mid-Atlantic and migrating slowly as immature fish toward the coast, where they find their way into rivers and streams. Even butterflies migrate; one species emerges from cocoons in North Africa, and the individuals fly north and west across western Europe as far as the British Isles and even Iceland.

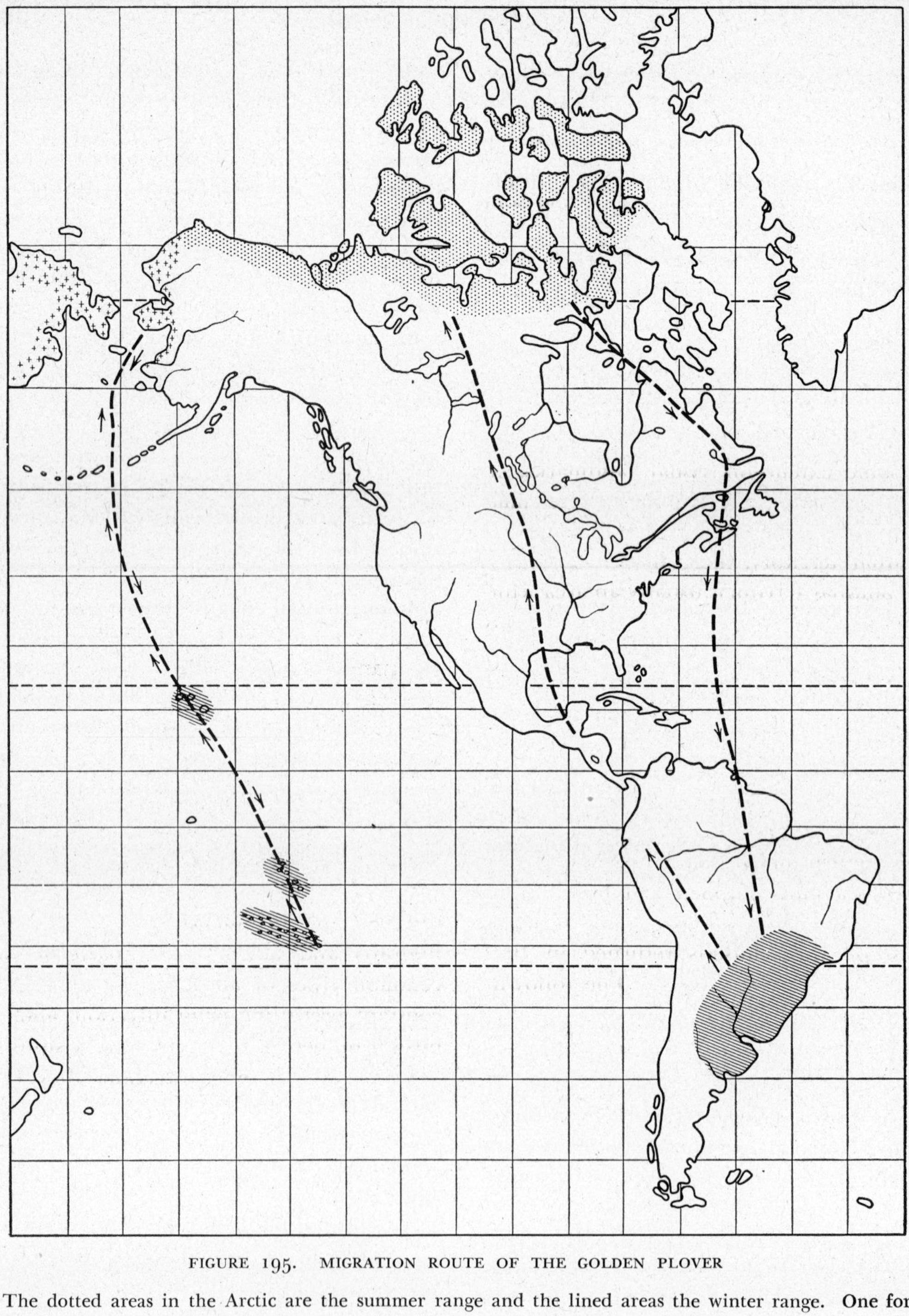

FIGURE 195. MIGRATION ROUTE OF THE GOLDEN PLOVER

The dotted areas in the Arctic are the summer range and the lined areas the winter range. One form migrates across Canada to South America. The other goes from Alaska to Hawaii and the South Seas. [Reproduced by permission of the U. S. Department of Agriculture, *Circular* 363, Fig. 22.]

The Sensory Basis of Migration

To date no truly satisfactory answer can be given to the question, "How do animals find their way about?"

Birds have been most studied, and some information has been obtained from homing experiments in which a migratory flight is simulated by removing birds from their nests and releasing them at a distance. Many wild birds will return to their nests, like homing pigeons, from one thousand miles or more away. The results of such homing experiments show that birds rely to some extent on visual landmarks, for when experimental shipments are made over equal distances into familiar and unfamiliar territory, more birds return from the familiar territory, usually an area which they were known to have traversed previously during their natural migration. Also the speed of the return flight is higher, on the average, from familiar territory. Furthermore, birds which have returned from unfamiliar territory evidently learn new landmarks in the process; after a second shipment to the same release point, they return much sooner. For instance, three sea gulls shipped 250 miles inland from their nests on an island near the coast of Massachusetts returned in 10, 6 and 4½ *days* respectively. The following year they were shipped again to the same release point and returned in 29, 18 and 48 *hours*. The first two birds required only one-eighth as long to make the second trip as the first.

But something more than visual landmarks seems necessary to account for the longer homing flights and natural migrations. For instance, one strictly marine species, the shearwater, has been shipped from a nesting island off the coast of Wales to points in the Swiss Alps and to Venice, Italy. Shearwaters never normally fly any appreciable distance inland; only during the nesting season do they come to land at all (usually on small islands). The rest of their lives are spent at sea. Furthermore, this particular species is not found in the Mediterranean. Clearly both Venice and the Swiss Alps lie in totally unfamiliar territory, yet both of the shearwaters shipped to Venice returned, one in 14 days, and three out of twelve came back from the Alps after 13 to 17 days.

Sensitivity to the earth's magnetic field has been postulated as a means by which birds might navigate over these long distances, but there is no physiological evidence that birds have such sensitivity any more than men. In some cases the direction of the sun may be used as a clue to direction, yet some birds migrate at night, in overcast weather and in fog. Another possibility is that birds are aware of the prevailing wind direction when various types of air mass cover the region through which they are traveling. Air masses are bodies of air several hundred miles in extent which are characterized by temperature, degree of visibility (the distance we can see) and turbulence (the presence of updrafts and downdrafts). Each of the common types of air mass has a roughly constant prevailing wind direction, and, if birds can perceive temperature, visibility, turbulence and wind direction, they can perhaps find their way over long distances with considerable success by flying upwind, downwind, crosswind or quartering, whichever is appropriate to the situation. Some migrating birds have actually been observed to change the direction of their flight with shifts in the direction of the wind. This hypothesis of navigation, based on atmospheric clues, is, however, largely speculative at present, and it is obviously not applicable to the migration of fish.

Some men have also developed an ability to navigate without obvious sensory clues. Among the best examples, so far studied only casually, are certain fishermen who spend much of their time sailing in small boats through foggy waters. Often they can steer a course for several miles, from one island to another, through thick fog, without benefit of compass or other instrumental aid, allowing for the effects of wind and strong tidal currents, and striking the desired landfall with an angular error of only a very few degrees. The sensory basis of their ability is as obscure as the migratory birds'.

REFERENCES

1. Boring, E. G. (Ed.). *Psychology for the armed services.* Washington: Infantry Journal, 1945. Chap. 8.

   A twelve-page chapter on how to get to strange places, how to get home and how to find your way when lost.

2. Hayes, S. P. *Contributions to a psychology of blindness.* New York: American Foundation for the Blind, 1941. Chap. 3.

   A chapter which gives a good account of the early experiments on 'facial vision' and the avoidance of obstacles by the blind.

3. Lincoln, F. C. *The migration of American birds.* New York: Doubleday Doran, 1939.

   A well-known classic study of bird migrations written by an ornithologist. It contains numerous maps showing the courses of the migrations.

4. Thompson, A. L. *The problems of bird migration.* London: Witherby, 1926.

   A descriptive study of the problems involved in bird migration.

5. Warden, C. J., Jenkins, T. N., and Warner, L. H. *Comparative psychology, a comprehensive treatise: vertebrates.* New York: Ronald Press, 1936.

   Brief discussions of homing in animals. See pp. 236-249 *et passim,* using the index.

6. Watson, J. B., and Lashley, K. S. *Homing and related activities of birds.* Washington: Carnegie Institute, 1915. Pp. 9–60.

   An account of some experiments on homing, a review of the theories, a sound discussion which is now out of date but dispenses with many current mysteries.

CHAPTER 18

Individual Differences

INDIVIDUAL differences in behavior are characteristic of all living organisms. Casual or superficial acquaintance with a group, even within our own species, often creates an erroneous impression of uniformity and leads to the false generalizations at the basis of many of our social stereotypes. "All cats look gray at night," but upon closer acquaintance each becomes an individual in his own right. Not only within the human species, but also among lower forms, wide variations in individual capacity and behavior are to be found.

Every laboratory investigation employing more than one animal subject reveals extensive individual variation. Such variation has been observed in amount of spontaneous activity, in relative strengths of needs, in speed of movement, in speed of learning and in problem solving. In experiments on conditioning, for example, the number of trials required to establish a given conditioned response ranged from 79 to 284 in a group of 82 protozoa; in a similar conditioning experiment with 14 crustaceans, the range of trials was from 34 to 1112; in a group of 59 fish, from 3 to 35; among 13 pigeons, from 30 to 40; and among 11 sheep, from 3 to 17.

MEASUREMENT OF INDIVIDUAL DIFFERENCES

It has become increasingly evident in recent years that the more we know about individual differences in intelligence, in aptitudes for particular tasks and in the ability to make good adjustments in social living, the better able we shall be to train and guide the individual in making the most of his physical and mental equipment.

It is not enough to know the ways in which a single person differs from others. We must also know how in a particular way a number of persons differ with respect to one another. Only then can we properly judge the capacity of any one person relative to that of his fellows. The one reliable method of obtaining this knowledge is by measurement.

We have already considered some of the basic problems of psychological measurement in Chapter 11. We have seen that, in order to measure sensibility, special methods of measurement had to be invented and a unit of measurement found. In this chapter we shall see that many other methods have been devised to measure psychological capacities, abilities and aptitudes.

This chapter was prepared by Anne Anastasi of Fordham University.

They differ widely among themselves, but in principle they are all alike. They are called *psychological tests.*

Characteristics of a Psychological Test

Basically every psychological test is an objective and standardized measure of a sample of the individual's behavior. Such a test is merely a small sample of the type of behavior being explored. The psychologist proceeds in much the same way as, for example, the chemist who 'tests' a quantity of milk or iron by analyzing one or more samples of it and deducing from his results the approximate characteristics of the entire quantity. Similarly, when the psychologist wishes to measure an individual's vocabulary, arithmetic ability or hand coordination, he observes the person's performance with only a limited number of words, arithmetic problems or hand movements, carefully chosen so as to be typical of the total behavior he wishes to assess.

Standardization

If the results of a psychological test are to have value in diagnosing or predicting behavior, the testing procedure must be standardized. The standardization of a test consists in the establishment of *uniform conditions* for administering the test to all individuals, as well as a uniform method for evaluating responses. The one variable in a test situation is the person being tested. If all other conditions are kept rigidly constant, then (and then only) can differences in score be correctly attributed to the individual himself, who should be the sole variable.

Norms

When the testee has taken the test, the psychologist has for him a score, the total number of correct items, the time required to complete the task or some other objective index of response suited to the specific test content. That is the testee's *raw score.*

Such a raw score has little meaning in itself, however, because a psychological test imposes no arbitrary, predetermined standards of 'passing' or 'failing.' Thus a score of 78 items correct out of 100 on a particular test of arithmetic reasoning could indicate an excellent performance, or it could be just fair, or quite inferior. The evaluation of the raw score depends upon *norms,* which must be objectively determined for each test before it can be put to practical use. A norm is simply the normal or average performance on the test in question. If we are designing a test for 8-year-olds, we must first administer it to a large, representative group of 8-year-olds in order to determine what is the average 8-year-old performance. Then if we find, for example, that the average 8-year-old completes 6 out of 15 problems correctly, a raw score of 6 becomes the 8-year norm on this test. Such a norm can then be used in the future in evaluating the performance of any 8-year-old child we wish to examine.

Raw scores are frequently translated into *percentile norms* in order to express their relationship to the performance of the group used for standardization. A percentile is the percentage of individuals who fall below the given score. Thus if 65 per cent of the subjects in the standardization group score below 20 in a vocabulary test, a raw score of 20 on this test corresponds to a percentile of 65. Thus to know that an individual has received a percentile score of 65 *on any test* enables us to conclude immediately that his performance excels that of the lower 65 per cent of the standardization group on that test.

The fiftieth percentile score is obviously the midpoint or average score. The zero percentile signifies a score below the lowest of any in the standardization group; the one hundredth percentile is above the best score obtained by anyone in the group. The former does not usually represent a zero raw score, nor the latter a perfect score. Percentile scores are expressed in terms of *people,* not the number of items passed. In a good test or examination the zero percentile should be above zero score, for a test on which anyone tested can get zero fails to show how much less than zero he might have got, had he but had the chance. Similarly every test and examination should have the one hundredth percentile below the perfect score, for the person who gets a perfect score has lost the chance to show how much better than perfect he can be in his performance. He is the victim of too easy a test.

Reliability

A test is said to have *reliability* if it gives the same results on different occasions. The reliability of a test refers to the consistency of the subjects' scores when they are tested again. You do not, of course, expect to get identically the same result on a second trial. The testee may have changed or the test may be working differently. You can rule out variation in the testee's ability by taking a large number of subjects. If the test then seems not to give consistent results, it lacks reliability and cannot be used for accurate measurement. You can measure the length of a room by a yardstick or by pacing the distance off. Which is more reliable? You can tell by seeing which method gives you more variability when you repeat the measurement. If the yardstick gives results varying between 23 feet 2 inches and 23 feet 2½ inches, and if pacing gives results varying between 22½ feet and 23½ feet, it is plain that your yardstick is more reliable than your stride as a measuring instrument.

There are three ways in which the reliability of a test may be measured. (1) A large number of persons may be tested and then retested, and their scores on the test and the retest compared. (2) A test, which consists of many items, may be divided in half, and scores obtained from one half the items taken alone compared with scores from the other half. (3) Different forms of the test may be constructed, as is necessary if experience with one form makes retesting unfair, and the scores of many persons on each of the forms can be compared. A coefficient of correlation (see below) may be used to measure these relationships and thus the reliability.

Validity

The degree to which the test actually succeeds in measuring what it sets out to measure is called its *validity.* In order to determine test validity, it is necessary to have an independent *criterion* of the trait being measured, so that the results of the test can be compared with the criterion, validated against it. For example, in validating a test of musical aptitude, actual performance by the testees in music schools was used as the criterion. A test designed for the selection of taxicab drivers would be validated against subsequent job performance of a sample of the group of drivers—for example, against the numbers of their accidents. A scholastic aptitude test for college freshmen would be checked against the students' grades in college courses. If a test has high validity, those persons scoring high on the test will do well in their subsequent performance on the job, in school or in whatever activity the test ought to predict; and conversely for those with low scores.

Two illustrations of test validation taken from the military use of tests in the Second World War are to be found in Figs. 196 and 197. Both are concerned with the validity of the Army General Classification Test (AGCT). Figure 196 indicates the degree to which this test could be used to predict the success of officer candidates. The actual commissioning of the men at the completion of their officer-training course was the criterion. The data on 5520 officer candidates distributed in fourteen schools suggest a fairly close correspondence between test score and criterion. Thus, of the men scoring 140 or higher on the test, over 90 per cent received commissions. Of those scoring under 110, on the other hand, less than 50 per cent succeeded in obtaining the commission, although they had gone through the same training course.

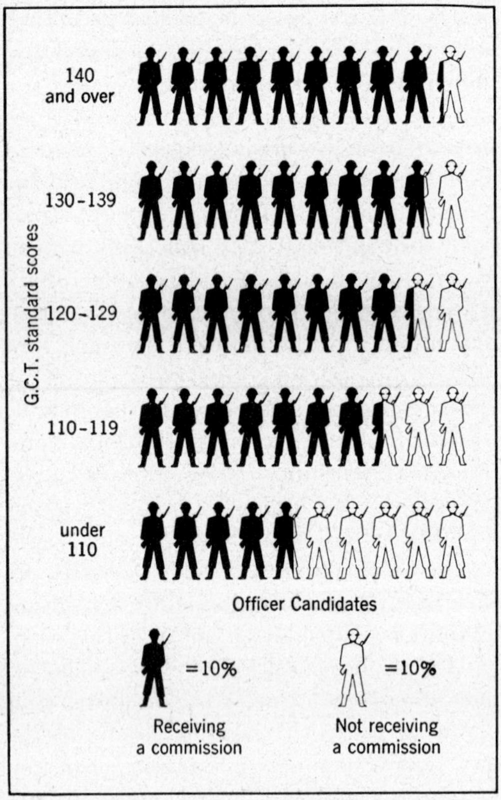

FIGURE 196. TEST VALIDATION WITH OFFICER CANDIDATES

Shows the percentage of officer candidates in the U. S. Army who received their commissions in relation to their scores on the Army General Classification Test (14 schools, 5520 men). [From E. G. Boring (Ed.), *Psychology for the armed services,* Infantry Journal, 1945, p. 242.]

Similar data for tank mechanics are given in Fig. 197. Grades obtained in a tank mechanics course constituted the criterion for this group. The figure shows that the AGCT score (lower half of the figure) predicts success well. It is hardly worth while to train men in groups III, IV or V. The upper half of the figure shows that the amount of schooling which the men had is not so good a criterion in predicting success as the AGCT score.

The Correlation Coefficient

In measuring either the reliablity or the validity of a test, the *closeness of correspondence* between two sets of measures must be ascertained. A single index of such correspondence is furnished by the coefficient of correlation (r), a value which can vary numerically from $+1.00$, a perfect positive correlation, through 0, to -1.00, a perfect negative or inverse correlation.

A correlation of $+1.00$ between the results of two tests means that all the persons tested on the two tests rank in the same order on each, and that their scores are proportionally spaced in the same way on the scale of each test. If you measure the heights of people in inches and in centimeters, you should find a perfect correlation between the two measurements, $r = +1.00$. Usually a perfect correlation is

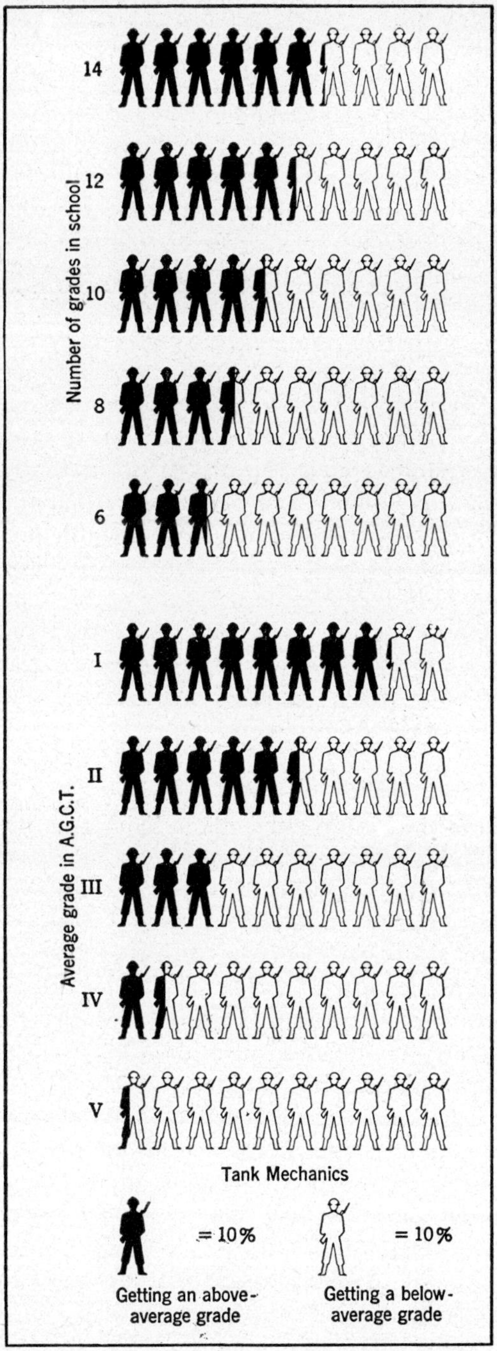

FIGURE 197. TEST VALIDATION WITH TANK MECHANICS

taken to mean that the tests correlated are measuring the same thing.

A good example of a perfect negative correlation, $r = -1.00$, comes from physics. If you can keep the temperature of an amount of air constant, you can halve the volume by doubling the pressure, or you can halve the pressure by doubling the volume. $r = -1.00$. Negative correlations sometimes mean, however, that the scale of measurement should be reversed. If industry and poverty were to be found negatively correlated, undoubtedly industry and wealth would be positively correlated, since wealth is the opposite of poverty.

A zero correlation means that there is no relationship at all. You would expect a zero correlation between the heights of adults and their intelligences. Zero correlation is the indicator of complete independence. Tall adults are neither brighter nor duller than short ones, but you would not get zero correlation with children, for the children grow both brighter and taller at the same time.

The meaning of a correlation coefficient may be further clarified by reference to Table XX, which shows, by means of a *scatter diagram,* the relationship between intelligence test scores and school grades in a group of 480 students. The numbers in each box or *cell* of the scatter diagram represent the *number of people* who fall within each category or *class interval* with reference both to intelligence score and to school grades. We can see at once from the

---

Shows the percentage of men receiving an above-average grade in tank mechanics course in relation to score on the Army General Classification Test. The relationship between school grade and performance in tank mechanics course is included for comparative purposes. [From E. G. Boring (Ed.), *Psychology for the armed services,* Infantry Journal, 1945, p. 251.]

diagram that correlation is positive and neither zero nor +1.00. The upper left and lower right corners of the table are empty. There are no children with very high school grades and very low intelligence, nor with very low grades and very high intelligence. Still there is a great deal of scattering; we could not predict school grades accurately from intelligence scores, nor conversely. Actually the coefficient of correlation for this table is $r = +0.460$. That is moderately high, yet far from perfect.

A glance at Table XX as a whole immediately reveals the fact that the subjects tend to cluster in an area of the table which extends diagonally from lower left to upper right. This means that, in gen-

TABLE XIX

Scatter Diagram for a Low Correlation

$r = +0.128$ $N = 216$ cases

Mechanical Skill	Mental Age: 4	5	6	7	8	9	10	11	12	13	14	15
43–45										1		
40–42												
37–39					1				1			
34–36		1		2	1							
31–33					1	1						
28–30				2	2	1						
25–27		1	2	2	3		1		2			
22–24		1		2	1	1	2		2			
19–21			1	4	3	4		1				
16–18		1	2	3	4	2	2	1				
13–15			2	3	4	6		1	1			
10–12		1	2	7	6	7	4	1				
7– 9		1	7	6	11	7	3		1	1		
4– 6	1	1	11	13	12	7	4		1			1
0– 3	1		5	4	4	4		1	1	1		

TABLE XX

SCATTER DIAGRAM FOR A CORRELATION OF INTERMEDIATE VALUE

$r = +0.460$ $N = 480$ cases

School Grades	Intelligence Test Scores									
	Below 85	85–89	90–94	95–99	100–104	105–109	110–114	115–119	120–124	Above 124
90 and over				3	3	15	12	9	9	5
85–89				8	17	15	24	13	6	6
80–84			4	6	22	21	20	10	5	1
75–79			7	25	33	23	10	7	4	
70–74		4	10	18	14	22	12	1	1	
65–69	1	3	3	12	7	8	8	1		
60–64			2	5	3	1	1			

eral, those students who received poorer grades (lower part of the table) also had relatively low intelligence test scores (left part of the table), and those receiving good grades tended to score higher on the intelligence test. For the correlation to be a perfect +1.00, however, all entries would be in a single diagonal row, a relation approximated in Table XXI, where the correlation is +0.994.

Further light on the meaning of a coefficient of correlation is obtained by comparing Tables XIX, XX and XXI, which show the scatter diagrams for correlations of +0.128, +0.460 and +0.994, respectively. The correlation between mental age and mechanical skill shown in Table XIX is only a little removed from a random scatter. We do not take such a correlation seriously unless it is for a very large number of cases, or its lowness as such has significance. Table XX, as we have just seen, shows a definite positive relation between school grades and intelligence scores. This is the sort of relationship that keeps turning up; two measures of ability vary together, yet are by no means identical. You can say of such abilities that they have a common factor and that each also has a specific factor. Table XXI shows a correlation that is nearly +1.00. It means that the two measures are measuring practically the same thing. We can see how that is, when we note that the table gives the correlation between raw Alpha test scores and weighted Alpha test scores. The scores were supposed to have been improved by the use of statistical weights, but the table shows that the weights did little good.

The coefficient of correlation is negative when high rank in one ability is related to low rank in a second ability (see Fig. 199).

Figure 198 shows five scatter diagrams for different degrees of correlation varying from $r = 0$ to $r = 1.00$. These are actual photographs of the way a beam of electrons varies at random right and left, and also up and down, when the variation is controlled by the random movements of elec-

TABLE XXI

Scatter Diagram for a High Correlation

$r = +0.994$ $N = 2856$ cases

Alpha Test: Weighted Scores

Alpha Test: Raw Scores	0–9	10–19	20–29	30–39	40–49	50–59	60–69	70–79	80–89	90–99	100–109	110–119	120–129	130–139	140–149	150–159	160–169	170–179	180–189	190–199	200–209	210–219	220–229	230–239	240–249	250–259	260–269	270–279	280–289	290–299	300–309	310–319	320–329	330–339	340–349	350–359
180																																			1	1
175																																	1			
170																																				
165																																	1			
160																																3	1			
155																														1	2					
150																																				
145																											1	1	2	1						
140																											1	3	1							
135																											2	5								
130																									1	4	4	1								
125																								1	4	2										
120																							2	3	9		1									
115																							2	2	2											
110																						4	2	4	2											
105																				1	1	5	1													
100																				2	5	2	1													
95																			1	9	3															
90																		5	10	7	2															
85																		6	7		2															
80															1	4	8	5	3																	
75															4	14	11	4																		
70															4	6	4																			
65												2	3	11	6	2																				
60												1	10	15	3																					
55												7	13	4																						
50										2	7	6	4																							
45									3	4	9	3																								
40							1	2	6	12	3																									
35							2	8	13	6																										
30						3	10	16	3																											
25					1	17	10	8																												
20				4	12	15	2																													
15			3	10	9	2																														
10			21	15																																
5	1	22	10																																	
0–4	40	9																																		

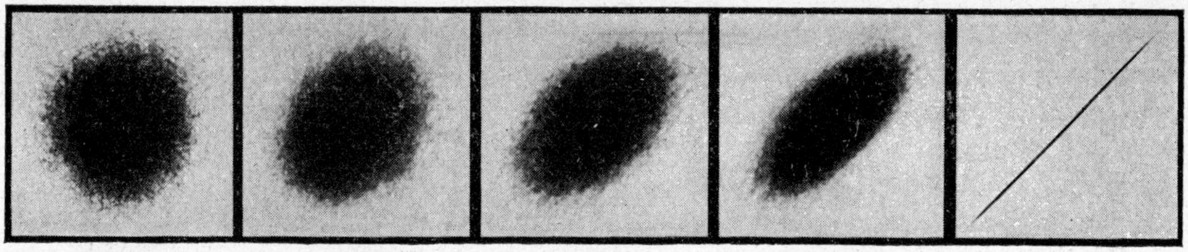

FIGURE 198. SCATTER DIAGRAMS FOR CORRELATIONS FROM $r = 0$ TO $r = 1.00$

Photographs of a beam of electrons impinging on the screen of an oscilloscope. A voltage with random variation (the kind used to produce white noises; see p. 315) is used to make the beam vary at random horizontally. You would then see a horizontal line. Similarly another random voltage makes the beam vary vertically. If the two voltages, each varying randomly and having no relation to each other, act simultaneously, the projected beam will fill the field, producing the circular scatter diagram for $r = 0$. If the same random voltage is used at the same time for both horizontal and vertical variation, you get the line for the perfect correlation, $r = 1.00$. The intermediate diagrams are obtained by keeping some of the variation in the two voltages independent, while making the remainder of the variation common to both voltages. [Courtesy of J. C. R. Licklider.]

trons in another stream. The correlation is zero when the right-left and up-down variations have nothing in common. It is perfect (+1.00) when the same random variation controls both the right-left and up-down movement of the beam. It is intermediate when the two variations are partly the same and partly different.

The uses of correlation coefficients in psychology are many. In test construction, the *validity coefficient* is the correlation between test scores and the criterion measure on a group of subjects. Similarly, the *reliability coefficient* is the correlation between two scores on the same test, obtained by retesting, parallel forms, or split-half procedures. The chief use of the correlation coefficient is, however, the determination of the relationship between two abilities. Will ability to pass a certain test predict ability to do a certain job? Are the skills required in two different jobs the same, similar or different? When a man has learned one of the jobs, how much of the other one has he learned? It will be by answering many such questions that the inventory of human abilities will finally be made out.

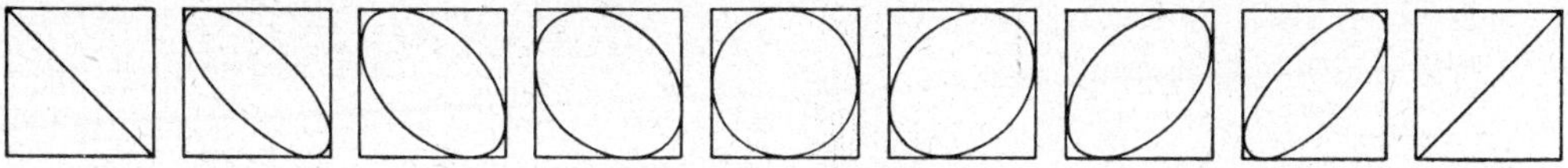

FIGURE 199. COEFFICIENTS OF CORRELATION AND SCATTER DIAGRAMS

The lines and ellipses of scatter diagrams which show the relationships between two variables for coefficients of correlation from $r = -1.00$ through $r = 0$ to $r = +1.00$. Figure 198 shows the correlations for the actual photographed scatter of electrons for different degrees of correlation. This figure shows the same relation with the ellipses computed mathematically and indicates further the relation between negative and positive correlations. [Courtesy of J. C. R. Licklider.]

INTELLIGENCE TESTING

During the last forty years the concept of intelligence has grown and changed with the development of the intelligence tests. In general intelligence is thought of as *general ability,* a *common factor* in a wide variety of *special aptitudes.* The concept becomes clearer as the discussion continues.

The Binet Tests

The first intelligence test was prepared by the French psychologist, Alfred Binet. In 1904 the French Minister of Public Instruction appointed a committee to investigate the causes of retardation among public school children. Binet was a member of this committee. As a direct outgrowth of his work on this committee, Binet published (with a collaborator) the 1905 scale for measuring intelligence. This scale consisted of thirty problems arranged in an approximate order of difficulty. In 1908 appeared Binet's first revision of the scale, in which the tests were grouped into age levels, and he introduced the concept of *mental age.* In such a scale, the tests are assigned to 'year levels' on the basis of the performance of representative groups of children of different ages. Thus tests passed as often as not by the 8-year-olds are grouped into the 8-year level, those passed as often as not by the 9-year-olds into the 9-year level, etc. A child's score on the scale is then expressed as the mental age (M.A.) that he is able to reach. If, for example, he passes all tests assigned to the 10-year level and none at the 11-year level, he has a mental age of 10, regardless of what his chronological age (C.A.) may be, because he has succeeded as well as the average 10-year-old and no better. If his C.A. is 8, such a child would be two years accelerated in his intellectual performance; if he is 11 years old, he would be one year retarded.

The Binet tests have been translated into more than a dozen languages, and their use has spread to every continent. In America five independent revisions have appeared, of which the best known is the Stanford-Binet, prepared by L. M. Terman and his associates at Stanford University. In his first revision of the Binet scale, appearing in 1916, Terman increased the number of tests, substituted some new tests for less suitable ones in the original scale, and revised others. The scale was readjusted on the basis of American norms. The most far-reaching innovation in this revision, however, was the introduction of the concept of the *Intelligence Quotient* (IQ). The IQ is the ratio of Mental Age to Chronological Age, multiplied by 100 to get rid of decimals. IQ = 100 M.A./C.A. Thus, if a child of 10 passes the 12-year level, he will have an IQ of $100 \times 12/10 = 120$. If he just passes his normal level for 10 years, his IQ will be $100 \times 10/10 = 100$. If he can pass the 9-year level and no more, then he is retarded with an IQ of $100 \times 9/10 = 90$.

The chief advantage of the IQ, as contrasted with a statement of mental-age retardation or acceleration as used by Binet, is its comparability at different ages. An IQ of 100 means a normal performance regardless of the child's age; IQ's of 80 or 120 represent comparable degrees of retardation and acceleration, respectively, at all ages. In terms of M.A., however, a retardation of one year in a 4-year-old child (IQ = 75) is a more serious degree of backwardness than a retardation of one year in a 12-year-old (IQ = 92). This follows from the fact that intellectual development is more rapid during early life and exhibits a gradual slowing down with increasing age. There is a more marked difference between the behavior of the average 3-year-olds and 4-year-olds than there is between 11-year-olds and 12-year-olds. Actually, the child who is retarded one year at the age of 4, is likely, when retested at age 12, to be found to be three years retarded (IQ =75). Under these circumstances, the IQ, being a relative measure, remains constant. It is clear that mental-age deviations from the norm increase with age and that the IQ tends to remain approximately constant throughout life, provided that the individual is not subjected to drastic environmental changes or other unusual conditions.

On most intelligence scales of the Binet type, the average individual does not improve in performance with age beyond 15 years. The average 22-year-old or 30-year-old would thus do no better on the Stanford-Binet test than the average 15-year-old. For this reason, in computing the IQ of an adult on such a test, the C.A. is taken arbitrarily as 15. That is because the M.A. of the average adult is 15. That creates a complication. An M.A. of 12 is the average performance for persons 12 years old. An M.A. of 18 is *not* the average performance of persons 18 years old. Persons 18 years old have an M.A. of 15, the M.A. of the average adult. An M.A. of 18 means merely that statistical analysis indicates such a person to be about as much brighter than a person with an M.A. of 15, as the M.A. = 15 is brighter than M.A. = 12.

There are, in these scales, three "Superior Adult" levels (S.A. I, S.A. II and S.A. III) of increasing difficulty. Mental ages—and the IQ's derived from them—are not, however, well suited to testing adults. Other types of scores, such as percentiles, and other specially designed tests, are more commonly used in the testing of adults. The Stanford-Binet itself has undergone repeated revision. Its latest revision, the Terman-Merrill Scale, appeared in 1937.

The content of the Stanford-Binet examination samples a wide variety of intellectual functions in the effort to arrive at the subject's 'general mental level.' A few examples will suggest the range covered. At the lower age levels many of the tests involve the manipulation or identification of objects; the standard materials employed in such tests are reproduced in Fig. 200. For example, at the 2-year level the child identifies, by pointing, small toy objects such as cat, button, thimble and cup, as the examiner names each object. At a slightly higher level, similar objects (toy cup, shoe, penny) are identified in terms of use, the examiner saying, "Show me what we drink out of," "Show me what goes on our feet," etc. Identification of pictures of objects in terms of use or other characteristics occurs at the 4-year level. Memory tests are included at several levels, involving objects, pictures, numbers, words, sentences and the content of a passage. A vocabulary test, consisting of 45 words steeply graded in difficulty, from *orange* and *envelope* to *homunculus, sudorific* and *parterre,* extends from the 6-year level to Superior Adult level III. Naming similarities among objects is also found at several levels; for example, "In what way are wood and coal alike?" (year VII); "In what way are a teacher, a book and a newspaper alike?" (year XI); "What is the principal way in which farming and manufacturing are alike?" (S.A. I). The detection of absurdities in pictures and in short passages likewise appears at various year levels. For example, a 9-year-old should be able to say

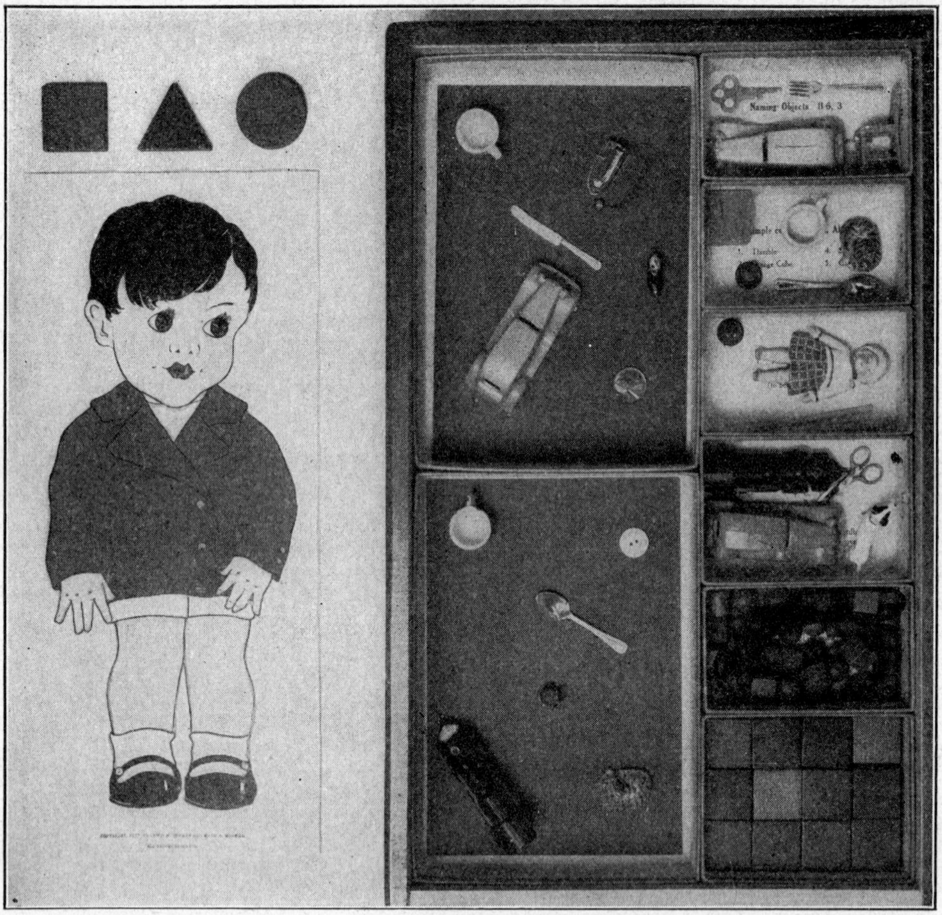

FIGURE 200. SOME MATERIALS USED IN ADMINISTERING THE STANFORD-BINET INTELLIGENCE SCALE AT THE YOUNGER AGE LEVELS

[Materials used by L. M. Terman and M. A. Merrill, *The new revised Stanford-Binet tests of intelligence,* Houghton Mifflin, 1937.]

what is foolish about this statement: "In an old graveyard in Spain they have discovered a small skull which they believe to be that of Christopher Columbus when he was about ten years old." Similarly, an 11-year-old should be able to detect the absurdity in the following: "When there is a collision the last car of the train is usually damaged most. So they have decided that it will be best if the last car is always taken off before the train starts."

Group Testing

The Binet type of test is known as an *individual test* since only one subject can be tested at a time. Because of the complexity of directions and scoring, furthermore, the administration of such tests requires a highly trained examiner. As long as this was the only type of available intelligence test, large-scale testing programs were not feasible. It is undoubtedly the development of *group tests* of intelligence which is largely responsible for the widespread popularity of mental testing. Group tests are not only designed for the simultaneous testing of large groups, but their administration has also been so simplified as to require relatively little training for the examiner. Scoring has also been highly simplified, some of the tests being adapted for scoring by electrical machine.

The immediate stimulus which led to the development of the first group test of intelligence was furnished by the urgent need for testing soldiers in the United States Army during the First World War. A quick, rough classification of the men with respect to intelligence was needed for many purposes, including discharge for mental defect, assignment to special battalions demanding a relatively low level of ability and selection for officer training. The test designed to meet this need was the well-known Army Alpha. Many revisions of this test have been prepared in the intervening years, and its latest revisions are still used today for civilian testing.

Alpha established a pattern, in both procedure and content, which has been closely followed in most group intelligence tests. On Alpha, as well as on most other group scales, performance is usually expressed in terms of percentiles or some other similar score which indicates in a convenient and comparable unit the subject's position relative to a group average.

Among the best-known intelligence tests for general adults is the Otis Self-Administering Test of Mental Ability (Otis S.A.). In this test the role of the examiner is reduced to a minimum since all necessary directions are printed on the test booklet. The examiner is needed only to see that proper testing conditions are maintained and to give the starting and stopping signals for the entire test.

The student is probably already familiar with at least one of the tests which have been especially designed for college freshmen. The American Council Psychological Examination, prepared under the auspices of the American Council on Education, and the Scholastic Aptitude Test of the College Entrance Examination Board are among the most widely used. A new form of such tests is prepared each year, and norms are computed for the several thousand college freshmen who are tested throughout the country every year.

During the Second World War, the United States Army developed the Army General Classification Test (AGCT), which was used in place of Alpha of the First World War. This test provided a means of classifying the men roughly according to their general ability to learn the various duties required in military life. It was prepared in four equivalent interchangeable forms, each requiring about one hour, including preliminary instructions, a fore-exercise and the test proper given with a 40-minute time limit. The test involved verbal, numerical and spatial skills, having its items arranged in order of difficulty. Upon arrival at a reception center, each man who could read English was given one of the four forms of the AGCT. On the basis of his performance, he was classified into one of five Army Grades. His score was also recorded on his Qualification Card in terms of a standard scale in which 100 represents the average score of men of military age. The scores on this scale corresponding to each of the five grades are as follows:

I	130 and over
II	110–129
III	90–109
IV	70–89
V	below 70

A more analytical score could be obtained by means of a later form of the AGCT test, requiring two hours and yielding separate scores in (1) verbal ability, (2) spatial comprehension, (3) arithmetic computation and (4) arithmetic reasoning.

Performance and Nonlanguage Tests

Early in the history of intelligence testing, psychologists began to realize that the Binet type of test, depending so largely upon language, is not suited to all types of persons. The testing of illiterates, the foreign-speaking, the deaf or those who have speech disabilities requires a different kind of test. *Performance tests* were designed to meet this need. Among the earliest was the Pintner-Paterson Scale (Fig. 201), consisting of fifteen tests which can be administered without the use of language, oral or written, on the part of either examiner or subject. Blocks, pictures of simple objects or scenes and geometric forms are the principal materials of these tests. In picture completion tests, for example, the subject inserts irregularly shaped blocks into a board to complete a picture, much in the manner of a jig-saw puzzle. Form-board tests, involving the insertion and assembling of variously shaped blocks to fill in recesses, vary from those simple enough for a preschool child to some which will baffle the average college student. Most of these tests are scored in terms of time required to complete the task, as well as number of errors. The scores can be interpreted as M.A. and IQ or as percentiles.

A more recently standardized performance test is the Arthur Performance Scale, consisting of ten of the original Pintner-Paterson tests, a series of paper maze tests and a block design test in which the subject duplicates with colored blocks the designs on a series of printed cards. All performance tests are by their very nature individual tests. Besides their usefulness in testing subjects with a language handicap, they are also sometimes employed to supplement the Binet type of test in order to achieve a better-rounded picture of the individual's abilities.

Nonlanguage scales are group scales for testing persons incapable of taking the usual intelligence scales. Unlike performance tests, they involve the use of paper and pencil rather than the manipulation of objects. They do not, however, require the ability to read or write anything but single digits. The subject uses a pencil merely to underline, cross out or connect items, or to make other nonlinguistic marks. The directions are given by blackboard demonstrations, charts, gestures and pantomime. As with the Alpha, speed of performance contributes to the score, since each test is given with a time limit too short to permit any but the very fastest to complete it. Special nonlanguage tests for the illiterate and foreign-speaking soldiers were also developed for use in the Second World War.

No one has as yet succeeded in creating a good international or so-called *culture-free test.* All the tests depend upon language and other ideas peculiar to the particular culture for which the test was constructed. Until such tests are made, however, it is not possible safely to use test results to compare the 'intelligence' of different nations or 'races.'

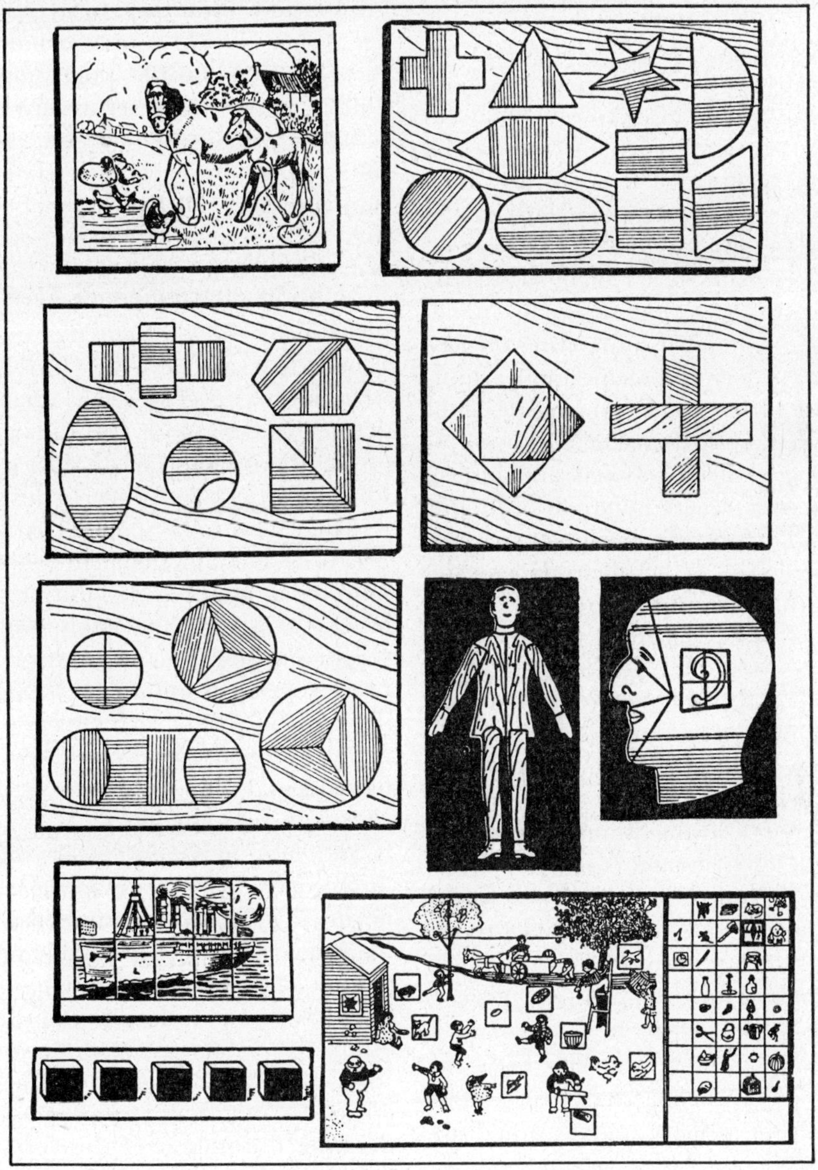

FIGURE 201. MATERIALS FOR ADMINISTERING THE PINTNER-PATERSON PERFORMANCE SCALE

[From C. H. Stoelting, *Catalogue of apparatus, tests and supplies,* 1939, p. 172.]

Testing Infants and Preschool Children

A recent development in mental testing is the construction of scales for measuring the intelligence of very young children, some scales extending down almost to birth. Infant tests, covering the period from birth to about 1½ years, are often essentially a series of developmental norms which can be applied to an evaluation of the child's everyday behavior in such activities as crawling, walking, sitting up, standing, picking up and manipulating objects, recognizing colors and shapes and acquiring the use of language. Among the most accurately established and extensive norms are those prepared by Gesell and his coworkers at Yale, where hundreds of infants have been periodically examined in practically every type of behavior under carefully controlled conditions (p. 78).

Preschool tests, generally designed for children between the ages of 1½ and 5, present the child with simple, standardized tasks. Many involve motor coordination, as in throwing a ball, folding paper, cutting with scissors, inserting buttons in buttonholes and copying simple geometric figures such as circles and crosses. Some of them test the development of perceptual skills, as in color and form matching, recognizing oneself in a mirror, identification of pictures and picture completion. Executing simple commissions, as in response to the directions to "take the box from the table and put it on the chair," as well as simple tests of memory and learning, are also used.

Infant and preschool tests have proved highly sensitive in detecting individual differences in behavior, wide differences in score being revealed even among the youngest subjects tested. These tests furnish an effective practical technique for the comparison of the developmental status of any given child with the norms for his own age. The use of scores obtained below the age of 6 for the prediction of later 'intelligence' is, however, regarded as questionable by most psychologists. In general, follow-up studies have as yet failed to substantiate the predictive value of such measures.

Evaluation of Intelligence Tests

To make the most effective use of intelligence tests, we must be clearly aware of what not to expect as well as what to expect of them. Only with the full recognition of such limitations can we determine when to use the tests and how to interpret the results. The rapid popularization resulting from the development of easily administered group scales during the First World War was inevitably followed by skepticism since many fantastic expectations remained unfulfilled. Nevertheless the proved value of such tests as the AGCT in the Second World War attested to the fundamental soundness of intelligence tests when properly applied.

The first consideration in interpreting intelligence test scores is to remember that no intelligence test measures native capacity independently of the individual's background of experience. Only insofar as the testees have had common opportunities for acquiring the same general information and skills can the differences in test scores be diagnostic of future performance. An interesting illustration of this fact is offered by some of the results obtained with the United States Army's Special Training Units in the Second World War. Following an intensive twelve-week course of instruction in these units, many men whose initial AGCT score placed them in Army Grade V were able to raise their standing to Army Grade IV or even higher. Most of the men selected for such training were either illiterate or had a very inferior educational background. Had the initial classification of these men been regarded as an index of their 'native intellectual capacity' without reference to their poor education and other experiences, the possibility of raising them to Grade IV level would have been overlooked.

In constructing any intelligence test, the effort is made to include only materials which are common to the experience of all individuals to be tested, so that everyone will at least have had the opportunity to acquire the necessary information in the course of his everyday experiences. Care is exercised to avoid special information or skills which are not available to all subjects. On the other hand, it is obvious that the common knowledge upon which intelligence tests are based is common only within certain limits. It follows that, to have full diagnostic significance, intelligence tests should be given only to persons whose backgrounds are similar to the background of the group by which the test was standardized. Only in that way can the effect of previous experience be held sufficiently constant or be ruled out for practical purposes. It follows also that in interpreting any intelligence test score, knowledge of the subject's education, socioeconomic level and similar environmental conditions is essential.

A second consideration is that no intelligence test samples all intellectual functions to an equal degree. Most tests are overloaded by one or two types of ability. Tests, such as the Binet, the National Intelligence Test and the Otis, are predominantly verbal or linguistic in content, with some dependence on numerical ability, but making little if any use of spatial or mechanical insight. It is for this reason that routine clerical workers, for example, frequently do better on such tests of 'intelligence' than persons in high-grade mechanical jobs which require considerable judgment and originality. In brief, most of the 'intelligence' tests are in large measure, though not entirely, tests of verbal aptitude.

An examination of the criteria against which intelligence tests are validated provides illuminating data on what it is that such tests are actually measuring. One of the most common criteria is school achievement. If those individuals receiving high test scores do well in school and those receiving low test scores do relatively poorly, we conclude that the intelligence test in question has high validity. This means, of course, that the test is effective in predicting scholastic aptitude or those abilities which are important for success in school work. The verbal nature of so much of our school instruction is undoubtedly an important factor in this correlation.

We should also note that not all tests labeled 'intelligence' measure the same combination of abilities. Performance and nonlanguage tests, for example, stress spatial insight to a greater extent. It is not enough to know a child's IQ. We must also know on what test it was obtained. It is entirely possible for the same child to receive a high IQ on one occasion and a considerably lower one on another, not because the tests are unreliable or because the individual's intellect fluctuates haphazardly, but because different abilities were measured on the two occasions by different tests.

Finally, we may ask why intelligence tests are not designed to cover equally *all* the individual's abilities. Would this not give us the 'general mental level' which would enable us to make predictions in all situations? To a certain extent, as more information was acquired regarding the organization of abilities, this has been done. For example, the inclusion of equal parts of materials for assessing verbal, numerical and spatial abilities in the AGCT, as contrasted with the predominantly verbal content of the old Army Alpha, was a move in this direction. The solution, however, is not so simple as it might seem. In the first place, for a number of purposes an intelligence test which is overloaded with certain functions, such as verbal ability, is more diagnostic than one which samples all functions equally. The classification of school children, the selection of college applicants, the evaluation of probable employee success in many types of positions, for example, are themselves largely dependent upon a knowledge of the individual's verbal ability. A test which reflects the same disproportionate representation of abilities will have higher validity in such situations.

A further point is that a single score indicating the average or general level of all the individual's abilities is not enough. For the most effective educational or vocational guidance, for selection of employees and in similar practical problems, it is necessary to know also the individual's strong and weak points. Two testees with identical IQ's or percentile scores may have very different patterns of abilities and disabilities, since the differences balance out and disappear in the total score. The increasing use of intelligence tests which yield partial scores is one solution for this problem. For example, both the American Council's Psychological Examination and the Scholastic Aptitude Test of the College Entrance Examination Board now report separate scores for verbal and numerical abilities for each student. The development of the later AGCT, which yields four separate scores, has already been described.

Another solution is the use of special aptitude tests to supplement the preliminary screening and classification provided by the intelligence tests. These tests are discussed in the following section.

MEASUREMENT OF SPECIAL APTITUDES

Tests of special aptitudes are now regularly employed in individual guidance as well as in industrial personnel selection. Although a general intelligence test is given as a preliminary instrument of classification for most jobs, such a measure is nearly always supplemented with more specific testing in especially relevant areas. Many of these tests are tailor-made for the particular job and are validated locally through a direct follow-up of a typical group of new employees. The United States Army and Navy also made much more extensive use of special ability tests in the Second World War than in the First, when such tests were almost nonexistent. Special *batteries* or combinations of tests were constructed for pilots, bombardiers, range-finder operators, radio operators and scores of the other specialized occupations of modern warfare. Tests of mechanical aptitude, clerical aptitude, motor dexterity, speed of reaction, visual and auditory acuity under different conditions, perception of distance or depth and radio code learning were among the special areas covered in such batteries.

Trait Variability

We have seen that the recognition of specialized abilities, or differences *within* the individual from trait to trait, has important practical implications in the interpretation of intelligence test scores as well as in the separate testing of special aptitudes. Such variation within the individual is known as *trait variability*. It can be readily seen by the examination of any individual's *psychograph*, that is to say, a graph showing the subject's relative standing in a series of different tests, with all scores reduced to such comparable units as percentiles or mental ages.

A more precise way of gauging the extent of such variability is illustrated in the following study. A group of 107 high school freshmen were given a series of 35 tests, some being parts of standardized intelligence tests and others being special tests of motor abilities, perception, attention and emotional characteristics. All scores were transmuted into the same kind of units, making direct comparison possible from one test to another. The extent of trait variability, based upon the differences between each person's own average and each of his 35 scores, was computed and was found to be almost as great as the variations in score from one person to another in any one test.

The study of individual cases exhibiting striking irregularities of mental development suggests the extremes of trait variability which may occur. From time to time, persons have been found who were so deficient in general intelligence that they had to be confined in institutions for the feebleminded but who were, nevertheless, remarkably gifted in some one trait. Mechanical aptitude, ability in drawing or painting, a phenomenal memory, arithmetic proficiency and musical talent have all been found as exceptional abilities of persons who seemed in every other respect to be feebleminded. There are also available descriptions of persons who are not in institutions, who are dull or mediocre in most respects, but who have a special gift along one particular line. It is also true that a pronounced deficiency in any one of these characteristics can occur in combination with superior general intelligence. It is noteworthy that verbal or linguistic abilities are conspicuously absent from these lists of special talents and defects. Good verbal ability does not occur in individuals of very low intelligence, or deficient verbal ability in those of high intelligence, for the reason that verbal ability is closely associated with general intelligence, as assessed by intelligence tests developed in and for our own culture.

Factor Analysis

The method of correlation is especially well adapted for the study of the relationships among traits. Suppose you have under consideration two abilities, like the capacities to perceive verbal analogies and spatial relations, and you have for each a particular test. You wish to find out whether the particular abilities which each test measures are related to each other or independent of each other. What do you do? You give both tests to a large number of persons whom you would expect to vary considerably among themselves in each of these abilities, and then you compute r, the coefficient of correlation. If r were to come out near zero, you would conclude that you had been testing two independent abilities. If r were very high (in this case it would not be), you would conclude that the two abilities were closely related, probably that they both depended principally on some common factor like general intelligence. If r were an intermediate value—say, 0.20 to 0.80—you would see that the two abilities that your two tests test are related; that they involve, perhaps, more or less of some factor common to both and, in addition, two specific factors, each of them involved in one test and not in the other. This is the simplest and usual correlational analysis of two test abilities: one common factor and two specific factors.

Usually, however, we are interested in many more tested abilities than two. In that case we can perform a general *factor analysis*. The tests are paired, and r is worked out for every pair. If there are n tests, there will be $n(n - 1)/2$ pairs of them —10 r's of 5 tests, 45 r's of 10 tests, 190 r's of 20 tests. If every test shows some significant positive correlation with every other test—not at all an unusual finding—we have evidence of the existence of a *general factor*, one which is common to all the abilities tested, as 'intelligence' has been thought to be. If several tests show intercorrelations with one another and not with the remaining tests, we have evidence of the existence of a *group factor* common to this group of tests. A battery of tests may involve quite a number of group factors. A test which stands off by itself and has only low correlations with the other tests gives evidence of a *specific factor*. The principal result of much work with factor analysis is finding that the tested abilities form groups or clusters because they involve common group factors.

The most clearly demonstrated group factors are the *verbal, numerical* and *spatial*. Tests of any one of these skills or insights show low correlations with the other two, whereas two tests in the same category show a high correlation. The verbal factor is, as we have seen, the most important in 'intelligence' tests, although the numerical and space-perceiving abilities may also be included, as they were by design in Army Alpha and in the AGCT.

Dynamic Organization of Mental Traits

The pattern of trait relationships is not fixed and static but changes with age and probably with other conditions. Preschool children, for instance, depend largely on a general factor for their performance in widely different tests. With advancing age, however, they show more and more specialization. In other words, they use the general factor first, and then improve in test performance by adding group factors to the general factor.

In one investigation, three groups of school children aged 9, 12 and 15, respectively, were given tests of memory, verbal, numerical and spatial aptitudes and of motor speed. The correlations among all these tests tended to decrease with their age, as is indicated by the average r's of 0.29 for the 9-year-olds, 0.26 for the 12-year-olds and 0.14 for the 15-year-olds. Factor pattern analyses showed a large general factor whose relative importance decreased consistently from ages 9 to 15. In a second study, a single group of school children was retested after three years with eight tests covering verbal, numerical and spatial tasks. The correlation coefficients dropped from the first to the second testing, and the decrease was greater between groups of tests than within groups. Factor pattern analyses corroborated these results. A large general factor was found at both ages, but its magnitude decreased over the three-year period.

Tests of college students have repeatedly brought out large independent group factors, with little or no general factor common to all the tests.

Some evidence is also available to indicate that these age changes in factor pattern are not a phenomenon of maturation but the result of the type of training which the individual receives. Thus it has been found that in trait organization adults with only an elementary school education resemble school children more closely than college students. Educational level rather than age appears to have determined the pattern.

Further evidence is furnished by the fact that it is possible to alter the pattern of trait relationship experimentally within a short period. Such a change occurred in one investigation in which five tests (vocabulary, memory for digits, verbal reasoning of the syllogistic type, code multiplication and spatial pattern analysis) were administered to two hundred sixth-grade school children. Instruction was then given them in the use of special techniques which would facilitate performance on the last three tests only. This instruction was similar, in general, to that received in the course of school work—for example, they were taught computation short-cuts in arithmetic. After thirteen days, equivalent forms of all five tests were given them under the same conditions as in the initial testing. The intercorrelations among the five tests showed no changes between the two tests for which no special instruction had been given, a slight change between tests which had had special instruction and tests which had not had it and a marked change between the tests with the special aids. The relative importance of the group factors was altered.

This experiment represents a highly condensed version of the type of experience to which the child is exposed in the course of school work and other everyday activities. It is, therefore, entirely possible that factor patterns are determined in the first place by the nature of such experiences. Under existing cultural conditions, a certain degree of uniformity of factor patterns is found because of common environmental conditions. Traditional educational curricula and vocational classifications contribute to this uniformity. Thus in the young child we find a relatively large general factor occurring in all the types of activities taught in the schools, that is to say, the so-called higher mental processes. As the child grows older and specialization is encouraged, certain culturally determined differentiations begin to appear. Group factors are produced for linguistic, mathematical and mechanical skills and possibly for other functions. At the same time, the increasing identification of the linguistic or verbal group factor with 'general intelligence' as the individual grows older is quite understandable in a culture in which language plays so important a part in a wide variety of fields.

MEASUREMENT OF PERSONALITY CHARACTERISTICS

Now we must consider the ways of testing those human traits which are of special importance in determining how persons will act toward one another.

What Are Personality Tests?

The term *personality* is sometimes used in psychology to refer to the individual considered as a whole, the composite pattern of all his behavior characteristics. A narrower and more common meaning of the term restricts it to those traits which are of chief importance in the individual's relations to other people. It is in this latter sense that the term is used in connection with *personality tests*. (See pp. 487 f. for more on the meaning of personality.) Any trait may, of course, play an important part in the individual's social relations. To be exceptionally tall or short, handsome or ugly, or to have very poor motor coordination, an excellent memory for names and faces, a flair for dealing with mechanical gadgets or a genius for well-turned phrases—any of these attributes could be the determining factors in a person's relations to his fellows. In such traits, however, only extreme deviations play a significant role in social behavior. Those traits classified under *personality* in the more restricted sense, on the other hand, play a dominant part in the social behavior of all individuals, and in them even slight deviations from the norm are of paramount importance.

Among the traits most commonly assessed by personality tests is *emotional stability* or relative freedom from such neurotic symptoms as phobias (abnormal fears), compulsions, obsessions, frequent nightmares, insomnia, sleep walking, shifts of mood without apparent cause, uncontrolled outbursts of temper, excessive worries and many others. Although the average person has at some time experienced a mild degree of a few such symptoms, when their number or severity exceeds a certain 'normal' maximum, serious maladjustment is likely to result. Social traits such as *introversion-extraversion* and *dominance-submission* are also commonly considered in personality testing. The former refers to the tendency to be shut in or outgoing in your interests and social relations; the latter, to the tendency to dominate your associates in face-to-face situations or be dominated by them. Tests have also been devised to measure *character traits,* such as honesty, perseverance and cooperativeness. The measurement of *attitudes, interests* and *sense of values* represents another recent development in personality testing.

Construction of Personality Tests

The most widely popularized type of personality tests is the *questionnaire.* There are also the much-used *projection tests.* (These tests are described on pp. 495–497.)

Personality tests are constructed by essentially the same principles as all psychological tests. *Norms* are empirically established by giving the test to a large representative group of subjects and ascertaining the average score. A norm is, however, neither an ideal nor a perfect score, nor is it predetermined. Thus the norm in a neurotic inventory might be fifteen questions answered in the neurotic direction. That would show how normal neuroticism is. On the tests of introversion-extraversion and of ascendance-submission the norm generally falls at a point approximately midway between the extremes.

Besides adequately determined norms, personality tests must have demonstrated *reliability* in order to be of practical value.

The *validity* of personality tests is more difficult to establish than that of other types of tests because of the difficulty of finding a satisfactory independent measure, or criterion, for most personality traits. One technique for checking such validity is by correlating test scores with *ratings* by associates, teachers, job supervisors or others who have had an opportunity to observe the subjects over an adequate period of time. (See pp. 492 f.) In general, such criterion ratings should be made by more than one observer in order to guard against individual bias and other idiosyncrasies of the raters. Similarly, care should be exercised to make sure that the raters have had 'trait acquaintance,' that is, that they have had the opportunity to observe the subjects in those specific aspects of behavior covered by the test. Correlation with *psychiatric diagnosis* has been employed in validating certain tests of emotional maladjustment. Such a procedure is satisfactory if the criterion itself is based upon a careful and prolonged follow-up rather than upon a cursory psychiatric examination which may itself be no more valid than the test being validated. Correlations with *other personality tests* have sometimes been used as an index of validity, but this procedure presupposes that the criterion itself has previously been validated.

The method of *contrasted groups* is essentially based upon a variety of criteria which operate in the situations of everyday life. Suppose that occupational selection is taken as the 'criterion' and that a test of extraversion or sociability is given to, let us say, salesmen and engineers. If the salesmen's scores are clearly higher than the engineers' scores, some evidence will have been furnished that the test is valid, or some information will be gained about salesmen in relation to engineers, depending upon which way you think about the matter. If you are ready to define *sociability,* for instance, as what salesmen exceed engineers in, you can validate the test in this way. Delinquent and nondelinquent children have sometimes been used in a similar way to check the validity of certain character tests. Or the scores of neurotics under treatment can be compared with those of a matched normal group of persons who have never been under psychiatric care, in order to see whether a test or inventory really does indicate neuroticism.

In tests of neuroticism or emotional instability, the *frequency of a response* in a normal group is a further check on abnormality. If a particular 'symptom' or response occurs in a large percentage of normal persons, *ipso facto* it cannot be abnormal.

Finally, there is the method of *internal consistency.* It consists of a comparison of the subjects' performance on each item or part of the test with their performance on the test as a whole. For example, the 25 per cent most introverted and the 25 per cent most extraverted subjects in the group are selected *on the basis of* their total scores on an introversion-extraversion test. The responses of these two groups to each item on the test are then compared. If a supposed characteristic of introverted behavior occurs as often among the 'best' extraverts as among the 'best' introverts, obviously it should be discarded as not being correctly diagnostic. To be retained, an 'introversion' item must occur with significantly higher frequency in the introverted than in the extraverted group. The reader may have already perceived a difficulty with this method. To be of any value, such a check of validity must assume the complete, or at least high, validity of total scores on the test, since such scores actually constitute the criterion against which individual items are being checked. Actually all that the method does, as its name implies, is to increase the internal consistency of the test, to make sure that the different items are directed upon closely related characteristics. A consistent test, however, is more likely to be valid than an inconsistent one. At least it is easier to mistake the significance of a self-contradictory test than of a test which always points the same way. With a consistent test there is some meaning in defining the characteristic tested as being 'what the test tests.'

Evaluation of Personality Tests

There is considerable value in personality tests, but, as with all tests, there is need for caution in their use and interpretation. In the first place, most of the terms used in describing personality do not correspond to *clearly defined traits* in the sense of traits as independent group factors. In fact, when factor pattern analyses of personality test responses are made, the traits which emerge cut across the traditional classifications of introversion-extraversion, ascendance-submission, emotional adjustment and the like. These categories have, nevertheless, been retained for practical convenience in describing the social and emotional aspects of behavior. As such, however, they do not lend themselves to rigid and unambiguous definition. Somewhat different areas of behavior may therefore be designated when different investigators use the terms *introversion, dominance, honesty* or *sense of humor.*

The available evidence suggests, furthermore, a greater *specificity* of behavior in the realm of personality than among intellectual abilities. Thus a man may be quite extraverted toward his business associates and relatively introverted in his other social contacts. In the same way, in their studies on character traits, May and Hartshorne found honesty to be specific to the situation. The correlations between honesty in the classroom and in out-of-class situations, for example, were very low.

Personality characteristics are also *changeable* with time. The individual's shifting pattern of experience is reflected more readily in his emotional than in his intellectual behavior. Changes in ability do occur as a person's environment changes, but such alterations are slow and come only from drastic and prolonged modifications of environment. Personality characteristics, on the other hand, may show significant variations following such episodes as living away from home for the first time, taking a new job or going from high school to college. For this reason, retests of the same individual over fairly long periods of time may reflect actual changes in behavior, not merely poor test reliability. It is for this reason also that many questionnaires ask only about the subject's behavior during the past few months. Many persons would answer a particular question very differently when it refers to recent behavior from the way they would answer it with respect to their customary behavior up to, for example, a year before they took the test.

One of the chief practical difficulties, particularly in the use of questionnaires, is their susceptibility to *faking,* to deliberate deception on the part of the subject. It is undoubtedly possible on such tests for subjects, especially the brighter or better educated ones, to falsify their responses in the direction of the impression they wish to create. An individual could make himself appear more neurotic or less neurotic than he actually is, more dominant or more submissive, depending upon the exigencies of the situation. Various partial solutions to this problem have been attempted. One technique is to disguise the purpose and nature of the test. In practically every personality test this is done to a certain extent by careful wording of the instructions, by elimination of suggestive trait labels and by keeping the subject in ignorance of the way the responses will be scored. When only group results are needed, preserving the anonymity of individual papers is a way of reducing faking by eliminating the principal motive for misrepresentation. Similarly, when the test results are to form the basis for advice and guidance, the examiner can more often count upon the cooperation and truthfulness of the subject than when the test is being used to select employees. The individual will in general —but not always—be relatively truthful when he is himself seeking help in his personal adjustment or his educational or vocational planning.

Even when the subject is cooperative and frank, his *ability to report* his own personality characteristics may be questioned. This criticism obviously applies especially to the questionnaire. It should, however, be noted, first, that most personality test questions do not require the subject to judge or describe his characteristics but to report what he has actually done in certain situations in the immediate past. Furthermore, the questions in personality tests are not so much concerned with the apparent facts involved as with the individual's reactions to them. For example, if the subject is asked whether his associates generally treat him fairly, the real interest lies in knowing whether he *believes* that he is treated fairly.

It is not wise in the present day to rely on the results of personality tests alone when important decisions about human beings are to be made. The test scores aid the diagnostician—be he psychiatrist, psychologist or personnel expert. The results must be supplemented by all the other information which it is possible to obtain. A candidate for a job, a person seeking advice about choosing a profession or his personal problem, a patient who might conceivably turn out to need institutional care or at least temporary psychiatric treatment is interviewed. The technique of the *interview* is well worked out, and it supplies a great deal of information which supplements test results. When possible the *case history* is also worked up, the details of the person's past life being got from all available sources. (These techniques, which are beyond the scope of the present chapter, are considered on pp. 493–497; 539–541.)

DISTRIBUTION OF INDIVIDUAL DIFFERENCES

We may now turn our attention to understanding how individuals vary with respect to different traits, to the question of whether individual types exist and to a description of extreme degrees of intelligence.

Frequency Distributions

How are the various degrees of psychological traits distributed among the general population? Are individuals scattered uniformly over the entire range, or do they cluster at one or more points? With what relative frequency do the different traits, abilities and other human characteristics occur? These questions are answered for any particular case by drawing up a *frequency distribution.*

Table XXII shows a typical frequency distribution for the scores of 1000 college students on a simple learning test. The scores are divided into class intervals, in this test intervals of four points each. The frequency with which scores fall in each class interval is shown as number of cases and as percentage. In this instance, since there are 1000 cases altogether, the percentage frequency looks like the case frequency, but ordinarily you could not be sure about the percentages by merely inspecting the numbers of cases. It is often useful to change cases into percentages in order to make different curves comparable. Since no student obtained a score below 8 or above 55, extreme class intervals do not have to be shown. Higher and lower scores might have occurred if 10,000 or 100,000

TABLE XXII

Frequency Distribution of the Scores of One Thousand College Students on a Simple Learning Test

[Data from A. Anastasi]

Score	*Frequency*	
Class Intervals	*Cases*	*Per Cent*
52–55	1	0.1
48–51	1	0.1
44–47	20	2.0
40–43	73	7.3
36–39	156	15.6
32–35	328	32.8
28–31	244	24.4
24–27	136	13.6
20–23	28	2.8
16–19	8	0.8
12–15	3	0.3
8–11	2	0.2
	N = 1000	100.0

students had been tested instead of only 1000.

The data of Table XXII are plotted in Fig. 202, which shows the frequency distribution in two forms. The dotted lines form a *histogram,* the kind of graph in which the frequency for each class interval is drawn as a horizontal line and the resulting distribution curve appears stepped. If the frequency for each interval is plotted as a point in the middle of its interval and the points are then connected by straight lines, the resulting curve is called a *polygon* distribution.

Both table and curve show what a typical distribution is like. Some midpoint is its highest point, that is to say, some midvalue is the most frequent and thus the value you would be most likely to get if you had to pick out one at random. Frequencies decrease in both directions from the middle. Extreme values—very high and very low—are very infrequent, and there are practical limits to the curve in both directions, although you may get greater extremes when you have more cases. If the frequency with which college students will get a score of 3 (Table XXII) is only once in 10,000, more often than not you will get no score so low as 3 when you have only 1000 cases.

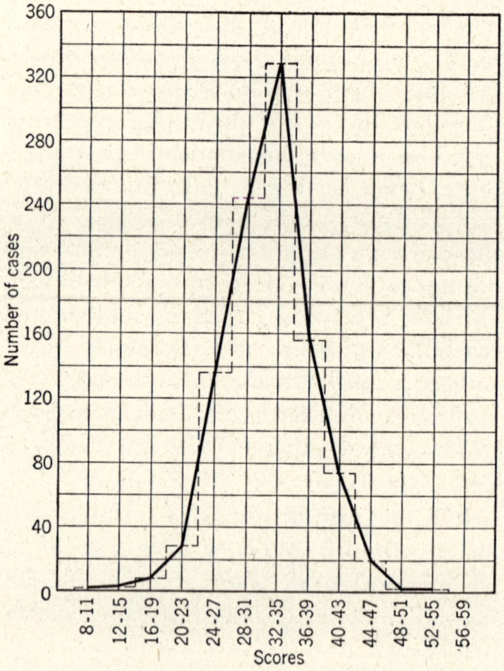

FIGURE 202. DISTRIBUTION CURVES: FREQUENCY POLYGON AND HISTOGRAM

[Data from Table XXII.]

The standard form of frequency distribution is the *normal distribution curve,* shown in Fig. 102 (p. 262) and already discussed. It is the symmetrical curve that you get when the positive and negative deviations from the average are made up of the sum of many small factors, and the positive and negative factors occur equally often, as they do when a coin is tossed without bias. Suppose you took 6 pennies, and tossed them all together 64 times, and every penny came equally often heads and tails, and every combination of heads and tails occurred equally often, which is to say *once* for each combination, since there are 64 possible combinations and only 64 tosses. Then suppose you counted up the numbers of heads in each throw of 6 pennies and tabulated the frequencies. You would have:

Number of heads	6	5	4	3	2	1	0
Frequency	1	6	15	20	15	6	1
(Total = 64)							

That makes sense. There is only one way in which all 6 pennies can turn up heads, but there are 6 ways of getting 5 heads, for any one of the 6 pennies might be tails. There are 15 ways of getting 4 heads and 2 tails, 20 ways of coming out 3 and 3, and of course the right half of the distribution must be symmetrical with the left because, if there are 6 ways of getting 5 heads, there must also be 6 ways of getting 5 tails (and one head). If you graph these frequencies as a histogram, you get approximately the normal curve. If you draw a smooth curve through the points, you get exactly the bell-shaped normal distribution curve, which is also the mathematicians' *normal probability curve* (Fig. 102).

The normal curve is 'normal' because it is what happens when everything is symmetrical, when 'more' is just as likely to happen as 'less,' when events vary in a random fashion. In fact the mathematicians define the term *random* as the kind of variation which gives normal distributions, as does penny tossing when it satisfies the conditions just enumerated. Mathematical statistics has been built up to apply more accurately—at least in its simpler forms—to normal distributions than to asymmetrical distributions. For this reason psychologists prefer distributions that are symmetrical enough to approximate normality. If they get distributions that are very much distorted, being much steeper on one side than the other, they look for some different scale of measurement or scoring, one that will expand the steep side and compress the gradual slope, making the distribution more symmetrical.

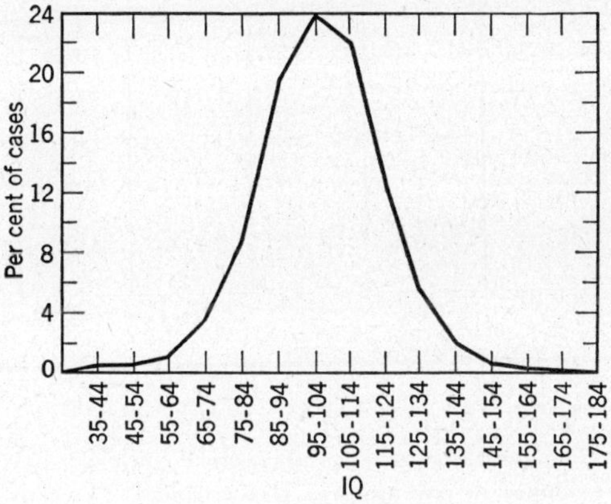

FIGURE 203. IQ'S OF 2904 UNSELECTED CHILDREN BETWEEN THE AGES OF 2 AND 18

[From L. M. Terman and M. A. Merrill, *Measuring intelligence,* Houghton Mifflin, 1933, p. 37.]

If they get two humps in the curve, a *bimodal distribution* (Fig. 207), they try to analyze the characteristic being measured into two factors, each of which will have a unimodal distribution. It is for this reason that we find so many approximately normal distributions of psychological data. The tests are, often unconsciously, adjusted to give symmetrical distributions in order that a common prejudice for symmetry may be satisfied and that statistical treatment of the results may be easier.

Figures 203 to 206 are examples of distribution curves based upon the test scores of large groups of subjects. Figure 203 is a frequency polygon of the Stanford-Binet

IQ's of 2904 children between the ages of 2 and 18. It will be noted that the largest percentage of cases receive IQ's in the middlemost class interval, from 95 to 104, the percentage tapering off gradually until only a small fraction of 1 per cent is found with

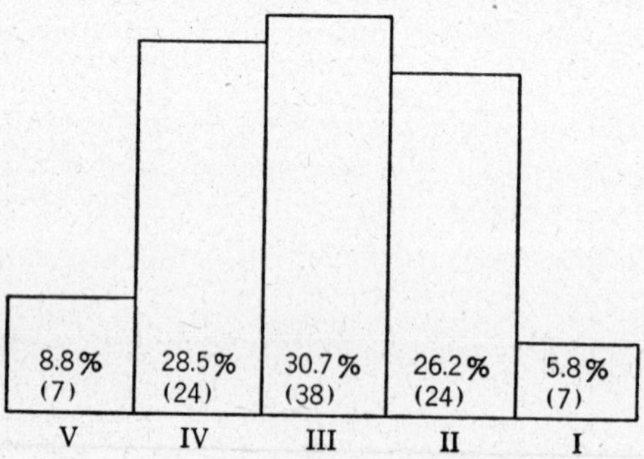

FIGURE 204. DISTRIBUTION OF ARMY GRADES OF THE ARMY GENERAL CLASSIFICATION TEST

The percentages for a theoretical normal curve are shown in parentheses. [Data from W. V. Bingham, *Science,* 1946, **104,** 148.]

IQ's from 35 to 44 and from 165 to 174. The scale is adjusted to have the average the most frequent value and to have it fall at IQ = 100.

Figure 204 is a histogram showing the percentage of men falling into the five Army grades on the basis of their AGCT scores. These percentages are based upon a group of nearly ten million men. For comparison, the percentages which would fall in each grade in a perfect normal curve are given in parentheses. It will be seen that the correspondence is fairly close but not exact. The test was constructed with the intention of getting exact correspondence, but it is impossible to predict exactly just what will happen with frequencies.

Figure 205 is a frequency polygon of the scores obtained by 400 college men on the Allport Ascendance-Submission Test. The peak falls approximately midway between the ascendant and submissive extremes, the number of cases tapering off gradually as these extremes are approached. Similarly, the scores of 801 school children on one of the May and Hartshorne tests for measuring cooperativeness, as shown in Fig. 206, are symmetrically distributed in accordance with normal expectation for a unitary trait. If the curve had been asymmetrical or bimodal, the authors of the test would probably have done something to the test to make it more 'normal' or else have discarded it and tried to invent something 'better.'

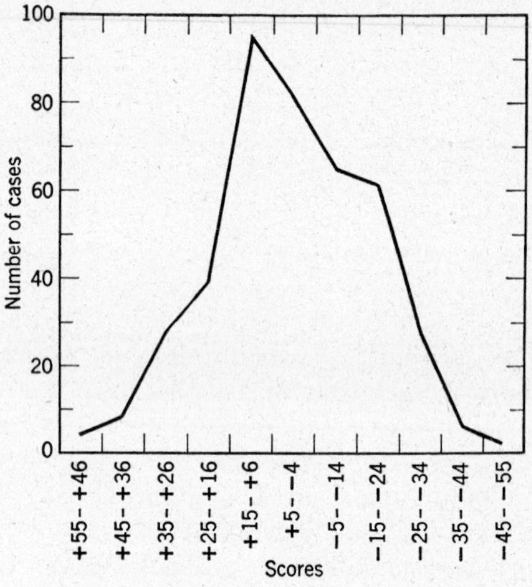

FIGURE 205. SCORES OF 400 COLLEGE MEN ON THE ASCENDANCE-SUBMISSION TEST

[From G. W. Allport, *J. abn. soc. Psychol.,* 1928, 23, 129.]

In a number of behavior characteristics indicative of social conformity, a type of distribution known as the *J-curve* is often found. This curve, named after its resemblance to the letter J, is in reality a greatly distorted distribution curve, with the majority of people falling at the end which represents complete or nearly complete conformity. A favorite example is the behavior of motorists. At an ordinary intersection with no traffic signal, drivers' behavior will probably be symmetrically distributed. The majority will exhibit a moderate amount of caution, very few will come to a

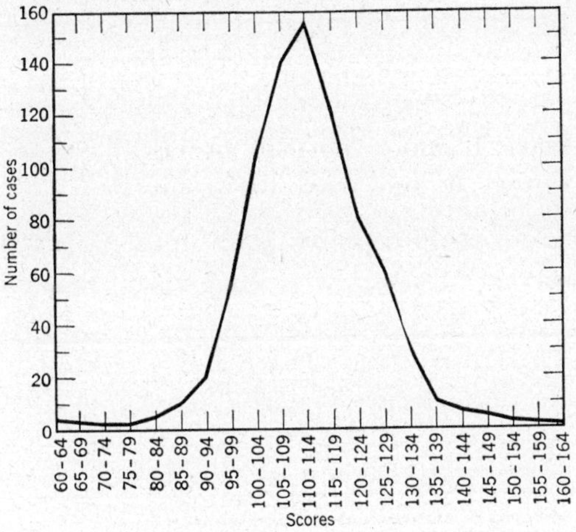

FIGURE 206. DISTRIBUTION OF COOPERATIVENESS: TEST SCORES AMONG 801 SCHOOL CHILDREN

[After unpublished data of H. Hartshorne, M. A. May and J. B. Moller. From A. Anastasi, *Differential psychology,* Macmillan, 1937, p. 51.]

full stop, and equally few will continue at the same rate of speed with no observation of oncoming traffic. If, however, a stop light and a policeman are installed at the intersection, these external constraints will pull the distribution into a J-curve. In this situation over ninety per cent of the drivers will come, as they should, to a full stop; of the remaining small percentage, a few will slow down markedly, still fewer will slow down slightly, and a very small number will continue at the same rate of speed. Such a J-curve could, of course, be turned back into a symmetrical curve by stretching the full-stop class interval. For instance, you could divide the full-stop interval into several, according to the drivers' attitudes that produced the full stop. You might be able to separate out and plot separately *almost-did-not-stop, stopped-but-resented-having-to, stopped-as-a-matter-of-course* and *always-stop-whenever-there-is-any-possible-reason-for-it.*

Types

In popular characterizations, people are often classified into distinct types. The sheep are clearly separated from the goats, the honest from the dishonest, the brilliant from the dull, the meek from the aggressive. Our language usage is undoubtedly an important factor in this tendency toward twofold categorizing. Such categories imply a *bimodal distribution,* with two distinct peaks, or modes, and perhaps a few mixed or intermediate cases falling between the peaks (Fig. 207). We have already seen that studies of the actual distributions of traits almost never have more than one mode. Individuals cluster around a single peak, usually located near the center of the scale. The majority of persons seem to fall in the intermediate or 'mixed' area, and

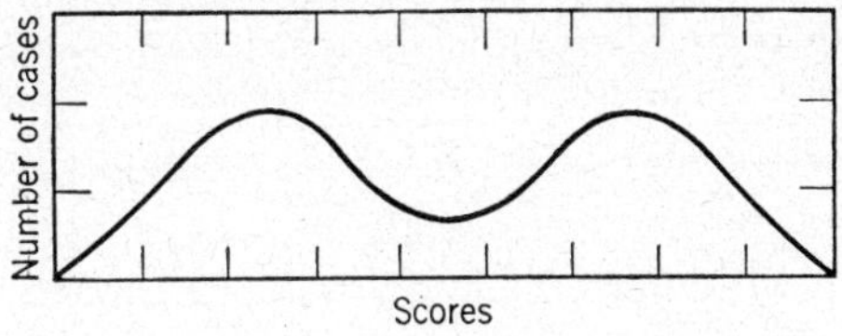

FIGURE 207. A BIMODAL DISTRIBUTION

there is no sharp line of demarcation between different degrees of a trait. People do not fit into separate groups without intermediates—not very often. Continuity is the rule, and all-or-none typing is rare.

Is the biology of sex an exception? Is sex bimodal? It is if you take overall sexuality and count frequencies. Most persons are either male or female, and the hermaphrodites—some verging toward male, some toward female, some half and half—are the infrequent intermediates. Hair-on-chin would be bimodally distributed in a total population of men and women. You could take as a measure the average growth of a hair in one month on one square centimeter of initially shaved skin. It has never been done, but it is clear that a bimodal distribution would result. There would be variable amounts of very little growth (the women mostly, a few men), variable amounts of heavy growth (the men mostly, the bearded women) and a sparse sprinkling of men and women in between. There are some biological types in this sense of differences existing with but few intermediates. Continuity, is, however, the rule in biology, largely because characteristics and traits are so complexly determined that it is not so often that all the predisposing factors are present together or absent together. If you consider the heights of men and women, you find that the men's heights are distributed according to a smooth unimodal curve, the women's according to another smooth unimodal curve, and that, when you add the two curves together, you have still another smooth unimodal curve. Yet the fact remains that women are shorter than men, *on the average,* although the tallest woman is ever so much taller than the average man, and conversely.

It is the same way with the other secondary sexual characteristics. You can find traits that are properly called masculine and others that are properly labeled feminine, and you can measure both men and women in respect of them. The result is like the one for human statures; on the average men are more masculine than women, but the most masculine woman is more masculine than the average man, and conversely.

One might expect color sensitivity to be bimodally distributed, but it is not except when the method of testing for color blindness makes it so. True, there are two types of people, those who can pass a certain test for color blindness and those who cannot. But careful measurement of color sensitivity soon reveals the fact that there are intermediates, persons with diminished sensitivity who see all the colors and color-blind persons who are no longer color-blind when the stimuli are made very effective.

Whereas the all-or-none types are rare, *bipolar continuity* is common. That is what you usually find instead of types. There is red, and there is yellow, and there are also all the oranges between the red and yellow poles. There are color normality and color blindness and many stages of color weakness in between. There are masculinity and femininity and all possible degrees between the two poles. When you know what your poles are, it becomes a matter of observation whether the poles are themselves approximated more frequently than their intermediates (bimodal distribution) or whether the poles are rarely reached and some midmixture is the most frequent case (unimodal distribution, presumably more or less symmetrical).

Constitutional Types

There has been a great deal of talk in psychology about *constitutional types,* each of which is distinguished by its own physical or psychological characteristics. This is an old theory and many commonplaces of language attest the favor it has enjoyed in the past. The jolly fat man, the square jaw of determination, the receding chin of the timid soul—all these are reminders of ancient systems of typology.

Psychologists have subjected to study many of the claims that have been put forth regarding the relation between behavior and physical traits. Three problems always present themselves: (1) how to measure and describe the human body, (2) how to select and evaluate the basic traits of personality or temperament and (3) how to determine, if there seems to be a relationship between the two, just what aspects of physique, on the one hand, are related to just what aspects of human behavior, on the other.

That people differ in shape and appearance has always been obvious. Long ago an ancient Greek divided people into two categories: the short-thick and the long-thin. Many bodies fit one or the other of these descriptions and from time to time this two-category system has reappeared with modifications and elaborations. One well-known typologist distinguished between *pyknic* (short, thick) and *leptosome* (long, thin) body builds. Patients with manic-depressive psychosis tend to be pyknic, whereas schizophrenic patients are frequently leptosome. Continuity is, however, the rule. Neither height nor width of the human frame is bimodal in distribution. (For further criticism of the type theory, see pp. 488 f.)

Recognition of this fact has led recently to the abandonment of the notion of distinct *types* in favor of a description of human physiques in terms of mixtures of three *basic components*. A few individuals have one or another component developed to an extreme degree, but in most people the components tend toward a more balanced development. Accurate description is made possible by a system for measuring each component on a scale of 1 to 7, where 1 is the least and 7 is the greatest amount possible. These three components are described as follows.

(1) *Endomorphy*. The degree to which softness and roundness predominate. When high on the scale of endomorphy (near degree 7), a person is flabby, soft and rolypoly. He is usually 'fat,' in the ordinary sense, but not all people of large girth are predominantly endomorphic. Some 'fat' may be mainly muscle.

(2) *Mesomorphy*. The degree to which bone and muscle predominate. Weight lifters and professional strong men usually have 7 degrees in mesomorphy. They are neither fat nor thin; they are mostly bone and muscle.

(3) *Ectomorphy*. The degree to which linearity and fragility predominate. People extreme in ectomorphy are 'skinny,' with long, thin bones and stringy muscles.

A person is given a rating, which is called his *somatotype*. He is rated in each of the three components, in the order in which they are given above: endomorphy-mesomorphy-ectomorphy. If a man is rated a "2–6–1," that means that he is low (only 2) in endomorphy, very high (a 6) in mesomorphy and as low as anyone could be (1) in ectomorphy.

Figure 208 shows examples of physiques extreme in each of the three components and one case in which the components are nearly in balance. The extreme mesomorph has the somatotype 1–7–1½. The most common somatotype found among male college students is 3–4–4. There are about 58 of them in every thousand.

We have here a system for classifying human physiques. In itself it is an anthropometric system, not a psychological one. It shows, however, how to deal with the problem of types and polarities. When continuity is the rule you can still find poles and describe in terms of components. This is a tripolar system, and the individual cases are regarded as having three components. (The color system has four poles, and colors are describable in terms of four components: *R–G, Y–B, Wh–Bk, Gy*. See p. 270.)

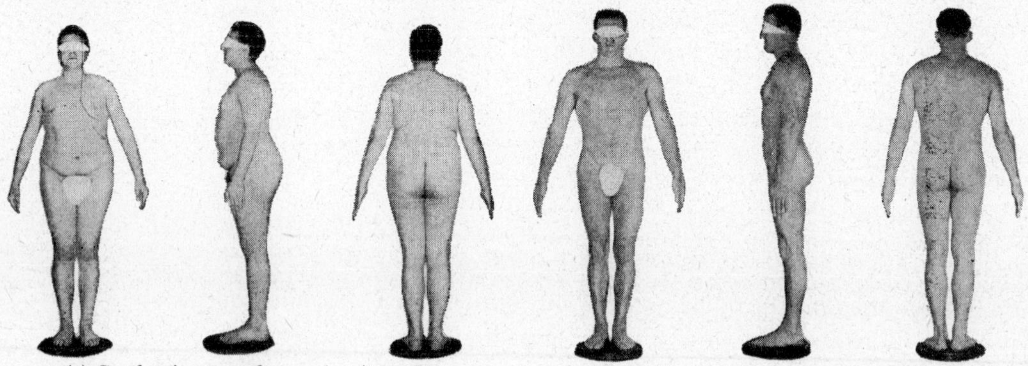

(*a*) Predominant endomorphy, 7–1–1½. (*b*) Predominant mesomorphy, 1–7–1½.

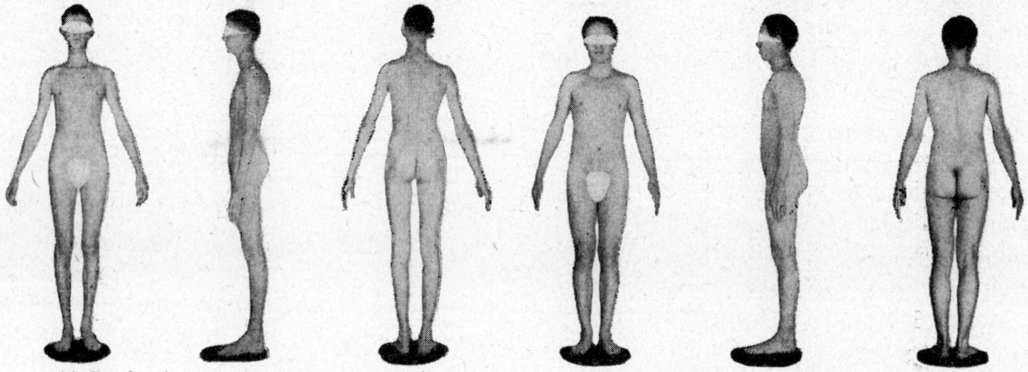

(*c*) Predominant ectomorphy, 1½–1½–7. (*d*) Balanced physique, 4–3½–4.

FIGURE 208. REPRESENTATIVE SOMATOTYPES

[From W. H. Sheldon and S. S. Stevens, *Varieties of human temperament*, Harper, 1942, pp. 8 f.]

Given this system the question comes up as to whether there is any psychological system associated with it. Would temperament, personality, intelligence, psychoses or any other psychological characteristic turn out to be related to physique? Some psychological variables have at best only a negligible relation to physique, such as acquired attitudes, for example. That is plain. Political persuasion and church membership probably have nothing to do with body build. Intelligence shows only a very slight relation: a low negative correlation with mesomorphy, a low positive correlation with ectomorphy. On the other hand, measures of physical strength and dexterity are correlated well with mesomorphy, as we might expect, and they show a moderate negative correlation with each of the other two components.

The most interesting relation thus far

demonstrated is between physique and temperament. Temperament refers to an individual's basic emotional nature, the quality of his mood, the direction of his deeper motivations, the stamp of his characteristic reactions. It would not be surprising that temperament so defined should be closely linked with man's physical constitution, including his physiology and his glandular functioning; but the task of demonstrating the linkage is not easy. The basic components of temperament must first be identified and measured.

In a recent study a group of 200 men was subjected to a temperament analysis in which each individual was rated on 60 traits of temperament. These 60 traits were divided into three groups, one for each of three components of temperament. The three components had been isolated by a process of correlational analysis. The components of temperament defined by these three clusters of traits were named and briefly characterized as follows.

(1) *Viscerotonia.* General relaxation, love of comfort, need for affection and approval, pleasure in eating and in digesting, indiscriminate amiability, easy emotional expression, complacent tolerance and need of people when troubled.

(2) *Somatotonia.* General assertiveness in posture and movement, energetic activity, love of power and risk, physical courage, directness of manner, psychological callousness, general noisiness and need of action when troubled.

(3) *Cerebrotonia.* General restraint and tightness in posture and movement, love of privacy, emotional restraint, sociophobia, unpredictability of attitude, vocal restraint, poor sleep habits and need of solitude when troubled.

Twenty traits were used to define each of these three components, and for each of the 60 traits the subject is rated on a 7-point scale. Then from the average rating on each group of 20 traits an index of temperament was derived. The procedure is analogous to that used for the designation of the somatotype. An extremely viscerotonic temperament scores 7–1–1; a perfectly balanced temperament scores 4–4–4. The parallel between the system for physique and the system for temperament is close and obvious.

For the 200 cases of this study, the relations between the components of physique and the components of temperament showed positive correlations near +0.80. These correlations are high, but they are not perfect, and they are based on but few cases.

Certainly it is not yet clear that there is a fixed, one-to-one relation between physique and temperament, nor is it in order to say that the one *causes* the other. All we can say as yet is that nature seems not to assemble physiques and temperaments in a purely chance or random fashion. It begins to look as if either the shape of a man has something to do—by and large—with the way he behaves, or the way he behaves has something to do with his shape.

The Subnormal Person

The subnormal should be regarded, not as a distinct class of persons, but as constituting the lower end of a continuous distribution of individual differences. Among the subnormal are included the *feebleminded,* who are deficient intellectually, and the mentally diseased, or *psychotics,* who deviate from the norm principally in emotional adjustment and other personality characteristics. The *neurotic* person displays a milder degree of emotional maladjustment, than the psychotic. (For the description of psychoses and neuroses, see pp. 531–537.)

For practical convenience in treatment and commitment to institutions, certain classifications of feebleminded persons are accepted. The most common among psychologists is in terms of IQ, thus:

Category	*IQ*
Normal	90–110
Dull	80– 90
Borderline	70– 80
Moron	50– 70
Imbecile	20– 50
Idiot	Below 20

The IQ's from 90 to 110 are classified as normal, because *normal* is thought of as a class with some range to it and not as limited to the point which is the average. In this case the average is, of course, an IQ of 100. The dull and borderline groups represent intermediate categories between the normal and the feebleminded levels, the feebleminded group generally including persons with IQ's of 70 and below. Within the feebleminded group, the three categories of *moron, imbecile* and *idiot* are commonly employed as subdivisions. Since the distribution curve is unimodal, there are fewer idiots than imbeciles, and fewer imbeciles than morons.

It is not possible to say in general what makes people feebleminded or, for that matter, what makes them geniuses. We have the unimodal distribution curve as a fact. It seems to be the sort of variation we should expect. We cannot explain the intellectual variability of mankind in terms of brain changes or of differences in motivation. On the other hand, there are certain known physical defects and diseases which cause feeblemindedness in some instances, though not all. The *microcephalic* is a mentally defective person. He has an abnormally small, pointed skull and a brain to fit his skull. The *hydrocephalic* has a very large skull, but with an excessive amount of cerebrospinal fluid between his skull and his undersized brain within it. *Cretinism* is due to insufficient secretion of the thyroid gland. It is a deficiency which produces both intellectual defect and characteristic physical symptoms, such as stunted growth, short and podgy limbs, dry rough skin and loss of hair. Other pathological varieties of feeblemindedness have been identified, but they remain exceptional. In most cases we know about the causes of mental deficiency only as much as we know about the causes of our own normality and —we all have them—our flashes of genius.

The Genius

Genius may be regarded as the upper end of the distribution of intelligence. Although the observation of isolated extreme cases may suggest that the genius is so unlike his fellows as to be qualitatively different, here again we find borderline instances of mental superiority which bridge the gap with the normal.

Investigations of adult geniuses have used three methods: biographical, statistical or historiometrical. In the first, all available printed material about a single genius is examined in the effort to understand the nature and origin of his genius. Statistical surveys are likewise based upon printed records but are more concerned with general trends in large groups of eminent men, the information being obtained from biographical dictionaries or questionnaires filled out by living men of great distinction. The method of historiometry attempts to evaluate biographical records, especially those dealing with childhood accomplishments, in terms of current mental test standards. On this basis an approximate estimate can be made of an eminent man's IQ in childhood.

Intellectually superior children are more readily available for direct psychological study than adult geniuses. A number of individual *child prodigies,* including some well-known juvenile writers, have been the subjects of detailed and prolonged observation by psychologists. In general, the results of such case studies are in agreement with the findings obtained by mental test surveys on large groups of superior children.

One of the most extensive of these investigations is by L. M. Terman and his associates on 643 California school children between the ages of 2 and 14, all of whose IQ's were 140 or above. These children were found, on the whole, to come from homes of higher-than-average social and cultural level. Parents' occupational and educational levels were likewise above average. A number of popular misconceptions regarding the child prodigy were disproved by this study. Thus gifted children as a group were equal to or better than the normal in health, physical development and emotional adjustment. They were not narrow and specialized in either abilities or interests, but showed wider breadth in both respects than the normal groups with which they were compared.

A six-year 'follow-up' of a large part of the original group and another 'follow-up' after sixteen years indicate that the group tended to retain its intellectual superiority and to make highly successful educational, vocational and personal adjustments, when it was compared with the general population. Within the group, however, the degree of adult success did not seem to depend on the degree of intellectual superiority. A detailed comparison of the 'most successful' and 'least successful' men in the reexamination after sixteen years led the investigators to conclude that "above the IQ level of 140, adult success is largely determined by such factors as social adjustment, emotional stability and drive to accomplish." The two groups—'most successful' and 'least successful'—did not differ significantly in initial IQ or in initial educational achievement.

GROUP DIFFERENCES

Sometimes the psychologist is more interested in differences between groups than in differences between the individuals who make up the group. He wants to compare old people with young, college graduates with those who left school after the eighth grade, men with women, white persons with Negroes. How do you go about the comparison?

Sampling

Not often, when you are interested in a possible difference between two groups of people, are you able to measure every member of each group and then draw your conclusion. You can do that sometimes, but only when the groups are small. If you want to compare the intelligence of the girls and the boys in a given class, you can, indeed, test them all and then see what you have; but, if you want to compare the intelligence of just girls and just boys, or even the intelligence of all girls and boys aged twelve in the United States in 1948, you have got to take *samples* and compare them. The correctness of your conclusion will depend upon whether your samples really represent your groups or whether they are biased.

The first thing you do is to measure your *sampling error,* and you do that very much as you measure the reliability of a test.

You take several samples, each as good as you know how to take, and compare them. You intended them to be the same. The amount that they differ is your sampling error. A small difference between your groups would not be regarded as significant if your sampling error were large. A small sampling error indicates the validity of your sampling, though the true validity you would never know unless you measured the entire group—and then you would not need a sample.

Mostly in interpreting measurements you deal with differences—individual differences, group differences, other differences. Nearly always the differences are between samples. You are comparing samples of adults when you say that some people are color-blind and others are not. You are comparing samples when you say 'intelligence' increases during childhood and not during adulthood—samples of ten-year-olds, twelve-year-olds, twenty-year-olds, forty-year-olds. When you compare two groups, you generally get the mean measurement of each, see what is the difference between these means, and then decide whether the difference is significant or merely what might have occurred by chance. How is that done?

There are three factors that affect the *significance of a difference:* (1) the size of the difference between the means of the samples, (2) the variability of the samples and (3) the number of cases in each sample. A large difference is more likely than a small difference to be due to something other than chance variability. The greater the variability of the samples, however, the less likely is it for the difference to be significant. It may have resulted merely from this variability. Still if the difference is maintained when the number of cases is very large, the probability that it is due to chance is greatly diminished. The larger the samples, the more reliable the difference.

It is possible by a very simple formula to compute the standard deviation of a difference between the means of two samples (σ_D). We get it from the standard deviations (σ) of the two samples and the numbers of cases measured. (For the meaning of the standard deviation, σ, see p. 263.) Then we determine what is called the *critical ratio,* the ratio of the difference to its standard deviation (D/σ_D). The larger the difference in relation to its standard deviation, the less likely is it to vary enough to be reversed. If, for instance, a conclusion from two samples were to be that high school girls of twelve are brighter than high school boys of twelve, we should want to know how likely it is that, in taking other samples, the difference might be reversed so as to show the boys brighter than the girls. A modern convention is to require the difference to be at least three times its standard deviation, to ask that the critical ratio equal at least 3. Then the difference is regarded as *significant enough* for use in important conclusions. There is, of course, no point at which significance begins nor any other point at which it is complete. Values less than 3 show low significance, and values greater than 3 do not mean 'certainty.' Forty years ago scientists were rejecting results when the critical ratio was less than 5, but nowadays they are satisfied with smaller samples. What has happened is that they have gained confidence in their ability to choose samples with few errors.

In choosing samples it is especially important to avoid special *selection.* Any group that is not a representative sample of the population from and for which it is drawn is said to be a *selected group.* Selection vitiates group comparison in exaggerated degree when it occurs differently in the two groups compared.

Immigrant groups furnish a good example of this differential operation of selective factors. Immigrants coming to the United States from different countries are usually neither fair samples of their home populations nor comparable selections for the different countries. If it could be shown that immigrants from all nations were drawn consistently from, let us say, the lower socio-economic and intellectual levels, such groups would at least be comparable with one another. But it is well known that, largely because of economic and political factors, the immigrants from certain nations at a given time may represent a relatively inferior sampling of their home population, from others a more nearly random sample, and from still others a fairly superior sample. You cannot say that the British are brighter than the Italians just because the British-born recruits in the First World War got, on the average, higher scores on Alpha than the Italian-born recruits. The samples for the United States Army were fair enough. The Italians *in it* were not so bright as the British. But the samples were selected as against the populations of Great Britain and Italy, selected by the economic conditions which controlled immigration differently for the two countries at the time when men of recruit age in 1917 were immigrating to America.

Selective factors can operate just as well in studies of sex differences. There are, for instance, two studies of sex differences in an intelligence test. One study, with a total sample of 2544 elementary school children, showed that the girls did better than the boys. The other, with 5929 high school students, came out in favor of the boys. Why? Do the boys mature faster than the girls? At some ages they do, but that is not the answer here. The groups were differently selected. The boys who do poorly in school work tend to drop out before high school and get jobs; the dull girls more often keep on. The sampling was not comparable in the two cases.

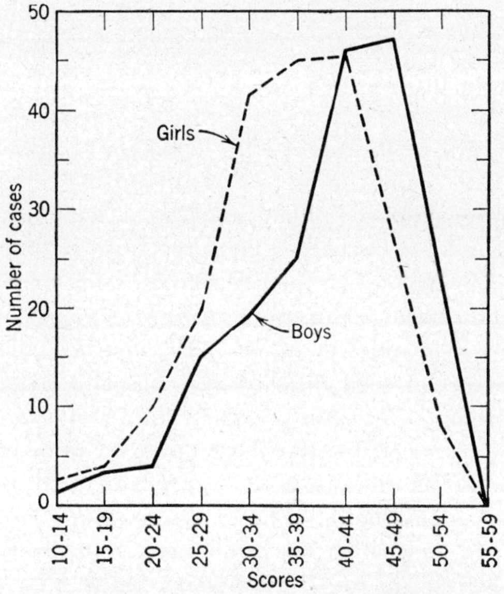

FIGURE 209. OVERLAPPING DISTRIBUTIONS

Shows the distribution of boys' and girls' scores on a test of arithmetic reasoning. [After data from B. Schiller. From A. Anastasi, *Differential psychology,* Macmillan, 1937, p. 403.]

It must be borne in mind that two distributions can *overlap* each other, and yet the difference between the means may be highly significant. See Fig. 209, which shows the overlap of the distributions for boys and girls in a test of arithmetic reasoning. The boys, with a mean score of 40.4, are better than the girls, with a mean score of 35.8. The difference is 4.6, and the critical ratio is found to be about 6. Certainly it is no chance variability that makes this sample of boys better than this sample of girls. Nevertheless, 38 per cent of the girls scored higher than the boys' average, and 24 per cent of the boys scored lower than the girls' average. The difference between the groups is significant, but you cannot safely predict about individual boys and girls. This point was succinctly put by Samuel Johnson who, when asked which was superior, man or woman, is said to have replied: "Which man? which woman?"

Psychological Sex Differences

A comparison of test results of men and women, even when interpreted with the cautions discussed in the preceding section, can only show sex differences under existing conditions in our *present* society. The tests cannot in themselves indicate the origin of such differences. It is, however, of practical value to ascertain the typical behavior characteristics of men and women, whatever the origin of such characteristics. In many fields definite assumptions are made regarding sex differences in abilities, interests, attitudes and similar traits. This discrimination between the sexes is noticeable in advertising and selling, political campaigning, the organization of newspapers and magazines, social work, crime prevention and the treatment of offenders, to name only a few outstanding examples. Insofar as cultural conditioning may have produced certain clear-cut sex differences, these cannot be ignored in the practical adjustments of everyday life.

Test results show with considerable consistency that men excel, on the average, in skill with numbers and the understanding of spatial relations, women in verbal aptitude and memory. These differences appear fairly early in life and tend to increase with age. Several studies on preschool children have brought out these characteristic differences in test performance. Among college students, the differences are large and clear-cut. For example, the results of the Scholastic Aptitude Test, given to 4394 men and 3318 women applying for admission to colleges throughout the country, showed a large and reliable difference in favor of the women on the verbal part of the test and an equally large difference in favor of the men on the numerical part. The critical ratios of these differences were 13.5 and 11.6, respectively.

Nearly all tests of 'spatial' or mechanical aptitude have shown male superiority. Among them are the puzzle boxes, form boards, slot mazes, paper-and-pencil mazes, construction tests and most of the tests which make up performance scales of 'intelligence.' In numerical aptitude and arithmetic reasoning (both the speed and accuracy of computation) the boys are favored, although the differences are not quite so consistent as in mechanical aptitude. This result might be expected from social tradition and environmental conditions, since the sex differentiation with regard to mathematical work is not so pronounced as it is for mechanical pursuits. Girls are given more opportunity for the development of numerical than space-perceptive functions. In both the elementary school and high school, for example, girls are taught arithmetic in the same classes as boys, but the boys are segregated for shop courses. The superiority of women on tests of memory is found with all types of material and all methods of testing memory. Women also excel in tests of association and in vividness of mental imagery. Their superiority in verbal ability is likewise evidenced in a variety of functions. Observations on normal as well as gifted and feebleminded children have shown that, on the average, girls begin to talk earlier than boys. Similarly girls of preschool age are known to have larger vocabularies than boys of the same age. Girls excel consistently in reading and in such tests as sentence completion and story completion. The large verbal content of most intelligence tests often results in a difference in favor of girls in total score.

The results of personality tests reflect the traditional sex stereotypes of our culture. Thus on such tests as Bernreuter's, men's scores indicate more extraversion, dominance and self-sufficiency, as well as fewer neurotic symptoms. On the Allport-Vernon Study of Values, men obtain high averages in theoretical, economic and political values; women in esthetic, social and religious values. The May and Hartshorne character tests indicated no sex difference in honesty, but a slight tendency for the girls to be more cooperative and more persistent, and a large, reliable difference in favor of the girls in 'inhibition' or self-control.

A comprehensive approach to the measurement of sex differences in personality traits is represented by the Terman-Miles Masculinity-Femininity Index (M/F index). This index is obtained from a series of tests in which each item was chosen because it differentiated significantly between the responses of men and women in our society. The M/F index thus shows the degree to which the individual's responses coincide with those typical of the majority of men or women in our culture. Plotting the distribution curves for men's and women's M/F ratios results in an extreme case of overlapping in the face of a significant average difference. The most masculine woman is much more masculine than the average man, and conversely.

A growing body of evidence suggests that the observed sex differences in psychological characteristics are chiefly traceable to certain environmental factors rather than to any innate tendencies associated with sex. Terman and Miles found, for example, that the M/F index for both sexes was significantly influenced by education, occupation, socio-economic level and familial pattern, such as number of brothers and sisters or death of one parent. Similarly, in an investigation of neurotic tendencies in children, it was found that ten-year-old boys manifested a greater average number of such tendencies than ten-year-old girls. The difference decreased sharply at age eleven and was reversed among twelve-year-olds. Thereafter the girls showed an increasingly greater number of neurotic tendencies. The increasing differentiation in the social environment of the two sexes after puberty and in the cultural pressures which come upon them at that time may explain these changes in emotional stability. It is also interesting to note that anthropologists have reported that, in certain primitive cultures, the traditional personality characteristics of the two sexes are very unlike those in our society. In some groups the pattern is nearly the reverse of ours.

Are There Racial Differences?

The classification of men into racial groups is essentially biological and corresponds to such divisions as breed, stock and strain in infrahuman organisms. In its simplest terms, the concept of race implies common physical characteristics deriving from a similar heredity.

The task of classifying people into races is far more difficult and complex than would appear from the glibness with which individuals are popularly assigned to one race or another. The essential problem in such classification is the identification of inheritable physical characteristics which differ clearly from one group to another and which can therefore serve as *criteria of race*. A wide variety of such criteria have been proposed, including skin color, eye color, hair color and texture, gross bodily dimensions, facial and cranial measure, blood groupings and endocrine gland activity.

In the application of any of these criteria of race, several difficulties appear at once. In the first place, there is wide variability in all these charatceristics within any one racial group. The overlapping between groups in respect of each of these criteria is likewise large. The indications of one criterion, moreover, are often contradicted by those of another. A person can have the skin color of one racial group, the bodily proportions of a second and the head dimensions of a third. Finally, there is the fact that several alleged racial characteristics, which were formerly regarded as innate, have proved to be changeable under the influence of environmental factors. Even such apparently hereditary traits as height, shape of the skull and facial conformation have been shown to depend in part upon environmental conditions in early life.

The study of racial differences is further complicated by the frequent confusion of racial with *national* or *linguistic* categories, as in speaking of a French 'race' or a Latin or Aryan 'race.' The extent of *race mixture* which has gone on for many generations makes any such simple classification impracticable. The psychological study of mixed or hybrid individuals is beset with more complications. On the one hand, the social disapproval of certain race mixtures creates an atmosphere which may produce characteristic personality deviations in the hybrid person. On the other hand, the hybrid may have opportunities for educational and social development not open to the relatively purer stock of certain racial groups. This is undoubtedly an important factor in the common finding that American Indians and Negroes, with considerable white mixture in their ancestry, tend to do better on our intelligence tests than the American Indians and Negroes with less white blood. The hybrid may get some of the advantages of both the cultures which he combines. The Indian-white hybrid, for example, gets the white man's schooling, which helps him with the white man's intelligence test; but he may be better than the white man and poorer than the purer Indian in woodcraft.

A serious barrier in the comparative testing of different racial or cultural groups is *language handicap*. It is obvious that in testing people who speak different languages, verbal tests cannot be employed. Nonlanguage tests and performance tests have been constructed for this purpose. It will be recalled, however, that the same traits are not measured by all these different tests of intelligence. Furthermore, difference of language makes the use of verbal tests impossible, and the range of functions which can be measured is greatly narrowed, for there is as yet no good substitute for verbal tests. You cannot eliminate the verbal content of a test without altering the abilities involved. The translation of an intelligence test into different languages does not solve this problem, for translation renders the original norms inapplicable and makes the test useless for intergroup comparisons.

The effect of language handicap upon test performance is actually most serious for those individuals with sufficient knowledge of English to admit them to the ordinary verbal tests. It has not generally been considered necessary to give these persons performance or nonlanguage tests, although it is now known that even mild degrees of language handicap will significantly lower test scores. In studies made of the American-born children of immigrant parents, the bilingual children who spoke English in school but a foreign language at home made consistently poorer scores on 'intelligence' tests than the 'monoglots' who spoke English at home as well as in school. It might be argued that the more intelligent, adaptable and progressive families are more likely to learn and adopt English and that these initial differences in intelligence—rather than language handicap—account for the differences in test scores. Such an explanation is contradicted, however, by studies which reveal that, on nonlanguage and performance tests, the bilingual children do not show a clear-cut inferiority. In some studies they actually excel the performances of the monoglots and even the norms for American children.

It is apparent, also, that immigrant groups in America, as well as the American Indians and Negroes, frequently differ from the native white American in *educational* and *occupational opportunities,* in *socio-economic level* and in other circumstances which undoubtedly influence intelligence test performance. *Customs* and *traditions* must likewise be taken into consideration in evaluating test scores. The emphasis placed upon speed of performance as a desirable objective varies widely in different cultures and is thus a case in point. In one investigation with a performance scale used with groups of American Indians, Negroes and white boys, the average IQ's placed the white group first, the Indians second and the Negroes third. An analysis of total scores into errors and times, however, showed that, in accuracy of performance, the whites and Negroes had approximately equal scores, whereas the Indians excelled both groups in this respect.

There is, therefore, no answer to the question: Are there racial differences? There is too much intermixture of races to get pure strains. You cannot test accurately for differences in 'intelligence,' when there are language differences or even broad cultural differences. In the few cases where this difficulty is not encountered, as with white persons and Negroes in the United States, there are socio-economic differences which vitiate a difference in scores on intelligence tests. Social and cultural differences obviously create personality differences. A minority group, which is discriminated against by the majority, will develop certain defensive attitudes and traits. So may the majority if the minority is strong and dangerous. There are ever so many demonstrable differences between groups, but they are not between races. Races scarcely exist any more.

The basic scientific question that is raised here, however, is this: *Are psychological characteristics inherited?* That is the topic of the next chapter.

REFERENCES

1. Anastasi, A. *Differential psychology.* New York: Macmillan, 1937.

   An introduction to the problems, methods and results of the study of individual and group differences in behavior.

2. Carmichael, L. (Ed.). *Manual of child psychology.* New York: Wiley, 1947. Chaps. 9 to 19.

   Eleven chapters by eleven authors on differences in children and adolescents in respect of culture, language, intelligence, emotions and sex.

3. Freeman, F. S. *Individual differences.* New York: Holt, 1934.

A textbook on the psychology of individual differences.

4. Garrett, H. E. *Statistics in psychology and education.* (2nd ed.) New York: Longmans, Green, 1937.

A standard textbook on psychological measurement and statistics, covering distribution, variability, sampling, reliability, validity and correlation.

5. Garrett, H. E., and Schneck, M. M. R. *Psychological tests, methods and results.* New York: Harper, 1933.

A survey of common psychological tests, including sensory and motor functions, special aptitudes, general intelligence and personality characteristics, together with some of the problems involved in their construction and use.

6. Gilliland, A. R., and Clark, E. L. *Psychology of individual differences.* New York: Prentice-Hall, 1939.

Another textbook on the psychology of individual differences.

7. Greene, E. B. *Measurements of human behavior.* New York: Odyssey, 1941.

A text on psychological testing, covering the topics of intelligence, special aptitude and personality tests, and including several chapters on the more technical problems of test construction.

8. Huxley, J. S., and Haddon, A. C. *We Europeans: a survey of "racial" problems.* London: Cape, 1935.

A sound, popular introduction to the critical evaluation of studies on race differences in psychological characteristics.

9. Klineberg, O. *Race differences.* New York: Harper, 1935.

A comprehensive survey of psychological data on race differences, discussed from the biological, psychological and cultural approach.

10. Lindquist, E. F. *A first course in statistics.* Boston: Houghton Mifflin, 1938.

Another standard textbook on psychological statistical methods, discussing distribution, variability, sampling, reliability, validity and correlation.

11. Mead, M. *Sex and temperament in three primitive societies.* New York: Morrow, 1935.

An anthropologist's field observations in three primitive cultures, which have a bearing on the problem of sex differences in personality characteristics.

12. Paterson, D. G. *Physique and intellect.* New York: Appleton-Century, 1930.

A standard textbook, somewhat out of date, discussing the relation of physique to intelligence, mental efficiency and temperament.

13. Penrose, L. S. *Mental defect.* New York: Farrar and Rinehart, 1934.

A systematic treatise on feeblemindedness, its diagnosis, varieties and treatment.

14. Scheinfeld, A. *Women and men.* New York: Harcourt, Brace, 1943.

A popularly written but thorough review of the whole problem of sex differences.

15. Sheldon, W. H., and Stevens, S. S. *The varieties of temperament.* New York: Harper, 1942.

The case for the relation of temperament to physique—the relation of viscerotonia, somatotonia and cerebrotonia to endomorphy, mesomorphy and ectomorphy.

16. Sheldon, W. H., Stevens, S. S., and Tucker, W. B. *The varieties of human physique.* New York: Harper, 1940.

The system for the characterization of human physiques in respect to endomorphy, mesomorphy and ectomorphy, with some psychology thrown in on the side.

17. Terman, L. M., and Miles, C. C. *Sex and personality.* New York: McGraw-Hill, 1936.

Report of an extensive research project on sex differences in personality characteristics in our culture; the most comprehensive treatment of this question to date.

18. Terman, L. M., and Oden, M. H. *The gifted child grows up.* Stanford, Calif.: Stanford University Press, 1947.

The fourth volume, a follow-up after twenty-five years, of Terman's well-known study of a thousand very gifted children.

19. Tyler, L. E. *Psychology of human differences.* New York: Appleton-Century, 1947.

A recent textbook which considers the general problems of measuring individual differences and summarizes the evidence for differences dependent on sex, race, social class, age and intelligence, and the present status of attitudes and traits.

20. Wellman, B. L. Sex differences. In C. Murchison (Ed.), *A handbook of child psychology.* Worcester, Mass.: Clark University Press, 1933. Chap. 15.

A summary of the major findings on sex differences in psychological characteristics prior to 1933.

CHAPTER 19

Heredity and Environment

THE underlying causes of individual differences in behavior are to be found in the subjects' varied hereditary backgrounds and in the differing environmental conditions to which they have been exposed. Besides its basic theoretical significance, the question of the causation of individual differences has important practical applications. Any procedure concerned with the control or modification of human development must be based upon an understanding of the factors which influence such development. All educational methods, for example, make some assumption, tacitly or explicitly, regarding the causes of human traits. Is it the function of education to produce certain desirable traits or merely to offer opportunities for the development of the individual's inborn potentialities?

For instance, what causes sex differences? Biologically sex is inherited, for it depends upon the characters in the germ cells that unite to form the new individual. How much of the psychological sex differences depend also on the germ cells or on other differences which in their turn are dependent on the germ cells, and how much do they result from experience and social pressure? Can you, do you, *learn* to be a man? or a woman? The beliefs about what is the right answer to this question affect the answer, for they determine the types of educational programs, vocations and many other activities that are assigned traditionally to men and to women, and which thus help to make masculinity and femininity what they are today.

It is the same way with the problems that concern racial or national groups. If you think that the characteristics of such a group are inherited, you will be recommending one kind of action about the group. If you think the characteristics are gained through formal education or through the informal education of living, you may have a different set of recommendations. You cannot deal wisely with such problems unless you know what has caused the differences that create the problems.

FUNDAMENTAL CONCEPTS

Every trait of the individual and every reaction which he manifests depend both upon his heredity and upon his environment. We have already met that truth in our study of the facts of maturation (Chapter 4). Traits or activities cannot be divided into those which are inherited and those which are acquired. Since it is now recognized, however, that hereditary and environmental influences interact in the production of all the characteristics

This chapter was prepared by Anne Anastasi of Fordham University.

of the individual, the problem resolves itself into a determination of the relative contribution of each in the development of any given function. How much is *nature* and how much *nurture?* we may ask, using the pair of words that Francis Galton introduced when he discussed this problem. To what extent can the development of a function be altered by the control of environmental conditions, and to what extent is such modification limited by hereditary factors? Individual differences occurring under the same heredity may be attributed to the operation of different environmental factors. Similarly, when the environments are sufficiently alike, dissimilarities of behavior indicate differing heredity.

What Is Heredity?

It should be borne in mind that the term *heredity* signifies biological heredity. It is only figuratively that we speak of 'social heredity,' as in such expressions as 'the cultural heritage of the twentieth century' or 'the inheritance of the family fortune.' Society is in the environment, and social inheritance is actually a kind of environmental influence.

The hereditary factors which contribute to the development of the individual are referable to the *genes,* minute structures occurring within the nucleus of all living cells. The genes are grouped into *chromosomes,* 'colored bodies,' so named because they become visible when the cell is stained by certain dyes for observation. These chromosomes occur in pairs, the two members of each pair being similar in appearance. The number of chromosomes in each cell is, in general, constant for every species, but differs from one species to another. Each human cell, for example, contains 48 chromosomes (24 pairs); in each cell of the mosquito, there are 6 (3 pairs); and in each cell of a certain species of crayfish, 200 (100 pairs). (See Fig. 210.)

Growth takes place by cell division. One cell divides into two; later these two into four, and so on. When a cell divides, the 48 chromosomes split longitudinally, presumably splitting each gene in two, and one half of each chromosome goes to each daughter cell. Thus the daughter cells—and what we might call the granddaughter and great-granddaughter cells, all down the line—have exactly the same constitution as to chromosomes and genes as the original parent cell which started the individual off in life.

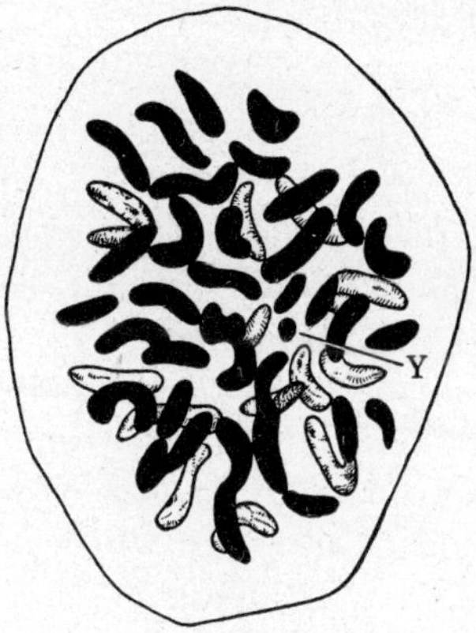

FIGURE 210. MICROSCOPIC VIEW OF HUMAN CHROMOSOMES

Shows the 48 human chromosomes. The Y-chromosome determines sex. Sex is hereditary, depending on the genes of the father. [From H. M. Evans and O. Swezy, *Mem. Univ. Calif.*, 1929, **9**, No. 1.]

At puberty the *germ cells* are formed, *ova* in the female and *sperms* in the male. They are formed from other cells by a different kind of division, known as *reduction division,* because the chromosomes do not split longitudinally in two, but pass one set of 24 to one cell and the other set to the other cell. An ovum or a sperm has, thereafter, only 24 chromosomes, half the equipment of a normal cell, and that means only half of the normal cell's double set of genes. Although the chromosomes do not split longitudinally in this division, they may divide transversely, recombining genes in new combinations in a single one of the new chromosomes. The parent cell, it will be seen, has many pairs of genes, ever so many of them, although we do not know just how many genes are in one chromosome. Every germ cell gets one gene from each pair of genes in the parent cell, but, since there is some crossing over, a new chromosome may contain some genes from a given parent chromosome and the other genes from the mate of that chromosome.

When a new individual is begun at conception, an ovum and a sperm combine to make the first parent cell which *is* the new organism. It will have 24 chromosomes that came from the ovum and 24 that came from the sperm. Together they make up the normal complement of 48 chromosomes in 24 pairs. Half the genes are from one parent, and half from the other. When this single cell has, by repeated division, grown into a mature individual, it will pass half its genes to its ova or its sperms and thus to its progeny. There is, however, no way of predicting which genes of any pair will be the ones included in any one germ cell and thus be the ones inherited by the new individual.

Chromosomes are visible under a microscope, appearing as rodlike, sausage-shaped, or V-shaped bodies. A microscopic view of human chromosomes is shown in Fig. 210. Within each chromosome are the genes, particles so minute that they are invisible, even with a high-power microscope. Recent observations of the giant chromosomes in the salivary glands of the fruit fly have, however, opened a way for the study of the internal structure of chromosomes and may thus lead to a direct knowledge of the genes. Figure 211 is a photograph of such a giant chromosome, with its characteristic pattern of transverse bands. It has been suggested that the bands may bear some relation to the theoretically inferred genes. A gene is the carrier of a *unit character,* an hereditary factor which is always transmitted as a unit in all-or-none fashion. The unit characters carried by the genes are not to be confused with traits, for the genes are of a much more elementary nature. Thus, even such a relatively simple characteristic as the eye color of the fruit fly depends upon more than fifty separate genes. Such complex hereditary determination will of course produce varying degrees of a trait, even though each individual gene is transmitted in an all-or-none manner.

Any attempt to identify psychological characteristics, and especially such complex and vaguely defined behavior phenomena as 'intelligence,' with unit characters is wholly unjustified when we know so little about the genes. So simple a relation is also highly improbable. The experimental identification of the specific genes which influence the development of observable characteristics of the organism is an extremely difficult task. In recent years some progress has been made in this work by geneticists. T. H. Morgan has mapped genes on the chromosomes of the fruit fly. No one, however, expects to find a gene or even a simple set of genes for the mental diseases or other complex human behavior characteristics, the incidence of which we should like to control by eugenics.

The hereditary basis of individual differences lies in the almost unlimited variety of possible gene combinations which may occur, especially in so complex an organism as man. Here you are. Could your parents, knowing themselves, have predicted what you would be like? Could they even have predicted your complement of genes? No, of course they could not. If you got only a thousand genes from one parent and a complementary thousand from the other parent, the number of possible combinations of genes is so large that it makes the number of electrons you could pack into a sphere with the diameter of the stellar universe (10^{110}) seem like a very small number indeed. Of course not every gene combination makes a difference. Nevertheless, the wonder is that, in spite of the fact that everyone has only half the genes that his parents had and many of them have no apparent effect, the resemblances due to heredity are as recognizable as they are.

It is clear that two *siblings* (brothers or sisters or a brother and sister) will not have identical heredity. They will not get the same genes from each parent. *Fraternal twins,* born of the same parents at the same time but from different pairs of germ cells, will also not have the same complement of genes. On the other hand, *identical twins,* which develop from the same sperm-and-ovum will have exactly the same set of genes, for they get their genes by division of the common set. For this reason there has been a great deal of study of identical twins, because they constitute cases where, heredity being the same, differences of environment can be found acting alone.

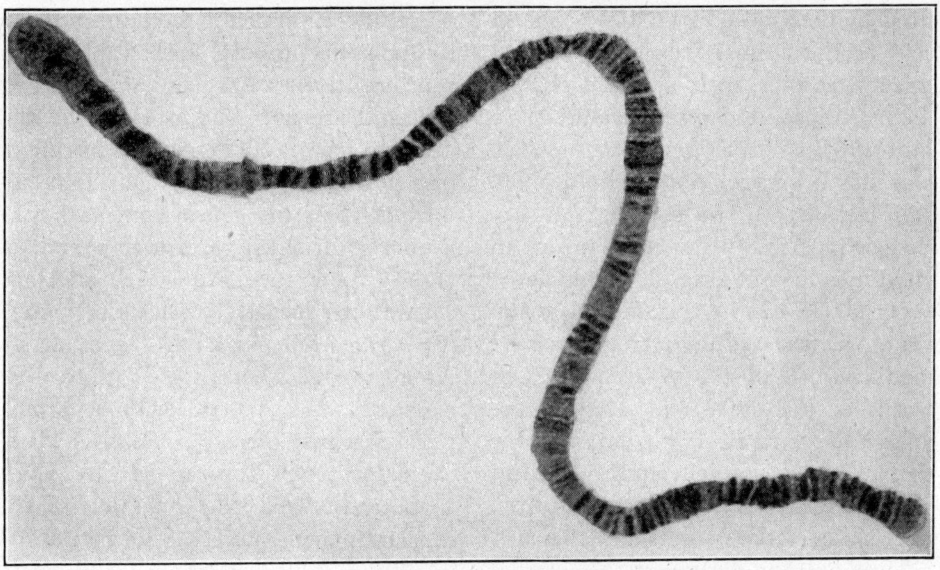

FIGURE 211. MICROSCOPIC VIEW OF GIANT CHROMOSOME FROM THE SALIVARY GLAND OF THE FRUIT FLY

[From T. S. Painter, *J. Heredity,* 1934, **25,** 464.]

Popular Misconceptions Regarding Heredity

(1) In the early part of the nineteenth century, the naturalist Lamarck put forth

the theory of the *inheritance of acquired characteristics.* This theory claimed that the evolution of species characteristics through successive generations resulted from the transmission of the effects of use or disuse of functions by the parent organism. A classical example was the assertion that the long neck and legs of the giraffe were produced by the gradual stretching of neck and legs as the animals reached for food among the tree tops, such acquired elongation being transmitted by each successive generation to its offspring. No acceptable evidence has ever been found to support such an hypothesis. In fact, present-day knowledge regarding the mechanism of heredity tends to contradict it. Only genes in the germ cells can be transmitted to the offspring, whereas acquired characteristics are modifications of the nonreproductive body cells of the organism. Despite the lack of scientific support, the popular belief that children can inherit the musical training, artistic sophistication or acquired muscular skills of the parents still survives.

(2) A related popular superstition, even farther removed from the known facts of heredity, is that experiences of the mother during pregnancy exert *prenatal influences* upon the developing offspring. Birthmarks, as well as numerous other abnormalities of appearance or behavior, have from time to time been erroneously attributed to such maternal experiences. One is told, for example, that a disfiguring hairy mole on the chin resulted from the subject's mother having touched her chin when frightened by a shaggy-haired Airedale. Or a child's agility in climbing will be ascribed to his mother's frequent visits to the monkey house at the zoo during her pregnancy. Although there is no possible way in which such experiences of the parent can affect the developing embryo, hopeful mothers can still be found who frequent art museums or concerts during their pregnancies in the fond expectation of developing their children's interests along these socially esteemed lines!

(3) Another popular misconception is that the inheritance of a characteristic is indicated only by *resemblance to parents.* A consideration of the mechanism of heredity fails to support such a belief. The genes continue from generation to generation and are not produced new by the individual parent. The parents merely transmit genes to their offspring. Thus a person gets half his genes from each parent, a quarter of them from each grandparent, and $1/_{1024}$ of them from each ancestor ten generations back. He has no genes that his parents did not have. Many genes are latent or *recessive* in that they are not effective when paired with a *dominant* gene, yet may become effective when, in the later generations to which they have been transmitted, the operation of chance in gene pairing may have taken away the dominant inhibitor. When a person gets two recessive genes from his parents, both of whom were hybrids with their observable characteristics determined by dominant genes, he will resemble neither parent. He may, however, resemble an ancestor, for he is still what his genes make him so far as hereditary characteristics go, and his ancestors were also what their genes made them, and it was from his ancestors that he got his genes.

These facts become clearer when we understand the Mendelian scheme of inheritance, which shows how dominant and recessive genes interact to give different observable characteristics in offspring. Figure 212 shows how inheritance of black and white coat color in guinea pigs works out. Black being dominant, a black guinea pig may be either pure black or a hybrid. Figure 213 shows the same relations schematically, with recessive white hidden under dominant black in the hybrids. In other words, when both parents are hybrids, about one-fourth of the children resemble neither parent.

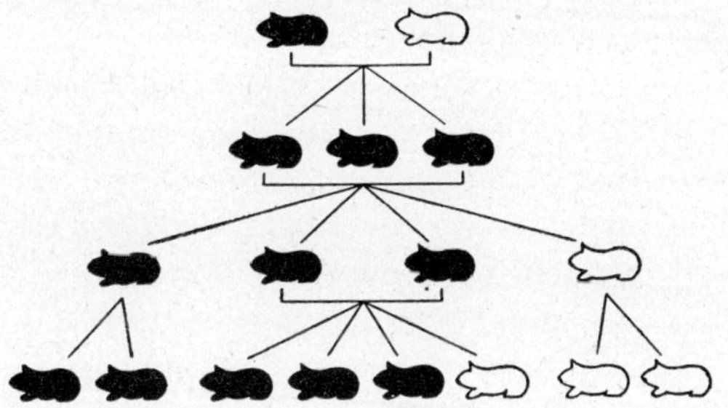

FIGURE 212. MENDELIAN INHERITANCE OF COAT COLOR IN THE GUINEA PIG

The black coat is dominant over the recessive white coat. The first pair here shows the mating of an animal from a pure black strain with one from a pure white strain. All guinea pigs of the second generation are hybrids, but they look black because black is dominant over white. In the third generation you get pure blacks, black hybrids and pure whites in the ratios shown in Fig. 213.

Not all characteristics follow the rule of dominance and recession. Some hybrids are intermediate between their parents. Thus the white and Negro genes combine to give mulattoes of varying degrees of whiteness and blackness.

(4) Still another popular misconception about inheritance is that *whatever is present at birth is inherited and whatever develops subsequently is acquired.* Taken as it stands, this statement is inconsistent with the concept of development as an interaction of heredity and environment. Even if reformulated to state that hereditary influences cease at birth, however, it is still incorrect. Hereditary factors may influence the development of the individual long after birth, and in fact throughout his life span. Even the onset of death itself may be determined partly by hereditary factors, as is suggested by the observation that longevity tends to run in families. Hereditary influences may first become manifest at any age. Similarly, environmental influences begin to operate upon the organism before birth and from the moment of conception. Birth is not to be regarded as a beginning in the life of the individual, but as one important event which occurs in a long life history extending from conception to death.

What specifically, then, do the genes accomplish? In an earlier chapter we have seen that heredity, working in an adequate environment, determines the growth and development not only of all the structures of the body, but also their organization into a functional whole, and in particular the neuromuscular coordinations that occur before any unlearned form of behavior can take place. These coordinations of un-

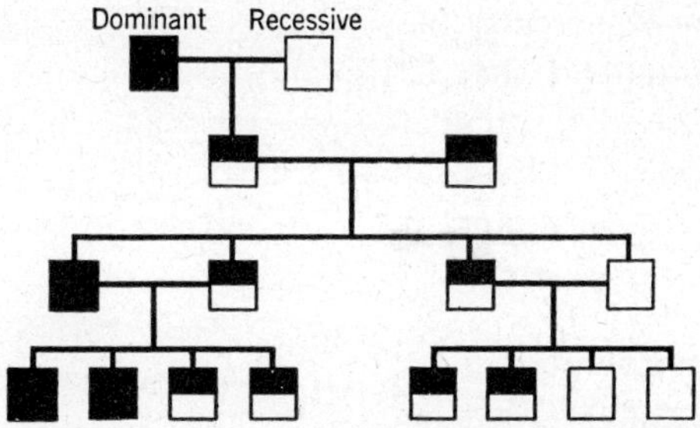

FIG. 213. MENDELIAN INHERITANCE: SCHEMATIC

Comparable to Fig. 212. Black is dominant, white is recessive. Hybrids are shown with black on top of white. Pure dominants and pure recessives are solid black and solid white, respectively. The figure shows the ratios of progeny that different matings would yield. For example, two hybrids mated should have progeny in the ratio 1 pure dominant : 2 hybrids : 1 pure recessive, but to observation the 1 : 2 : 1 ratio looks like 3 : 1.

learned behavior are common to every normal human being of whatever race or culture.

A large proportion of man's behavior, however, is learned. What part does heredity play in learning? In the first place, man's bodily structure determines some things that he cannot learn to do. He cannot learn to fly like a bird because he has no wings. He cannot learn to breathe under water because he has no gills. In learning he is limited by the equipment which the genes have provided. He can develop muscles he already has, but he cannot create new ones. He can strengthen nerve connections and perhaps open new paths through the synapses, but he cannot create new connectors or paths. In other words, heredity has furnished him with an equipment that is capable of doing many more things than are necessary for the maintenance of his life and the reproduction of his species, and man in learning utilizes this equipment.

Environment

Now environment. What is it? The concept of environment also requires some clarification. Psychologically, a person's environment consists of the sum total of the stimulation which he receives from his conception until his death. Physical objects are in the environment only when they serve to stimulate. There are many kinds of stimulators, situations as well as energy changes, objects and events, light radiations and sound waves, as well as a teacher's command, a friend's request, an emotion or the result of a bit of thinking. The environment is *everything* that affects the individual *except his genes.* The genes have furnished the mechanisms of behavior. Only the environment can actuate it, can set it going. Only the environment can start the learning of new forms of behavior which, when established, must in turn be actuated by stimulation.

The popular definition of environment is a geographical or residential one. A child is said to have a 'poor environment,' for example, because he lives in the slums. Or his 'environment' is specified as a French village, an American small town or a British mining community. Psychologically these are inadequate characterizations of environment. We cannot even conclude, for example, that an eight-year-old boy and his five-year-old brother standing in the same room at the same time have identical psychological environments at that moment. The very fact that the immediate environment of the former includes the presence of a younger sibling and that of the latter the presence of an older sibling constitutes a significant psychological difference. Furthermore, the differing backgrounds of previous experience of the two siblings will in turn cause a difference in what each gets out of the present situation. For such reasons it is possible for differences in abilities, emotional characteristics, interests and other psychological characteristics to be found in siblings and to result from different environmental influences, even though the siblings have been brought up in the same home.

Structure and Function

It is a mistake to speak of functions and activities as if they were directly inherited. As we have seen, functions, activities and all forms of behavior result from the interaction of heredity (the structures and their organization) with environment. Functions as such cannot possibly be inherited. Can abilities? An ability is the potentiality which you possess for producing a certain result, and the measure of the result—your performance—is the measure of your ability. It is almost impossible, however, to determine how much of an ability is the result of heredity. Consider, for example, a race horse. Horses are, of course, bred for speed. There must, therefore, be unit characters that make for a body conformation that in turn makes for speed. A horse, thus bred, must demonstrate his ability by performance. He must show what he can do in a race. But, before the race, he goes through a long period of training (environment) and in the race he runs in competition with other horses (more environment) under the guidance of a jockey (still more environment). If he wins his race he has turned in a good performance, but not even the breeders themselves can accurately evaluate his performance in terms of heredity and environment.

The breeding of animals for some particular ability has thrown some light on the influence of heredity, but in man breeding still goes by natural selection. Since men and women mate for a wide variety of reasons we have no way of knowing for certain whether there are in fact unit characters for some abilities, for example, intelligence. Consequently many experimental techniques have been devised for the study of the problem. Some of these together with their results we shall now consider.

THE STUDY OF HEREDITARY AND ENVIRONMENTAL INFLUENCES

The difficulty of isolating the influence of heredity from that of environment is the chief problem which must be met by investigators in this field. If heredity can be assumed to be constant, as in identical twins, differences can be attributed to environment. Similarly, if environment could be held constant, any observed differences would be the result of hereditary influences. In view of our discussion of what, psychologically, constitutes environment, it should be apparent that it is impossible to hold environment wholly constant for any two individuals, especially for human subjects. Nevertheless there have been many efforts to distinguish between the effects of heredity and environment, and to the chief techniques employed we may properly turn our attention now.

Selective Breeding

Since the famous experiments of Mendel, geneticists have made constant use of selective breeding to investigate the inheritance of the characteristics of bodily structure. So far, however, the experimental mating of animals selected on the basis of psychological characteristics has been infrequent. One such investigation has, however, dealt with maze learning in white rats. An initial group of 142 rats were given 19 trials in running a maze, and the number of errors was determined for each animal. The group exhibited wide individual differences in maze-learning ability, the total number of blind-alley entrances in 19 trials ranging from 7 to 214. On the basis of these scores, a group of the brightest and a group of the dullest rats were selected for experimental mating. The bright rats in this parent generation (P) were mated with each other and the dull were likewise mated together. This procedure was followed through 22 successive filial generations (F_1 to F_{22}). In each successive generation, the brightest rats were selected and were bred together, the dullest were selected and interbred. Environment—food, lighting, temperature and living

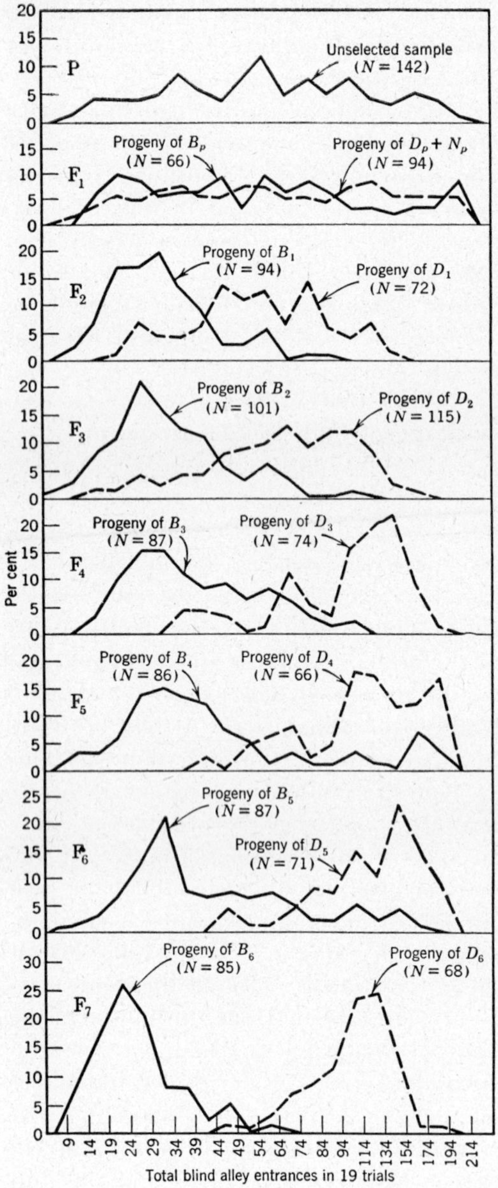

FIGURE 214. EFFECT OF SELECTIVE BREEDING FOR A PSYCHOLOGICAL TRAIT

Number of errors (blind-alley entrances) in maze learning of white rats when brightest rats (*B*, solid line) are bred together and dullest rats (*D*, dotted line) are bred together in each successive generation. Many errors = dullness; and conversely. After 7 selections and 7 generations the distribution curves hardly overlap at all. [From R. C. Tryon, *Thirty-ninth Yearbook of the National Society for the Study of Education,* 1940, Part I, p. 113.]

quarters—was kept constant for all rats in the different generations.

The effect of such selective breeding upon maze performance is illustrated in Fig. 214. The distribution curves indicate the percentage of rats in each group who made the number of errors given on the baseline. It will be noted that the distributions of the bright and dull subgroups gradually separate until there is virtually no overlapping between them when the seventh generation is reached. Beyond the seventh generation, the effects of further selective breeding were negligible; individual differences within the bright and dull groups remained virtually unchanged and the differentiation between the two groups showed no appreciable increase. When groups of bright and dull rats were bred with each other, a distribution similar to that of the original parental group resulted; most of the animals obtained intermediate scores, with relatively few at the dull and bright extremes. The distributions of the bright and dull parental groups and of two such crossbred filial generations are given in Fig. 215. No simple relation of dominance and recession holds for the ability of rats to learn mazes. Here brightness and dullness mix like white and black in the mulatto.

Such an experiment demonstrates that hereditary factors play an important part in the maze performance of rats. Through what specific structural characteristics the hereditary influences operated is not, however, indicated. It cannot be concluded that there is a specific gene or combination of genes *directly* concerned with the transmission of any such characteristic as maze-learning ability. The learning of a maze was a performance employed as a measure of the general ability called intelligence.

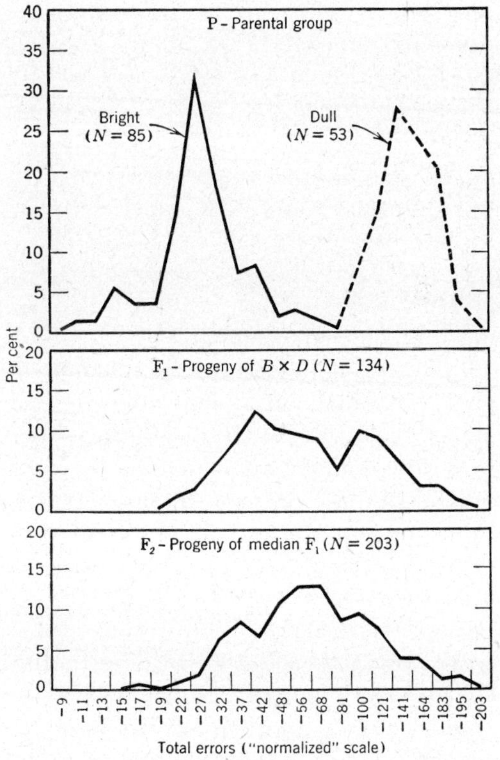

FIGURE 215. THE EFFECT OF MATING BRIGHT AND DULL RATS

Reversing the selection shown in Fig. 214. The bright and dull maze-learning rats were mated, and at once the progeny spread over the entire range of maze-learning ability, with the average brightness more frequent than either extreme. [From R. C. Tryon, *Thirty-ninth Yearbook of the National Society for the Study of Education,* 1940, Part I, p. 115.]

The results may be regarded as showing that this ability may perhaps be inherited, but it is also possible that hereditary factors may influence a number of characteristics, such as health, physical vigor, brain development, endocrine balance, intensity of the hunger drive, activity level, which in turn affect *indirectly* the maze learning of white rats. For example, in the experiment just described, clear-cut differences in emotionality were observed between the bright and dull groups.

Family Resemblances

It is a common belief that family resemblances in psychological characteristics furnish direct evidence of the influence of heredity. Thus a child may be described as having his father's flair for public speaking, his aunt's musical sensitivity, 'taking after' his paternal grandfather in obstinacy and inheriting his sense of humor from an Irish grandmother on his mother's side! Nor is this type of interpretation to be found exclusively in naive popular discussions. Many otherwise accurate and well-conducted studies on family resemblances contain the same fallacy in that they fail to consider the fact that close relatives commonly live together. The environment of individuals who share the same home is certainly more similar than that of persons chosen at random. The closer the hereditary relationship, furthermore, the greater, in general, will be the environmental similarity. Siblings usually live in the same home, but more distant relatives —uncles, nephews, grandparents, cousins— come into less frequent contact and may vary more widely in socio-economic background and in other environmental conditions. Persons who live together or are associated in the same community also constitute in part each other's environment and may become more alike by such interaction.

The two principal methods employed in the study of family resemblances are *family history* and *correlation.* In the family history method, genealogies are traced and pedigree charts constructed for families selected as outstanding either in their talents or in their deficiencies. This method was launched by Francis Galton in 1869 in his book *Hereditary Genius,* where he summarized data on 997 eminent men in a total of 300 British families. Later studies in different countries have, in general, corroborated Galton's findings. All show that eminence tends to run in families. In some families there is even a succession of persons of similar talents, as in science, or literature, or engineering. Similarly, the investigations of degenerate and feebleminded families, of which the most widely quoted in the psychological literature are known by the pseudonyms of the *Jukes* and the *Kallikaks,* show that such characteristics as crime, pauperism and other social ills also tend to run in families. To argue from such results to hereditary causation, however, is not justified. The operation of environmental family influences in such instances is too obvious to be ignored.

Investigations by the correlation method are based upon the mental test scores of a group of individuals bearing a certain family relationship to each other. For example, pairs of siblings from one hundred different families may be given the Stanford-Binet Intelligence Test. The IQ's of the two siblings in each family are then paired off and a correlation coefficient computed between these two sets of IQ's. The size of the correlation indicates the degree of resemblance or correspondence in the performance of siblings within the group.

The trend of results in such mental test studies is illustrated in the correlations reproduced in Table XXIII. It will be noted that the coefficients fall into a hierarchy which parallels closely both the degree of family relationship and the extent of environmental community and contact. Thus a correlation of +0.90 is found for identical twins, who have identical heredity and are also exposed to more nearly identical environmental influences than any other type of siblings. Fraternal twins, including both like-sex and unlike-sex pairs, yield a correlation of 0.70, which drops to 0.59 when only unlike-sex pairs are included. In interpreting this drop we must recall the traditional differences in training and play activities and in attitudes of parents and associates toward boys and girls. Such differences in the environments of the two sexes would serve to increase the discrepancy in ability between unlike-sex fraternal twins as contrasted to the twins of like sex. Another interesting comparison is that between the total fraternal-twin correlation of 0.70 and the sibling correlation of 0.50. The degree of hereditary resemblance within these two types of family relationship is the same, since all develop from different germ cells of the same parents. The difference between these two correlations can therefore be attributed primarily to the greater environmental similarity of twins as compared to siblings born at different times.

TABLE XXIII

HIERARCHY OF CORRELATION COEFFICIENTS INDICATING FAMILY RESEMBLANCES IN INTELLIGENCE TEST SCORES

[From A. N. Wingfield, *Twins and orphans: the inheritance of intelligence*, Dent, 1928, p. 106.]

Type of Relationship	*Correlation Coefficient*
Identical twins	0.90
All fraternal twins (both sexes)	0.70
Fraternal twins of unlike sex	0.59
Siblings	0.50
Parent and child	0.31
Cousins	0.27
Grandparent and grandchild	0.16
Unrelated children	0.00

On the other hand, the difference between the 0.90 correlation of identical twins and the 0.70 of fraternals is more commonly attributed to heredity. A word of caution should, however, be added here. Because of their closer physical resemblance, identical twins generally receive more similar treatment than fraternal twins. Fraternal twins may be children who vary as much in health, physical vigor and attractiveness as two ordinary siblings. Such physical differences may in turn lead to differences in social acceptance and in attitudes, interests, motivation and habitual activities. Furthermore, it should be noted that if only like-sex fraternal twins had been considered, the correlation would undoubtedly have been considerably higher than 0.70. The identical-twin correlation is, of course, derived only from like-sex pairs, for all identical twins are of the same sex. Sex is inherited; it depends on a gene.

Further reference to Table XXIII shows that the correlations between parents-and-children, cousins and grandparents-and-grandchildren follow in decreasing order of magnitude. The correlation between unrelated children is zero by definition, since to compute a correlation in such a group the children would have to be paired off by chance.

Foster Family Relationships

Foster children, as well as orphans reared in institutions, offer a special opportunity to isolate, to a certain extent, the influence of heredity from that of environment, since such children are not in contact with persons related to them by heredity. Such isolation is not, however, perfect. When the children have spent the first few years with their natural parents, an uncontrolled environmental influence is introduced which tends to heighten resemblance to parents. Nor can we ignore the role of prenatal environment, with possible differences in the nutrition of the mother and the adequacy of prenatal medical care which usually occurs with difference in socio-economic level. At best the isolation of hereditary and environmental factors in such investigations is only partial.

Foster children, nevertheless, show a rise in IQ after adoption into a foster home. The rise is greater the younger the child at the time of adoption and the higher the socio-economic level of the foster home. Usually adoption means increase of socio-economic level, although there may be exceptions in the adoption of illegitimate children shortly after birth. The resemblance between siblings living in different foster homes, furthermore, is much less than that ordinarily found between siblings in the same home. For example, in one group of 125 siblings, each of whom was adopted into a different foster home and separated for a period ranging from 4 to 13 years, the sibling correlation in Stanford-Binet IQ was only 0.25, in contrast to the correlation of about 0.50 usually found between siblings living together. Foster siblings who are unrelated by heredity but live in the same home, on the other hand, yield correlations even higher than 0.25. Significant and moderately high correlations are also found between the IQ's of foster children and the intelligence test scores of their foster parents. The children's IQ's also show good correlation with indices of the cultural level of the foster home. All these findings indicate how important is the role which environment plays in the development of intelligence.

On the other hand, certain investigators have stressed the influence of heredity on the grounds that the correlation between the intelligence of foster parents and foster children is appreciably lower than between children and their own parents when the latter are living together. Thus in one study 194 foster children, adopted under the age of 6 months, were compared with a matched control group of 194 children living with their own parents. The children in the foster and control group were paired off in sex, mental age, father's occupation and father's and mother's schooling. The socio-economic levels of both groups were similar and quite homogeneous. The children were 5 to 14 years of age at the time of testing; thus the foster children had lived in their adopted homes for many years. The correlations between foster children's Stanford-Binet IQ and foster father's score on the Otis Intelligence Test was 0.19, with the foster mother's Otis score, 0.24, and with the cultural index of the foster home, 0.26. In the control group, all three correlations were 0.51.

A similar emphasis upon hereditary factors is found in an investigation on illegitimate children placed in an orphanage under the age of one year and reared there together, without home contacts. Such children developed large differences in intelligence which were found to be correlated significantly with the socio-economic level of their own parents. Orphans of merchants and professional men, for example, scored on the average about 10 points higher in IQ than the orphans of laborers in the same institution. Such differences may result in part from prenatal care and in part from hereditary factors which affect health, stamina, physical vigor and other characteristics and thus influence 'intelligence' indirectly.

An even more crucial isolation of factors may be achieved in the study of identical twins who have been separated in infancy or early childhood and reared in different foster homes. In one investigation 19 such pairs of twins were studied intensively through psychological tests, interviews with the twins and their associates and visits to the foster homes. The interpair difference in IQ ranged from 1 to 24 points, with an average of 8.2. A fairly close correspondence was found between difference in educational opportunities and difference in IQ from one twin to the other in each pair. Differences in personality characteristics tended to be larger, but they also showed the same variation as the IQ's, some pairs being closely alike and others very different. Such variations in interpair differences, both in intelligence and personality, are not surprising. The accidental separations of everyday life, which any one pair of twins may undergo, cannot be regarded in the same light as an experimentally controlled segregation. In the latter every effort is made to choose environments which are as unlike as possible, in order to make the test more crucial and the results more distinct. In the 19 pairs under consideration, however, a certain element of chance entered into the allocation of the twins in each pair to specific foster homes. Thus certain pairs may have been adventitiously adopted into homes which differed markedly, other pairs reared in surroundings which shared a few important features, and still others put in environments which, although geographically remote, may have been fundamentally alike in their influence upon the growing child. Let us examine a sample case, showing a relatively large discrepancy between the twins.

The case of M and R. These twin girls were fifteen years old when examined, having been separated at the age of three months and reared, one of them in the home of a maternal uncle and the other with the uncle's brother-in-law. M lived in a small town where she knew nearly everybody and had many friends and playmates. Her foster father was well educated and had a cultured home, with good books, good music, etc. R was brought up in a large city but was kept closely at home and had few friends. Her home environment is described as narrow and unstimulating. Neither of her foster parents had received much education. Formal schooling differed little for the twins; M was in grade 10A and R in grade 10B at the time of examination. The physical environment was reported to be about the same for both girls. When examined, the twins showed remarkable similarity in physical characteristics. Mentally, however, there was a large difference, M doing consistently better on all the tests. The Stanford-Binet IQ's were 92 and 77, respectively, for M and R. In temperament their differences were also large, as indicated both by personality tests and by general observation. R was described as timid and retiring, with a marked lisp in her speech, and apparently unhappy. M, on the other hand, seemed quite normal in emotional adjustment. One might expect a girl with few friends not to be very happy; the point here is that she also had a lower IQ. The IQ is favored by a high level of motivational alertness which may in turn arise from environmental stimulation.

Evidence from Maturation

We have already seen how the maturation of the organism depends both on the contribution of the genes in heredity and on the effect of the environment and experience as maturation proceeds. In both children and infrahuman animals new items of behavior are added to the repertoire when certain levels of development have been reached. The child must have usable legs to walk on before it can walk, but it also needs a certain development of its nervous system. The embryo and the fetus develop regularly, dependent largely on heredity for what happens to them, but also to some extent upon the environment as they meet it in the uterus. A baby born one month prematurely needs one month of development before it is able to do what can be expected of a child born at the normal term; and a baby born one month late is found to have matured beyond the level normal for a neonate. Psychological age at this period is better measured from the time of conception than from the time of birth.

Further evidence on this nature-nurture problem has been gained by controlling the environment and noting whether maturation takes place without the aid of nurture. How far, the question is asked, can the flying or singing of birds, the swimming of tadpoles or the sexual behavior of monkeys develop in the absence of relevant environmental stimulation? We have seen that preparation for them may develop without practice or exercise, that the unpracticed organism quickly picks up the new behavior when it has matured enough and when it is at last provided with the situations that call for the use of the behavior (pp. 79 f.).

Sometimes normal maturation is altered by environmental change. An example of this process occurs in the sexual behavior of animals who are reared in isolation from other members of their species or in exclusive association with individuals of their own sex. They often develop sexual perversions which persist after a normal environment has been provided for them. Although the causes of the comparable development in human beings have been much disputed, there seems to be little doubt that environmental factors have played an important role in the development of many, perhaps all, human sexual perversions.

Of special interest for the problem of heredity and environment are the experiments by the method of *co-twin control.* This technique uses pairs of identical twins. One member of each pair is given intensive training in certain functions; the other is used as the control subject, being allowed to continue his normal everyday life without special training. In general, such studies have shown that the effects of specific environmental stimulation are either slight or temporary in the development of motor and sensory behavior in young children. For example, a pair of 46-week-old identical-twin girls were examined for stair climbing and for behavior toward play cubes, including their ability to reach for and grasp the cubes, to manipulate them and to play constructively with them. The trained twin (T) received 20 minutes of training daily for 6 weeks. At the end of this period, the control twin (C), having had no specific training in either function, proved equal to the trained twin in her behavior with cubes. In stair climbing, T excelled, but this difference disappeared after C had received only 2 weeks of training. Thus, because she was 53 weeks old when she began the training, twin C was able to accomplish in 2 weeks what had required 6 weeks of training for T, who began when only 46 weeks old. (On the development of the twins, Johnny and Jimmy, see pp. 80 f.)

Experiments with human infants who have been artificially prevented from exercising such motor functions as standing, sitting or reaching for objects show at first considerable retardation in the development of these functions as compared with the norms. After only a short unrestricted period, however, the normal activities appear.

A natural experiment of this type is furnished by the cradling practices prevalent in certain cultures. Among the Hopi Indians, for example, the newborn child is bundled tightly in a blanket and then tied securely to a stiff board. In such a position the infant cannot move his arms or legs or even turn his body. For the first three months he is kept in these wrappings except for about one hour each day, when he is cleaned and bathed. Despite this extreme early restriction of movement, Hopi children when released later show the same sitting, creeping and walking behavior and in the same sequence as white American children. During the short daily periods when they are freed of their wrappings, furthermore, they assume the usual flexed position, reach for objects and carry them to the mouth, reach for their toes and put them into the mouth, and manifest the other characteristic motor behavior of an unrestricted infant. No significant difference has been found between the average walking age of Hopi infants cradled in the traditional manner and other Hopi children who were reared in the manner of white American children.

Effect of an Unusual Environment

There are some instances of children who have grown up wild with animals and then have been brought into civilization. The results do not indicate that this is a good way to prepare children for modern civilization, but the accounts of what the children were like contain so many vague interpretations that they cannot be reduced to the status of scientific data. Besides there was no control, no identical twin who was not brought up by wolves and went to grammar school instead!

There is, however, on record the case of a human infant and a chimpanzee infant who were for nine months reared together. (A similar case has already found place in this book; p. 81.) The chimpanzee infant, Gua, was isolated from her mother at the age of $7\frac{1}{2}$ months and lived in the psychologist's home, together with his 10-months-old son. The chimpanzee was treated, not as a pet, but as a child, and the two infants were given as nearly identical care as possible. A photograph of them is reproduced in Fig. 216. Gua wore the same articles of clothing as the child and manifested no difficulty in keeping on her shoes, stockings and other clothing. She slept in her own bed equipped with pillow, sheets and blankets. She learned upright locomotion quickly, although that is not normal to chimpanzees. Gua also made excellent progress in learning to eat with a spoon and drink out of a glass. She was able to manipulate pencil, crayons and paper to produce simple scribblings. She also learned to respond correctly to oral language, and by the end of the experimental period understood over fifty words or simple phrases, such as "Show me your nose," "Take it out of your mouth," "Do you want to go bye-bye?" and "Blow the horn." The degree to which it proved possible to 'humanize' the behavior of this ape is especially significant in view of the shortness of its residence—nine months—in a human environment.

Let there be no mistake, however, about this matter. Environment was not the only influence effective on Gua's behavior. Gua could not have been made into a homely child, sent to high school and college or put to work in a store. Heredity was limiting her, not only in personal beauty as judged by human standards, but also in intelligence and many other psychological characteristics, while at the same time it was giving her superhuman strength. The boy soon outstripped the ape in verbal facility, and the ape the boy in ability to climb and jump.

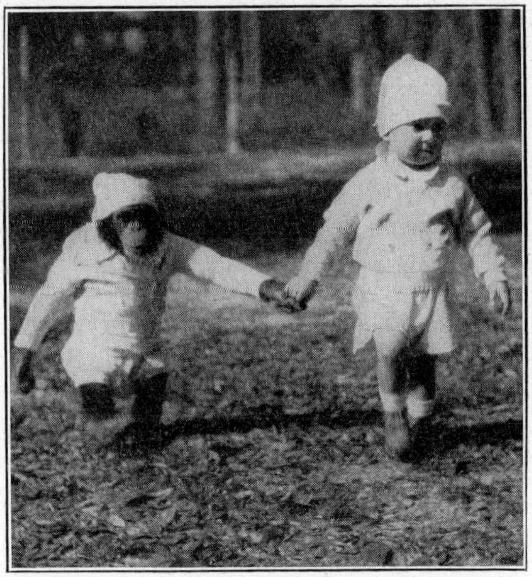

FIGURE 216. HUMAN INFANT AND CHIMPANZEE INFANT REARED TOGETHER

For nine months the two infants were reared together. In Fig. 36, p. 81, another such pair is shown. [From W. N. Kellogg and L. A. Kellogg, *The ape and the child,* McGraw-Hill, 1933, p. 275.]

Effect of Parents' Socio-economic and Occupational Status

Comparison of the intelligence test scores of children reared in different socio-economic levels presents less dramatically the same type of environmental dissimilarities and concomitant behavior differences observed in wild children. Although overlapping is large, as in most group comparisons, it can be said that the average IQ of children shows a consistent relationship to their father's occupational level. In an investigation on 380 preschool children between the ages of 18 and 54 months, for example, the average Kuhlman-Binet IQ's of the children of unskilled laborers was 95.8, that of the children of professional men 125.0. The average IQ's of the intermediate occupational groups fell consistently between these two extreme values. In another study, a group scale of intelligence was administered to 6688 elementary school children and 1433 high school students. The results were similar. The number of children in each occupational group, together with the median and range of IQ, are given in Table XXIV.

TABLE XXIV

IQ of Children in Relation to Father's Occupation Level

[From M. E. Haggerty and H. B. Nash, *J. educ. Psychol.*, 1924, **15**, 569 f.]

Father's Occupational Level	Elementary School Children			High School Students		
	No. Cases	Median IQ	Range in IQ	No. Cases	Median IQ	Range in IQ
1. Professional	349	116	70–177	201	121	80–167
2. Business and clerical	944	107	54–169	374	112	60–168
3. Skilled	1028	98	54–177	54	111	69–139
4. Semiskilled	524	95	53–152	267	108	78–149
5. Farmer	3098	91	50–161	48	108	90–159
6. Unskilled	745	89	51–146	489	106	72–155

We note there that the occupational group differences tend to be smaller in the older groups—the high school groups as compared with the elementary school groups. This difference may result in part from selection, the duller children in all occupational groups having left school before reaching the high school level, and in part from the equalizing influence of the common school environment. The association between father's occupational level and children's IQ in itself could be interpreted as the result of either hereditary or environmental influences, or both. Thus it might be argued that the brighter fathers are more likely to qualify for higher level occupations and are likewise more likely to have brighter children. On the other hand, the superior home environment furnished by fathers in the higher occupational levels may have determined the higher IQ's of the children in these levels.

The testing of children reared in isolated rural communities and other environments, which provide but limited opportunities for intellectual development, furnishes data bearing upon these two interpretations. Children living under these conditions are not exposed to equalizing school influences as they grow older, since their formal schooling is itself inferior. Their other contacts outside the home are usually few and of the same general level as those within the home. In such groups the average IQ's of young children is close to the normal, but it decreases sharply in the older groups. Thus in one investigation of children living in an isolated mountain community in Kentucky, the median IQ dropped steadily from 83.5 at age 7 to 60.6 at age 15. It would hardly be heredity producing that change. Presently we shall see how rural and urban children compare in intelligence.

A survey conducted in England on a group of children living on canal boats and a group of gypsy children showed similar trends. Both groups of children had very inferior schooling, being able to attend school only during short periods of each year. Home environment was also intellectually inferior, many of the parents being illiterate.

The average IQ of all the canal boat

children, whose school attendance was estimated to be only about 5 per cent of that of ordinary elementary school children, was 69.6. An analysis of the IQ's by age level, however, shows a marked negative correlation (−0.75) between IQ and age. Most of the youngest children had IQ's between 90 and 100. Among the eldest, on the other hand, were several IQ's which, at face value, would have led to the diagnosis of feeblemindedness. A comparison of siblings again revealed a consistent drop in IQ from the youngest to the oldest child in the same family.

The scores of the gypsy children corroborated in general the conclusions reached with the canal boat children, although the gypsy children as a group obtained somewhat higher IQ's. This finding is understandable in view of the better schooling of this group, their school attendance being approximately 35 per cent of the normal in contrast to the canal boat children's 5 per cent.

The decline in IQ with age in these groups suggests the influence of environment. Under normal conditions the IQ remains very nearly constant at different ages. In these atypical environments, however, the inadequate education and reduced opportunities for intellectual development become increasingly influential with age. The intellectual requirements of a three-year-old child can be satisfied about as adequately on a canal boat or in an isolated mountain community as in a prosperous urban home. The older child, however, with his broadening intellectual needs, will be seriously affected by these environmental limitations.

At the other extreme, we may note that gifted children generally come from homes whose social and cultural level is above average. Terman, you will recall, in his study of California school children with IQ's of 140 or above, found that the cultural rating of the homes, as well as the educational level reached by parents and grandparents, were well above the average of the general population, although income level was not. An analysis of the fathers' occupations showed nearly one-third (31 per cent) to be in professions, 50 per cent in semiprofessional or higher business occupations, 11.8 per cent in skilled labor and less than 7 per cent in semiskilled or unskilled labor (see p. 427).

Urban, Rural and Regional Influences

In most current intelligence tests, children in rural areas receive lower average scores than those living in cities. This difference is greater in those districts with poorer school facilities, as, for example, those having only one-room schools. The difference between rural and urban children is larger in verbal than in performance tests, and larger in individual than in group scales. A possible explanation of the latter finding is the rural child's greater shyness with strangers, which may handicap his performance in tests administered by an outside examiner. In the administration of an individual test, this difficulty should be in part overcome by the examiner's tact and skill.

We should also note that the majority of intelligence tests have been standardized largely or even exclusively with city children. Thus the selection of content, allocation of items to difficulty levels or age levels and the establishment of norms have been based primarily upon the performance of children reared in urban environments. The influence of such a selection is indicated in a few investigations in which the process was reversed, the choice and placement of items being determined with rural samplings. In a test so constructed, the urban children as a group turned out to make the poorer showing.

The comparison of rural children of different ages reveals the same trend in intelligence test scores observed in isolated or educationally limited environments. In an intensive study of farm children in Iowa, for example, the older children were found to be farther below the urban norm than the younger. Thus a group of 123 infants between the ages of 4 and 40 months showed no noticeable inferiority to urban norms on the Iowa Baby Tests. Nor could this lack of urban-rural difference be attributed to inadequate discriminative power of the tests, since wide individual differences were revealed by these tests. In a preschool group of 163 children between the ages of 3 and 6 years tested with the Detroit Kindergarten Test, an inferiority of the rural children appeared at ages 5 and 6, but no significant difference was found in the lower age levels. A group of 871 rural school children, however, showed a clear mental retardation which increased with age.

In addition to this difference between urban and rural groups, other regional influences have been found. In the United States, for example, differences in intelligence test performance occur among different states, paralleling closely the educational opportunities available in each state. Similarly, clear-cut differences in average intelligence test score have been noted between northern and southern Negroes. On Army Alpha, for example, the median scores of northern and southern Negroes were 38.6 and 12.4, respectively, and on Beta (a performance test) 32.5 and 19.8. Similar results have been obtained in studies with Negro school children. So large are the regional differences among both Negroes and whites, in fact, that the 'racial difference' may be completely reversed when comparing samples from different regions. For example, the median Alpha score of Negro soldiers from certain northern states was higher than that of white soldiers from some southern states which were poor in educational facilities.

The poorer performance of rural and other regional groups on intelligence tests, *per se,* could be interpreted in terms of either *selective migration* or *environmental handicap*. The former hypothesis maintains that the more progressive, intelligent or energetic families are attracted to the more favorable localities, whereas the duller and less ambitious remain in the poorer areas. The action of such a selective process for several generations would, according to this hypothesis, eventually produce a segregation of the inferior stock in the regions which offer fewer opportunities. Urban-rural and other regional differences in intelligence would thus be attributed primarily to an hereditary basis. The hypothesis of environmental handicap, on the other hand, attributes regional inferiority to the poorer facilities for schooling and other educational opportunities, as well as differences in home environment, parental education, play activities, traditions and other cultural factors.

Many of these results on urban-rural differences in 'intelligence' suggest the environmental explanation, although the explanation by heredity is not ruled out. There are, however, a few other studies which furnish direct evidence in support of the environmental explanation. Thus among Negro children who had migrated from the country to the city, it was found that the longer the period of their residence in the urban environment, the higher was their average intelligence test score.

Another technique consisted of the examination of the previous rural school records of both white and Negro children who had subsequently migrated to cities. In no case was the migrating group superior to the nonmigrating at the time when both were living in the same area. Studies of Negro children who had moved from the South to the North yielded results similar to those for rural-urban migrations.

Cross-comparisons of Cultural and Biological Groups

Another fruitful approach to this analysis of the hereditary and environmental contributions to the psychological repertoire is the comparison of overlapping biological and environmental groupings. The same individuals, for example, may be classified according to nationality and 'racial' category. The former is a cultural and environmental classification, the latter a biological category based upon physical characteristics. This approach is illustrated by an investigation conducted on boys from ten to twelve years old in rural areas of Germany, France and Italy. Each of these countries contains more than one of the subgroups of the Caucasian race in its population. In Germany, Nordic and Alpine samples were obtained; in France, Nordic, Alpine and Mediterranean samples; and in Italy, Alpine and Mediterranean samples. The boys were selected from those areas in which 'pure types' of each of these physical subgroups were supposed to be most likely to be found. Only boys born in each specified area, whose parents had also been born in that area, were included. The boys were further chosen on the basis of their eye color, hair color and cephalic index so as to fall within the specified limits of Nordic, Alpine or Mediterranean stocks. Six tests from the Pintner-Paterson Performance Scale were administered with brief oral instructions in the child's own language. When the boys were classified as Nordic, Alpine and Mediterranean, without regard to nationality, no reliable difference in average score was found. Larger and reliable differences appeared, on the other hand, among the three national groups, when the three racial groups were combined. Marked variation was observed, furthermore, within a single racial group when samples of different nationalities were compared. The difference between two Nordic groups of different nationality, for example, was larger than that between the Nordic and Mediterranean groups as a whole.

The major role played by environmental, rather than biological, factors in determining group differences is also indicated in a study of Indian, Negro and white school boys in the United States. Selected tests from the Pintner-Paterson Scale were also used in this investigation. The Indian boys included a group attending a government school and a group living on an Indian reservation. Similarly, two groups were Negro boys, one from New York City and another from rural West Virginia. The white boys were taken from New York City, rural West Virginia and a rural district near the Indian reservation. A comparison of average scores, especially in speed of performance, yielded much larger differences between two groups of the same race living in different regions than between different racial groups in the same region. Thus the New York City Negro boys did better than those in rural West Virginia, and the government school Indians scored higher than the reservation Indians. These differences were larger than the differences among white, Indian and Negro boys as a whole or in comparable areas.

You now have a fair sample of the evidence.

THE HEREDITY-ENVIRONMENT QUESTION: PRESENT STATUS

So what makes the adult? Heredity or environment? His genes or the life he has lived since he was conceived? Obviously both. Both in general, and both in particular. There is no item of the behavior repertoire, no intellectual trait nor personality characteristic that is wholly independent of the genes of its possessor or of the events which have altered him since he began living. Those events include, of course, all his learning, but besides learning, and genes, there are the effects upon the organism of health and disease and accidents. They too help to make the adult what he is.

If we are so sure about this answer, why do we say that this question of heredity and environment is a problem, a controversial problem? Because we want to know how much of each factor is effective. Actually what we are after is knowledge of how to change people, knowledge of how much they can be changed. The solutions of all the great social problems, all social progress, depend on that. Is our behavior as fixed and stereotyped as the behavior of bees and ants, who have a very well-organized totalitarian and socialistic order, or can present experience and learning undo what the genes and past experience seem to have fixed? No wonder everyone is curious about the answer to this question.

Present-day psychologists are not in agreement on this matter. Some lean more heavily upon heredity, others upon environment, in their explanations of behavior. Even when all the approaches are taken into consideration, the available data are still inadequate for a conclusive answer. As in all experimental design, the essential prerequisite is the control of conditions in such a way that all variables shall be constant except the one whose influence is being investigated. Since in nearly all investigations of individual and group differences, the two variables—heredity and environment—have operated together though differentially, the resulting data are usually ambiguous and incapable of definitive interpretation. The crucial experiment is yet to be performed.

It is correct to state that general agreement exists regarding the *interaction* of hereditary and environmental influences in the development of all characteristics, structural as well as behavioral. It is the degree to which any one aspect of behavior depends upon structural limitations traceable to heredity and the degree to which it depends upon the accumulated effects of environment that is the area of controversy.

In the development of *motor* and *sensory* capacities, the role of hereditary factors is commonly emphasized. The results of developmental studies on young children and animals are cited in support of such a view. The close dependence of motor and sensory functions upon physical structures makes such functions more directly susceptible to hereditary determination although both capacities depend in part on environmental influences. In *intellectual* functions, extreme deviations in either direction from the norm often reflect, in part, the influence of health, stamina, endurance, glandular activity or pathological conditions which make normal intellectual development impossible. Insofar as these influences are effective, heredity is playing a part. Within the broad range of intermediate deviations, the range which includes most persons, the role of heredity is, however, much less apparent. It is in regard to such minor individual differences in intellectual functions that one finds the greatest divergence of opinion among psychologists. In respect of emotional and social characteristics, attitudes, moral standards and other aspects of *personality,* most psychologists recognize a major contribution by environmental factors.

To those whose chief concern is with social progress, who fear that heredity may make the human race as unprogressive as the ants, the answer is this: There is plenty of opportunity for change and development. The genes may have been altered little since the dawn of history, yet look at what civilization has accomplished! Even intelligence, as the tests test it, is not beyond improvement. And the personality traits, the psychological items that worry the social planners most, are notoriously dependent on learning and not on the genes. The trouble with the traits is that they tend to get fixed in childhood, so that we turn up with an adult society that is almost as unalterable as if it were gene-determined. Infantile fixations, however, are not gene-determined. The matter of their adjustment belongs in a later chapter (pp. 516–523).

REFERENCES

1. Anastasi, A. *Differential psychology.* New York: Macmillan, 1937.

   An introduction to the psychology of individual and group differences, with considerable attention to the problem of heredity and environment.

2. Freeman, F. S. *Individual differences.* New York: Holt, 1934.

   An elementary treatment of individual and group differences, including many studies on the effects of heredity and environment.

3. Gilliland, A. R., and Clark, E. L. *Psychology of individual differences.* New York: Prentice-Hall, 1939.

   Another more recent textbook on individual and group differences, including some of the heredity-environment data.

4. Hegner, R. W. *College zoology.* (5th ed.) New York: Macmillan, 1943. Chap. 35.

   This chapter is a good orientation in the biological mechanism of heredity for those students who have not had courses in biology at the college level.

5. Jennings, H. S. *The biological basis of human nature.* New York: Norton, 1930.

   A famous biologist's discussion of the roles of genes and environment in human development and of the social implications for eugenics, the family and intermarriage.

6. Kellogg, W. N., and Kellogg, L. A. *The ape and the child.* New York: McGraw-Hill, 1933.

   Report of the widely quoted experiment in which a young chimpanzee was reared in the manner of a human child.

7. National Society for the Study of Education, *Thirty-ninth yearbook: Intelligence, its nature and nurture.* Chicago, 1940. Parts I and II.

   The two volumes of this yearbook constitute a rich source of research data on the roles of heredity and environment through the analysis of mental test scores. Topical surveys, critical articles and original studies are included.

8. Newman, H. H., Freeman, F. N., and Holzinger, K. J. *Twins: a study of heredity and environment.* Chicago: University of Chicago Press, 1937.

   Survey of research on nineteen pairs of identical twins who had been reared apart.

9. Schwesinger, G. C. *Heredity and environment.* New York: Macmillan, 1933.

   A critical survey of the psychological literature prior to 1933 on the effect of heredity and environment.

10. Snyder, L. S. *The principles of heredity.* (3rd ed.) Boston: Heath, 1946.

The latest revision of one of the most widely known standard textbooks on genetics.

11. Woodworth, R. S. Heredity and environment. *Soc. Sci. Res. Council Bull.,* 1941, No. 47.

A clear presentation and critical analysis of recent material on twins and foster children, with reference to its implications for the relation of heredity to environment.

CHAPTER 20

Efficiency

CONSIDERATION of the conditions for efficient human action constitutes an important chapter of psychology. These are the sort of questions put to psychologists: "What are the most efficient conditions of study?" "Is efficiency impaired by the use of alcohol and tobacco?" Such questions have known answers, but to state the answers we shall have first to come to a clear understanding of what is meant by *efficiency*.

The psychologist's and the physiologist's notion of human efficiency is derived from the concept of mechanical efficiency. In order to get a machine to work we must supply it with energy, and the efficiency of a machine is defined as the ratio of the useful work it performs (output) to the amount of energy it consumes (input). Efficiency = Output/Input. For example, the efficiency of a good automobile engine is said to be about twenty-five per cent because only about one quarter of the energy of the gasoline is converted into useful work, the rest being lost as heat. In general, the greater the output per unit of input, or, conversely, the smaller the input per unit of output, the greater is the efficiency of the machine.

In a similar manner we conceive of human efficiency as the ratio between *achievement* (output) and the *cost of work to the organism* (input), and we set ourselves the task of determining the methods and conditions of work which will lead to maximum achievement at a minimum cost.

Research upon the practical control of human efficiency has been developed extensively in the past few decades. There are two major phases of this research. One major advance has occurred in the area of vocational selection and guidance, which is the subject of a subsequent chapter. The invention of techniques for the measurement of skill, aptitude, interest and temperament makes it possible to assign men to jobs for which their individual characteristics best suit them. It is obvious that a man who is working at a job for which he has little aptitude, or which does not interest him, is working inefficiently. His level of production will be low, and the cost of his output will be unnecessarily high.

The other major phase of this research, and the subject of the present chapter, is the discovery of the most efficient methods and conditions of work. Even if a man has the right job, he does not necessarily work as efficiently as he might. The way he performs his task and the conditions under which he works are important variables. Progress toward a solution of these practical problems depends, however, on

This chapter was prepared by M. E. Bitterman and T. A. Ryan of Cornell University.

the development of dependable measures of efficiency. To that problem we turn our attention first.

MEASUREMENT OF HUMAN EFFICIENCY

Since efficiency is output divided by input, to measure efficiency we have to measure both these factors.

Output: Evaluation of Performance

Output is measured by the amount of the product produced—the number of pages read, the number of bricks laid, the number of pieces assembled on the assembly line. You cannot compare a page read with a brick laid, but seldom do you wish to. What you want to know is whether certain conditions get more pages read or more bricks laid than other conditions. Is it more efficient to read under direct or indirect illumination? How do outdoor temperature and humidity affect the efficiency of brick laying?

The problem seems simple enough with pages and bricks, but it becomes difficult when the product is a complicated high-level activity. How do you measure amount of good piloting of an airplane? In the Second World War the Army was reduced to the use of a rating scale which was of doubtful reliability; yet it was important that it know what training methods produced good results, and how good the product was.

A better method than the rating scale is to set up some standard test of pilot performance. You arrange to have every pilot whose efficiency is being measured fly a bomber from one predetermined point to another at a fixed speed under specified weather conditions. You set up this task as a constant standard. Then you see, not how much you get out of the pilot, but how much you have to put into him to get him trained to this required standard of expertness. In other words, you measure efficiency by input instead of output.

Input: Expenditure of Bodily Resources

Input is best regarded as the cost of work to the organism. In general the cost is known by fatigue. For how much fatigue can you get this amount of the product?

Fatigue is not easily measured, yet it is a common experience. Any continued work involves effort, even reading a detective story. You can note when you are done, how much the reading has tired you. Often you are aware of effort while you are making it. It is easier to lift a 50-pound bar-bell with two hands than with one. It is easier to read by the light of a 100-watt lamp than by the light of a candle. It is easier to study in a room at 70° F than in one at 45°. Effort is different in the different cases, and so, after the work is done, is fatigue.

Fatigue of some sort is characteristic of all continued effort or activity. The organism wants change, at least eventually. As the need for change increases, the organism's effort increases. If it does not, the quality and rate of its performance suffer.

Fatigue is best defined as reduction in efficiency resulting from continuous work. There are two ways of measuring it. (1) If a suitable index of effort is available, fatigue can be taken as the increase in effort per unit of accomplishment when work is continued. (2) Or fatigue may be regarded as the physiological changes which produce this loss in efficiency with continued work.

The initial efficiency of a given method

is not necessarily its later efficiency. Fatigue may come on faster with one method than with another. If you have five letters to sign, you had best sit down and do it quickly without any fuss, for that way of doing the job is most efficient. You can even do it while standing. On the other hand, if you have a hundred letters to sign, you had better fuss a little—make yourself comfortable, get the best pen, arrange the letters systematically, for you will tire less and thus turn out to be more efficient in the long run, even though you are less efficient on the first five letters.

Physiological Indicators of Effort and Fatigue

At the present time we do not know a great deal about the physiology of effort. We should like to know what bodily changes go on when effort is expended; then we could measure effort by measuring these changes. Let us see exactly what is the extent of our knowledge in this field.

(1) *Oxygen consumption.* Since the body is a machine which converts food energy into useful work, it is reasonable to assume that the energy released in the body during work should provide a good index of effort expenditure. We cannot, however, use food consumption as a measure of energy cost for any given period of time, because the body stores up food without consuming it. On the other hand, using the food consumes oxygen, which cannot be stored, and thus oxygen consumption itself can be used as a measure of energy expenditure. For each liter of oxygen consumed, about five calories of energy are liberated in the body, although this value varies to some extent with diet.

Figure 217 illustrates a technique for measuring oxygen consumption which is employed when freedom of locomotion is desirable. The subject inhales the surrounding air but exhales into a sack attached to his person. By comparing the oxygen content of the inspired and expired air it is possible to compute the amount of oxygen consumed. Other more convenient and accurate devices are available for ex-

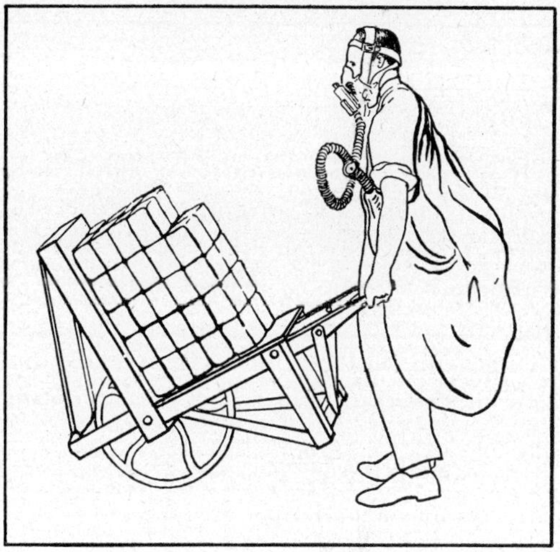

FIGURE 217. THE MEASUREMENT OF OXYGEN CONSUMPTION DURING PHYSICAL WORK

[After A. V. Hill, *Muscular movement in man*, McGraw-Hill, 1927, p. 9.]

periments in which the subject can remain attached to a stationary apparatus.

This technique was used to compare the efficiency of pushing a load with that of pulling it. A number of different loads were used. The work was measured in meter-kilograms (mkg). This unit is the amount of work required to push or pull one kilogram through a distance of one meter. The oxygen was measured and the consumed calories computed. Table XXV gives the results. At each of the four loads pushing is more efficient (uses less oxygen) than pulling, and both pushing and pulling are most efficient at 13.6 kilograms.

TABLE XXV

RELATIVE ENERGY COST OF PUSHING AND PULLING

Input is energy or oxygen consumed in calories. Output is work in meter-kilograms pushed or pulled. Thus efficiency is output/input in mkg/cal. [Data from E. Atzler, *Ergebnisse der Physiol.*, 1928, **27**, 742.]

	EFFICIENCY: MKG/CAL	
Load, kg	*Pushing*	*Pulling*
10.3	0.109	0.094
11.6	0.111	0.098
13.6	0.115	0.102
16.1	0.112	0.101

If oxygen consumption is a valid indicator of effort, and prolonged effort produces fatigue, we should expect oxygen consumption to be related to fatigue. Figure 218 presents sample curves that show changes in the rate of oxygen consumption in the course of work in a printing factory. The increasing rate of oxygen utilization indicates a decrease in efficiency with the passage of time.

The use of oxygen consumption as a measure of the cost of work is limited largely to those activities which involve the gross bodily musculature. Sedentary activities—often called 'mental'—such as reading a book or solving an arithmetic problem require the expenditure of physical energies which are so minute that it is almost impossible to measure them reliably by methods now available.

(2) *Cardiovascular indicators.* The functioning of the cardiovascular or circulatory system—the heart and the blood vessels—gives evidence of being related to energy expenditure. It is possible, for example, by combining measures of blood pressure and heart rate to derive an index known as pulse product which is correlated with oxygen consumption in muscular work. The measurement of blood pressure is a rather cumbersome procedure, however, and very often requires the interruption of

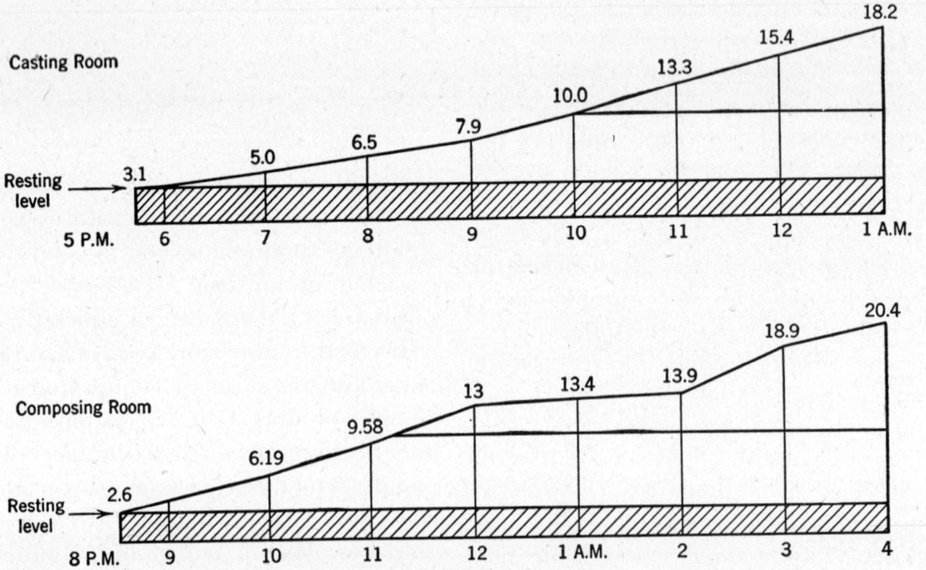

FIGURE 218. INCREASING RATE OF OXYGEN CONSUMPTION DURING WORK IN PRINTING FACTORY

Shows oxygen consumption for 7½ hours work in casting room and composing room for 12 nights. [After A. D. Waller and G. DeDecker, *J. Physiol.*, 1919, **53**, cvi.]

activities in progress. Heart rate, on the other hand, can be recorded very easily. The small electrical changes which spread through the body during each 'beat' of the heart are amplified and used to activate a pen writing on a moving sheet of paper. The procedure requires only that two small metal disks (called electrodes) be taped firmly to the body of the subject. These electrodes may be connected to the amplifiers by wires long enough to permit freedom of activity. In Fig. 219 there is a record of heart rate.

Heart rate is usually higher during sedentary work than during rest, and frequently it is found to rise as work continues. If we compare two conditions of work which we can assume to be different in difficulty, we find that heart rate is sometimes higher, and never lower, for the more difficult task. For example, in one recent experiment heart rate was found to be greater during mental work done in the presence of intense distraction than during work under conditions of comparative silence, despite the fact that the quality of performance was the same in both cases. Heart rate is not, however, as certain an indicator as would be desirable.

(3) *Muscular tension.* There is reason to believe that muscular tension will ultimately furnish us with a sensitive and convenient index of effort expenditure. The muscles of the body always show a certain minimal level of activity or tension, and tension seems to be a function of the difficulty of a task and the adequacy of the conditions under which the work is done. In one early experiment, for example, a group of subjects was set to work translating code. The typewriters used for the task were so constructed that it was possible to record the pressure exerted on the keys. When work was done in the presence of loud noise, much more pressure was exerted than under the control conditions of quiet. It has also been demonstrated that tension and restlessness increase in the course of sedentary work as the subjects become fatigued.

In modern experiments very sensitive electrical measurements of tension are made. All muscular activity gives rise to very small changes of electrical potential (voltage) which can be picked up through a pair of small silver electrodes taped to the skin over the muscle in question, and suitably amplified and recorded. Figure 219 shows a sample of the kind of record which is obtained. In one experiment the subjects were asked to relax upon a couch and potentials arising from the muscles of their arms were recorded. When the subjects were given simple arithmetic problems to do 'in their heads,' the recording apparatus indicated a significant increase in muscle tension. The more difficult the

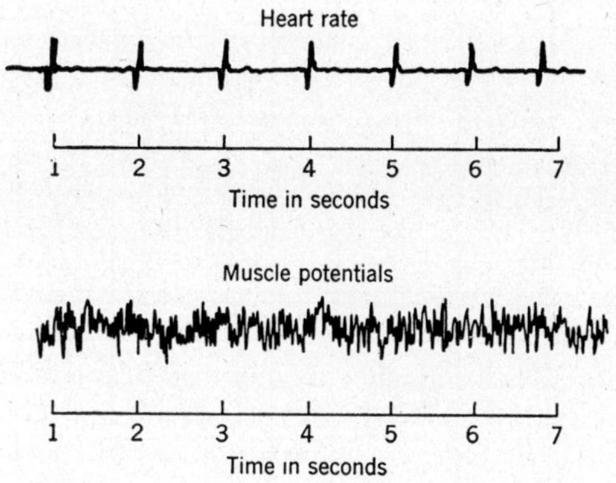

FIGURE 219. GRAPHIC RECORDS OF HEART BEATS AND MUSCLE POTENTIALS

The upper figure is the graphic record of the heart rate. The lower figure is the graphic record of the electrical potentials arising from tension in the triceps muscle of the arm.

problems, the greater were the potential changes registered.

There is some evidence that muscle tensions facilitate 'mental' work and help the organism to compensate for and overcome resistances encountered in its course. For example, it has been discovered that tensions artificially induced by instructing the

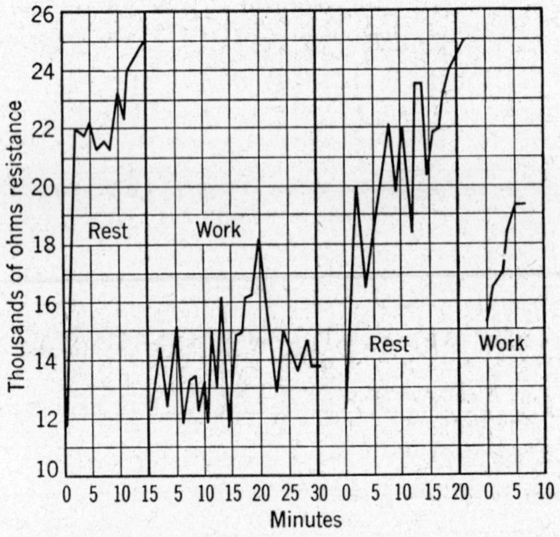

FIGURE 220. ELECTRICAL RESISTANCE OF THE SKIN DURING REST AND DURING MENTAL WORK

[After T. K. Kirby, in A. G. Bills, *The psychology of efficiency,* Harper, 1943, p. 119.]

subject to pull on a weight speed up the learning of nonsense syllables. Perhaps furrowing the brow really does help thinking. It is quite often that the feeling of effort in 'exerting one's will' comes from tension in the facial muscles.

(4) *Skin resistance.* The electrical resistance of the skin is another indicator of exertion. As muscle tension increases, skin resistance decreases, that is to say, the skin becomes more conductive. Measurement of this resistance requires much less technical skill than is needed for the measurement of muscle potentials. Figure 220 shows how skin resistance falls rapidly at the onset of mental work and remains low, rising rapidly again at the termination of the work. The fact that emotion has an effect on the electrical resistance of the skin must be taken into account in the use of this method in the measurement of exertion.

(5) *Fatigue products.* Muscular activity gives rise to certain chemical end products, notably lactic acid, which probably are responsible in part for fatigue effects. These products may be found in the muscles themselves or in the blood stream which carries them from the muscles of origin to the organs of excretion. The importance of this function of the blood is suggested by the fact that muscle groups deprived of their blood supply become fatigued and lose the power of contraction long before those whose blood supply is intact. The adverse effect of fatigue products is demonstrated by the fact that the symptoms of fatigue can be produced in a rested animal if it is injected with a quantity of blood taken from a fatigued one.

Attempts to discover fatigue products resulting from activities other than gross muscular work have thus far been largely unsuccessful. Recent studies of pilot fatigue, however, suggest that some chemical measure of fatigue may presently be found.

Measuring Efficiency and Fatigue by Performance

The worker turns effort into the product of his work. If he keeps at work he also turns effort into fatigue.

Effort is important. You cannot measure efficiency and fatigue unless you can measure effort or at least keep it constant. Too often in industry a change of conditions, which increases production, is supposed to increase efficiency. That conclusion follows only if there is control of the effort which the workers put into the production.

There is a well-known experiment which illustrates this point. The workers were engaged in assembling electrical fixtures, and records of their production were kept as the illumination under which they worked was increased. They worked first at 24 foot-candles, then at 46 and finally at 70. With each increase in illumination production increased. Do not such results show that increased illumination increases efficiency? No, they do not, for in a second part of the experiment production was found to increase regularly when illumination was *decreased*. This experiment was begun at an illumination of 10 foot-candles which was then regularly decreased until finally at 3 foot-candles the workers began to complain that they could not see what they were doing. Why did *any* change in illumination, up or down, increase production? Because the change increased the workers' motivation, and increase of motivation increases effort. The workers were responding not to the improved visual acuity which goes with greater illumination, but to the seeming interest of management in their welfare. They were prepared to work harder, to put more effort into their jobs because they believed that working conditions had been bettered.

The question can be raised as to whether management did not really get increased efficiency with lowered illumination. Certainly it got greater production—at the start. The output was increased and the input, in terms of workers' pay, was constant. The input in terms of workers' effort was not, however, constant. It cost the workers more effort to assemble parts at lowered illumination, even if at first it cost management the same number of dollars. Had the low illumination been continued, fatigue would have been greater, and the increased motivation would not have remained high. Management was fooling the workers. making the work harder and letting them suppose that it was trying to make the work easier. The factory's efficiency was up temporarily, but the worker's efficiency was not, for he had increased his input of effort.

It is not often the case that any change in working conditions by management leads to increased output merely because the workers have confidence that management is acting in their interests. Too often an 'efficiency expert' devises a new method for doing a job and then, with no evidence that he has cut effort in half, asks for double production. Piece rates are then cut, and the worker must increase his total effort or accept less pay. At first production may gain at the expense of the worker, but usually there is no permanent gain, not even for the factory. The demand for greater effort presently results in greater waste, poorer quality, increased rates of turnover, absenteeism, sickness, accident and unfavorable public relations. The workers suspect that management is trying to make the work harder and the effort greater, and they build up their own standards of what constitutes a fair day's work. These standards they maintain by social pressure. A violator is labeled a 'rate buster' and subjected to scorn and ostracism. In this way labor builds up its defense against the 'efficiency expert' and the 'speed-up,' all because the 'efficiency expert' is developing a false increase in efficiency. The true efficiency expert—the *methods engineer* or *industrial engineer,* as they like to be called—knows that the way to increase efficiency is to reduce effort. If the engineer aims at increase of individual efficiency by decreasing the necessary input of effort, he may find that the workers respond by maintaining effort constant and giving the factory more production. In that case both personal and industrial efficiency are increased together, and efficiency remains high because it is supported by good morale.

Laboratory Tests of Efficiency

Since many of the conditions of work can be duplicated in the experimental laboratory, efficiency has been measured there. The *speed test* is one of the more common techniques. In it the subject is asked to work at maximal effort, and the experimenter undertakes to see how much he can produce under different conditions. Illumination, temperature, humidity, distraction, distribution of rest periods can all be varied and the effect of the changes on production noted. Such speed tests are not, however, as reliable as they would be if effort could be satisfactorily controlled. Merely telling a man to use maximal effort does not make sure that he will. Nor does the worker's conscious intent to use maximal effort insure his doing so.

For instance, you can measure strength of grip with a hand dynamometer. You ask your subject to squeeze the handles each time as hard as he possibly can, and you hope to measure his fatigue by keeping effort constant and noting how strength diminishes in successive squeezes. But effort, intended to be maximal, is not constant. If you tell your subject that he is to make fifteen successive contractions, each as strong as he possibly can make it, he will give you fifteen contractions diminishing in strength, but the first contraction will not be so strong as it is when you ask him to give you but a single contraction as strong as possible. His knowledge that he has fifteen efforts to make reduces his 'maximal' effort on the first trial.

It is also true that when a muscle becomes so fatigued that its owner 'can no longer move it,' a sudden increase in motivation, like pride in showing off before an important person, will often result in movement of the 'exhausted' muscle. Great feats of strength performed in emergencies are partly due to this ability of motivation to command reserves of effort, although also to the more fully understood ways in which emotion increases efficiency by endocrine secretion (pp. 95 f.).

There are other experiments which show how unpredictable degree of effort in the input may be. Ordinarily you would expect a distraction to reduce efficiency, but actually potential distractors often work in the opposite way. Persons may be working at what they think is maximal speed on an intelligence test. A loud noise is sounded in the room. It bothers them. They screw themselves up in their chairs, grit their teeth, grasp their pencils harder and go determinedly on, with the result that they do more work within the time limits than they would have done without the potential distractor, which really acted as a stimulator to effort. Measurement of heart rate and muscle tension show that the 'bothered' subject is truly giving more to his task than he was able to give by 'voluntary intention.'

Work Decrement

The attempt has often been made to measure fatigue by plotting production against the duration of continued work. This method uses *work decrement* as a measure. If we could assume that effort remained constant during the day, the work decrement would be a very satisfactory measure of fatigue. A typical work curve for a day in a factory shows production increasing at first as the worker warms up, then decreasing steadily throughout the morning, rising a little as the lunch hour approaches, falling further throughout the afternoon, rising again in anticipation of the quitting time. These irregularities in the curve obviously are not due to fatigue alone. They are the result of a mixture of fatigue and the variations of effort due to boredom and the anticipation of release from work. It shows what management can normally expect from workers, but not the efficiency of the worker.

When a work curve actually rises as work is continued, it is likely that the worker is exerting greater effort. Often a worker consciously tries to compensate for his fatigue, attempting to keep his output constant. He may succeed for a while or even overcompensate, doing better as he gets more fatigued. Sooner or later, of course, a decrement will appear, because the worker cannot or 'will' not exert the amount of effort required to maintain his previous level of performance.

Summary

We may summarize our discussion of the various means and methods of measuring efficiency by saying that we could study efficiency much better if we knew how to control input. Output by itself tells nothing about efficiency, which depends upon output's relation to input. Input is what the worker puts into the work, his effort. We ought to be able to measure it, or at least to keep the worker's contribution constant, so that we can discover the effect of changing other conditions upon the output. At present attempts at accurate measurement of efficiency remain unsatisfactory because we are so uncertain of the cost of work to the working organism. As we turn next in this chapter to some of the practical generalizations, we must remember that word of caution. Exact knowledge in the field of human efficiency waits upon more knowledge of the physiology of work and effort.

METHODS OF WORKING

Any given task can usually be accomplished in a variety of ways, some of which are more efficient than others. This consideration is extremely important even in so simple a job as carrying a load, as Fig. 221 shows. The development of the best methods of work is one of the most important problems in the field of human efficiency.

The 'Natural' Way versus the 'One Best' Way

A worker who is given a job but not given any information as to how it should be done is not likely to work out the most adequate method. Even after years of experience, he may still be using inadequate methods. To appreciate this fact it is only necessary to compare the performance of an athlete trained by a skillful coach with that of an athlete who had no benefit of coaching, or the performance of a trained typist with that of a person who has learned by trial-and-error. That the 'natural' or spontaneous method of doing a job is not necessarily the best method is further demonstrated by the following example taken from industrial practice.

The work in question was the inspection of tin plates for imperfections. The inspector's task was to leaf through a pile of plates in much the same way as a reader leafs through the pages of a book and to remove any defective plates from the pile. The natural tendency of the untrained

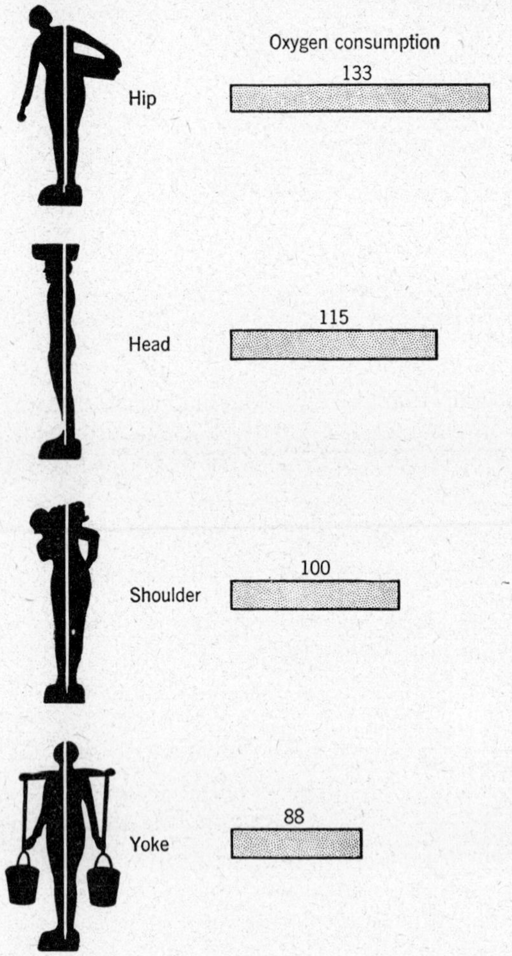

FIGURE 221. RELATIVE EFFICIENCY OF FOUR DIFFERENT METHODS OF CARRYING A 30-POUND LOAD

Bars show oxygen consumption per horizontal kilogram-meter. [Adapted from E. M. Bedale, *Industrial Fatigue Research Board Report,* No. 29, His Majesty's Stationery Office, 1924, p. 37.]

worker was to inspect each plate as she turned it from one pile to the second (Fig. 222, *left*), just as if turning the pages of a book. As the first sheet was being turned, side 1*a* and then side 1*b* were examined; then the next sheet was turned, and, while it was being turned, sides 2*a* and then 2*b* (the two sides of the second sheet) were examined. This method made for inaccuracy since it required the inspection of moving surfaces. Investigation led to the development of a new method which required the worker to ignore the plate in motion and inspect the one at rest. First side 1*a* would be inspected; then side 2*a* would be inspected as the first sheet was being turned; then as the second sheet was being turned, first side 1*b* and then side 3*a* would be examined; as the third sheet was being turned, sides 2*b* and 4*a* would be examined, and so on (Fig. 222, *right*). Adoption of the new method led to a considerable improvement in accuracy.

While studies of this sort indicate that the problem of developing suitable methods should not be left entirely to the worker, there is a question as to how far standardization can be pushed. Many investigators proceed on the principle that there is 'one best' way of doing any given job and that all workers should be required to adopt this method with no variation in detail. On the other hand, the facts of individual differences suggest the possibility that a method which is best for one individual may not be best for another. This problem, however, does not have a great deal of practical importance. First, the procedures employed for selecting workers usually narrow the range of individual differences to a very great extent. Second, we are usually more interested in the efficiency of groups than in the efficiency of individuals, and a new method may be regarded as more efficient than the old if it increases the efficiency of most members of a group, despite the fact that it may reduce the efficiency of certain individual workers. The workers adversely affected can be transferred to new jobs for which they are better suited.

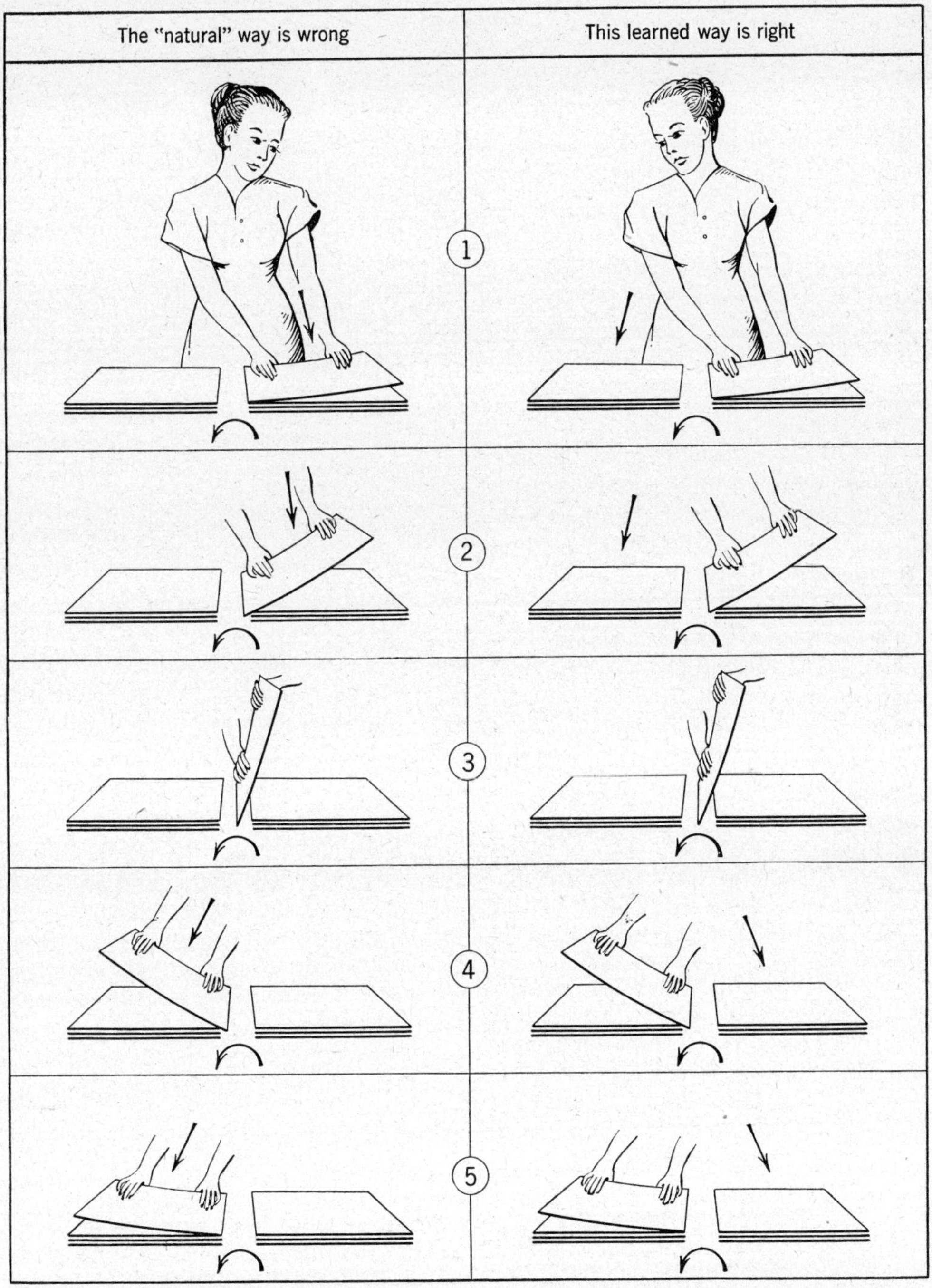

FIGURE 222. ANALYSIS OF TWO METHODS OF INSPECTING TIN PLATES

Five successive phases of the 'natural' way and of the better learned way. The sheets are turned over (semicircular arrow) from the inspector's left to her right. The upper arrow in each sketch shows where she directs her eyes. See text. [Adapted from J. Tiffin, *Industrial psychology* (2nd ed.), 1947, p. 312.]

Motion Study

In modern industry the development of efficient working methods and procedures is more often the concern of engineers than of psychologists. The reason is in part historical; engineers first drew the attention of management to the potentialities of methods research. Important, too, is the fact that the working out of new methods usually involves the redesign of machinery and equipment, work for which the engineer is specifically trained. This development within the field of engineering is commonly known as *motion study* or *methods engineering.*

The first step in the process of working out new methods is to make a careful study of present methods of doing a job. Often motion pictures are made, each phase of the work being carefully timed, and these data are then studied in order to determine whether time or effort is being wasted at any particular point. In recommending changes the motion analyst is guided by a set of general rules relating to the proper use of the body, the arrangement of working materials and the design of tools and equipment, most of which seem to be very sensible. One rule states, for example, that wherever possible the hands should be relieved of holding operations by the introduction of mechanical devices so that the hands can be used instead for more complex operations which cannot easily be performed mechanically. Another rule states that tools, materials and controls should have definite fixed stations so that the worker will not have to search for them each time they are required. Still another rule suggests that wherever possible the two arms should be used simultaneously and symmetrically.

To illustrate the changes which result from the application of rules of this sort, we shall consider the modification of one routine industrial job. The task of the worker was to coat the ends of small blocks with solder so that wires could be attached to them later on in the manufacturing process. Originally the job was done according to the diagram in Fig. 223*A*. The left hand selected a block from the supply pan and passed it to the right hand. Then the left hand remained idle while the right hand dipped the block first into the flux pot and then into the solder pot, knocked it against the knock-off plate to remove the excess solder, and dropped the block into the box of completed pieces. Figure 223*B* shows a diagram of the new method. There are two supply pans, two knock-off plates, and one pan for finished stock. Each cycle of movement now results in two finished pieces, the two hands working symmetrically and simultaneously.

Time Study

When the new method has been devised, some estimate of its advantage over the old method must be obtained. For this purpose, a technique known as *time study* is used, a method of establishing standards of performance for any given job. The result of a time study is a *standard time* which is used for determining piece rates of pay, working out schedules, estimating costs and the like, as well as for evaluating the results of a motion study. Standard time is defined as the time required for the job by a person of 'average' skill working with 'average' effort under 'average' conditions.

One widely used method for determining this time value is the following. A single worker, preferably one who is above average, is selected for study. His performance is timed by the engineer, who also makes a rating of his skill and effort as well as of the adequacy of working conditions. The measured time is then modified in the light of these ratings in order to obtain the standard time. For example, the measured time is increased if the worker is superior in skill to the average worker and this increase is in proportion to his rated superiority. If the worker is thought to be expending more than average effort, a certain amount is added to the measured time; if he is thought to be expending less than average effort, a certain amount is subtracted. Other amounts are added or subtracted depending upon how adequate the rater considers the conditions of work to be.

The final time value which is arrived at by the engineer is thus in one sense a performance measure of efficiency. It is an estimate of the relation between method of work and output, with the influence of all other variables, including effort expenditure, ruled out. The method is based upon a complex series of subjective judgments and the results which it gives can be only as accurate as these judgments.

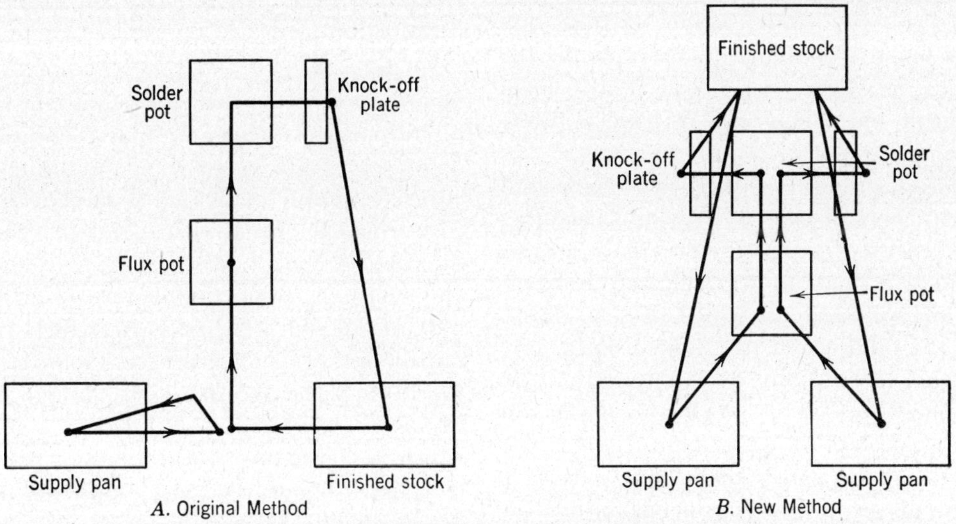

FIGURE 223. TWO METHODS OF DOING A SIMPLE REPETITIVE JOB

[After Mogensen, *Common Sense Applied to Motion and Time Study*, 1932, p. 58, McGraw-Hill Co.]

Evaluation of Motion and Time Study

There is little doubt that many of the principles upon which methods engineering is based are fundamentally sound and that their application has led to considerable improvement in working efficiency. In any given instance, however, it is hard to say just how much improvement, if any at all, has been made, since standard times are derived from subjective judgments and no attempts are made to check them against objective measures of the cost of work. At present, motion study should not be used as a basis for cutting piece rates or speeding up production belts if the evidence for improvement is based only on standard times.

One major criticism of time and motion

study, which is really a criticism of an important trend in modern industry, has been that it results in the breaking up of complex jobs into simpler ones. This process of simplification, so the argument runs, deprives the worker of the opportunity to exercise judgment and initiative and consequently leads to boredom, loss of interest and discontent. This criticism must be given careful consideration because job satisfaction is extremely important for the well-being of the worker as well as to management for whom it may have a direct economic import.

It is certainly true that most people find it extremely boring to perform a meaningless repetitive task for more than a short period of time. They welcome any possibility for variation which presents itself. On the other hand, the more routine the activity, the less attention it requires, and the more free is the worker to engage in conversation or to listen to music. It is also clear that the nature of the job activity is by no means the only factor responsible for the development of monotony in industry. The emotional problems of the worker, his attitude toward the company, the supervisor, his fellow workers, and his conception of the importance of his job—these factors and many others are related to reports of boredom. It is safe to conclude that mass production methods do not inevitably produce discontent.

THE WORKING ENVIRONMENT

There have been numerous investigations of the relation between the efficiency of work and certain important environmental variables, such as atmospheric conditions, illumination and noise. We may now review the current status of research with respect to these factors.

Atmospheric Conditions

Atmospheric conditions—the chemical composition of the air, barometric pressure, air temperature, humidity and so forth—are principally related to human efficiency only insofar as they affect two vital physiological functions—respiration and the maintenance of body temperature.

Respiration

In order to live and function normally, man must be provided with a sufficient supply of oxygen. Under ordinary conditions of life on earth, however, maintaining an adequate supply of oxygen is rarely a difficult problem. Atmospheric air, the chemical composition of which remains remarkably constant, contains about 20 or 21 per cent of oxygen. Actually air which contained only 14 or 15 per cent of oxygen would be perfectly suitable for human use. Of course, if a man is enclosed in a space which is sealed off from the rest of the atmosphere, sooner or later his supply of oxygen will fall below the level necessary for his normal functioning, which is about 14 per cent. But even in the most poorly ventilated rooms which contain large numbers of people the oxygen content of the air is well above that level. The feeling of suffocation and the other ill effects that we experience in such places may be attributed, not to inadequate oxygen supply, but to the high temperature and humidity. This interpretation is supported by the results of an experiment in which it was found that people enclosed in a small sealed room were not relieved when they were permitted to breathe through a tube 'fresh air' from the outside, whereas other people, stationed outside the room but breathing the air of the room by means of tubes, did not suffer any discomfort.

Under special conditions, however, oxygen deficiency—*anoxia,* as it is called—does become a problem of special interest. The development of modern aviation has stimulated a great deal of research on the relation between anoxia and efficiency. At high altitudes the percentage of oxygen in the air remains constant, but the decreased barometric pressure results in a decreased passage of oxygen from the lungs to the blood. Breathing atmospheric air at an altitude of 10,000 feet is about the equivalent of breathing air which contains only 14 per cent of oxygen at sea level. Above this altitude, unless steps are taken to increase the oxygen supply, the first signs of anoxia will appear. One solution is to increase the percentage of oxygen in the air which the pilot inspires by the use of an oxygen mask, but this solution is satisfactory only at altitudes below about 40,000 feet. Above this level, barometric pressure is so low that, even if pure oxygen is breathed, there will be an insufficient passage of oxygen into the blood stream. Prolonged flying at very high altitudes is possible only in sealed cabins in which normal air pressure is maintained.

During the Second World War many investigations of the effects of anoxia were conducted. It was for the most part unnecessary to risk studying the phenomenon under actual flight conditions, because high altitudes could be simulated by the use of controlled-pressure chambers in ground laboratories. One of the earliest symptoms of anoxia to appear, usually at about the pressure equivalent to 10,000 feet altitude, is an unmistakable *euphoria*—a pronounced experience of well-being and self-confidence similar to that often produced by small amounts of alcohol. As altitude—real or simulated, it makes no difference—increases, further marked emotional changes occur. The individual may be intensely happy, angry or depressed, and he has usually become quite delirious before he finally loses consciousness at about 20,000 feet. Psychological tests administered at various altitudes show many other pronounced functional changes. Muscular coordination becomes very poor, reaction time is lengthened, visual and auditory acuity are reduced, range of attention becomes restricted, and intellectual capacities are impaired.

Temperature Regulation

Under ordinary circumstances atmospheric conditions are important because they affect the maintenance of body temperature. The temperature of the body varies about a mean of approximately 98.6° F, and the body is provided with mechanisms which maintain this level of temperature in the face of wide variations in atmospheric conditions. If the environment cools the body, the oxidative processes of the body will be speeded up to produce more heat. There is a further control of body temperature which can operate without changing bodily heat production. If the air is cool, the skin cools down, constricting the blood vessels and thus cooling the skin even more. Less heat is transported from the inside of the body to its surface, and the cool skin radiates less heat to the surrounding air than it would had the skin remained warm while the air was cool. On the other hand, when the surroundings are warm the blood vessels of the skin dilate, and more heat is transferred to the surface of the body for radiation to the air. In addition, sweating begins, and its evaporation takes additional heat from the skin surface.

The ease with which optimal body temperature can be maintained is a function, not of one, but of a number of environmental variables. Air temperature is important because, depending on the difference between air temperature and skin temperature, the air conducts heat away from or to the body. But humidity, rate of air movement and the temperature of surrounding objects also are important

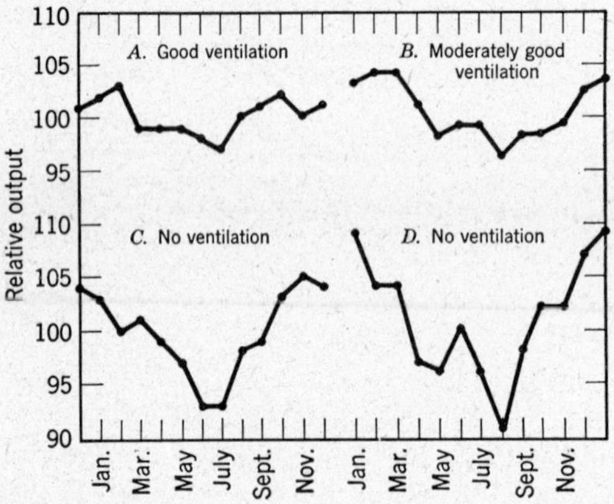

FIGURE 224. SEASONAL VARIATION IN PRODUCTION AS AFFECTED BY VENTILATION

[After H. M. Vernon, *Industrial fatigue and efficiency,* Dutton, 1921, p. 242.]

variables. Humidity affects the rate of evaporation of sweat from the skin; air movement serves to carry warm moist air away from the skin and to replace it with cooler, drier air; and the temperature of surrounding objects is important because much heat exchange between organism and environment occurs as radiation. This exchange of radiant energy is largely independent of the air temperature; we can be cool when the air is hot provided we are surrounded by cool walls. Any study of the efficiency of atmospheric conditions must therefore take all these variables into account. At a given air temperature a person may feel very warm, very cold or quite comfortable depending on whether his body is losing too much or not enough heat to keep its own temperature close to normal.

The principal method of experimental study of the effects of these environmental factors has been the speed test rather than the complete analysis of efficiency. Temperature has a marked influence upon amount of muscular work as measured by speed of performance. In one experiment the amount of work done was 40 per cent less at 86° F and 80 per cent relative humidity than it was at 68° F and 50 per cent relative humidity. The first condition was experienced as uncomfortably warm, and the second as comfortable. It has also been found that factory production is much lower in the summer than in the winter, and that this variation can be partially controlled by improved methods of ventilation (Fig. 224).

For tasks which require little muscular exertion, however, speed tests do not show any consistent effect of temperature variation over a wide range. (See Table XXVI.)

TABLE XXVI

EFFECT OF VENTILATION ON MENTAL WORK

[Adapted from *Ventilation*, Report of the New York State Commission on Ventilation, Dutton, 1923, p. 102.]

	RELATIVE PERFORMANCE	
Mental Test	*Comfortable* (68° F; 50 per cent relative humidity; good air circulation)	*Uncomfortably Warm* (86° F; 80 per cent relative humidity; poor air circulation)
Number cancellation		
Test 1	100	93.6
Test 2	100	99.8
Addition	100	106.1
Multiplication	100	102.4
Typewriting	100	101.1

Although this result is important in itself, it does not necessarily mean that efficiency is also unaffected. Discomfort and disinclination to work are themselves indications that efficiency is down, although we cannot be sure that the temperature which we prefer is necessarily the most advantageous from the point of view of health and well-being. The chief difficulty here lies in the influence of acclimatization and adaptation. In summer warmer temperatures are preferred than in winter, and, in general, the temperatures to which an individual has become accustomed determine to a large extent what his preferences will be.

Illumination

The light which is available for visual work is a function of the light source and of the reflecting surfaces in the environment of the work. It can be described in terms of three important variables—amount, spectral composition and distribution. In practice a change in one of these aspects of lighting often produces a change in one or both of the others, but theoretically at least each aspect can be considered independently. Each of the three variables has been shown to be related in an important way to the efficiency of visual work.

Amount of illumination. Amount of illumination has for the most part been studied in terms of performance. In a wide variety of industrial and laboratory situations it has been possible to demonstrate increases in output owing to increases in intensity of light. Table XXVII shows representative examples of such changes for a number of factory jobs. Further investigation indicates, however, that output does not continue to rise indefinitely as brightness is progressively increased. For every task thus far studied an intensity level is found—often called the 'critical' level—beyond which there is no further improvement in performance. The critical level varies with the nature of the task.

TABLE XXVII

EFFECT OF INCREASED ILLUMINATION ON INDUSTRIAL PRODUCTION

[After L. T. Troland, in M. A. Tinker, Illumination standards for effective and comfortable vision, *J. consult. Psychol.*, 1939, **3**, 17.]

Factory	*Initial Level (foot-candles)*	*New Level (foot-candles)*	*Increase in Production (per cent)*
Electrical	3.8	11.4	8.5
Piston ring	1.2	6.5	13.0
Piston ring	1.2	9.0	17.9
Piston ring	1.2	14.0	25.8
Roller bearing	5.0	6.0	4.0
Roller bearing	5.0	13.0	8.0
Roller bearing	5.0	20.0	12.5

For speed of reading easy passages printed in good-sized type it is about 3 or 4 foot-candles, which is relatively low illumination. (Three foot-candles is the amount of light which is thrown on a surface 52 inches away by a 50-watt bulb in an ordinary bridge-lamp shade.) For general study 15 foot-candles is about the critical level; for speed of threading needles, 30 foot-candles; and for certain tests of visual acuity the critical level may be above 100 foot-candles, provided the illumination is fairly uniform throughout the visual field.

The effect of illumination level upon performance is, as usual, better known than its effect upon efficiency. Increases in industrial production resulting from changed conditions of illumination may perhaps be attributed to better morale as often as to greater efficiency. On the whole, however, the opinion has more often been given that performance indices point to optimal illuminations which are too low rather than too high. This suspicion arises from the fact that, since critical levels derived from speed tests are often only a small fraction of daylight levels, there is the possibility that *ease* of seeing may continue to increase with increasing illumination far beyond the point at which there are no further gains in speed of work. There is some evidence for this point of view from studies of muscular tension, at least in the case of reading. Although speed of reading does not increase as intensity is raised be-

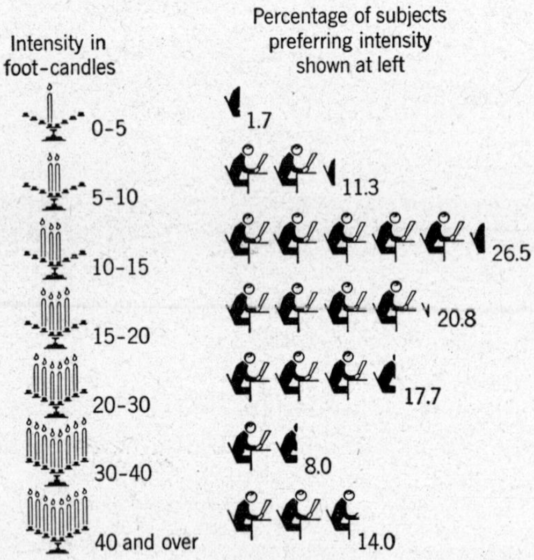

FIGURE 225. DISTRIBUTION OF ILLUMINATION LEVELS PREFERRED FOR READING

[Adapted from C. E. Ferree and G. Rand, *Good Working Conditions for the Eyes,* Personnel Jr., 1936, 15, 330–340 by F. K. Berrien in *Practical Psychology,* Macmillan, 1944.]

yond 3 or 4 foot-candles, tension developed in the course of reading appears to be reduced significantly by increases in intensity up to 10 or 20 foot-candles.

Another approach to the problem of best illumination has been to determine what intensities people prefer for work of various sorts. In most of these experiments the subject is allowed to select any intensity within a wide range by means of a control knob. Distributions of choices obtained under such conditions show a great deal of variability, probably reflecting differences in personal experience that need have no relation to efficiency (Fig. 225). Furthermore, it can be shown that the average level of illumination selected by a group of subjects is to a large extent determined by the level to which they are light-adapted at the time they made the choice. Thus there is danger in recommending illumination for factories, offices or schoolrooms on the basis of preferences.

Certain investigators have issued recommendations for lighting in schools, factories, offices and homes which are no better than good guesses. Some of these recommendations have been high, for the 'experts' assume that light is cheap in comparison with the value of good eyesight and that we can never have too much light. One investigator has gone so far as to suggest the use of 100 or more foot-candles for ordinary reading. This extravagant approach to the problem of lighting may be dangerous. For one thing, although the visual mechanism can adjust to a wide variety of illumination levels, anybody who has tried to read by the light of the summer sun will be able to conceive of the possibility of *too much* light for a given purpose. Then again, these recommendations assume that special precautions have been taken to prevent glare and bad distribution, whereas the layman, attempting to follow instructions, may easily overlook these precautions and thus make reading more difficult than with less light.

Distribution of light. It is generally agreed that the distribution of light in the visual field should be as uniform as possible —that areas of relatively high or relatively low brightness should be avoided. Uneven illumination produces *glare;* the transmitting media within and without the eye (fog, dirty windshields, cloudy media within the eye) diffuse the light and blur the retinal images. Glare spots are especially harmful because they produce conflicts in the mechanisms of fixation and accommodation. There is a reflex tendency to look toward points of high brightness which occur in peripheral vision, and this tendency must be inhibited if the visual task is to be uninterrupted. Such a competition of reac-

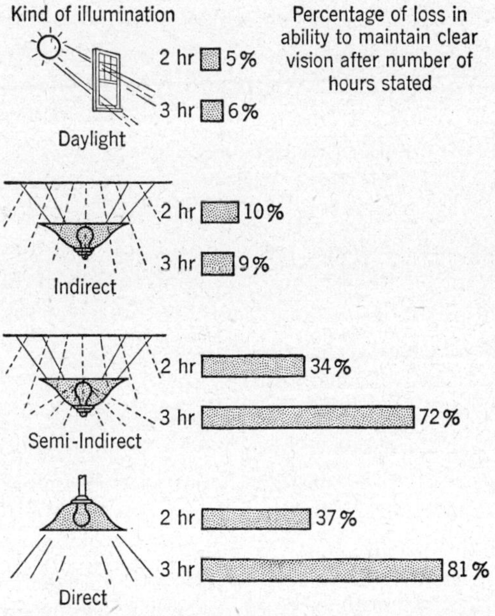

FIGURE 226. DECREMENTS IN ABILITY TO MAINTAIN CLEAR VISION AFTER SEVERAL HOURS OF READING UNDER DIFFERENT TYPES OF ILLUMINATION

[After C. E. Ferree and G. Rand, from F. K. Berrien, *Practical psychology,* Macmillan, 1944, p. 251.]

tion systems produces muscular tension, discomfort and fatigue, although it may not affect performance measures such as speed-of-reading tests.

Unshaded or only partially shaded light sources are probably the commonest cause of glare, and the superiority of indirect lighting is attributable to the fact that the light sources are never directly visible. Figure 226 shows the relative adequacy of these different types of lighting in terms of decrements in ability to maintain clear vision after several hours of work under the various conditions.

Spectral composition. Since modern illuminating engineers have developed illuminants of many different spectral compositions, the relation between this variable and visual efficiency presents a problem. Certain general relationships have already been established. When lights of various colors are compared, yellow is found to make for the greatest initial acuity and the least impairment of clear vision after several hours of reading. This result still holds even after the intensities are adjusted for the differential sensitivity of the eye; that is to say, even if the blue light is made as bright as the yellow, the yellow is still more satisfactory.

Because of the phenomenon of chromatic aberration (unequal refraction of lights of different wave lengths), it might be expected that monochromatic sources, such as the sodium vapor lamp, would be superior to more complex sources, such as ordinary tungsten lamps; but in practice the differences in performance have not been large, and in some studies they have been in favor of the tungsten. Among complex sources, those whose spectral composition approximates that of daylight seem to be superior to the yellower tungsten illuminants.

Noise

The principal experimental studies of the effect of noise upon efficiency have been laboratory investigations of relatively short duration. Industrial studies have consistently shown increases in production when noise is reduced. Performance in speed tests given under laboratory conditions, however, has not been found to be very markedly affected by noise. The introduction of noise often produces short term decrements, but performance soon returns to approximately the original level, sometimes a little lower and sometimes even somewhat higher. Despite this fact there is some evidence to show that heart rate, muscular tension and oxygen consumption are all somewhat higher during the noise, indicating increased effort. As we have already noted, performance may even be increased by noise because it spurs effort. Airplane noise tires pilots but does not seem to reduce the quality of their work. Most persons seem to become rapidly accustomed to noise, and the effects of noise both upon bodily tension and upon skilled performance usually disappear in time.

REST AND SLEEP

What is the best distribution of work and rest from the point of view of overall efficiency in any given activity? Study of this problem has been carried out both in industrial and in laboratory settings, and in each case output indices have been relied upon almost exclusively.

Hours of Work

It is fairly easy to demonstrate that efficiency is a function of the rate of work. Studies of speed of walking indicate, for example, that it is more efficient in terms of oxygen consumption to walk at the rate of four miles per hour than at three or five miles per hour. Because of the relation of efficiency to rate of work, the length of the working day becomes an important problem. If a worker is expected to produce a certain amount on a given day, over how many hours shall the work be distributed (at what rate shall it be done) so that the total cost will be minimal? Conversely, if the worker comes prepared to expend a given amount of effort, over how many hours shall this effort be distributed so that the total achievement will be maximal?

The earliest systematic studies of the length of the working day were conducted during the First World War. In that period of manpower shortage and high-production requirements, hours of work were very long, often seventy or more per week, and it soon became apparent that total production could actually be increased by *reducing* working hours. In other words, the increases in rate of production which resulted more than compensated for the decrease in number of hours worked (Fig. 227). Financial incentives were not responsible for the results, which held for the workers paid by the hour as well as for the piece workers. As the investigators continued to reduce the number of hours worked, however, production eventually fell off because rate of work did not increase so rapidly as before. The optimal length of the working day or week varied considerably from job to job.

Although interest in these studies was largely centered in production, there was some reason for believing that the differences in production which were found represented real differences in efficiency. It seemed that the workers came to their jobs prepared to expend a fixed amount of effort irrespective of the length of the work spell. The gradual manner in which increases in production appeared after a reduction in working hours—often the full effects of the change were not realized for several months—suggested that the workers were learning to redistribute the amount of effort which they were ready to expend.

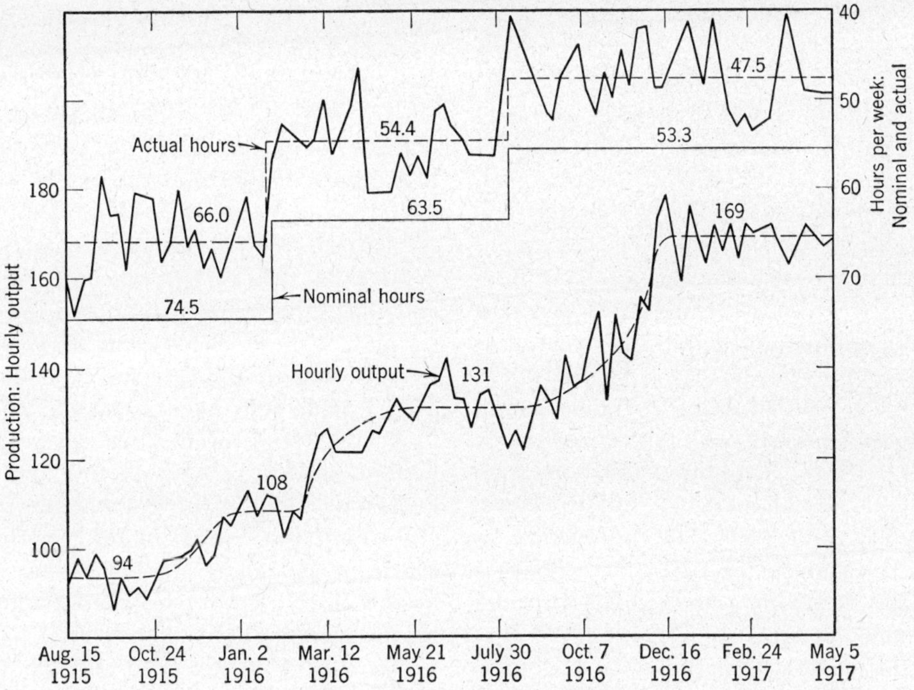

FIGURE 227. RATE OF PRODUCTION IN RELATION TO LENGTH OF WORKING WEEK

Shows how increase of production during pressure of war emergency was secured by decreasing working hours per week. "Nominal hours" are those present in the plant. "Actual hours" represent actual working time. The upper curve (scale reversed) shows decrease in working hours that accompanied the increase in output shown on the lower curve. [From H. M. Vernon, *Industrial fatigue and efficiency*, Dutton, 1921, p. 39.]

Rest Periods

The efficiency of prolonged work can be notably increased by the introduction of periodic rest pauses which permit a certain amount of recovery from fatigue. Industrial observations show clearly that, when there are no regularly scheduled rest pauses, workers manage to find many reasons for stopping work in the course of the working day. These 'unofficial' rests are less efficient than regularly scheduled ones because they may not come at the proper times and because they are usually furtive and incomplete.

The effectiveness of regularly scheduled rest periods has been demonstrated in terms of production. It has also been shown that rest intervals should be brief and frequent, although the optimal schedule varies from job to job. Frequency is important because of the relation between duration of work and the development of fatigue. Fatigue develops slowly at first and then more and more rapidly; if one unit of work produces one unit of fatigue, two successive units of work may produce three or even four units of fatigue. In one experiment it was shown, for example, that it takes four times as long to recover from the effects of lifting a weight thirty times as it does to recover from the effects of lifting it fifteen times.

In addition, short rest periods are more efficient than longer ones because recovery from fatigue is also rapid at first and then more and more gradual. In another experiment on weight lifting, it was found that there was 72 per cent recovery 5 minutes after a period of work, 75 per cent after 10 minutes and only 77 per cent after twenty minutes.

The so-called warming-up phenomenon also suggests that rest periods be kept fairly short. At the beginning of the work spell a certain amount of time usually elapses before a stable level of production is reached. During this time the worker is gradually developing the proper attitudes and muscular sets. If rest pauses are too long this process of warming-up or getting into the swing of activity must be repeated all over again.

It should be noted, however, that increases in production after the introduction of regularly scheduled rest periods may often represent changes in motivation rather than changes in efficiency. Although studies of oxygen consumption have demonstrated genuine increases in efficiency under such conditions, other evidence indicates that production increments are to some extent a function of improved employee morale and resulting additional exertion. Only through a measurement of effort expenditure would it be possible to distinguish between the effects of these two variables.

Sleep

Since the average individual may spend anywhere from a quarter to a third of his life in sleep, it is a phenomenon of considerable importance. As yet, however, we know very little about the efficiency of our sleeping habits; we cannot tell how much sleep a given individual requires or under what conditions sleep is most beneficial.

Investigations of the need for sleep have been based largely on the use of fatigue tests, the usual procedure being to administer batteries of physical and mental tests before and after certain schedules of sleep and wakefulness and to compare the effectiveness of these schedules in terms of differences in performance. In general, however, fatigue tests have proved to be very insensitive, and even after several days without sleep a person's performance may be just as good as it was when he was rested. Only those tests which require continuous attention and effort are much affected by loss of sleep. Of course, the person who has been awake for a long period of time knows that he needs sleep and has to try very hard to keep awake, but performance scores give little indication of his condition. There is some evidence to show, nevertheless, that performance levels are maintained under such conditions only at the expense of additional expenditure of effort.

EFFECTS OF COMMON DRUGS

The widespread use of alcohol, coffee, tea and tobacco has given rise to much speculation concerning their effects upon the organism. The usual experimental procedure has been to administer batteries of physical and mental tests before and after the administration of various quantities of the substance in question and to study the effects on performance. The data of such experiments must be interpreted cautiously for a number of reasons. For one thing the insensitivity of performance measures, when effort is not controlled, makes it dangerous to conclude that a given substance has no effect upon efficiency when test scores are unchanged. When test scores do change after administration of a drug, the drug itself is not necessarily the responsible factor. The change may have stemmed from the subject's expectation that the drug would have some effect—either facilitating or detrimental—upon his behavior. For this reason it is always necessary to arrange the conditions so that the subjects never know when they have taken the substance in question or how much they have had. We should also bear in mind in evaluating available information that most experimental studies deal only with the short-term effects of the various drugs and tell us nothing about the consequences of the continued use of these substances over a period of years.

Alcohol

Alcohol is not a stimulant but a depressant. Moderate doses have an apparently stimulating effect presumably because the higher neural centers are most easily affected and the inhibitory control which they ordinarily exert on the lower centers is impaired. It is difficult to administer alcohol without the subject's knowledge. Its presence can be partly disguised by giving it in mixed drinks or injecting it directly into the blood stream, but the subject can usually detect the presence of more than very small quantities from its 'warming' effect.

It is well recognized that alcohol taken in fairly large quantities leads to serious impairment in motor and intellectual functions. When the level of alcohol in the blood stream has reached about three or four tenths of one per cent, the individual is usually in a comatose state. It is difficult to be specific about the consequences of moderate doses, however, since people vary considerably with respect to their susceptibility to alcohol, their 'tolerance' of it. Experiments nevertheless indicate that, whenever alcohol is found to influence performance at all, the effect is consistently adverse.

The deleterious effects of relatively small quantities of alcohol have been demonstrated for a wide variety of functions including muscular coordination and control, speed of muscular reactions, simple arithmetic operations, memory and intelligence test performance. Although it is not possible to rule out completely the influence of suggestion in these results, the fact that these effects vary in a consistent manner with the amount of the dose indicates that it is the alcohol in the blood stream which is responsible. It should be noted that the effects disappear in a few hours as the alcohol is absorbed and excreted.

This type of experimentation does not, of course, answer the question as to whether the continued use of alcohol in moderate amounts produces a permanent impairment of efficiency.

Tobacco

It is well known that tobacco contains a substance known as nicotine which has certain toxic effects on the body. Actually, however, very little nicotine enters the body during smoking because, as the tobacco burns, the nicotine which it contains is broken down into less harmful substances.

At present time there is very little dependable evidence concerning the relation between the use of tobacco and efficiency. The only well-controlled investigation that has been reported is limited to the period of an hour and forty-five minutes directly after the smoking of a single pipeful of tobacco. The important feature of this experiment is that the subjects could not tell whether they were smoking tobacco or not. The investigator invented a bogus pipe through which the subjects could draw warm moist air. When they were blindfolded the subjects could not distinguish between the real pipe and the control device since the odor of smoke was present in the air from the experimenter's pipe. The results of the experiment showed that smoking unmistakably increased pulse rate and unsteadiness of the hands in both experienced and inexperienced smokers. For inexperienced smokers speed of addition was decreased slightly by tobacco but increased slightly for habitual smokers. A variety of other motor and intellectual functions could not be shown to be affected by the tobacco.

Caffeine

Caffeine, which is found in various 'soft' drinks as well as in coffee and tea, has significant stimulating properties. Although the average cup of coffee does not contain enough caffeine to interfere with sleep, larger doses may do so. A number of controlled laboratory investigations demonstrate the facilitating effects of moderate amounts of caffeine on a variety of muscular and simple mental performances, although adverse effects upon muscular steadiness have also been found. Larger amounts of caffeine often reverse these favorable effects. It has also been demonstrated that tolerance for caffeine develops very rapidly, so that the effectiveness of a given dose varies inversely with the amount that any given individual is accustomed to using.

JOB SATISFACTION

In any discussion of working efficiency we must not fail to consider the attitude of the worker toward his job. Not only is psychological well-being as important to the worker himself as his physiological well-being, but it is also clear that the discontented worker expends more effort for the same result than the worker who likes his job. The resentful, antagonistic employee, who goes through the motions of working, yet slacks at every opportunity, may actually be putting in more energy for a given accomplishment than the worker whose morale is good and whose rate of production is relatively high. Certainly, from the point of view of management, discontent among employees is costly. It may be responsible not only for low production levels, but also for wasted materials, deterioration of plant and equipment, absenteeism, excessive turnover and work stoppages.

Although many theories have been advanced as to why men work and the conditions which make them satisfied or dissatisfied with their jobs, reliable information can be obtained only from a direct study of the worker himself. One nationwide study shows that there may be very little relation between what the worker wants from his job and what his employer thinks he wants. The eight factors listed in Table XXVIII were ranked with respect to their relative importance as factors in morale by three thousand employees and several hundred employers. The rank of 1 indicates that a given factor was considered to be most important, and the rank of 8 that it was considered least important. The table lists the average ranks assigned to each item by the two groups of raters. The correlation between these

TABLE XXVIII

RANK ASSIGNED VARIOUS FACTORS IN MORALE BY EMPLOYERS AND EMPLOYEES

The correlation between the two rankings is approximately zero. [After S. J. Fosdick, in *Industrial conflict: a psychological interpretation*, First Yearbook of the Society for the Psychological Study of Social Issues, Cordon, 1939, p. 119.]

Morale Item	*Employee Ranking*	*Employer Ranking*
Credit for all work done	1	7
Interesting work	2	3
Fair pay	3	1
Understanding and appreciation	4	5
Counsel on personal problems	5	8
Promotion on merit	6	4
Good physical working conditions	7	6
Job security	8	2

two sets of rankings is practically zero. (The coefficient of correlation is actually −0.10.) Certainly the employers did not know what their workers wanted, even though the table does not prove that the workers would have been best satisfied by having their preferences accepted as the basis for improved working conditions.

In recent years much use has been made of questionnaire and rating techniques of this sort in the study of industrial morale. The information obtained from these investigations has been useful both for getting at the general principles of worker motivation and for uncovering specific sources of discontent in particular industrial organizations. One of the most general conclusions to be drawn from these studies relates to the importance of financial incentives. Good pay, it appears, is not the only important factor in job satisfaction, nor is it the most important factor. The worker must be treated with consideration and respect; he must be made to feel that his contributions are valued; he must be encouraged both to offer suggestions and to seek advice in case of need; and his supervisors must be leaders rather than 'bosses.' In other words, what seems to be essential is that the worker be dealt with as an entire person rather than as a pair of hands.

ACCIDENT CONTROL

Accidents represent an important factor in the personal and social cost of work, much more important than is commonly realized. For example, during the period of the Second World War accidental deaths in the United States numbered about 355,000, and there were approximately 36,000,000 accidental injuries. War casualties in the United States, on the other hand, totaled only about 295,000 killed or missing and 652,000 wounded. Research in accident prevention has centered largely about industrial and highway accidents, the kinds which account for a large portion of the toll.

The problem of accident control has been approached from two principal directions. One approach is the search for general factors influencing the accident rates of an entire group—motorists, miners, factory workers—and the attempt to reduce the incidence of accidents by controlling these factors. It has been found, however, that in any group there is a minority of so-called accident-prone individuals who are responsible for a major share of the group's accidents. Thus the other approach to the problem of accident control consists of the attempt to identify these persons, to determine the principal reasons for their high liability to accident, and either to correct the conditions which endanger their safety or to reduce their exposure to hazardous situations.

General Causes of Accidents

There are a number of general factors which affect overall accident rates regardless of individual differences in liability. The earliest phase of accident research centered about the hazards inherent in particular activities such as driving an automobile, mining coal or operating a drill

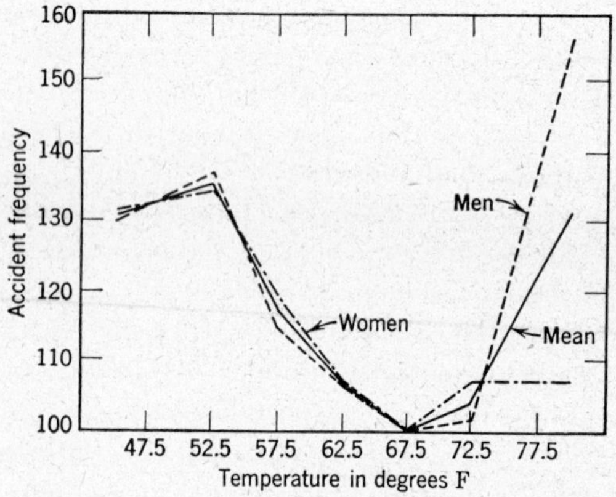

FIGURE 228. ACCIDENT FREQUENCY IN RELATION TO TEMPERATURE

The best temperature is near 68° F. [From H. M. Vernon, *Accidents and their prevention*, Macmillan, 1936, p. 76.]

press. The reduction of these hazards, which usually requires the redesign of processes and equipment, has largely been the work of safety engineers, but the problem has not been entirely an engineering one. Surprising as it may seem, people are often reluctant to observe safety regulations. We are all familiar with the kind of educational campaigns which have been developed for the purpose of persuading drivers and workers of the necessity for protecting themselves.

Many conditions that affect accident rate are found in the working environment. Illumination is extremely important; a stairwell which is relatively dimly illuminated, a source of glare in the visual field of a worker who is tending a dangerous machine, the blinding headlights of an approaching automobile, all may take a heavy toll. Temperature is another significant factor (see Fig. 228). Accidents increase when it is too hot and when it is too cold. Many factors determine what temperature is optimal, but the value is likely to lie in the region of 65 to 70° F. There is good reason to believe, therefore, that in many industrial plants the introduction of air-conditioning equipment would result in considerable decreases in accident rates. Indeed, it seems likely that any condition of work which makes for the elimination of excessive fatigue will tend to decrease the likelihood of accident.

In industry, the eight-hour day does not usually produce enough fatigue to have a significant effect upon accident rates. Accident rates fluctuate during the day and are primarily a function of the rate of work. During peak performance, accidents reach their highest hourly rate. In longer working days, however, there is some evidence that fatigue increases the frequency of accidents toward the end of the day. The number of accidents in relation to the amount of production is found to be highest in the tenth hour of a ten-hour day. On the highway the large number of accidents involving a driver asleep is another instance of the role of fatigue.

Accident Proneness

With general factors such as we have been discussing held constant, there are still wide individual differences in liability to accident. Statistics for any randomly selected group always show a minority of people who have consistently high accident records over long periods of time. The majority, of course, are just average, and the average does not make a great deal of trouble. It is these people at the extreme end of the distribution curve of accidents that need special attention. Figure 229 shows that the men who had to go to the hospital often in 1938 had, on the average, to go often in 1939; and conversely. The men who got along without any hospital visits in 1938 averaged only 0.85 visit in

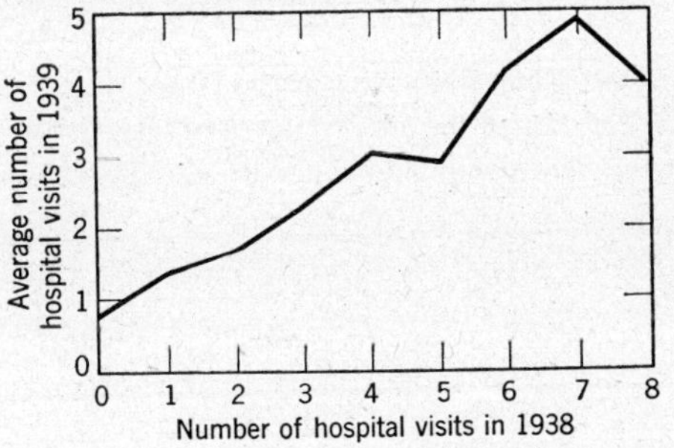

FIGURE 229. CONSISTENCY IN ACCIDENT TENDENCIES AMONG A GROUP OF 9000 STEEL WORKERS

Average numbers of hospital visits in 1939 for men who had, respectively, 1, 2, 3,···8 hospital visits in 1938. Accident hazards were similar for all. [From J. Tiffin, *Industrial psychology*, Prentice-Hall, 1943, p. 290.]

1939, whereas the men with 8 visits in 1938 averaged almost 4 in 1939. There are two kinks in this curve, but the relationship is unmistakable.

In recent years many attempts have been made to develop psychological tests which would make it possible to identify accident-prone individuals in various kinds of work. Tests of reaction time, motor coordination, distractability and visual functioning have been employed for this purpose with some success. Research of this sort will eventually enable us to determine the extent to which accident proneness is a generalized characteristic of the individual and to what extent it varies with the activity in which he is engaged. It ought eventually to be possible to keep people from engaging in pursuits in which they are particularly prone to accident or at least to provide them in advance with special training or equipment designed to reduce their accident liability.

Although these tests point to the possibility of detecting accident-prone individuals before they have had serious accidents, the past accident history of the individual is still the most reliable indicator we have of accident tendencies. For one thing the tests measure only some of the factors which make an individual accident-prone, and for this reason a person can be accident-prone even though his test performance is good. On the other hand, a person can very often compensate for his deficiencies and consequently can have a good safety record although his test scores are not at all satisfactory. At present, therefore, best results are obtained when the diagnosis is based both upon test scores and upon previous accident history.

REFERENCES

1. Bartley, S. H., and Chute, E. *Fatigue and impairment in man.* New York: McGraw-Hill, 1947.

   A recent book on the psychology and physiology of fatigue, reporting researches and clearly written. It stresses the role of psychological factors in fatigue, especially of frustration.

2. Berrien, F. K. *Practical psychology.* New York: Macmillan, 1944. Part 3.

   A well-written survey of applied psychology with some useful chapters on efficiency.

3. Carmichael, L., and Dearborn, W. F. *Reading and visual fatigue.* Boston: Houghton Mifflin, 1947.

   An experimental study of prolonged reading which failed to find visual fatigue or a decrement in the eye's performance.

4. DeSilva, H. R. *Why we have automobile accidents.* New York: Wiley, 1942.

Some interesting statistics and a program for research into the causes of highway accidents.

5. Poffenberger, A. T. *Principles of applied psychology.* New York: Appleton-Century, 1942.

A mature presentation containing fairly detailed accounts of important experiments on efficiency.

6. Roethlisberger, F. J., and Dickson, W. J. *Management and the worker.* Cambridge, Mass.: Harvard University Press, 1939.

A detailed description of the well-known Western Electric experiments which bear primarily upon the problem of industrial motivation and morale.

7. Ryan, T. A. *Work and effort.* New York: Ronald Press, 1947.

Another recent book, an extensive analysis of theory and experiment in the field of efficiency by one of the authors of the present chapter.

8. Tiffin, J. *Industrial psychology.* (2nd ed.) New York: Prentice-Hall, 1947.

A new and enlarged edition of a standard textbook dealing with the applications of psychology in industry with a relatively brief discussion of fatigue and efficiency.

9. Vernon, H. M. *Industrial fatigue and efficiency.* New York: Dutton, 1921.

A description of British experiments conducted during the First World War.

10. Vernon, H. M. *Accidents and their prevention.* New York: Cambridge University Press and Macmillan, 1936.

A statistical and psychological analysis of industrial, domestic and highway accidents.

11. Viteles, M. S. *Industrial psychology.* New York: Norton, 1932.

A good general account of industrial psychology which presents detailed discussions of research up to 1932.

CHAPTER 21

Personality

IN our culture, with its emphasis on the importance of being liked by people, nothing is more important than 'personality.' In this popular sense, personality is conceived by most people as an intangible quality that makes an individual attractive or unattractive to his fellows. Psychology uses the word *personality* in a much broader meaning. Every human being has characteristics which are shown in his typical ways of reacting to common situations; they make up his personality.

Personality differences are evident in every classroom. Some students are confident of their own ideas, readily contributing to the discussion; others are inhibited and seem afraid to raise their voices. One student may be rigid and inflexible in his thinking so that nothing can alter his preconceptions. At the opposite and no more desirable extreme, another student may be swayed by every passing fad, may lack independence and decisiveness.

Classroom behavior is highly conventionalized and is governed by certain social rules, thus minimizing the expressions of individuality. Personality differences are demonstrated more clearly in freer situations which are less bound by custom. When a group of college students come together informally, each one is more at liberty to 'be himself.' Student A is vigorously assertive, trying to dominate the others. B is easy-going, adaptable, tending to agree with the majority. C is sensitive, regarding opposition to his opinions as a personal injury. These characteristics do not, of course, always occur in the same combinations. One student whose actions are calm and secure may yet be friendly and warm-hearted, whereas another equally calm and stable person may be coldly critical of his associates. If enough observations can be made of each person, it becomes possible to make a word picture of him, a description of his typical style of behavior in interpersonal relationships. This total picture is what we call his *personality.*

PSYCHOLOGICAL CONCEPTS OF PERSONALITY

So we begin with the definition of *personality* and the consideration of what is meant by *personality types* and *personality traits.*

Definitions of Personality

The word personality comes from the Latin *persona,* which was the mask worn by players in the theater.[1] Thus at its very

This chapter was prepared by Laurance F. Shaffer of Teachers College, Columbia University.

beginning, the word implied a *false appearance,* which in today's slang might be termed a 'front,' showy but deceptive. Then, even in Roman times, an interesting shift of meaning occurred, so that *persona* came to mean the player himself, as an individual with distinct qualities. This is almost the opposite of the first meaning, for it makes personality signify the *true character* of the individual, rather than merely his appearance.

The ancient contradiction in the definitions of personality is of continued interest because it throws light on the difference between the popular and psychological usages. Popular speech still tends toward the meaning of 'mask' or appearance in its concept of personality. This kind of *personality* is the individual's superficial attractiveness or his social effect upon others. At the opposite extreme, certain philosophers have used the word for the *inner essence* of the individual, the ultimate reality that organizes and controls his observable behavior. This is a development of the 'true-character' definition; personality is viewed as a first cause, and everything about the individual is explained as due to his personality.

To the psychologist, however, personality is neither a false appearance nor an ultimate cause. Since people are products of their biological structures and their environments, personality has come to be regarded as the individuality that emerges from the interaction between a biological organism and a social and physical world. Personality can be described only in terms of the behavior of the individual—his acts, postures, words and thoughts. It is therefore an appearance, as are all phenomena of nature, but not a false appearance. In this conception the 'mask' and 'substance' views of personality are fused. Personality consists of observable behavior, and it is also individual and intrinsic. It is defined as an individual's *typical or consistent adjustments to his environment.*

Personality Types

The complex phenomena of personality can be understood only if they are described in detail. One of the earlier approaches to the description of personality, formerly much used, was the division of people into *types.* According to this usage, one individual would be said to be of a dominating type, another of a sociable type, and a third of a seclusive type. Type theories have persisted because they appeal to a long-standing habit of popular thinking. There is a very common tendency to speak of people as being tall or short, good or bad, blond or brunet. On more careful consideration, everyone will recognize that the extremes are exceptional and that most people are not tall or short, nor entirely good or bad. (See pp. 421–425.)

In spite of their serious shortcomings, type theories of personality have contributed to psychology concepts and terms that have had a wide influence. One of the best known is the classification of *introvert* and *extravert.* The introvert is one who turns from active participation in the objective world to an inner world of thought and fantasy. The extravert, on the other hand, is more directly governed by objective data and by a perception of necessity and social expediency. This bipolar classification is seen to be closely related to the popular distinction between the practical man and the visionary. The usual concept of extraversion also has other implications. An extravert is supposed to be thick-skinned and relatively insensitive to criticism, spontaneous in his emotional expression, impersonal in argument, neither deeply affected by his failures nor much occupied with self-analysis or self-criticism. Introversion is associated with opposite tendencies: sensitivity to criticism, inhibition of emotional expression, personalization in discussion, magnification of failures and preoccupation with self-analysis and self-criticism.

Another widely discussed pair of personality types is the *schizoid* and *cycloid*. These concepts are based on the characteristics of the two most common types of serious mental disorder, schizophrenia and manic-depressive psychosis. The schizoid type is thought of as a normal person whose behavior tends toward that of the schizophrenic. The schizoid is therefore self-centered, given to fantasy, shyly withdrawn from social participation, highly strung and sensitive. The cycloid personality is characterized as emotional, active, readily responsive to external stimulation and given to instability of mood. The schizoid-cycloid classification is not entirely independent of the introvert-extravert 'types.' Although based on different approaches to the problem of personality, the two systems use many of the same descriptive terms.

The type theories are unacceptable because they oversimplify the description of personality. First, as we have just seen, they assume that all persons will fit into one or the other of two categories. This is contrary to the facts of observation and measurement, which indicate that most persons lie between the two extremes, and that there is a continuous gradation from one pole of a bipolar continuum to the other. Second, the type theories throw together characteristics that are not always associated in real persons. For example, the concept of an introvert demands that he be both seclusive and emotionally sensitive. These qualities may or may not actually occur together. An emotionally sensitive person may be either withdrawing or gregarious; an aloof individual may be either emotionally self-critical or coldly independent. Experimental studies of personality characteristics show that the 'types' are composites, and not pure or fundamental components.

Another objection to type theories is their tendency to give rise to a confusion between cause and effect. To say that an individual adjusts by withdrawing *because* he is an introvert is a superficial and circular explanation. The person's typical adjustments are the result of many factors, the most important of which are found in his life history. His introversion is the result of these same causes. Classifying an individual as belonging to a certain psychological type does not explain why he acts as he does, but only describes his behavior.

Personality Traits

The description of personality in terms of *traits* is clearly superior to its classification into types. A trait may be regarded as a dimension of personality, as a scale along which one characteristic or aspect of personality may be measured. For example, *dominance-submission* is a trait that a person may show in any degree. It is conceived quantitatively, as a continuous scale of measurement from the greatest dominance to the most abject submission. Few people lie at either extreme; most show the characteristic in a moderate or intermediate degree. As a trait, dominance-submission is regarded as only one dimension of personality. People also vary in other dimensions, and as many traits may be identified as are required to account for observations of behavior. Unlike the type theories, the analysis of traits does not require that all people be cast into a small number of molds.

Although a trait is a description of human behavior, not every word that describes behavior defines a trait. That is indeed fortunate, since one study has shown that there are approximately eighteen thousand words in the English language that designate forms of behavior. These words specify behaviors that may be observed in large numbers of people, such as *accurate, active, agile, alert* and *assertive,* and also rarer qualities, including *agnostical, alarmist, anarchistic* and *atavistic.* Designations such as these are traits only if they fulfill certain conditions. The most important requirement is that the trait must describe the *consistent behavior of an individual.* Thus, in order for *accuracy* to be a trait, an individual must consistently display about the same degree of accuracy, which may be at any point on a scale from very accurate to very inaccurate, in a great variety of situations. If his accuracy fluctuates widely from one time to another, or if it depends on the situation instead of on his own quality, accuracy is not a trait. It can, therefore, be seen that a trait such as accuracy-inaccuracy may exist in some persons and not in others. This fact places limitations on the quantitative investigation of some traits, especially on rare qualities such as those of being an alarmist, being anarchistic or being Machiavellian. These characteristics cannot be discovered at all in most people, but, when they do occur, they may be the most significant personal quality in the individual.

Common traits, which exist in some degree in almost all people, can be studied statistically. The usual method of investigation is to discover characteristics that *vary together.* It may be found, for example, that people who are idealistic are also cooperative, and friendly, and cheerful, and trustful, and that the opposites of these qualities also go together. This cluster of characteristics, then, defines a trait that has a broader meaning and is therefore more useful for description than the component qualities taken separately. We have already seen that the statistical method that has been applied for this purpose is factor analysis, which makes use of intercorrelations to reduce to group factors those measures which vary together. (See pp. 411 f.)

As a result of factor analysis, psychologists now agree that *introversion-extraversion* is not a trait. It is a collection of a number of imperfectly correlated traits. One research made a factor analysis of a large number of questionnaire items originally intended to measure introversion-extraversion. By studying the questions that fell into groups as defined by factors, it was found that introversion-extraversion consisted of five separate traits. They were identified as *social introversion* (shyness, withdrawal), *thinking introversion* (meditation, philosophizing), *depression* (unworthiness, guilt), *cycloid tendencies* (ups and downs of mood) and *rhathymia* (happy-go-lucky or carefree disposition). This factorial study clarified the concept of introversion, showing, for example, that a person who is shy need not be meditative or moody.

Many writers have attempted to make lists of the common traits of human personality. When prepared by arm-chair speculation, these lists often have been in disagreement. Some were short and obviously incomplete, others were long and repetitive. An application of factor analysis to the identification of the common human traits has given a solution that is a marked advance over unsupported opin-

TABLE XXIX

PRIMARY TRAITS OF PERSONALITY

[After R. B. Cattell, *Description and measurement of personality*, World Book Co., 1946, pp. 313–336.]

I. *Cyclothymia*	*vs.*	*Schizothymia*
Outgoing		Withdrawn
Good-natured		Surly
Adaptable		Inflexible
II. *Intelligence*	*vs.*	*Mental defect*
Intelligent		Stupid
Conscientious		Slipshod
Thoughtful		Unreflective
III. *Emotionally mature*	*vs.*	*Demoralized emotionality*
Realistic		Subjective
Stable		Uncontrolled
Patient		Excitable
IV. *Dominance*	*vs.*	*Submissiveness*
Boastful		Modest
Egotistic		Self-effacing
Tough		Sensitive
V. *Surgency*	*vs.*	*Melancholic desurgency*
Cheerful		Unhappy
Optimistic		Pessimistic
Sociable		Aloof
VI. *Sensitive, imaginative*	*vs.*	*Rigid, tough, poised*
Idealistic		Cynical
Intuitive		Logical
Friendly		Hardhearted
VII. *Trained, socialized*	*vs.*	*Boorish*
Thoughtful		Narrow
Sophisticated		Simple
Aesthetic		Coarse
VIII. *Positive integration*	*vs.*	*Immature, dependent*
Independent		Dependent
Persevering		Slipshod
Practical		Unrealistic
IX. *Charitable, adventurous*	*vs.*	*Obstructive, withdrawn*
Kindly		Cynical
Cooperative		Obstructive
Frank		Secretive
X. *Neurasthenia*	*vs.*	*Vigorous character*
Languid		Alert
Quitting		Painstaking
Incoherent		Strong-willed
XI. *Hypersensitive, infantile*	*vs.*	*Frustration tolerance*
Infantile		Adjusting
Restless		Calm
Impatient		Phlegmatic
XII. *Surgent cyclothymia*	*vs.*	*Paranoia*
Enthusiastic		Frustrated
Friendly		Hostile
Trustful		Suspicious

ion, although it can undoubtedly be improved by additional research. Starting with a list of some 4000 trait terms, the number was reduced to 171 descriptive concepts by eliminating near-synonyms and rare characteristics. A preliminary study of the relationships of the 171 concepts further reduced the list to 35 'clusters' of traits. A substantial group of adult men was then rated on each of the 35 personality variables. The correlation of each characteristic with each other characteristic was calculated, and the underlying factors were extracted statistically. The twelve factors specified in Table XXIX were found. Below each factor in the table three descriptive words are given to help define the area of personality indicated.

By thus identifying and defining traits, psychology has made considerable progress toward a specific and objective understanding of personality. Instead of a vague and philosophically defined concept, personality has become an observable and potentially measurable system of characteristics. There is a danger, however, that the wholeness and uniqueness of the human being may be lost in the enumeration of his separate qualities. This fault should be overcome, not by a return to obscure generalities but by increasingly penetrating research on the interdependences and integrations of the characteristics of personality.

MEASUREMENT OF PERSONALITY

The measurement of personality serves both theoretical and practical purposes. Many of the problems concerning the nature and development of personality could be solved satisfactorily if we had more precise methods for measuring traits. Measurements could be made of aspects of personality and also of relevant factors that might affect personal development. The relationships could then be examined to reveal the sources of personality. This ideal program of research lies chiefly in the future, but useful beginnings have been made, and much of our present knowledge of personality has come through quantitative measurement.

Personality measurement also has many practical applications. When an individual who has difficulties of personal adjustment comes for help to a psychiatrist or to a psychological clinic, it is valuable to assess his personality. An appraisal of his personality deficiencies indicates the degree of disturbance present and the handicaps that he will have to overcome. A study of his assets reveals the sources of his strength that can be used in helping him overcome his troubles. Another common use of personality measurement is in the *screening* of large groups of students, military personnel and others, to discover individuals who need psychological assistance in dealing with their personal adjustments. Personality measurement has also been attempted for positive aspects of individual diagnosis, as in the selection of leaders and of stable persons for responsible positions. At least moderate success has been achieved in all these applications.

Informal Diagnosis

The original method of personality appraisal, and still a basic one, is the *interview.* In using this type of evaluation, the psychologist usually starts by listening to the subject's own story, hearing his problems or complaints, his interpretation of their meanings and his account of his past experiences. By accepting the subject's story without condemnation, the psychologist frees him to talk of more intimate and emotionally tinged matters and draws out from him a full picture of his personality. Sometimes he questions the subject in order to probe attitudes and areas of experience which are suppressed. In some instances, especially when working with children, facts about the subject's life history are gathered from parents, teachers and other observers.

A highly skilled interviewer gains impressions from this procedure far beyond those conveyed by the subject's words. Observation is an integral part of the method. The subject's manner of speaking, his hesitations, his averted glances, his signs of emotional response, provide clues that are as valuable as his story or even more valuable. Because of the opportunity that it provides for making observations and because of its flexible adaptability to various circumstances, the interview will continue to be an indispensable technique for personality study.

Nevertheless, in spite of all its merits, the interview has serious limitations. People vary greatly in their skill as interviewers, so that the conclusions obtained by this method are not uniformly valid. Moreover, skill in interviewing is difficult to teach. An excellent interviewer rarely can describe just how he accomplishes his task. The skill has to be acquired by a trial-and-error process of learning. The results of interviews, clear to the interviewer, are difficult to communicate. They are not readily expressed in quantitative terms or by precise description. For these reasons, psychologists have made many attempts to develop more refined methods for assessing personality.

Rating Methods

A rating scale is a technique for quantifying observations based on acquaintance or on interviews. In the most usual form, a rating scale consists of a question defining an aspect of personality, followed by four or five alternative descriptions. Here is an example.

Is the subject at ease or self-conscious?

•	•	•	•	•
Always at ease.	Seldom flustered by actions or remarks of others.	Self-conscious on occasions.	Frequently embarrassed.	Painfully self-conscious and ill at ease.

The rater places a mark above the most appropriate descriptive phrase, or between phrases, and his rating is easily converted into a numerical score on a scale of 1 to 5, or 1 to 9 if the line is checked between the phrases as well as at them. Another valuable method of rating requires the observer to rank a group of persons in the order in which they show a characteristic, as, for example, from the most dominant individual to the most submissive one.

A rating scale is not a substitute for lack of information. You cannot rate another man unless you know him and have also observed in him the trait on which you are rating him. There has been ample demonstration of this point. Teachers can rate their students well in scholarship but not on some other characteristics, like adaptability or impulsiveness. Enlisted men do a better job in rating each other on leadership than the officers in charge of the men. The men know each other intimately from constant mutual observation under a wide variety of circumstances. Similarly students can rate the teaching ability of their teachers better than the supervisors who do not see the teachers constantly in action.

Sometimes a trait can be brought into use for special observation by raters. For instance, a man may be required to build a small bridge, being provided with several helpers and a very limited supply of materials. By watching his behavior in this situation, practiced observers can rate his leadership, ingenuity, tolerance of frustration, etc., more validly than they could from less specific evidence.

Questionnaires

In an interview conducted for the purpose of assessing personality, much information is gained by asking questions and evaluating the subject's answers. Usually the questions are printed, and the subject is instructed to mark or write his responses. Such a set of questions is known as a *personality questionnaire.* A questionnaire obtains more uniform information than an interview, since all examinees are asked the same questions. That permits the quantitative study of the results and the comparison of one person with others. The questionnaire saves time, for it is a group test.

The printed questionnaire was first used in the First World War for the detection of recruits who were emotionally unstable. A large number of questions were assembled from the case histories of persons who suffered from maladjustments of all kinds. The typical style of questions is shown by the following samples.*

Do you usually sleep well?	yes	no
Do you ever walk in your sleep?	yes	no
Do you feel tired most of the time?	yes	no
Did you have a happy childhood?	yes	no
Were you shy with other boys?	yes	no
Do you make friends easily?	yes	no
Are you ever bothered by a feeling that things are not real?	yes	no
Do you get rattled easily?	yes	no

* R. S. Woodworth's Psychoneurotic Inventory, in S. I. Franz, *Handbook of mental examination methods* (2nd ed.), 1919, by permission of The Macmillan Co.

This questionnaire was a 'blunderbuss,' intended to detect all sorts of maladjusted behavior. It did not attempt to measure any personality traits separately. It was assumed that a greater number of symptoms indicated a more severe degree of maladjustment, so the score was the number of questions answered in the unfavorable direction.

Many recent personality questionnaires have limited themselves to a specified trait or to a series of defined traits, and have made some effort to validate the score. An example is the *Allport Ascendance-Submission Reaction Study,* from which the following items are taken.*

At church, a lecture, or an entertainment, if you arrive after the program has commenced and find that there are people standing but also that there are front seats available which might be secured without 'piggishness' or discourtesy, but with considerable conspicuousness, do you take the seats?

habitually ______
occasionally ______
never ______

When you see someone in a public place or crowd whom you think you have met or known, do you inquire of him whether vou have met before?

sometimes ______
rarely ______
never ______

The validity of this questionnaire was established by comparing its results with ratings on college students made by themselves and their close associates. Only the significant items were retained. Such a combination of the questionnaire and rating methods reduces the author's dependence on his unsupported opinion in the construction of a questionnaire.

Another method used in the construction of personality questionnaires is to make up a very large number of questions and then to determine by experimental study which items will distinguish between normal persons and definite groups of individuals that deviate from normal. For example, if certain questions are answered *no* by normal persons, and *yes* by depressed persons, these questions constitute a scale for measuring depression. The *Minnesota Multiphasic Personality Inventory* is a questionnaire prepared by this method. It consists of 550 statements, phrased in simple language, to which the examinee responds by indicating whether or not the statement is true for him. Examples of statements are: "I do not tire quickly"; "Someone has it in for me"; "At times I think I am no good at all." By comparing the answers of normal people with groups having psychiatric diagnoses, keys have been constructed to measure *hypochondriasis* (undue concern about bodily complaints), *depression, hysteria, psychopathic tendency* (disregard of social motives), *paranoia* (suspiciousness and delusion), *psychasthenia* (phobias and compulsive behavior), *schizophrenia* and *hypomania* (excessive level of activity). There is also a *masculinity-femininity* scale, consisting of the items on which the responses of men and women differ. Each of these traits is scored by means of a separate key, and the results may be expressed as a *profile* that shows the individual's relative standing in each characteristic (Fig. 230). Several studies have shown that this questionnaire is an aid to the diagnosis of disturbances of personality.

Performance Tests

Performance tests have been devised for certain traits, some of the best-known being the May and Hartshorne tests for measuring character traits in school children.

* G. W. Allport, *J. abn. soc. Psychol.,* 1928, **23,** 125.

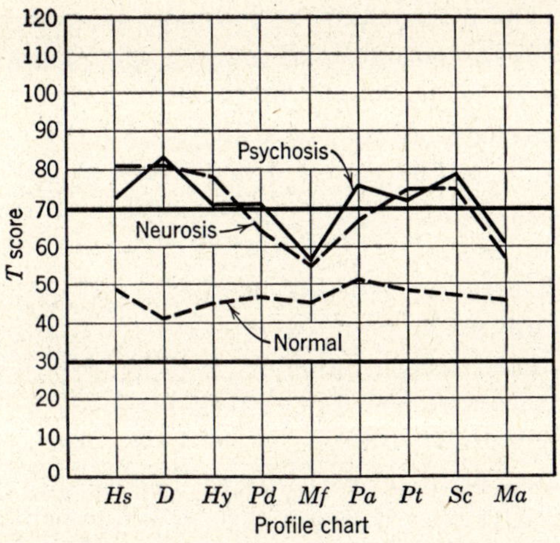

FIGURE 230. THREE PROFILES FROM THE MINNESOTA MULTIPHASIC PERSONALITY INVENTORY

The symbols of the profile identify these scores: *Hs,* hypochondriasis; *D,* depression; *Hy,* hysteria; *Pd,* psychopathic deviate; *Mf,* masculinity-femininity; *Pa,* paranoia; *Pt,* psychasthenia; *Sc,* schizophrenia; and *Ma,* hypomania. The defined normal score is 50, and scores above 70 are regarded as abnormal. The lowest line represents the scores of 98 normal soldiers. The dashed line shows 64 cases of severe psychoneurosis (note typically high *Hs, D* and *Hy*). The solid line is the scores of 13 cases of psychosis (note high *D, Pa* and *Sc*). [After H. O. Schmidt, *J. appl. Psychol.,* 1945, **29,** 115–131.]

They comprise an extensive series of tests, covering such behavior as cheating, lying, stealing, cooperation, persistence and inhibition. All the tests are administered in everyday-life situations, including classwork, assigned 'homework,' athletics or party games. The children are not aware that they are being tested or that their behavior can be detected or identified with them.

An example of one of the cheating tests is the 'self-scoring' technique, in which children are given a test of arithmetic, spelling or some other regular school subject. The papers are collected, and a record is made of each child's answers. Then the papers, which have not been marked in any way, are returned to the children together with the correct answers. The children are now told to grade their own papers, after which the papers are again collected. Any change which the child has made in his answers can of course be detected by checking against the previous records.

Several of the May and Hartshorne tests use the 'improbable achievement' technique. For example, the subject is given seven pill boxes to arrange in order of weight, the correct rank order being printed on the bottom of each pill box. The discriminations required are very fine and, if the child achieves a perfect or nearly perfect arrangement, it is clear that he must have cheated by looking at the printed weights despite instructions not to do so.

Projective Methods

A new approach to the exploration of personality has received much attention from psychologists in recent years. The new methods are called *projective,* because in them the subject tends to project his own characteristics into a response to a situation that is vague and undefined.

The use of projective methods is based on the hypothesis that the mechanism of projection (p. 521) is operating, and that an individual reveals his own characteristics by what he sees in his environment. The indefinite character of the material used in the projective tests frees the person from social conventions and from reality, so that he can 'be himself.' These techniques are subtle, because the examinee, not knowing what is a 'good' answer, is less able to distort his responses deliberately to make a favorable impression.

The *Rorschach test* is the most widely used projective method. In its present form, it was first described in 1921 by Hermann Rorschach, a Swiss psychiatrist. The material consists of ten ink-blot patterns, similar in character to Fig. 231. Five of the blots are in black only, two are black and red, and three are entirely in colors. The cards are presented to the subject one at a time, the examiner saying only, "What might this be?" The examiner writes

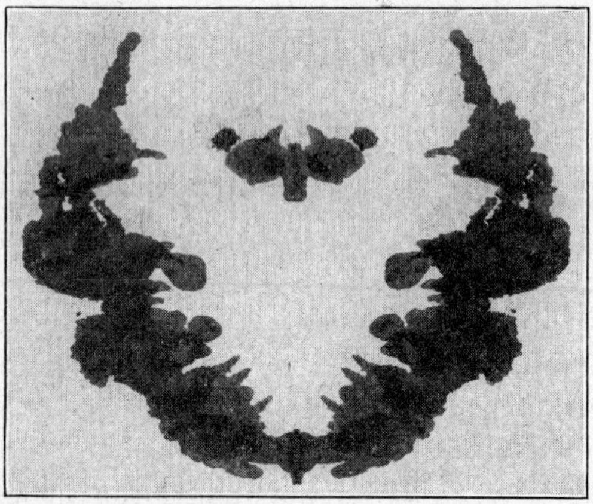

FIGURE 231. AN INK BLOT SIMILAR TO THOSE EMPLOYED IN THE RORSCHACH TEST

the subject's responses in full. After the ten cards are completed, the examiner goes through them a second time to make a record of *where* the subject saw each thing that he mentioned.

Each response is scored with respect to three principal features:

1. *Location.* Whether the response was based on the whole blot or on a detail.

2. *Determining quality.* Whether the response was determined by the form of the blot, by color, by shading or by movement. (The latter is assumed if figures are seen in motion, for instance, "two bears dancing.")

3. *Content.* This refers to what is seen, as human figures, animals, objects, landscapes, maps, anatomical details.

The scores from the ten blots are added, so as to give the total number of responses referring to whole blots, determined by movement, concerned with animals and the like. A number of other scores are also noted, such as the total number of responses, the reaction time to each card, and whether or not the responses are commonly made ones.

The interpretation of a Rorschach test is a complicated task. Most of the conclusions drawn from a subject's responses are based on logic and on psychiatric 'experience,' rather than on formal experimental proof. For example, a person with an unduly large number of 'whole' responses is described as theoretical rather than practical, and given to expansive generalities. If he gives notably more responses based on small details than most people, that shows a preoccupation with minor matters, a petty person or even a compulsive one. Movement responses are supposed to indicate introversion or fantasy, and color responses to show warmth of emotional tone. In general, however, no interpretation is based on a single sign. Responses are compared to one another, ratios are calculated, and an elaborate system of checking and balancing factors is employed.

Although much work has been done with the Rorschach test, its validity is not firmly established, largely because it is so difficult to find other good measures of personality against which to check the Rorschach results. Some of the Rorschach ratings have been validated against other test results, but the final decision about the validity of the test, in spite of the enthusiasm of some of the specialists who use it, waits upon the future.

Another widely used projective method is the *Thematic Apperception Test.* It consists of a series of standard pictures, almost all of which contain human figures, but which are sufficiently ambiguous to permit a variety of interpretations in terms of desires, threats and emotional responses. The subject is told to make up a story about each picture. The examiner may ask, "What is happening? What led up to it? What will be the outcome? What are the feelings and thoughts of the characters?" It has been found that persons taking this test usually identify themselves with one of the characters in a picture, and that the stories become implicitly autobiographical.

One of these pictures, reproduced in Fig. 232, shows the head of a young woman with a very wrinkled old woman behind her shoulder. The older woman has her chin resting on her bony hand. The following story was told about this picture by a middle-aged woman who was diagnosed as a case of conversion hysteria. Prominent in her history was an unfortunate relationship with her mother which is reflected in this account.

"A younger woman and an older woman, very, very old, weatherbeaten. They certainly don't do justice to women in this, do they? The older woman looks as if she might have said something to the younger woman to hurt her . . . make her feel bad or something. She looks sort of pleased with herself to see that she could hurt her. Makes me think of a witch. Well, maybe this woman has some sort of power over the girl—as if she's afraid to break away from her. She has a sort of sly smile on her face. Oh, I can't say anything more."

Unlike the Rorschach test, the Thematic Apperception Test has no quantitative scoring. The value of the method is that it induces the subject to verbalize his thoughts, attitudes and feelings behind the thin disguise of making up a story. Themes that recur in more than one picture are noted, and analyses are made of the prevailing emotional tone of the narratives, of the subject's identifications with characters, of his strivings or needs, of his thwartings and conflicts and of his defenses. The experienced clinical psychologist can gain a conception of the subject's personality that is rich and suggestive, even though it is lacking in quantitative precision.

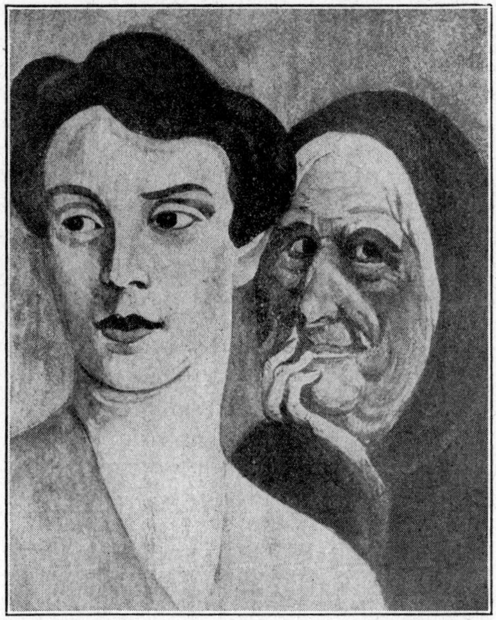

FIG. 232. THEMATIC APPERCEPTION TEST

One of the series of pictures used. [From H. A. Murray, *Thematic Apperception Test,* Harvard University Press, 1943.]

THE ORIGINS OF PERSONALITY

Thus far our analysis and description of personality are representative of the *cross-sectional* approach which seeks to determine the status of the personality at a given time in the individual's life. Another and probably more valuable approach is the *longitudinal* one, which traces the development of a personality and tries to identify the influences that contribute to its formation. The longitudinal point of view is genetic and developmental, seeing a person as a continuously growing and learning organism.

The variety of influences that contribute to the formation of personality can be seen quite clearly by case studies of individual development. As an example, we may trace, by means of a hypothetical case, the factors that could produce a *dominant* or *ascendant* person. Suppose that a boy develops with better than average size, strength and skill. His activity level is high, owing, in part, to the excellence of his glandular balances, to his high metabolism and to his freedom from hampering diseases. In his infancy he was given loving acceptance by his parents, so that he developed a basic sense of security and belonging. He readily identified himself with his father, who is a large, secure, dominant person. He has had ample opportunity for contacts with other children. He is the largest boy in his particular play group and has become accustomed to the role of initiating and leading their activities. His parents encourage his independence of action and give him responsibilities in keeping with his developing ability to fulfill them. Although he is bright enough, bookish accomplishments are not highly regarded in his family or in his social group, so he never becomes distinguished for scholarship. He is, however, rewarded for proficiency in sports and for taking an assertive part in school activities. The end result of such a development is very likely to be a man with a dominant personality, sure of himself, accustomed to being liked by others, and with values based on vigorous physical and social activities.

The personality just sketched is by no means an ideal one. If other traits were favorable, he could become a successful executive, salesman and golfer. Suppose, however, that he is also insensitive to the weaknesses and troubles of others, and obtuse to aesthetic values and intellectual interests. Then he will probably be a bore. He is also poorly prepared for catastrophe. If failure should overtake him later in life, he will be unprepared for it, inexperienced in it.

More than one pattern of conditions may lead to approximately the same result in the development of a personality. Another individual may be reared in a home in which he evolves aspirations for dominance. Some qualities or circumstances may frustrate the direct realization of these motives. He may be overprotected by his parents, or unable to compete physically with other boys, or lacking in skill or intelligence. Such circumstances may lead him to acquire a *compensatory dominance,* which can be recognized in its earlier stages by excessive striving, by emotional reactions to threats or competition and by other evidences of insecurity. If his attempted compensation is unsuccessful, he may become sour, obstructive and hostile. Some compensations are very successful adjustments, however, and this person as an adult may seem as genuinely ascendant as our first hypothetical example. It may take a very penetrating psychological investigation to discover the differences in their origins.

Both these illustrations show the effects of a great number of factors on the growth of an aspect of personality. Physique, glandular and metabolic processes, health, the pattern of the culture, social contacts and opportunities, parental models, abilities and skills, all contribute. Above all, adjustive learning is important, for an individual's personality is the residual of all the behavior that he has found successful in satisfaction of his needs and in the resolution of his frustrations and conflicts. These factors do not act separately, but are interdependent, so that a change in one of the causal factors not only changes the resulting personality directly but also modifies some of the other determining influences as well.

BIOLOGICAL FACTORS IN PERSONALITY

Personality emerges from the interactions of a biological organism with a social world. Before beginning a detailed consideration of the social development of personality, it is necessary for us to investigate the influence of some of the most significant biological factors.

A division of developmental factors into biological and social is like the old opposition between heredity and environment which we have already studied. According to it an individual's attainments, capacity and character are regarded as the result of both nature and nurture. Whatever cannot be ascribed to learning and training is attributed to the genes, the carriers of inheritance. In this division between heredity and environment, however, certain types of environmental factors are omitted. Such environmental forces as temperature and the chemistry of nutrition contribute to the growth of the nervous system, of the glands and of man's physical structure in general, and to the functioning of these structures. The genes likewise make their contribution, of course, but it is a common error to classify as inherited all those characteristics of man which are not due to learning. The strength and quickness of the vigorous child, for example, are not wholly a matter of his good luck in drawing the right pattern of genes. They depend also upon a fortunate interaction of the right genes with favorable environmental forces. (See pp. 441–443.)

Evidence on this point from anthropological studies is fairly conclusive. The physical measurements of American-born children of southeastern European peoples have been compared with measurements of their parents. East European Hebrews are below the American norms in height and skeletal structure; yet their children, reared in a more favorable environment, deviate from their parents in the direction of the American norms. Even the form of the head undergoes change. The south Italian has an exceedingly long head, but his American-born children are more short-headed. The east European Hebrew has a very round head, but his American-born children are more long-headed. In this country these immigrant groups approach a uniform type with respect to head form.

Since even biological factors are not wholly the effects of inheritance, personality can no longer be considered, as was formerly the case, the progressive unfolding of an innate constitution. The blue-blooded aristocrat does not owe his polished tastes and manners to his genes. Nor does the thief come by his antisocial habits through genes which make for thieving.

The role of biological factors is to set the limits within which the individual's personality will develop. Their influence is general and indirect as compared with the influence of social and psychological forces. This fact will appear more clearly if we consider specific biological factors in development. Three such factors are (1) body chemistry, (2) physique and (3) the nervous system.

Body Chemistry and the Endocrine Glands

Most of us are aware of differences in mood and behavior due to physical well-being or ill-being. At times we are sluggish and despondent; at other times we feel alert and animated. And we are sometimes correct in attributing these changes to diet, sleep, toxins and infections. In addition, however, the body contains within itself a mechanism of chemical control in its endocrine organs, or glands of internal secretion. These glands release chemical substances, or hormones, into the blood stream, which carries them to all parts of the body. The hormones sensitize or desensitize nervous and muscular tissue, the particular effect depending upon the chemical composition of the hormone. Hence our responses to external objects are facilitated or retarded by the activity of the endocrine organs. Thus, though the primary function of these glands is concerned with the growth and metabolism of the body, they also influence behavior. Clearly the endocrine glands are important! We have already learned something about them in Chapter 4 in their relation to development, in Chapter 5 in their relation to emotion, and in Chapter 6 in their relation to motivation. Now we have to examine their relation to personality, reviewing some of the facts which we have already learned, so that we may have the whole picture clearly in mind.

The *thyroid gland* is directly related to the metabolism of the body, that is to say, the destructive and constructive changes in body tissues. Its hormone acts as a catalyzer to facilitate the breaking down of waste products so that they can be readily eliminated from the body. If the thyroid gland is underactive, partially decomposed proteins are retained in the tissues and further cell destruction is diminished. Oxidation is lessened and blood pressure falls. With the metabolic processes slowed up in this manner, the individual becomes lethargic and despondent. Easily fatigued, he often suffers from states of depression. If the thyroid gland is overactive, on the other hand, metabolism is increased and body tissues are overstimulated. An increase in muscular tension follows, and the person appears excitable, restless, worried.

The thyroid gland is balanced by the *parathyroids.* An overactive parathyroid tends to quiet and slow down the individual. The mechanism involved is the regulation of the calcium balance of the body; a lowered supply of calcium in the blood stream sensitizes nerves and muscles and makes the individual overexcitable. This supply of calcium is associated with the parathyroid hormone. An excess of the hormone means an excess of calcium salts; a diminution means a lowered calcium supply. The removal of the parathyroids produces muscular tremors, spasms and cramps—an indication that the nervous system is oversensitive. An underactive parathyroid may thus be one determinant of an excessively high activity level.

The *pituitary gland* is important in its contribution to body growth. Impaired functioning of the pituitary in childhood is related to a generally deficient bony structure, weakened skeletal muscles and underdeveloped sex organs. The child thus afflicted lacks aggressiveness, gives up easily, cries readily and is regarded as cowardly. Overactivity of this gland (specifically of its anterior lobe) results in gigantism, thick skin and precocious sex development. The behavior picture in this case may be one of aggressiveness and pugnacity.

The development of the secondary sex characteristics is a function of the *gonadal glands.* These secondary characteristics include height, weight, the distribution of hair over the body, subcutaneous fat and the mammary glands. Experimenters have transplanted ovaries from female rats and guinea pigs to castrated male rats and guinea pigs. The result has been that the male animals have taken on the characteristics of the female both in physical and in behavioral traits. Similarly, the transplantation of interstitial tissue from the male testes to female animals whose ovaries had been removed, has produced male characteristics. These experiments indicate that the sex hormones are a contributing factor to masculine and feminine traits of personality.

Extreme instances of glandular malfunctioning have been mentioned to illustrate the importance of the endocrine organs. Normal individuals, however, may vary slightly in either direction from the norm of glandular balance. For example, the sensitivity of the excessively timid child is sometimes a matter of body chemistry. Observations of children show great differences in personality from infancy on, differences which cannot be explained entirely on the basis of experience. In general, however, the endocrines do not have direct effects upon personality. Rather they initiate physiological changes, the final results of which are complicated by habit and experience. Not infrequently the physiological state, produced by abnormal endocrine functioning, seriously affects the individual through his realization of his condition. The depression caused by an underactive thyroid condition is generally accentuated by a knowledge of the deficiency.

Physique and Physical Health

The most obvious aspects of the individual are his physical characteristics, his height, weight, bodily proportions, coloring and physical beauty. Their importance in the development of personality is generally misconstrued. Since they are easily noticed, they have been unduly emphasized as indicators of personality. Popular opinion persists in evaluating people according to physical appearance, although phrenology and related arts of character reading have long been thoroughly discredited. For the most part physical characteristics are not so much significant as external signs of the internal man, as that they play a part in the development of personality. Their effect is likely to be mediated through the social reception accorded to various types of physical appearance. The undersized child, for example, may acquire a feeling of inferiority if both adults and children react differently to him than to his fellows.

Before parents can compare their children with other children on the basis of intellectual attainment, they can and do consult height and weight norms and pronounce judgment accordingly. Their constant attention to physical growth means that the youngster builds up a notion of himself as a normal or an abnormal person physically. This concept of himself is also fostered by the competitive advantage or disadvantage of his size and weight. Most individuals tend to place themselves nearer the desirable norm than they really are. Most men a little under average in height, for example, think of themselves as taller than they are.

Actual deformity handicaps the child

both physically and psychologically. Fewer physically handicapped children develop into normal personalities than physically well-favored children. One study of this problem compared the responses of crippled girls with the responses of normal girls of the same age on a test of emotional stability. The average score for the crippled group was 75 per cent greater in the direction of instability than the score of the normal group.

Sheer size and weight are less important in the development of personality than strength and agility. It is not so often the undersized child who is pushed around by other children as it is the physically weak youngster. Health and vigor are significant in the formative years, since contacts and competition among children are often on the physical level. Even in adult years the man with a rugged constitution is at an advantage in maintaining an aggressive attitude toward life and in preserving his emotional balance.

The particular way in which a given person is affected by his physical constitution is further shaped by social experience. In general the physically inferior child follows one of two courses of development. If he is pampered and humored at every turn, he *under-reacts* toward his world. He never acquires the ability to solve his own problems. If, however, his inferiority bars him from the center of the stage, he may *over-react* to compensate for his deficiency. It is characteristic of compensation that the individual exceeds the normal person in striving for perfection or for power. One of the most famous track athletes of our time owes his career to an accident in which his legs were badly burned. He persevered in his running to develop the injured leg muscles until he outran all competitors.

It is true that there is current a theory of three constitutional bodily components which are held to be diagnostic of three patterns of personality. This theory of constitutional types, one which still awaits confirmation, has, however, already been outlined on pages 422–425.

The Nervous System

In enumerating the biological factors that contribute to personality, it is easy to overlook the most obvious of all—the quality and effectiveness of the individual's nervous system. In addition to their dependence on environmental influences and training, a person's mental ability, manipulative and motor skills, and special talents are due in some degree to the structure and properties of his nervous system. In particular instances it is usually impossible to distinguish the exact contribution of such biological factors to performance. It seems probable, however, that a person's neural equipment sets certain limits beyond which training is ineffective. No amount of special teaching will enable a moron to handle adequately problems of symbolic logic. Similar limitations affect the development of special motor and manipulative skills. Each athletic coach knows that certain tricks can be taught and certain techniques perfected, but that motor coordination, speed of response and physical alertness are in good measure determined by a man's biological equipment.

Although they are truly important, the limitations set by the properties of the nervous system are frequently exaggerated. Most people do not develop their abilities as far as their biological endowment permits. It is also true that limitations of capacity usually affect personality more strikingly through indirect social interaction than by direct hindrance. Failure is more important psychologically when others can succeed than when no one is successful. Even when a person can accomplish an end by strenuous effort, it is not comforting to see another reach the same goal easily.

INFLUENCE OF CULTURE ON PERSONALITY

The culture in which an individual is reared exerts the broadest kind of social influence upon his personality traits. Ancient man is not like modern man, and primitive peoples are not like civilized peoples, because of the interactions between individual personalities and their cultural backgrounds.

For instance, modern Western man contrasts strikingly with the Greek of classical times. The orientation toward time and space in the classical period is quite foreign to the modern mind. Classical man lived completely in the present. The calendar and the clock, those dread symbols of the flow of time, did not regulate his life. He had no conception of historical development. So completely did classical writers lack historical feeling that their fine pieces of history writing were confined to events occurring within their own memories. Thucydides, it has been said, would have been unable to handle even the Persian Wars, let alone the general history of Greece, and the history of Egypt would have utterly confounded him. Likewise the spatial world of classical man was limited to his own narrow experience. Olympus to him represented extreme distance, and even the Gods were no farther away. As against the unhistorical, timeless, spatially restricted mind of the classical Greek stands modern man with his sensitive consciousness of temporal distinctions, his historical perspective, his appreciation of distances beyond his immediate horizon and his orientation to an ever-expanding spatial world.

These differences between classical man and modern men are not to be explained, as some historians have attempted, as the difference between the Appollonian soul and the Faustian soul. Modern man is what he is because he develops in a certain social environment. He grows up in a mechanical world. He learns to adjust his problems by machines which annihilate space. Collective adjustments in a mechanized age call for specialization of labor and synchronization of effort. Trains run according to schedule and factories according to the timeclock, and schools open and close their doors by the bell. The pure present of the classical mind becomes transmuted into a finely discriminating time sense which relates each moment as it passes to the future and to the past.

Or consider the personalities of people in primitive societies. The Mountain Arapesh of New Guinea are said to lack egotism. These people are by and large peaceful, friendly, genuine, cooperative, but lacking in foresight and ambition. Among them there is no definite hierarchy of leaders. They recognize no single scale by which success may be socially measured. The admired personality is the all-round man. In contrast to these mild people of New Guinea are the Eskimos of Greenland. They are rampant individualists. The cardinal traits of personality in their society are initiative, self-reliance and aggression.

Again these differences in personality grow, in part, out of different conditions of life to which the Arapesh and the Eskimos have been compelled to adjust, although they also depend in part upon the way in which each tribe treats its young children. The Arapesh occupy a mountainous terrain which guarantees their safety from invasion and at the same time yields them a dependable though a meager living. They eke out a bare existence through agriculture, trading and hunting. Not menaced by danger from without and not facing actual starvation, the Arapesh have never developed a strong social organization. The tortuous nature of the country with its narrow paths and slippery rocks, moreover, makes standardization of complicated cooperative group activity difficult. Social relationships are consequently personal in nature. Though common ownership of property is not the usual practice, there are exceptions, such as the communal sharing of food through gifts to friends and the giving of public feasts.

The personality of the Arapesh is thus partly the product of these material and social conditions of life. Their enemies are natural forces so much beyond their control that it seems to them useless to work very hard to produce a bumper crop. Their friends are their fellowmen, and they all help one another in the work of living. Both the absence of organized pressure upon the individual to spur his competitiveness and the lack of social approval for the aggressive individual make for a mild, unambitious personality.

The Eskimos of Greenland, on the other hand, face such rigorous conditions of life that only strong individuals can survive. Any individual who, through infirmity or other physical handicap, cannot make his economic contribution perishes, commits suicide or is killed. The technology of the group is highly individualistic. Every man hunts for himself and manufactures his own tools and weapons. For open-sea hunting each man uses his own kayak. Should he capsize, he must be prepared to right it without help from others. The Eskimo couple is a self-sufficient economic unit. In addition to her other household tasks, the wife converts animal skins into clothing and equipment—an arduous procedure.

This type of individualism is favored by the difficulty of surviving in the frigid zone with the aid of only a very primitive cultural heritage. Simple individual adjustment rather than cooperative group activity is the first adaptation to such a situation. For example, even when a number of families live together in one house during the winter season, each woman cooks the food for her family in her own pot over her own lamp. Communal cooking is impractical, because it would take too long to heat the food for the group over blubber lamps and because it would be difficult to transport from summer to winter quarters a pot large enough for the group.

Adaptation to environmental demands is, however, not the only important determiner of the personality pattern of a culture. Other factors may enter in. In New Guinea, not far from the peaceful and unaggressive Arapesh, live the Mundagumor, a tribe whose typical personality is quite different. They are described as arrogant, impatient, suspicious and extremely quarrelsome. These characteristics do not seem to arise from economic hardships, as they live in a fertile lowland. One hypothesis that accounts for the difference between these two peoples arises from observations of their treatment of children. The Arapesh nurse their infants frequently and affectionately, wean them late and offer few frustrations to their young children. The Mundagumor, on the contrary, nurse their children briefly, slap them when they cry and even let some infants die from neglect. It is not hard to see that the former type of treatment would lead to a secure and peaceful personality, and the latter to insecurity and aggressiveness.

Studies of a number of other primitive cultures have shown a similar trend toward a marked relationship between the treatment of children and the resulting typical personality. The interesting further question as to *why* these tribes differ in their attitudes toward children has not yet been answered.

DEVELOPMENT OF PERSONALITY

The development of personality does not mean the automatic unfolding of intrinsic characteristics. It refers to a continuous process of learning through which individuals acquire their typical modes of response. Aside from the biological factors that have been described, the major determiners of personality seem to be the individual's adjustments—the ways in which he has learned to cope with his conflicts and frustrations. Unfortunately for our knowledge, there are relatively few satisfactory experiments on personality development. It has not been possible to subject children to experimental procedures to determine what experiences make a person sociable, or hostile, or outgoing, or shy, and, indeed, it would probably be highly undesirable to carry out such researches. Most of our hypotheses come from case studies of persons with strikingly deviant personalities. The background factors, the presumed causes of the personality traits, often have to be determined in retrospect. They are therefore subject to many errors of observation, and usually are not susceptible to quantitative treatment. For these reasons, the study of personality development is one of the least certain areas of psychological knowledge, although it is one of the most important.

If personality traits arise from the ways in which persons solve their conflicts, it will be important to examine the conflict situations to which adjustments must be made. Some conflicts occur in the lives of all persons in our culture, and therefore are the common background of personality. These conflicts arise from situations that occur at all periods of life, in infancy, childhood, adolescence and maturity. They include the experiences of weaning, group socialization, breaking away from parents, becoming economically sufficient and marriage. How an individual adjusts to these critical situations in part determines his personality. In addition to the adjustive conflicts that are common to all people, there are many less universal adjustive situations that influence individual personalities, such as rejection by parents, being less favored than his brothers and sisters, social isolation and physical disabilities. Adjustments to such difficulties also leave their residua in personality traits.

Infancy

The importance of early infancy in the development of personality has been recognized for about forty years. It is believed that the primary psychological need of the infant is for affection and security, which are provided by mothering and nursing. Nursing is interrupted by weaning, which is often regarded as the first critical frustration in every person's life.

An experiment with puppies has shown that they too have a need for suckling beyond the requirements of nutrition. Those puppies whose need for suckling was frustrated tended to suck other objects between meals and to show evidences of emotional upset. Evidence from case studies tends to show that this need is also felt by human infants. A study of rats has demonstrated that feeding frustration in infancy may have an enduring effect on the behavior of adults of the species. The rats which were frustrated early in life by being deprived of food, hoarded food to a much greater degree, when again kept hungry as adults, than those rats which had not experienced the infantile food deprivation.

We have already noted that differences in the care of young children in different cultures may cause variations in adult personality. The same hypothesis has been advanced to account for differences between individuals in our own culture.

A group of college students were tested with a questionnaire designed to measure *security-insecurity,* and they also obtained from their mothers information about the age at which they were weaned. A very striking relationship was found. Those who were weaned rather early (at six to nine months) had an average security score significantly lower than those who were breast-fed nine months or more. It was found, however, that those not nursed at all or who were weaned at a very early age (at three to six months) did not suffer from insecurity. This result was interpreted in terms of the other observation that, in the cultural group of first-generation Americans from which these students were drawn, the failure to nurse the child at all or its extremely early weaning arises from the inability of the mother to nurse and not from her unwillingness to do so. The study suggests that early weaning is perhaps not the basic causal factor, but that it is a symptom of the mother's unwillingness to be bothered with the child, which also manifests itself in many other ways that affect the infant's adjustments.

Although the evidence is incomplete, it favors the view that the character of the parent-child relationship in infancy is of permanent significance in the formation of personality. Children who have acquired feelings of insecurity or anxiety during this period have to adjust to conflict, and they may do so by developing traits that range from the depressed and withdrawing to the compensatingly hostile and aggressive, according to the other circumstances that shape the trials, errors and successes of adjustive effort.

Nursing and weaning have been described at length as one area of infant adjustment. There are many others, including later feeding problems, toilet training, displacement by a new baby in the family and the beginnings of social contacts with other children.

Childhood

Entering school at five or six years of age is another critical point in the life of a child, as he is then confronted with a new world of strange children and strange adults. He has to relinquish the specially privileged and protected position that he enjoyed at home and to learn the meanings of equality and fairness. The extent to which he is prepared to meet this conflict depends on the somewhat opposed factors of his personal security as established by earlier experiences and his readiness to assume independence. The protective mother that seems to be good for infancy is not necessarily beneficial at this time. She, too, has an adjustment to make to the child's increasing range of individual action.

A little later, approximately at seven to twelve years of age, the youngster encounters a new social situation in the demands of his own group. Whether the boy becomes a member of a 'gang' or only associates with his school friends, in most cases he does enter a group of his own age that has its own standards. To win approbation in this group, he must show his independence of adult control. The youngster who fails to make this adjustment may be ridiculed as a 'sissy' or may be excluded or avoided. Inability to adjust to a social group in later childhood may arise from a number of causes. A youngster may not have solved the problems of earlier development constructively, or, conversely, he may be so thoroughly satisfied with his dependent infantile adjustments that he is unable to relinquish them. The latter difficulty almost always arises when the parents have overprotected their child, a relationship which makes dependence satisfying to the child because it is satisfying to the parent.

Because the first important social adjustments are made in the childhood period, the individual most often forms his pattern of social traits at this time. On the positive side, he learns leadership, friendliness, sympathy and social adaptability or carries them over from earlier experience. It is now that compensating factors in one phase may overcome handicaps that originated in earlier development. Children who are insecure in their relationships with their parents may find satisfactions for their needs in their associations with contemporaries. Thus each developmental period presents corrective opportunities in the development of personality, as well as new hurdles to be overcome.

Frustration or conflict in the social relations of childhood is a frequent cause of a feeling of inferiority or inadequacy. It may arise directly from the social evaluation of the youngster by his fellows, and indirectly from his shortcomings in physique, skill, cooperation or other traits that his fellows assess. In the initial adjustments to a sense of inadequacy, a boy or a girl may seem to show inconsistent traits of personality, being shy and full of worry at one time and overaggressive or excessively eager at other times. These superficial inconsistencies are understandable in terms of an underlying real consistency, the need to adjust to the demands of the group. If the young person's withdrawing reactions are more rewarded, he will learn them. In other instances he will become assertive, or hostile, or independent because external circumstances combine to make these attitudes more satisfying to him. The fixed social adjustments of many adults, often not very appropriate to their mature abilities and opportunities, may frequently be traced to such childhood origins.

Adolescence

Adolescence has been defined in two ways, as a physiological event dependent on the maturing of the sex functions and as a social period bridging the interval from childhood to maturity. There is some evidence that physiological adolescence has some effect on personality traits but that this is less extensive than popular opinion believes. Sex interests, although by no means absent in infancy and childhood, become more intense and more specific after puberty. Several studies have shown that boys and girls after puberty have greater social maturity than those of the same age who have not yet reached puberty. The interpretation of this finding is not altogether clear. It may be due to physiological factors, or it may only reflect the individual's conception of himself as a more mature person according to his own social norms, since the fact of his or her own puberty is not unknown to the youngster.

The social problems of adolescent adjustment vary greatly from one culture to another. Adolescence hardly exists in a society such as that of Samoa, in which children do not form strongly dependent attachments to their parents, sex behavior is relatively uninhibited, and self-support is possible at an early age in a primitive economic structure. The Samoan boy or girl slips from childhood into maturity with little or no transition, and certainly without revolt, conflict or 'storm and stress.'

The main social problems of adolescent adjustment in our culture have been defined as emancipation from psychological dependence on parents, sex adjustment, self-support, including the choice of a vocation, and the development of an adult philosophy of life. If adolescence is a difficult period, it is so because of the conflicts involved in the solution of these adjustments, not because of any inherent quality of adolescent youngsters themselves. Parents often add to the complexity of the adjustments by refusing to recognize that the child is growing to maturity. The adolescent is often still a child, in the eyes of his father and mother, and is treated accordingly. The result may be either a thoroughgoing rebellion or an acquiescence that makes for arrested personality development.

The neglect of sex training in our culture makes adolescence often a critical period of development, for both boys and girls are rarely prepared for the physical and psychological changes in sex functions that occur at and after puberty. They learn the meaning of these changes through their own groups, often with more misinformation than truth, rather than from their parents or through constructively planned education. Consequently they regard their inevitable sex interests and feelings as private and guilty, finding themselves in conflict because their past training is not integrated with their present concepts of social values. Since most adolescents feel that they cannot discuss sex problems with their parents or with other experienced adults, conflicts of this sort are likely to remain unresolved, causing much needless anxiety and other disturbances of personality.

The impact of the economic realities of life hits most persons in late adolescence, when they face the choice of a career and the necessity for self-support. Getting a job, and thereby becoming an economically independent person, is a highly critical stage of development. Because of the standards of education and experience that are required for superior positions, many young people find a serious gap between their aspirations and what they can realize. Their inability to earn a living, or to hold a position that is felt to be significant and creative, often creates in them attitudes of inadequacy and inferiority. Many of the irresponsible and aggressive personality characteristics of youth are compensatory responses to the frustrations of economic adjustments.

There is a popular belief that a sweeping reorganization of personality occurs in adolescence and that the individual becomes a 'new person' at that time. This belief is unfounded. There is a continuity of personal development from infancy through childhood and adolescence to maturity, and the foundations of any one period may be found in the preceding ones. At the same time, it is true that undesirable personality traits, brought along from childhood, are sometimes modified by adolescent adjustments. For example, a youngster who could not gain childhood recognition because of physical weakness may readjust as an adolescent by success in scholarship, in debating or in other activities that are more valued by adolescents than by children. Adolescence has no magic qualities, but personality changes can occur then as at any period, according to the experiences and learnings of the individual.

Personality in Maturity

Recently psychologists have paid increasing attention to the problems of maturity and old age, formerly a neglected period. The new interest is due to a recognition that mature people do most of the work of the world and that the elderly, who are becoming an increasing proportion of the population, present special problems of adjustment.

Several questionnaire studies of adults over a wide age range confirm the conclusion that early maturity and old age are periods of stress, with a long interval of relatively stable adjustment in between. This finding agrees with an analysis of the causal factors. In the early adult years, usually in the twenties, the typical individual completes his adolescent adjustments by finding his permanent life work, marrying and becoming a parent. These three major adjustments inevitably demand some modifications of personality traits. The following thirty years—the thirties, forties and fifties—are the most stable period of life, with little incentive or need for change. With this stability usually come gradually the personality trends toward greater conservatism, tolerance and breadth of social outlook. There are individual exceptions, to be sure, which can be understood by a psychological study of the persons who show them.

The personality changes of older people are in a very large degree due to the adjustment problems of senescence. The elderly begin to have anxieties about their health, their earning power and their social acceptability in a world dominated by those who are younger. The mother whose children are grown finds her vocation gone and may begin to doubt her real usefulness. Unless she achieves more successful adjustments, she may acquire such compensatory interests as meddlesome or suspicious interference with the lives of others. The older man who is unable to work may find himself returned to a dependence unpleasantly reminiscent of his adolescence. Those fortunate enough to retire with a living income often do not have enough to do, unless they have maintained strong avocational interests through their adult years. In response to the needs of the increasing number of elderly persons, social and educational programs are being developed in many centers to assist their adjustments. (See also pp. 83–87 for changes with age.)

The drama of personality has the same broad pattern from the nursing infant to the lonely senile person. It consists of making adjustments to needs, frustrations and conflicts, which give rise to learning processes by which the individual acquires the characteristics of his personality.

REFERENCES

1. Allport, G. W. *Personality, a psychological interpretation.* New York: Holt, 1937.

   A comprehensive treatise on personality that takes up the definition of personality, its development, structure and measurement.

2. Cattell, R. B. *Description and measurement of personality.* Yonkers-on-Hudson, N. Y.: World Book Co., 1946.

   A report of a research study, leading to a factor analysis of personality traits.

3. Dennis, W. The adolescent. In L. Carmichael (Ed.), *Manual of child psychology.* New York: Wiley, 1946. Chap. 12.

   A review of research up to 1940 on adolescence, which is defined in terms of its biological meaning.

4. Greene, E. B. *Measurements of human behavior.* New York: Odyssey Press, 1941.

An excellent survey of all types of psychological and educational measurement, including measures of abilities, personality and educational achievement.

5. Hunt, J. McV. (Ed.). *Personality and the behavior disorders.* 2 vols. New York: Ronald Press, 1944.

These two volumes, the work of forty collaborators from psychology, medicine, anthropology and other fields, give the most comprehensive survey of personality and its abnormalities.

6. Lawton, G. *New goals for old age.* New York: Columbia University Press, 1943.

A popular presentation of the adjustment problems of older persons.

7. Mead, M. *Cooperation and competition among primitive peoples.* New York: McGraw-Hill, 1937.

An anthropological study that illustrates the dependence of personality upon culture.

8. Mead, M. Research on primitive children. In L. Carmichael (Ed.), *Manual of child psychology.* New York: Wiley, 1946. Chap. 13.

A summary of anthropological research methods that contribute to an understanding of human personality.

9. Murphy, G., and Jensen, F. *Approaches to personality.* New York: Coward-McCann, 1933.

One of the clearest presentations of various theories of personality—the behaviorist, Gestalt, psychoanalytic and genetic theories.

10. Murphy, G., Murphy, L. B., and Newcomb, T. M. *Experimental social psychology.* New York: Harper, 1937.

Contains important material on motivation, personality and development.

11. Murray, H. A. *Explorations in personality.* New York: Oxford University Press, 1938.

A classic, intensive, research study of the personalities of a group of normal men. The Thematic Apperception Test is described in this volume.

12. Rorschach, H. *Psychodiagnostics.* Berne, Switzerland: Hans Huber, 1942.

The description of the use of the Rorschach ink-blot test.

13. Stagner, R. *Psychology of personality.* New York: McGraw-Hill, 1937.

An excellent textbook, recommended as the first reference for students interested in further study of personality.

14. Tomkins, S. S. *The thematic apperception test.* New York: Grune and Stratton, 1947.

The manual on the theory and technique of the interpretation of this test.

CHAPTER 22

Personal Adjustment

THROUGHOUT their lives all living organisms, from amoeba to man, meet situations in which they are unable to satisfy their motives promptly or completely. A hungry wild animal may not find food in the accustomed places. A college student, hampered by the competitive activities of other persons and by his own limitations, may not be able to achieve as much prestige, approval or success as he feels he needs. All these situations call for adjustment, that is to say, for persistent activities directed toward the realization of goals in the face of difficulties.

It is fortunate that the frustration of needs is most often followed by successful adjustment. There is special psychological interest, however, in instances in which a person is unable to reach his original goal. In such cases, since the needs persist, individuals do not usually give up their motives entirely, but instead tend to make inferior or substitute adjustments. If even these substitute goals prove unattainable, the person may remain in a tense and unadjusted state, showing anxiety and other varieties of behavior that are commonly known as *psychoneurotic* or 'nervous.'

The psychological study of *personal adjustments* is an examination of the processes by which people cope with their needs, limitations and thwartings. It tries to throw light on the conditions which lead to solutions of superior or inferior quality. No other topic in psychology contributes more directly to an individual's understanding of his own life problems.

THE ADJUSTMENT PROCESS

Adjustment is the process by which a living organism maintains a balance between its needs and the circumstances that influence the satisfaction of these needs. Many of the simpler and more common adjustments can be described by the pattern shown in Fig. 233. An individual is proceeding in a course of action (1) that tends toward some end result (4), representing the satisfaction of a need. An obstacle blocks or thwarts the activity, leading (2) to varied and usually intensified behavior. At length, some response (3) circumvents the obstacle and readjustment is accomplished. This analysis indicates that the essential aspects of the adjustment process are the existence of a *motive,* circumstances leading to its *thwarting,* resulting in *varied responses,* which may eventually lead to the discovery of a *solution.* You will notice that this process is basically similar to the one which describes adjustment as learn-

This chapter was prepared by Laurance F. Shaffer of Teachers College, Columbia University.

ing and as thinking, both of which are special means for accomplishing personal adjustment.

The adjustment process is a universal sequence that can be identified in the behavior of organisms from the lowest species up to man. If a paramecium, a single-celled animal, meets an obstruction while swimming, it will back up, turn through a small angle and swim forward again. If

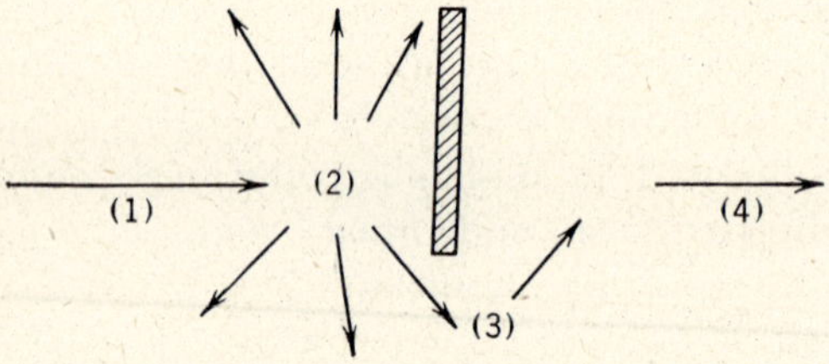

FIGURE 233. SEQUENCE OF ADJUSTMENT

The individual is proceeding (1) in the direction of the goal (4), when he is blocked by an obstacle. He makes varied responses (2), until he discovers some response (3) that gets around the obstacle. [From J. F. Dashiell, *Fundamentals of general psychology*, Houghton Mifflin, 1937.]

the change of angle is enough to avoid the obstacle, its problem is solved. If the angle is not enough, the paramecium goes through the act again. If it is constrained by being confined in a little bit of water in a fine capillary tube, whose diameter is hardly more than the length of the paramecium, it will try to turn again and again when it gets to the end of the water in the tube, and will finally succeed by making one great 'superparamecium' effort, turning half way around in a single try. The same process is illustrated by many experiments in animal learning. A hungry rat placed in a maze is stirred to varied activity until its frustration is overcome by finding the food. We do not have to look to the behavior of lower animals for illustrations, however. Human responses to the lost collar button, the stalled automobile or the failed examination are examples of normal adjustment processes.

Motives in Adjustment

In its broadest sense adjustment may be evoked by any motives whatsoever. Vital physiological needs for air, water, food, warmth and the like, when thwarted, arouse repeated adjustive behavior, but they are not of wide psychological interest for two reasons. First, they are reasonably well satisfied under the usual conditions of civilized culture. Second, the thwarting of the most vital needs may lead, not to substitute adjustments, but to death. There can be no continued satisfactory adjustment to lack of air, water or food, except breathing, drinking or eating.

Of greater significance in human adjustments are the social motives that are learned from the culture in which an individual develops, or at least are greatly modified by it. In our culture the needs for affection, security, approval, recognition, mastery, prestige and self-realization are among the strongest social motives. This group also includes the sex motives which, although fundamentally biological, are strongly influenced by cultural learning.

All strong motives are persistent. Once aroused, they continue to operate until reduced by some adjustive act. In this respect they resemble an appetitive desire like hunger, which persists until the drive stimulus has been removed by the ingestion of food. The principal physiological mechanism of social motives seems to be *tension*. (On tension in relation to needs, see p. 114.) When confronted by a motivating circumstance, as for example a competitive situation that calls forth a need for mastery, a person becomes alert, ready to react and selective in making responses that are pertinent to his motivation. His set is evidenced by a persistent muscular and visceral tension that continues until adjustment has been accomplished. Developmentally, the tensions of strong motivation are related to the physiological changes that occur in emotional states.

Thwarting

The second aspect of an adjustment process is the thwarting or nonfulfillment of an aroused motive. Thwarting may occur in a number of ways. A simple and common type of thwarting is the blocking of an adjustment by a material obstacle or by the opposition of other people. This is often called *frustration.* If a man is late for an important engagement because his alarm clock fails to operate, or because his train is not on time, he usually regards his frustration as environmental and external to his own character. Many man-made thwartings, due to laws, customs and competitive activities, are also viewed objectively. The usual response to frustration is an intensification of activity and effort. If the frustrator is a person, an aggressive attack against him is a common reaction, and this attitude is often shown against inanimate things also, as when a man kicks a stool over which he has tripped. Uncomplicated frustration evokes vigorous behavior but, as will be shown later, is not likely to result in serious personal maladjustment.

A second general type of thwarting is *conflict.* A conflict situation evokes two or more motives, the satisfactions of which are incompatible. For example, it is normal for a boy to be motivated to engage in rough-and-tumble play with his contemporaries, for this is one of the most approved ways of satisfying his needs for mastery, prestige and recognition. If a certain youngster has developed a fear of being hurt, he has conflicting motives when confronted with a group of playing boys. He simultaneously wants something, and fears the outcome of his want. That is the essence of conflict. An individual cannot fight against his conflicts directly, as he can against his simple frustrations. For that reason conflicts underlie most instances of futile and maladapted behavior.

There is a relationship between frustration and conflict. The usual first response to frustration is an aggressive attack on the person or thing that caused it. In a child, this aggression may be very direct and obvious, and usually meets with punishment or disapproval. After the connection between aggression and punishment has been learned, the overtly aggressive behavior may be inhibited and replaced by a fearful and insecure attitude. In his subsequent life, this person may respond to frustration not with aggression only, but also by a conflict between his impulses for aggression and his fear of retaliation. Simple obstructions may be sufficient stimuli under such circumstances for arousing strong conflicts in some individuals.

Adjustment by Trial and Error

The presence of thwarting implies that an individual's first or habitual response to a need is unsuccessful. The subsequent course of his activity is, therefore, to try another response, and then another, until some action is discovered that leads to adjustment (see Fig. 233). The early responses to thwartings are varied activities. The ones which are relatively more satisfying, the adjusting person retains. The less successful ones he discards as 'errors.'

If a boy is unable to compete with his fellows because he fears his own weakness or lack of skill, he is likely to exhibit a number of other adjustive attempts. He may bully younger children, daydream of imaginary accomplishments, develop skill in an unusual hobby or avoid his friends and sulk in his room. Superficially regarded, these actions seem to be inconsistent; the boy is a dreamer one moment and a bully the next. Psychologically they are not at all inconsistent, for they have a common meaning to the boy who is making the adjustments. They are varied trials that attempt to meet his needs by substitute or evasive behavior when the more usual forms of satisfaction are blocked.

As in all learning processes, the relatively more satisfying adjustments tend to be retained and used again, whereas the less successful ones tend to be extinguished. In later stages of adjustment to thwarting, the range of activities becomes narrower, and the thwarted person specializes in the kind of adjustment that he is most able to make. In this way the changeable adjustments of childhood crystallize into the less flexible traits of adults. Thus one man may be aggressive in most of his adjustment-demanding situations, another may be unduly suspicious, and a third habitually seclusive.

Adjustive Solutions

The concept of what constitutes 'success' or 'satisfaction' in the solution of an adjustment needs to be defined more specifically, since it is obvious that many cherished individual adjustments are not successful in the social sense. Psychologically an adjustive solution is an act that completes or reduces the motivation that started the sequence. When a need is unfulfilled, muscular or visceral tension keeps an individual stirred up and active, so that he makes one adjustive attempt after another. When this tension is reduced, the source of this self-stimulation has been eliminated. The criterion of an adjustive solution is, therefore, *tension reduction*. This is true whether the solution is socially 'good' or not. It is an adjustment if it satisfies a person's feeling of need. One of the most significant generalizations of psychology is that *all* behavior is satisfying to some motive of the individual, and that this rule holds even when the resulting actions are illogical, queer or socially unacceptable. That is another way of saying that all action is motivated and purposive. The general principle is a key to understanding a large part of human behavior.

RESPONSES TO THWARTING

To have one's motives thwarted is by no means an uncompensated evil. If human beings had no needs, or if all needs were easily satisfied, civilization might be reduced to an effortless Nirvana in which there might be neither maladjustments nor accomplishment. It is an accepted part of our cultural pattern for persons to be thwarted and to make adjustments that result in achievement.

Constructive Adjustments

Since constructive adjustments are assumed to be commonplace, no psychological techniques have been developed for assessing them in detail. Examples can be found in everyday life. College courses, for example, often present difficulties to individual students that thwart both their educational and vocational aims, as well as some of their basic social needs like the needs for prestige, approval and self-realization. Threatened with possible failure in college, most students adjust constructively by discovering the causes of the difficulty, by expending more time and effort on work, by getting help or, if the troubles are insurmountable, by changing their plans and accepting more attainable goals.

The normal thwartings of business executives and of research scientists, and of all of us in our social relationships, are most often met by similar procedures. The reasons why one person will make a constructive adjustment, whereas another person in the same situation will made an inadequate adjustment, are very intricate. This chapter seeks to clarify some of them. Two preliminary observations can be made now: (1) Mere frustration more often results in better adjustments than conflict; (2) a strong emotional reaction to difficulties is detrimental to good adjustment.

Substitute Adjustments

Constructive adjustments are not the only means for reducing individual tensions. The student who is faced with failure in his college work may adjust by making excuses that put the blame on his teachers or on irremediable causes, by giving an exaggerated emphasis to his accomplishments in athletics or other activities, by daydreaming about imagined success or by a host of other actions. He may even become ill as a way to explain his failure respectably and thus escape censure.

One may wonder why these events are considered to be adjustments at all, since they do not overcome the real difficulty at hand. The answer lies in an understanding of the motivation of the student. When he is in danger of failing, not only are his vocational and educational plans endangered, but, more importantly, his strongest social motives are thwarted. His adjustive attempts are not directed to the present situation, but they are means for coping with the tensions of his basic motives. The actions are therefore *substitute adjustments* to the dominant needs. They give indirect or partial satisfaction to strong motives, and hence tend to reduce tension and anxiety.

The chief shortcoming of substitute adjustments, however, is not their failure to remedy immediate and practical difficulties. Since a substitute adjustment usually is driven by an intense urge to satisfy one particularly strong need, it may end by thwarting other equally important motives. For example, showing off and excuse making may be satisfying to a person's drives for mastery and prestige, but these very forms of behavior invite scorn and criticism from others, and make it more difficult for him to satisfy another need, his need for social approval. Withdrawing from the company of other people may help a man to adjust to a fear of competition, but it thwarts his needs for companionship and security.

Another defect of substitute adjustments is that they are usually antagonistic to the well-being of other people. If a boy gains adjustive satisfaction by being a bully, or if a young woman asserts her feminine charms by stealing the men friends of her acquaintances, such adjustments create risks of retaliation, of isolation and of the loss of social cooperation.

While it is not possible to classify all adjustments as 'good' or 'bad,' there is undoubtedly a continuum from the most to the least effective ones. In general, the better adjustments satisfy an individual's motives as an integrated system, without the undue slighting of some needs at the expense of others. Good adjustments also facilitate the life processes of other persons, so that mutually helpful social relationships are encouraged.

Consciousness in Adjustment

It must not be thought that people adopt inferior forms of adjustment deliberately and maliciously. It is a universal finding that very few people, even quite normal persons, have a clear insight into their strong motives and typical adjustments. Persons who are making poor adjustments usually have less than average insight into their own behavior. An adjustive act is impulsive, and results in the reduction of tension. The individual feels vaguely relieved after an aggressive or evasive act, but he does not often understand why. Since learning can take place without full insight, the adjustive response is likely to be made again and to become habitual, still without a real understanding of its significance in the person's life.

The fact that people do many things without understanding why they do them is the basis of the psychological concept of *unconscious* processes. This is one of the great discoveries of modern psychology, but it is often misunderstood. It does not mean that there is a place or organ called *the unconscious* to which rejected motives and shameful adjustments are somehow relegated. In an earlier period of psychology, *the intellect* and *the will* were much discussed, as well as *the unconscious.* We now know that all these terms represent dynamic or functional concepts. They are descriptions of how people act, not of organs or faculties that people 'have.' *Intellect* is shown only by intelligent behavior, and *will* by voluntary behavior (p. 50). *Unconscious* has no different significance; its 'existence' is shown only by the fact that people do not know or understand their most basic motives or most habitual adjustments. (On the unconscious, see also p. 5.)

Unconscious aspects of individual behavior arise from two sources that are distinguishable, although closely related. (1) Much that is unconscious comes through learning processes that begin so early and are so gradual that they are never raised to perceptual clearness. Very small children learn to act so as to be approved, to fear scorn and criticism, and to seek prestige through mastering others. These derived needs continue to be strong motives even in adult life, but few people are clearly aware of the important part they play in determining behavior. (2) Another source of unconscious functioning is the adjustive forgetting of some motives and adjustments. This type of forgetting, called *repression,* will be described more fully later. One way of adjusting to a pain-producing memory is to forget about it. You can, if remembering the unpleasant item is very painful. Nevertheless, the experience may continue to influence your subsequent behavior, even though you cannot recall it consciously.

TYPICAL ADJUSTMENT MECHANISMS

To enumerate all the habits that even a single person uses adjustively would be an impossible task, because the number of such responses is so great. To a degree, it is adjustive to read the newspaper, to see a motion picture, to smoke a cigarette or to take a brisk walk around the block.

A few adjustive habits, however, are so widely and frequently used that they have been named and defined. These are known as *adjustment mechanisms,* or sometimes as *dynamisms,* a term that emphasizes the active or functional nature of such adjustments. Although the details of behavior differ considerably from one person to another, the named mechanisms provide useful conceptual points of reference for describing conduct. Thus, to designate a type of response as *compensation* or *rationalization* or the like, saves the necessity of a longer description of its nature and function.

The common adjustment mechanisms are found in the behavior of all people. They are used by the most normal of people. No one need be alarmed when he finds that the mechanisms are descriptive of his own conduct. At the same time, these same mechanisms are also the basis of some of the most bizarre symptoms of the serious mental disorders, in which they occur in exaggerated form. All people have a tendency to blame their shortcomings on others; that is normal. It is an extreme when persons with delusions believe that their families or associates are conspiring against them. A knowledge of these commoner adjustment mechanisms is essential to an understanding of both normal and abnormal behavior.

Compensation

In a culture such as ours that places a great premium on competitive achievement, adjustment mechanisms are needed to cope with feelings of failure and inferiority. Several mechanisms that serve this purpose are often grouped together as *defense mechanisms,* since they tend to defend an individual against a recognition of his inadequacies. *Compensation,* the most common of the defense mechanisms, consists of an excessive display of a characteristic, or an overemphasis of it, so as to balance or conceal a deficiency.

Since the concept of compensation is very broad, it covers a great variety of specific forms of behavior. The most obvious forms of compensation are found in childhood. Because of their lack of size and strength, their great dependence on others and their constant frustration by adults, children have especially strong needs for compensatory adjustment. Normally they achieve this end by aggressive play and noisy roughhouse, and by the inevitable teasing, taunting and quarreling that children do among themselves. Under some circumstances children are prevented or inhibited from using these normal outlets. A boy who has a very great need for expressing his adequacy, or who is afraid to assert himself in the common ways, may bully younger children, steal, destroy property and show other marked compensations. These maladjustments differ from normal compensatory behavior only in degree.

Adults also have their normal compensations that help them relieve the humdrum of ordinary existence. They include hobbies, sports, secret societies, card playing, gossip and scores of other activities that balance frustrations. Unfortunate compensations can be observed in persons who tyrannize over their business subordinates, or over their families, usually because they feel basically insecure of their own competence. Parents often seek compensation through the accomplishments of their children, pushing the youngsters at times toward achievements that are beyond their abilities or into occupations for which they are unfitted.

As in other substitute adjustments, the individual who compensates excessively satisfies a limited part of his motivation at the expense of thwarting his other needs, and sometimes at the risk of retaliation. His total tension is therefore not reduced fully, and his unacceptable behavior is likely to continue as a vicious circle, unless relieved by a favorable change of circumstances or by psychological counseling.

At one time defensive behavior was regarded as an adjustment to personal inferiority, and an individual who showed it was said to have an *inferiority complex*. More recent interpretations of the evidence show that this generalization is faulty. Inferior strength, skill, beauty or intelligence do not in themselves evoke defensive behavior. In fact many inferior persons show no compensations, whereas many really adequate individuals do. The important factor is the individual's conception of his own characteristics, which he learns from the evaluations made by his social group. A child of average intelligence whose brothers or sisters are brilliant may be so much criticized, because he fails to reach their level of achievement, that he accepts the conception of himself as an inferior. He may then develop a fear of competition and resort to defensive behavior in order to maintain some degree of satisfaction of his motives.

Rationalization

Persons may defend themselves by words or thoughts as well as by actions. *Rationalization* is a defense mechanism in which persons justify their behavior by giving socially acceptable reasons for it, with the effect of concealing motives and impulses that they have learned to regard as inferior or shameful. The rationalizer seldom understands the 'real' reasons underlying his conduct or else, sensing them vaguely, rejects them as unworthy. These rejected motives include the basic ones for mastery and prestige and the aggressive impulses directed against frustrating circumstances and persons. To deceive himself with a sense of virtue and to evade the recognition of his own antisocial tendencies, the rationalizer invents 'good' reasons to explain his conduct. They are his rationalizations.

A boy who is late for school finds many excuses. Perhaps the clock was slow, or breakfast late. These are the simple rationalizations of blaming impersonal or incidental factors for which the individual cannot be held responsible. Or perhaps the boy rationalizes his tardiness as due to has having taken time to do chores at home; thus he both places the blame on his parents and shows himself as a willing but unappreciated worker. His real reasons may be a fear of failure or scorn at school, or a need to show his hostility toward his parents who are pressing him to greater academic effort. These motives he recognizes vaguely or not at all. They are 'unconscious.'

Adults also rationalize. Indeed, almost all human beings make use of this mechanism every day in the year. The unpleasant task is not completed because more urgent matters have to be pursued. A job is done poorly because the right tools were not available. A promotion is not received because the employer is biased. The game is lost because the opponent has all the 'luck.'

Because of its common use, ordinary rationalization cannot be regarded as a serious maladjustment, but it assumes exaggerated proportions in some instances. If, through his past experiences, an individual has acquired a very strong need for success and an excessive fear of failure, his rationalizations can approach the intensity of delusions of persecution. A woman student once attempted a difficult subject while she was emotionally disturbed by other matters. She failed to meet the requirements of the course. Unable to acknowledge her failure or its causes, she placed the blame on the professor. She asserted that he was unfair, that he had singled her out for persecution, that he took a perverse delight in making a student miserable. This woman was able to cite many incidents that pointed to the professor's persecution of her. In the end she managed to transfer to another college, 'because' she could not be associated with an institution that had such a perverted character on its faculty. The severity of this student's adjustment problem is easily recognized. It accounts for the intensity of her rationalization.

Identification

Adjustive satisfaction can be gained through the accomplishments of other persons and of social groups. In using this mechanism, an individual is said to *identify* himself with the person or institution through which he fulfills his needs. A simple and almost universal type of identification is seen in the relationship of a child to his parents. Because of his own helplessness and the apparent omnipotence of a parent, the child adopts the parent's achievements as his own. Youngsters often show this by imitation. The boy's play follows his father's hobby or profession; the girl dresses up in adult clothes and mimics her mother's household or social activities. Less obviously, the child takes pride in the parents' status or strength, and adjusts to his own frustrations by accepting their superior attainments as in part his own. Since identification motivates the youngster in learning the manners, attitudes and interests of his parents and of his social group, it is a major factor in personality development.

Other identifications develop outside the family group, and act as adjustments to individual social thwartings. By hero worship, children, adolescents and not a few adults identify themselves with popular public figures, imitate their characteristics and vicariously enjoy their accomplishments. Identification with clubs, schools, cities, athletic teams and many other cultural units may result in as great a feeling of satisfaction in their victories as if the achievement were a personal one. On the whole, the mechanism of identification is constructive, with many values and few harmful effects. Harm comes when the parent, identifying himself with the child, puts pressure on the child to achieve what is impossible for him.

Seclusiveness

Compensation and rationalization are relatively aggressive and externally oriented types of substitute adjustment. Another means that a person may employ to cope with his difficulties is to run away from them. There are several varieties of these *escape mechanisms,* of which simple *seclusiveness* is the most basic. Withdrawing, timid or seclusive behavior is very direct evidence of a fearful response to social situations. In addition, withdrawing has a substitute adjustive value, since the withdrawer avoids failure by not attempting to place himself in competition with others. Seclusiveness is an incomplete adjustment, however, as it provides no satisfaction for the person's continuing social needs. Unless accompanied by other mechanisms, it usually results in attitudes of self-condemnation and anxiety.

Although everyone shows the seclusive adjustment to some extent, especially when in a new environment in which normal adjustive satisfactions have not been established, its continued or excessive use is unfortunate. Withdrawing is less often detected as a sign of adjustive need than the aggressive defenses, for the seclusive person is not troublesome. Indeed, some parents and teachers may encourage escape mechanisms in children, mistaking them for quiet and orderly adjustments. An habitually seclusive person is difficult to readjust, because he has not acquired the minor skills in dealing with people that most persons use in their social contacts. It is harder to break up a seclusive adjustment than an aggressive one.

Fantasy

Daydreaming, or fantasy, is both an escape and a compensatory mechanism. Released from the bounds of reality, a person can imagine any of the satisfactions that he does not attain more directly, including vocational success, money and possessions, sex satisfactions, intellectual brilliance, physical strength and beauty and all the other goals toward which he strives. Everyone daydreams. In one survey of college students, all reported that they had done so at one time or another, and ninety-eight per cent admitted fantasies during the preceding month. It is evident that this is a universal source of adjustive satisfaction.

A frequent type of daydream is the *conquering hero* pattern, in which the fantasy is of accomplishment, prestige or conquest. The *martyr* daydream, an expression of self-pity in which the dreamer pictures himself injured, is really satisfying even if superficially unpleasant, for it is an adjustment to a lack of appreciation from others.

The principal fault of daydreaming is the amount of time that it consumes. A student with a habit of daydreaming may take to compensatory revery whenever he meets a difficulty, and thereby take twice as long as necessary to complete his work. Fantasy occurs frequently in persons with markedly seclusive adjustments and is their principal means of tension reduction. In some of the serious mental disorders, fanciful delusions are found which correspond in content and function to the daydreams of normal persons. Obviously, fantasy is not the cause of these severe maladjustments, but only an incidental symptom.

Because of its common occurrence, daydreaming cannot be considered as a pathological condition, and no one should worry about the fact that he daydreams. Indeed, fantasy is only narrowly separated from imaginative planning. It has positive values in invention, literature and art.

Repression

Thoughts and impulses that are in conflict with the social values of an individual are unpleasant and troublesome. Satisfying these rejected motives, or even thinking about them, results in unpleasant feelings of guilt and anxiety. Consequently, an individual may adjust by inhibiting his responses to these needs and by keeping himself from even remembering their existence. This substitute adjustment is known as *repression*. The repression of response to certain motives does not remove the motives, however. Repression merely keeps them from being recognized and satisfied. They may still continue as tensions which are either partially reduced by other substitute mechanisms or remain to serve as a basis for vague anxiety.

Repression, like the other mechanisms, is found in the behavior of quite normal people as well as of the seriously maladjusted. As Freud pointed out long ago in his *Psychopathology of Everyday Life,* all persons have lapses of memory, make slips of the tongue or pen or have strange blind spots in their understanding of their environments that point to the existence of repression. A man wished to invite a couple to dinner. He greatly admired the wife. His note to the husband read: "I hope to see your wife and me at dinner tomorrow." A vain physician says, "The number of physicians who understand the nostril, even in this great city, can be counted *on one finger*—pardon me, I meant to say on the fingers of one hand." Secretly, he believes that he is the only authority, and his real but ordinarily inhibited vanity appears in an 'unintentional' slip of the tongue. (See p. 175.)

The basis of repression is the phenomenon of *inhibition,* which has already been described in connection with conditioning and learning (p. 142). It requires no occult explanation such as the 'damming up' of repressed memories in the 'unconscious.' One way to adjust to a situation is simply to fail to respond to it, and this failure may operate in the verbal or other symbolic behavior involved in recall, as well as in the case of motor responses. The chief danger in repression is that it hampers your reeducation. In order to learn a new response to a situation, often a more constructive adjustment, you have to recognize and respond to the problem. You cannot do that if the problem has been repressed.

Projection

A rejected or repressed motive is not recognized in your own behavior, yet you will still be excessively sensitive or defensive to evidences of it. This often leads to seeing your own inferior impulses in other people, and that is the mechanism of *projection.* An awkward person sees and criticizes awkwardness in others. Doing so has an adjustive value similar to that of rationalization, for it bolsters up his self-esteem by emphasizing that others are worse than he. A person with conflicts about his own honesty is more likely to see cheating and other forms of dishonesty in the world around him. By condemning such faults strongly, he expresses his own guilt and self-condemnation indirectly, with less anxiety than if he recognized his own shortcomings. Projection is especially noticeable in sexual conflicts. An individual with unsolved sex problems imputes sexual aims to others, and may be excessive in denouncing them or in guarding against them. Such is the traditional 'old maid's delusion,' though fortunately only a small proportion of unmarried older women really show it in appreciable degree.

The mechanism of projection is seen most clearly in delusions of persecution and in the less severe but similar attitudes of chronically suspicious people. Feeling thwarted, the individual has an impulse to attack the sources of his frustration aggressively. If the expression of his aggressions is inhibited because they conflict with his social training, the aggressiveness may be attributed to others. This leads a man to suspect his associates' motives and actions and, at the extreme, to have delusions that he is the victim of persecution or conspiracy. This kind of adjustment usually includes aspects of two mechanisms; it is rationalization in that it excuses failure, but it is also projection in attributing self-aggression to the external world.

Regression

Another form of escape from difficulties is to revert to solutions that were satisfying at an earlier period of personal development. Such return to the past has been termed *regression.* Its clearest manifestations are seen in the behavior of young children. When thwarted, they tend to regress to obviously infantile responses. A two-year-old who no longer gets his parents' undivided attention because of a new baby in the family may revert to crawling instead of walking or may demand that he be fed by hand. A number of experiments with animals have shown that they tend to return to earlier and simpler types of responses to problem situations, even though these are ineffective, when blocked by an excessive increase in the difficulty of the adjustment required. Experiments with children have shown that the quality of their play is likely to deteriorate to that typical of younger ages when they are thwarted by being deprived of attractive toys. Normal regression in adults is shown by the tendencies of men to revert to adolescent boisterousness at conventions and reunions. Every college has alumni who are perennial undergraduates, seeking to recapture the most satisfying period that came into their lives before fully adult responsibilities fell upon them.

In describing more serious maladjustments, the concept of regression is sometimes used in a broader sense, to imply a simplification of response to more rudimentary levels. An example is the psychological invalid, who takes to bed in order to escape a need for adjustment, demanding that others care for all his needs. Regression is even more striking in the serious mental disorders of the withdrawing types, in which a patient may long remain mute and unresponsive to adjustive demands. In this second sense, all maladjustments are somewhat regressive in that they are retreats from the intricate adaptations required in dealing effectively with reality. The two meanings of regression must not be confused. A withdrawn adjustment is oversimplified but it is not truly childlike, for normal children are active and outgoing in their behavior.

Sublimation

Since everyone is thwarted to some extent and yet is able to make a passably successful adjustment to life, there must be a mechanism or means of substitute satisfaction that is healthful. Perhaps it is sufficient to refer to such solutions merely as good adjustments, but they are often designated *sublimations.* A sublimation is a substitute response that is socially acceptable and does not interfere appreciably with the satisfaction of other motives. Examples of sublimation can be found in all persons' lives. Aggressive responses to thwarting are sublimated into interests in participant and spectator sports, especially those requiring physical force such as boxing or football. Anxieties concerning inferiorities may find constructive reduction in drives leading to achievement in business, professions or the arts. Thwarted needs to 'mother' people and to have them dependent may be sublimated into work in child welfare or social welfare.

Although sublimations are common adjustments, it is a mistake to suppose that they underlie all achievements. This hypothesis would assume that all personalities are essentially sick or inadequate, and that even good adjustment is a 'mechanism' or remedial measure to alleviate an infirmity. Most well-balanced adjustments are direct responses to motives. There is some experimental evidence that achievement is not usually due to sublimation. For example, it is often assumed that creativeness in the arts is a sublimation of sex motives. If this were true, the need for sexual gratification would be lessened in creative individuals. One study, of a group of creatively superior single men, found no evidence that their normal sex needs were replaced by their outlets in intellectual or artistic achievements.

CONFLICT

Among the various types of thwarting, conflict has the broadest significance, especially in contributing to an understanding of the more disabling maladjustments. Conflict has already been defined as a state of affairs in which two or more incompatible behavior trends are evoked that cannot be satisfied fully at the same time. In recent years psychology has given much attention to the problem of conflict by making theoretical analyses of various types of conflict, by performing experiments on conflict behavior and by studying its effects in men and animals.

An Analysis of Conflicts

Conflict can be described in terms of the interactions between an individual and his environment. This is the *field theory* of behavior, developed chiefly by Kurt Lewin and his associates, and named by analogy to a theory of electricity and magnetism. It emphasizes the observation that behavior does not depend on the organism alone or on the environment alone, but on what goes on between the two.

Tendencies to behavior may be represented by *vectors,* which show the direction and strength of the individual's striving. Most impulses can be described as directed toward or away from an environmental event. This is stated in terms of *valences,* of which positive (+) valences are tendencies to approach, and negative (−) valences are tendencies to withdraw and avoid (Fig. 234). It will be seen that valences and vectors are both field phenomena, and can be defined only in terms of both the character of the person and the environmental forces acting on him.

Approach-Approach Conflicts

Field theory shows that there can be only three basic types of conflict. A Type 1 conflict is between two positive valences that are about equal in strength. This is an *approach-approach* conflict (Fig. 235). A child may have to choose between reading an interesting book and going out to play football. A young man may have a conflict of this type when he can choose freely between two offered positions, or a young woman when faced with a decision between two equally qualified suitors.

FIGURE 234. VALENCES AND VECTORS

In *A,* the interaction of the individual (*I*) and the situation (*S*) may be described as a positive valence, in *B* as a negative valence. [After K. Lewin.]

Theoretical, experimental and practical observations all show that approach-approach conflicts rarely result in disturbances of behavior. For one reason, the absence of any negative valences means the lack of fear, anxiety or restraint, which are basic to maladjustment. Also, once a person starts in the direction of one alternative, its nearness adds to its strength, so that the vectors are no longer equal and a choice is found to have been made. Theory indicates that some vacillation may take place, however. If the person attains one goal, and if then satiation reduces the strength of the drive toward that goal, the opposite vector is now stronger and will attract. After tiring of the ball game, the boy returns to his book. Relinquished jobs and lovers sometimes seem more attractive in retrospect, and the grass is greener on the other side of the fence.

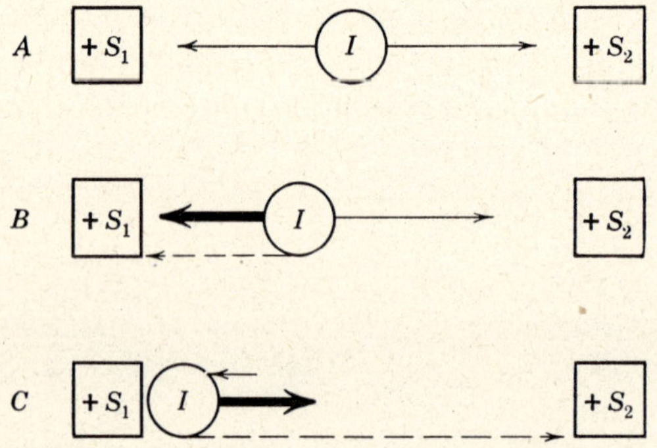

FIGURE 235. APPROACH-APPROACH CONFLICTS: TYPE 1

The approach-approach conflict, *A*, is solved easily. If some variation in behavior brings the individual a little closer, physically or psychologically, to the attracting situation S_1 and away from the other attracting situation S_2, the vector for S_1 is increased in strength because of the decreased distance, and the conflict is resolved by the individual's going in that direction (*B*). In *C*, satiation of the S_1 motive may weaken its vector. The individual then vacillates to the S_2 choice. The dotted vectors indicate actual movements and the solid vectors motivational forces. [After K. Lewin.]

Avoidance-Avoidance Conflicts

Conflicts of Type 2 are evoked by two negative valences. Both tendencies are to retreat from or to avoid something; this is being caught between the devil and the deep sea (Fig. 236). A youngster may want to avoid doing an unpleasant task and also want to escape the threat of parental punishment for his failure to perform. The soldier in battle has a conflict between his need to run away and save his skin and his need to avoid being scorned as a coward.

The most usual solution of an avoidance-avoidance conflict is *leaving the field,* that is to say, taking a third course of action which avoids both the threatening alternatives. That may be regarded as a response toward the resultant of the two vectors, as suggested by *B* of Fig. 236. Most escape mechanisms are methods for *leaving the field.* The boy just cited may develop a headache, thereby avoiding both the task and parental displeasure. Or he may apparently work at the job, but really be engaged in daydreaming, which is a common way to escape unpleasant alternatives. On

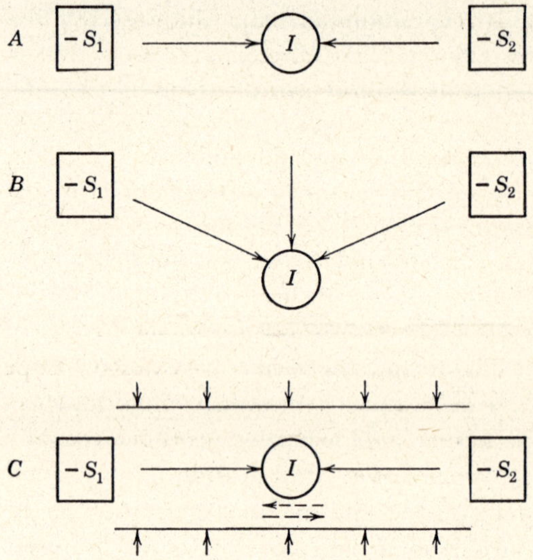

FIG. 236. AVOIDANCE-AVOIDANCE CONFLICTS: TYPE 2

The usual response to a Type 2 conflict in *A* is to leave the field, as shown by *B*. If material or psychological barriers prevent this, as in *C*, the individual shows vacillating behavior (two dotted vectors) at the choice point, and has unreduced tension. [After K. Lewin.]

the other hand, psychological, social or physical boundaries may keep the individual from leaving the field. Common boundaries include his social values acquired through learning ('conscience') and various other more direct social pressures. If unable to escape the dilemma, the individual may be forced to solve it by strengthening or weakening one of the vectors. For example, he may put off a disagreeable task until social pressure mounts so high that the penalty for nonperformance is greater than the unpleasantness of the duty. This pattern is often seen in students who put off studying until they are forced by the imminence of examinations.

If a person cannot solve an avoidance-avoidance conflict at all, he remains in a vacillating, insecure condition, usually with a strong emotional tone induced by the unremoved needs for escape (*C* of Fig. 236). He feels tension, which is often partially reduced by defense or escape mechanisms not directly related to the original conflict. If even this means of adjustment fails, the result is unreduced tension with its symptoms of anxiety, 'nervousness' and the like.

Approach-Avoidance Conflicts

The remaining variety of conflict, Type 3, is seen when a situation elicits both approaching and avoiding tendencies simultaneously (Fig. 237). The antagonistic valences may lie in the relationship of the individual to the situation, as for example, when a child wants to play football but is afraid of being hurt, or when he both loves and fears his mother (*A* of the figure). In other instances, one valence may be 'induced' by a psychological field set up by another person or by a cultural group. Thus, a child may want to take a forbidden piece of candy, but the parent's watchful eye surrounds the dish with negative valences (*B* of the figure). The opposite can also be observed, as when a person is in conflict toward an irksome duty, because it lies in a positive field representing the prospective approval of parents, teachers or associates.

Many serious conflicts that lead to substitute adjustments can be described in terms of the approach-avoidance situation. Feelings of personal inadequacy evoke this type of conflict. The individual is strongly motivated to achieve prestige and approval, but also has a fear of effort or competition because of his disbelief in his own competence. He may want to act aggressively against persons who thwart him yet be inhibited by fear of retaliation. Most serious of all is a conflict based on responses of love and fear, or of dependence and resentment, directed against the *same* person.

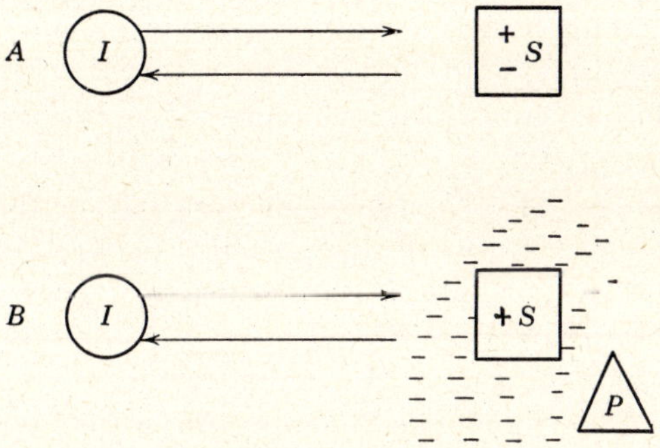

FIG. 237. APPROACH-AVOIDANCE CONFLICTS: TYPE 3

An unresolved approach-avoidance conflict in *A* results only in unreduced tension, since leaving the field is not a solution. In many instances this type of conflict results from induced valences, as shown in *B*, where a parent (*P*) forbids an approach, surrounding the desired goal (+*S*) with an atmosphere of negative valences. [After K. Lewin.]

Approach-avoidance conflicts cannot be solved by leaving the field, because the impulse for approach (positive valence) keeps the individual from retreating too far. The person in conflict thus tends to remain at a point of vacillating equilibrium, at which the strengths of the opposing forces are about equal. His impulses do not cancel each other, but leave him in a continued state of unreduced tension. More than either of the other two types, approach-avoidance conflicts are likely to underlie either inferior adjustment mechanisms or unreduced anxiety.

EXPERIMENTS ON CONFLICT

The study of conflicts can be explored experimentally by exposing subjects to situations in which two opposed needs are activated. Such experiments add to the knowledge that can be obtained from the clinical study of individuals, because of greater precision in the arrangement of the situations, in the control of other influences, and in the tabulation of the results. Some experiments on minor conflicts have been done with human beings as subjects, but the most revealing studies have used animals. You may not, merely for scientific purposes, create neuroses in human beings, but human welfare justifies the induction of neurosis in a cat or a sheep.

Conflicts in Cats

In an extensive series of experiments with cats, an investigator has studied the effects of conflict between a feeding response and an avoiding reaction to a fear-provoking stimulus. Hungry cats, placed in the apparatus (Fig. 238), learned to go to the feeding box when a light-and-buzzer signal was given. After this response was established, conflict was introduced by giving the cat a strong blast from a compressed air nozzle near the feeding box, or an electric shock from the floor grid, or both. This was an approach-avoidance, a Type 3, conflict.

The effects of the experimentally induced conflict were striking. Typically, cats that were normally quiet showed an inhibition of feeding responses, signs of emotional reaction such as the erection of hairs and the dilation of the pupils and extremely restless and agitated behavior that might properly be interpreted as evidence of tension and anxiety. Cats that were rather active and excitable in their normal condition tended to become passive and immobile, remaining in set postures over periods of ten to twenty minutes even while receiving electric shocks. Cats also developed 'phobic' reactions, cowering and showing signs of fear and avoidance when the feeding signals were given, even when the air blast or shock in a particular trial was being omitted. They showed the defense or tension reduction mechanisms in some cases, especially in continued cleaning, licking and preening of their fur.

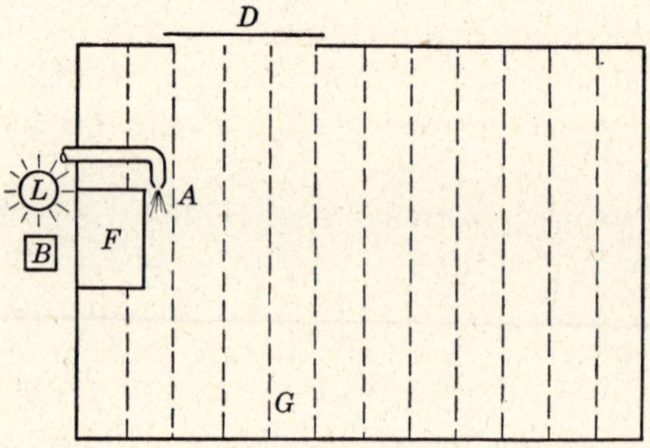

FIG. 238. APPARATUS FOR STUDYING CONFLICT IN CATS

The cat is introduced through the door *D*, and learns to feed at the food box *F* when light *L* and buzzer signal *B* are given. Conflict is introduced by stimulating the cat with an air blast *A* while he is feeding, or by an electric shock applied by the floor grid *G*, or by both. [After J. H. Masserman, *Behavior and neurosis*, Chicago University Press, 1943, Plate IV.]

The most striking findings of this series

of experiments concerned the duration and generalization of the effects of conflict. Conflicts set up by only two or three repetitions of the training situation remained unmodified for months. Also, the cats' behavior outside the experimental box was profoundly affected in almost every instance. Some cats who had been made 'neurotic' starved themselves until they had to be force-fed. Others became either excessively wild, or timid, or fearful, or aggressive. It was evident that the experimental conflict made profound and enduring changes in their ability to make their usual life adjustments.

Experimental Neurosis

Another experimental approach to the study of conflict was first made in Pavlov's laboratories by use of the conditioned response technique. Many experimenters have made further observations by this method, with dogs, sheep, pigs, rats and even with a few human subjects.

Most studies set up conflicts by requiring excessively fine discriminations of conditioned responses. In the first classic experiment, a dog was trained to salivate when a perfect circle was shown and not to salivate when the visual stimulus was an ellipse. Then the dog was given a series of ellipses, which approached nearer and nearer to the form of the circle. That produced the significant phenomenon. Instead of simply failing in discrimination, the dog 'broke down.' He showed frenzied emotional behavior, salivated for any stimulus even remotely connected with the experiment such as the sight of the experimenter and was unable to make easy discriminations that he formerly made without difficulty. He had developed what is now called an *experimental neurosis*.

It is evident that experimental neurosis can be regarded as a result of a conflict between excitatory and inhibitory tendencies evoked by the same situation. It is essentially a Type 3 conflict. Many studies have shown that not all animals are equally susceptible to this breakdown, some appearing to have higher conflict tolerance than others. Among those that do succumb, there is a tendency for formerly placid animals to show an excited neurosis, and for active ones to be overinhibited, just as happened with the cats. An experimental neurosis spreads to include the animals' behavior out of the laboratory, and it lasts for a long time. One sheep and one dog remained 'neurotic' for the rest of their lives, periods of thirteen and ten years respectively. One very important finding was that sheep, which were free to move about in a pen during the experiment could not be 'broken down,' whereas those strapped in the conditioning apparatus could be. The former were able to leave the field and escape the impact of the conflict. (Compare *B* with *C* in Fig. 236.)

Effects of Conflict

These experiments on conflict have made an invaluable contribution to the understanding of human adjustments. Conflicts are not only the precipitating causes of adjustive difficulties, but also have a relationship to the *ability to adjust* when confronted by new problems. The experiments show that strong, unsolved, early conflicts make enduring changes in personality, and case studies of people confirm these findings. If a person persists over a period of years in making inferior, excessively substituted or nonadjustive responses, it is very probable that earlier disabling influences have reduced his general ability to adjust.

COMMON SOURCES OF CONFLICT

In infancy and childhood the family, being the chief social background of the individual, is the scene of most of these conflicts. Later sex comes to determine many of the conflicts, for the reason that the demands of our culture have not been well adjusted to the sexual needs of the individual. And there are many other ways in which cultural values can give rise to conflicts.

Family Conflicts

The many interactions of personalities that take place within the family are of the greatest significance in determining reactions to conflict, because they are the most pervasive and intimate and are highly motivated. A child's relations with members of his family, moreover, mold his adjustive behavior when he is immature and least able to cope with difficulties independently.

Conflicts of *insecurity* are among the most common and, when severe, are among the most disabling. Insecurity results from a conflict between dependence and fear. A child is inevitably dependent on his parents not only for food and shelter but also for protection, approval and affection. The urgent nature of these latter needs has been recognized more fully in recent years. If parents are cold, disinterested or excessively demanding, or if they use scolding and punishment as the major technique for securing the child's compliance with domestic routines, the result, from the child's point of view, is *rejection*. Parents, of course, seldom reject a child intentionally or consciously, but the child feels rejected because he gets from them so much less than he needs. There are many reasons why parents fall short of their children's necessities. For some parents a child represents a frustration of their own needs, in that the care of an infant may prevent them from having their desired social recreations or, when both parents have professional ambitions, a child may interfere with the career of one of them—usually the mother. If the parents feel 'unconsciously' guilty about their relation to a child, they may project their guilt upon the child, finding fault with it or becoming angry with it. Or they may project other maladjustments of their own upon their children. Another difficulty arises when parents who have a strong need for social approval feel that their child's bad manners reflect adversely on them. They do not consciously admit the blame, but project it upon the child by nagging or punishing him. Rejecting parents defend their treatment of their children by rationalizations, making themselves believe that their actions are all for the child's good. So closely are the personalities of children dependent in these ways upon the personalities of their parents that a child guidance clinic, when asked to advise about a problem child, always studies the parents too. A problem child at once creates the presumption that there may also be a problem parent needing attention. In line with this reasoning, parents have been sentenced by the court for the delinquency of their children.

The relationships of a child with his brothers or sisters may also be the basis of conflicts which arise from *sibling rivalry*. Children in the family are always competitors, in some degree, for the attention and love of their parents. If one child succeeds more than another, because he has more approved traits or because the parents are 'partial' to him, the result may be the equivalent of rejection for the less favored youngster. Invidious comparisons of children with respect to their intelligence, willingness, strength or appearance may cause conflicts of inferiority.

In our culture, especially in urban families of the higher economic levels, parental *overprotection* is a common source of conflicts. It may take either of two forms. Parental *dominance* is found when the parents refuse to permit the child to bear responsibility for any decision or duty. Everything is done for him, because adults can carry out the tasks more quickly or efficiently than a child. The other form is parental *submissiveness.* The child is permitted to do as he wishes. The parents not only gratify every need that he expresses, but protect him from the consequences of his immature judgment. With either type of overprotection, the child may show no signs of conflict during the earlier years that are normally spent in the home. When he begins to have social contacts with other children, or when he starts attendance at school, the trouble is likely to begin. The overprotected child lacks independent social skills, and his demand for special consideration may lead to his persecution by his contemporaries. He is then likely to develop defense or escape mechanisms, or to regress to the protection of his family, leaving an even more difficult readjustment to be made in his adolescent or adult years.

Sex Conflicts

The sexual functions are often causes of severe conflicts because of the way they are regarded in our culture. Conflict is not inherent in sex, as studies of other cultures show very clearly. There are, however, a number of reasons why sex underlies so much conflict in our own particular pattern of civilization. One reason is found in the long time interval that separates physiological and social maturity. Young men and women are adults sexually from five to fifteen years before they can marry and support themselves and a family. This period of frustration is absent in primitive cultures in which occupational and educational demands for marriage are simpler. An even more important reason is the cultural standard that holds all sex desires, thoughts or acts to be indecent or guilty, and forbids open discussion or expression of them. Many parents effectively condition their children to regard anything sexual as clandestine and guilty. When sex drives occur, a conflict between the sexual need and the sense of guilt is likely. From a broad social point of view, the repression of sex has served the functions of reducing illegitimacy and the spread of venereal disease. From the standpoint of individual adjustment, it often achieves this end at the cost of conflict and anxiety.

Casual sexual relations among young unmarried persons are not, however, a good solution of the sex problem. The anxieties caused by the conflict with early training and with the dominant cultural ethics produce tensions that are greater than those relieved. Also, casual relationships are a poor substitute for the more broadly satisfying condition of marriage, which fulfills many needs besides the needs of sex. In general, it is the experience of psychological consultants that young people who are promiscuous create more conflicts than they solve. Sometimes the exaggerated sex needs are themselves substitutes for motives to prove one's manliness or attractiveness, a need which can be satisfied directly by other activities. In other instances, exaggerated behavior is evidence of an intercultural conflict, in which a smaller 'liberated' group feels a need to show its aggressive defiance of the larger culture by assaulting its standards.

It is the experience of many well-adjusted young people that sex desires can be recognized as normal, without fear or shame, but can be controlled by constructive substitute adjustments, chiefly of the type of sublimation. Among the sublimations that reduce sex needs are well-motivated work, adequate recreation and amusement, and opportunities for social contacts with the opposite sex. No psychological harm comes from sexual abstinence itself during the adolescent or young adult years, whereas disabling conflicts can indeed be induced by fears about the sex function, fears that may arise either in connection with sex fulfillment or with nonfulfillment.

Many young persons have grave conflicts over autoerotic practices (masturbation). This method of relieving sex tension is used by almost all adolescent boys and by many girls, and is often continued into the young adult years. Physiologically it is harmless and does not cause insanity or loss of virility, as are the common misconceptions. It does, however, involve psychological difficulties. Most persons have been so thoroughly taught that the act is harmful and wicked that they have strong feelings of guilt about masturbation. Also, masturbation is ridiculed by young people themselves, and one who is detected is subjected to humiliation. Guilt induced by masturbation does not reduce the practice, for the increased tension often causes a greater need for relief. Psychological counselors have found that the most effective treatment for masturbation anxieties is to reduce the feelings of unworthiness and to encourage sublimations that satisfy social motives broadly.

Other Cultural Conflicts

The pattern of values that exists in our culture is responsible for a number of other conflicts that may operate from childhood on through maturity. One of them is the conflict between the learned needs for *competitive achievement* and for *cooperation and submission.* From an early age rewards of approval by parents and community are given for competitive success in school marks, in sports and, later, in vocations. As a result, Americans learn to place a high evaluation on assertion and aggressiveness. At the same time an opposite set of values is taught equally vigorously. We learn to try to be popular, to be liked and to be appreciated. This demand places a strong emphasis on our needs for the approval and affection of others. The conflict between these two tendencies is one of the most common causes of tension and of substitute adjustments. It has been described as basic to "the neurotic personality of our time."

A somewhat related conflict, peculiar to the American culture and to others like it, arises from the need for *status.* Surveys of the occupational preferences of high school students show that a large majority want to enter the professions and white-collar occupations. They want to become physicians, lawyers, engineers and owners of businesses, in a proportion that is beyond their possible realization. In a few years most of these would-be professional men will be factory workers and clerks. This conflict does not occur in an old culture, in which a son expects to follow his father's occupation, or at the best not to rise much above his level. The good aspects of free opportunity are to some extent counterbalanced by these feelings of frustration and failure. Status conflicts are likely to continue throughout many people's lives, as they try to equal or excel their neighbors in houses, automobiles, clothes, entertainment and many other things. These conflicts underlie many financial worries and not a little of domestic discord.

Another variety of cultural conflict in America is found in the confusion of *group loyalties* and group identifications. This conflict is very evident in the children of immigrants, whose parents and whose own early home training represent one culture, and whose schooling and outside experiences are in another. Insecurity and anxiety often ensue. They may be reduced by aggressive defenses that relieve tensions but hinder social adjustment. (On conflict, see p. 570, and on group identification, see pp. 598 f.)

PSYCHONEUROSES

If an individual's adjustments are so inadequate that they cause him chronic discomfort, and interfere markedly with his efficiency in ordinary living, they may be characterized as *psychoneurotic* or *neurotic.* As used today, these two terms are synonymous. The psychoneuroses are not specific entities or diseases, but represent a certain range of severity in the continuum of maladjustments. They are more disabling than the reactions that can be classed as normal, but are less so than the psychoses, which are the most serious form of mental disturbance and will be described presently. Since there is a continuous gradation of quality of adjustment from the best-balanced person to the most obviously disturbed, no exact line can be drawn to separate normality from neurosis. Some writers have tended to use the term neurotic to characterize all adjustments short of the most excellent. There is even a "be-glad-you're-neurotic" school of thought which goes farther to ascribe all driving energies, and hence all achievement, to neurosis. According to this conception, everyone is neurotic at times, and many of us are neurotic most of the time, and the activity which builds civilization gets its power from the need to substitue readjustment for maladjustment. It seems best, however, to reject a definition that identifies neurosis with all imperfect adjustment and to restrict the use of the term to the more severe cases.

Although the psychoneuroses show a great variety of symptoms, there seem to be a number of common elements that constitute the psychoneurotic personality. The most striking characteristic is a low tolerance for conflict. Neurotic persons worry over matters that are not of immediate importance and show strong reactions to slight degrees of frustration. Furthermore, this pattern is persistent and chronic, often constituting a life style that can be observed from the individual's childhood. As to symptoms, a neurosis is distinguished either by a marked degree of anxiety that is out of proportion to the situation evoking it, or by certain typical mechanisms which serve to reduce strong anxiety but hamper social adjustments. This description of the characteristics of neurotic behavior, of course, again emphasizes the fact that it differs only in degree from the normal.

Anxiety

Fear is a 'catastrophic response' that all persons make when faced with a highly motivated situation to which they can make no effective adjustment (see p. 104). Anxiety is distinguished from fear in that it is a response to an anticipated danger, or to a symbol of one, rather than to the threatening situation itself. Normal anxiety is present when the anticipated peril is imminent and probable. It is sometimes called *situational anxiety,* for it is relieved when the situation that aroused it is past. For a military aviator in wartime to suffer a severe emotional disturbance when under enemy fire is normal fear. For him to show signs of emotion as he contemplates the next combat mission is normal anxiety. But if, in time of peace and in the safety of his own country, he trembles when an automobile backfires, or if he breaks into perspiration when someone slaps him on the back, he is showing *neurotic anxiety,* because these stimuli are only partial or inadequate symbols of the original fear-producing situation.

Anxiety manifests itself in three ways, which are the usual evidences of fear: through a conscious state of discomfort and apprehension, through visceral disturbances especially of the digestive and circulatory systems and through motor symptoms which include restlessness, trembling, irritability and the like. At one time, these symptoms were regarded as separate psychoneuroses. If a person showed mainly the signs of apprehension, he was diagnosed as having an *anxiety neurosis.* The visceral upsets were labeled *neurasthenia* or *hypochondria,* whereas the motor symptoms were ascribed to *nervousness.* It is now recognized that all anxious persons show all three of these effects of emotion, but that the intensity of a particular symptom may vary from one person to another. It is fruitless to try to classify anxiety states as if they were types of diseases. Real understanding can be achieved by regarding anxiety as an emotional and nonadjustive response which a person is making to his conflicts.

Sometimes anxiety is directed toward the real source of the conflict, as when a child who is reacting to a conflict between dependence and rejection fears that his parents do not love him or that they will leave him. More often the most important cause of the conflict is not identified, because the individual has repressed his responses to it. Such a repression is a partial adjustment, but it does not reduce the emotional tension of the conflict entirely. Anxiety may then take a generalized form, in which the individual shows dread, indecision and fear in many aspects of his life. The spread of anxiety to remote symbols of the original conflict is the same phenomenon as that found by the experimental studies of conflict in animals. When an intense conflict has not been solved, its effects are 'generalized' to many facets of behavior.

The visceral results of anxiety can be understood in terms of the physiological effects of emotion. Momentary fear inhibits digestion, accelerates heart beat, raises blood pressure and influences a number of glandular secretions (p. 104). The chronic anxiety often seen in psychoneurotic states has similar effects, but these are intensified because of the long duration of the fear. One of the most common symptoms is 'nervous indigestion.' The anxious person does not enjoy eating, suffers gastric distress after meals and may therefore be unable to assimilate food, even to the point of malnutrition. An extreme example of the effect of anxiety on the digestive system is the development of gastric ulcers. This 'psychosomatic' disorder results from disturbances of the gastric secretions and of the normal mucous lining of the stomach and seems clearly related to the emotional tensions resulting from conflicts. Chronic high blood pressure can also result from nonadjustment.

Since strong emotion is an emergency condition (p. 95), it rapidly exhausts the body's nutritional reserves. After a long period of anxiety, some people may show symptoms of 'nervous exhaustion,' including fatigue, weakness and lowered efficiency. This end result of chronic anxiety has an anomalous adjustive value, similar to that of an escape or withdrawal mechanism. If a person is ill, his failures are excused.

Common 'nervousness' is a very frequent symptom of anxiety. The nervous individual is irritable and 'jumpy.' He is given to random motor outlets, from pacing the floor to chewing his fingernails. The term also includes over-reaction to stimuli that do not disturb most people, such as startle responses for moderate sounds and undue irritation at petty annoyances. A common misconception of long standing has regarded nervousness as an organic condition due to 'weak nerves,' and countless bottles of 'nerve tonics' have been consumed futilely. Nervousness cannot be understood by itself, but is clearly explained as a diffused motor response under emotional tensions.

Phobias

In many instances a fear response is attached to a specific type of situation, and it is then known as a *phobia*. Mild phobias, which are very common, may be stimulated by almost every kind of situation imaginable. Among the more common phobias are fears of the dark, of small enclosed places, of heights, of animals, of crowds, of water and of thunderstorms. The list could be continued endlessly. A person with a phobia admits that his fear is groundless but he is unable to control it. Although many normal people have minor phobias, the condition is regarded as psychoneurotic when it is severe and of long duration, and when it interferes with ordinary life activities to an appreciable degree.

Some phobias have been traced to specific instances in the earlier life of the individual by which he learned to fear a certain type of situation. These are essentially conditioned fear reactions. In one classic case of phobia a British officer in the war of 1914-1918 was so afraid of small enclosed places that he could not enter a dugout. At first, he could not remember any cause for this phobia, but a long series of psychological consultations, probing his early experiences, eventually resulted in the recall of a pertinent childhood experience. When he was about three or four years of age, he had been caught in a narrow corridor with a vicious dog, from which he could not escape. He had never related this incident to anyone, for he had repressed a recall of it as a partial adjustment. When he finally was helped to remember the event, his phobia of enclosed places was cured. In another case a college girl's fear of eyes was traced to a childhood fright occasioned by finding a pair of glass eyes while she was guiltily peeping in the bureau drawers at the home of an aunt. As in the other case, memory of the event had been inhibited, but the conditioned emotional reaction remained to constitute the phobia.

Not all phobias have been traced to specific conditioned fears. In some instances, including the more severe and disabling ones, the feared situation is a symbol of the real cause of the emotion. For example, a young girl who had a phobia for open places and large rooms was found really to have a fear of death. These symbolic phobias are very similar to anxieties, except that the individual has displaced his fear to a specific kind of situation, instead of having it remain generalized.

The part that repression plays in many severe maladjustments is most clearly seen in the phobias. They show that a 'forgotten' event can continue to influence behavior. From a single experience, a person can acquire several responses that may be somewhat independent of one another. He may learn to represent the event by words or other symbols when an appropriate stimulus is presented in the future; that is *recall.* He may also learn to make certain emotional responses, and to have certain feelings or attitudes when a stimulus associated with the experience occurs. The recall can be repressed as an adjustment to its unpleasantness without the occurrence of a corresponding inhibition of the emotion or attitude. This is a factor worth understanding in the 'unconscious' determination of behavior. On the other hand, the inability to remember an experience inevitably makes it difficult or even impossible to readjust to it rationally. A phobia persists because an individual cannot learn to make a new, more constructive response to a past event which he cannot remember. The recall of the basic experience often cures a phobia, not because of any magic of 'getting a complex out of the unconscious' but because the individual is now able to work out a readjustment, using his more mature adult capacity to deal with the problem.

Compulsions and Obsessions

Most persons can remember normal, childish, compulsive acts and obsessive thoughts: not stepping on the cracks of the sidewalk, a silly phrase running through the head. Such affairs may be greatly exaggerated in some psychoneurotics.

When a compulsion occurs in connection with a phobia, its adjustive value is seen most clearly. To an individual who has a fear of being attacked in the night, tension is obviously reduced by examining all the bolts and locks repeatedly and by making several inspections of the closets and under the beds. A compulsion is a routine that gives a sense of security. It is exaggerated beyond the bounds of ordinary prudence because the anxiety that it reduces is itself not ordinary. A similar psychological function is served by the compulsive tendencies of persons who must always perform their common tasks in exactly the same way. Such a person is usually insecure, finding safety in living by rules and routines in a rigidly orderly manner. Persons with well-developed compulsions may reduce their anxieties so well that they have little consciousness of fear. Usually, however, compulsive behavior is accompanied by visceral upsets and 'nervous' mannerisms that reveal the existence of a strong tension.

An obsession is a compulsive thought that keeps recurring, even when the person tries to banish it. The obsessive thought is annoying, sometimes because it is distressing in itself and sometimes because it seems foolish and irrational. In one case a man had an obsessive thought that he would cut his wife's throat. He said that his relationship with his wife was excellent and that the unreal obsession troubled him seriously. In a long series of psychiatric interviews, it was discovered that the man's mother had been harsh and exacting. Recently he had given up activities in which he was interested on the demand of his wife. He transferred to his wife the resentment that he had felt toward his mother but had repressed any open hostility. The obsession was a substitute expression of this aggression, a thought which he was able to allow himself because he disowned any desire to harm her as absurd and unreal. The obsession disappeared after he had readjusted his attitudes toward his wife and his mother. Another common type of obsession is a compulsive worry lest some harm befall a member of the worrier's family. Often this fear has been found to be a defense against a rejected aggressiveness. What the worrier really fears is that he will himself bring harm to the person about whom he worries.

One should not generalize unduly from these few instances, for the meaning of any compulsion or obsession can be ascertained only by a careful study of the individual who shows the symptom. In all cases, however, a compulsion or obsession has some relationship to personal conflicts and anxieties.

Ailment Adjustments

Another way by which people can adjust to serious conflicts is by developing symptoms that give them the status of disabled persons, so that they receive sympathy and protection. Some very striking disabilities can be acquired adjustively, including pains, blindness, deafness and muscular paralysis. Historically, conditions of this sort have been called *conversion hysteria,* and the adjustive conflict is said to have been 'converted' into the physical symptom. Psychoneurotic reactions of this type are so bizarre that laymen are often skeptical of their existence, or else confuse them with malingering, the conscious faking of symptoms. It is possible, however, to understand them in terms of the psychological principles of learning and adjustment.

Suppose, for example, that a high school girl's social adjustment is so poor that she has a need to shun the company of other young people. One day, when she is particularly distressed by her basic conflict, her leg 'goes to sleep,' a temporary condition of numbness that is commonly experienced by normal people. This passing symptom is seized upon as a solution of her adjustment. If her leg is paralyzed, she cannot go to school, and will receive the sympathy that is extended to one who is ill. Since muscular responses are subject to learning and inhibition, 'learning to have a paralysis' as a solution to a conflict can be explained by the same psychological concepts that are used to account for other adjustments. Similar accounts can be given of cases of hysterical blindness, deafness, nausea and other symptoms.

Although severe cases of conversion hysteria are classed as psychoneuroses, because they are socially disabling and are responses to major conflicts, a similar mechanism can be found in a milder degree in normal people. It is not entirely a figure of speech that a disagreeable task 'gives you a pain.' The 'nine o'clock headache,' which disappears when it is too late to go to work or to school, is essentially a mild hysterical adjustment. Almost everyone becomes more fatigued when a given amount of effort is to be expended on a distasteful job than when it is to be devoted to play or to a hobby. There is a continuum from the defense mechanisms of normal people to the most severe hysterical psychoneuroses.

PSYCHOSES

The most seriously nonadjustive conditions are the *psychoses,* popularly known as insanities or mental disorders. Socially, a considerable gulf separates the psychoses from the maladjustments and psychoneuroses. A psychoneurotic person is a discomfort to himself and may be a nuisance to others, but a person with a fully developed psychosis is dangerous to himself and to society.

There is no continuity between psychoneurosis and psychosis. In fact, very few psychoneurotics ever develop a psychosis. Making an adjustment by developing anxiety and by reducing it with defense mechanisms, which is typical of neurosis, seems to be an alternative to the more serious psychotic response of adjusting by retreat from reality.

Psychoses are more common than is ordinarily realized. There are about half a million persons in mental hospitals in the United States. More hospital beds are devoted to the mentally ill than to all other kinds of patients together. Of every thousand persons born, approximately fifty will be admitted to a mental hospital at some time in their lives. On the brighter side of the picture, mental disorders are not as hopeless as uninformed popular opinion holds. A very large proportion of psychotic patients are discharged from hospitals as cured or as sufficiently improved to make a passable adjustment to everyday life. Recent developments in treatment seem to be increasing the proportion of successful outcomes.

Organic Psychoses

About one-half the patients in mental hospitals suffer from disorders that are caused by identified organic conditions. They include brain injuries, syphilis of the nervous system, chronic addiction to alcohol and other drugs and brain deterioration associated with old age. All except the senile conditions can be treated with some effectiveness if not in too advanced a stage.

Functional Psychoses

The remaining half of mental disorders are called *functional psychoses,* a term that implies that they are due to adjustive causes, that is to say, to the defective functioning of organically intact individuals. As a matter of fact, the causes of these psychoses are very inadequately known. The same adjustive mechanisms that are found in normal people occur in extravagant forms in these psychoses, which seems to support the interpretation that they are extreme reactions to conflict. Some case histories appear to explain a psychosis adequately as a response to a very severe conflict, but in other instances people break down under circumstances that do not ordinarily cause great difficulties. It may be supposed that all the functional psychoses are not due to the same causes, and that physiological conditions as yet undiscovered may be important factors in some or even in all cases.

Almost all patients with functional psychoses fall in one of the two main classes of such disorders, which are *schizophrenia* and *manic-depressive psychosis.* Classic cases of these two psychoses are clearly distinguishable, but there are also mixed or variable forms that cannot be classified so easily. Until we know more about the causes of the functional psychoses, even their diagnosis will remain uncertain.

The common behavior pattern of *schizophrenia,* which is also known as *dementia praecox,* is a lack of appreciation of reality, usually accompanied by apathy or a flat unresponsive emotional tone. This fundamental characteristic has associated with it a great variety of more specific symptoms. Some schizophrenics show little more than apathy, indifference and marked withdrawal from social demands. In extreme instances this withdrawal is so pronounced that the patient sits or lies for hours in the same posture, does not attend to his bodily needs or keep himself clean, and has to be fed by force. Other schizophrenic patients are more active but show the common loss of connection with reality. They may talk in a silly or incoherent manner, laugh or cry when there is no observable reason, destroy clothing and furniture and be difficult to care for without force or restraint. *Hallucinations,* especially of hearing accusing voices, are common.

Delusions, or false beliefs held without reference to reality, occur frequently in schizophrenia. In one type, called *paranoid schizophrenia,* the delusions are the most noticeable symptom. The most frequent delusion is persecution. The patient declares he has been robbed, cheated or imprisoned by his family, or that people have conspired to cause him to lose his position. Delusions of grandeur are less frequent and are believed to be secondary to those of persecution, arising because the patient has to build a false belief about his own importance to explain why he is singled out for oppression. Delusions in the mentally disordered serve the same purposes that rationalization and projection do in normal persons. Delusions help to explain defeats and to build a sense of importance. They are tolerated by the patient because his distorted perception of reality prevents their critical appraisal.

Schizophrenia is a psychosis typical of young persons. Although there are cases at all ages, the peak of hospital admissions with this diagnosis lies in the decade of the twenties. In most instances the disorder has been developing over a considerable period of time, having begun with seclusiveness and queer behavior. It becomes a full-blown psychosis when the individual is unable to make the adjustments that adult life demands.

Manic-depressive psychosis is the other frequent psychotic condition. It consists either of overactivity and an elated feeling tone in the *manic* phase or of retardation and sadness in the *depressed* condition. Usually a patient has an attack in one or the other of these forms, and then recovers. In some instances there may be a series of episodes, sometimes alternating between mania and depression. It is for this reason that the psychosis is regarded as one condition rather than as two separate disorders. Less is known about the psychological basis of the manic-depressive state than about that of schizophrenia. It has been suggested that manic-depressives are persons who have never learned how to compromise, who are either completely defeated by conflict or else deny it by an unreal elation. No hypothesis is very satisfactory, however, and the major factors underlying this psychosis remain to be discovered. Manic-depressive conditions are most frequent in middle life, the greatest frequency occurring in the decade from forty to fifty years.

The Treatment of the Psychoses

The functional psychoses have not been treated with great success in the past, although many cases show spontaneous improvement. The most promising method of treatment so far devised, developed in the 1930's, is known as *shock therapy*. In one technique, a drug (insulin, metrazol) is used to induce unconsciousness, convulsions or both in the patient. In another method, electric currents are passed through the brain to cause convulsions and unconsciousness. After a shock treatment the patient is found to be confused. When his confusion clears, his basic psychosis is often much improved. Insulin and metrazol have been used most successfully with schizophrenia and electric shock with depressed conditions, but treatments are not entirely specific.

Another very radical treatment is *prefrontal lobotomy* (p. 38), a surgical operation that severs the connection of a part of the frontal lobes from the rest of the brain. It has brought improvement to some cases of depression and of schizophrenia, but it results in permanent changes in personality. Topectomy is a recent operation more selective in the destruction of tissue.

The shock and surgical treatments are empirical and are not based on any generally accepted theory. Some hypotheses are that shock treatment stimulates the autonomic nervous system, leading to new adjustive attempts, or that it influences the metabolism of the brain. Other interpretations suggest that shock therapy, like lobotomy, damages the brain and destroys the pathways representing the nonadjustive reactions. The patient then has to learn new adjustments, using different neural connections. It is also argued that injury to the frontal lobes and their connections reduces the total integration of the brain and thus the patient's ability to relate to each other events that occur or are due to occur at different times. Thus the patient becomes thoughtless and his planning superficial. It is possible that a psychosis might get disrupted in this way along with a patient's 'time perspective.'

Psychotherapy is treatment carried out by consultations and interviews, that is to say, by psychological methods as distinguished from medical. Psychotherapy has not been of great value in treating fully developed psychoses, because of the patients' disturbed perception of reality and their inability to communicate with the psychiatrist as intelligibly as can a psychoneurotic person. It is effective with some incipient disorders that are not very severe and is of especial usefulness with patients whose psychoses have been terminated by shock therapy. In these cases, psychological consultation helps to work out the old conflicts and to establish more constructive adjustments to them.

All types of treatment have a greater chance of being effective if they are begun early in the development of a psychosis. Early treatment, however, requires the prompt recognition of symptoms of withdrawn, erratic or depressed behavior. The chief obstacle to such recognition is not ignorance but the superstitious fear of mental disorders that prevents families from recognizing the condition and seeking professional assistance. Educated persons can do much to aid mental hygiene in their communities by combatting the fear of mental disorders, by helping people to realize that psychoses are not more disgraceful than other illnesses and by promoting the development of psychiatric clinics at which reliable help can be obtained.

TECHNIQUES FOR READJUSTMENT

Persons who are worried about their social relationships or personal problems, or who recognize signs of maladjustment in themselves, can get substantial help from trained consultants whose profession is to assist anyone in working out his psychological problems. The qualifications for professional work in this area are not as yet well standardized. Many psychiatrists are excellently equipped to serve persons who need this kind of help. A psychiatrist is a medical doctor who has specialized in the care of mental disorders and psychological problems. Some psychiatrists are experienced only in the care and handling of the psychoses and are not interested in less severe conditions, but psychiatrists are now being trained whose major interest is in the psychoneuroses and maladjustments. Many clinical and consulting psychologists are also competent to give effective counseling on personal problems. Not all psychologists are included in this category, of course, as those with a primary interest in pure and experimental psychology, or in applications to industry, personnel selection, test construction and the like, may have no experience at all as counselors. In addition to psychiatrists and clinical psychologists, there are some social workers, teachers, school counselors and clergymen who can give adequate psychological guidance, but the majority of persons in these professions are not prepared to do so.

Counseling and Psychotherapy

Psychological treatment is usually called *counseling* when it deals with minor adjustments and *psychotherapy* when it treats psychoneuroses or psychoses. The aims of counseling and psychotherapy are essentially the same: to free the individual from inhibitions and repressions and to give him improved insight into his own conflicts and adjustments, so that he can work out a more satisfactory solution to his problems. In most instances, the objective is to relieve him of anxieties and to change his attitudes rather than to teach him better conduct. The person's distress is the main problem, not his specific behavior. When the tensions are reduced, social behavior usually rights itself.

Experience shows that *advice* is a poor tool for counseling. A maladjusted person usually knows what he should do, but finds himself unable to carry out his own best judgment. *Reassurance,* the technique of convincing the client that he is not badly off, is also of limited value. It may be serviceable in specific and limited problems, as in dealing with a boy who is worried about masturbation. A person with real anxiety, however, knows that something is the matter with him, and reassurance does not reduce his anxiety, but only discredits the counselor for his apparent lack of understanding. In general, counselors have found that they cannot solve a client's problems for him; they can only provide an atmosphere that aids the sufferer to work out his own solutions.

A universal technique in counseling and psychotherapy is to get the client to talk about his conflicts and feelings. After he has told about his complaint, the counselor often uses *questioning* to draw out further information. Questioning has limitations, however, as it may cause the client to become defensive and to resort to rationalizations. A superior method is *reflection of feelings.* When using this technique, the counselor responds to each statement of the client by showing that he understands it, is deeply interested in the client and appreciates how the client feels. This method, which is sometimes called *nondirective counseling* and sometimes *client-centered counseling,* is illustrated by the following fragment of an interview. The client, L. H., is a discharged serviceman, whose problem is restless and 'nervous' behavior.*

1. L. H. "I don't know what's the matter with me. I just can't seem to settle down. I don't like to stick to anything. This job I've got should be all right for me, but I can hardly stand it to keep on working."

2. COUNSELOR. "You're worried and upset because you can't buckle down to whatever you start to do."

3. L. H. "That's right—I get all upset—I—I always seem to remember what

* C. R. Rogers and J. L. Wallen, *Counseling with returned servicemen,* McGraw-Hill, 1946, pp. 62–64.

happened to me in the Army. I really went through hell!"

4. COUNSELOR. "You feel that you really had a very tough time while in the Army."

5. L. H. "I'll say I did. [Pause.] Well, the first few years weren't so bad, but the last year was terrible. I never want to go through that again as long as I live. The men didn't associate with me much. I wouldn't say I had any friends there. Nobody had any use for me, and my commanding officer rode me something awful—you can't imagine how it was."

6. COUNSELOR. "You feel that quite a few people had it in for you."

7. L. H. "Yes, that's putting it mildly. It got so bad that they were always calling me vile names and I had to fight for any rights I wanted, and then finally I was wounded and got away from all that."

8. COUNSELOR. "It was almost a relief to you to be wounded and get away from all the things you went through."

9. L. H. "Yes, it was. [Pause.] But the pay-off to all this came when an Army doctor got hold of me. I told him a lot of very, very personal things that had no concern with the Army. He betrayed my trust and told my commanding officer all that I had confided in him. I could have *killed* him for that! I had a bad time telling anybody anything after that. [Pause.] But for some reason it seems different with you—you know I wouldn't tell you all this if I didn't trust you."

10. COUNSELOR. "Although the doctor made it hard for you to talk about your feelings, you have some confidence in me."

11. L. H. "Yes. You know I hated those men so much I could kill them. I would just think of all the things I'd like to do to them. Maybe that's not right, but that's the way I felt."

12. COUNSELOR. "You feel a little guilty about these intense feelings of hatred, but they were there nevertheless."

13. L. H. "Yes—in fact [pause]—I just about did kill a fellow. We got in a fight [tells details of the quarrel], and I hit him with a wrench. I guess I went out of my head."

14. COUNSELOR. "You feel you lost all control of your emotions for a while."

15. L. H. "You know I seem to get relief by just getting this out. You're the first person I've ever told that to."

16. COUNSELOR. "It helps you to talk about these things that you have been keeping to yourself."

The remainder of the interview was concerned with other aspects of his problem.

In addition to the reflection of feeling, interpretation is sometimes used to speed insight, that is to say, the counselor explains to the client something of the meaning and origin of his conflicts. When done skillfully, interpretation may be of great value. If it is given prematurely, before the client is ready to admit the interpretation himself, it may produce anxiety or cause the client to discontinue the consultations. If it is incorrect, the client may be anxious and confused. For these reasons, many counselors avoid interpretation altogether, and trust the client to gain insight through his own recollections.

In successful counseling the client gains insight into the sources and meaning of his feelings and behavior, and no longer reacts emotionally to his problems. Sometimes the insight comes gradually, sometimes suddently after a considerable number of interviews. When his tensions are reduced, the client is able to attack his difficulties rationally instead of emotionally. He overcomes some of his limitations and accepts those that he cannot overcome. Such a mixed solution is regarded as a satisfactory outcome of psychotherapy.

Psychoanalysis is a particular form of psychotherapy and also a theory of the nature of the process of treatment. A standard psychoanalysis is a very lengthy type of treatment, usually requiring daily sessions for a period of a year to several years.

The psychoanalytic theory of treatment is based on the hypothesis that all maladjustments originate from the conflicts that a child has toward his parents. In the analysis, the client develops *transference* toward his analyst, that is to say, the analyst becomes an emotional substitute for the client's father or mother. The infantile conflicts are then reenacted and worked through, with the result that the client is freed of their effects. Many psychologists believe that psychoanalysis as a theory neglects immediate conflicts and cultural influences by its excessive emphasis on the influence of early childhood. It does, however, produce strikingly favorable results in some cases.

Interpretation of Psychotherapy

The explanation of how and why psychotherapy is effective does not require any far-fetched hypotheses, but can be made in terms of familiar psychological principles. Essentially it is a subtle kind of learning process.

The relationship between the client and the counselor is the first essential of psychotherapy. The therapist is warm and interested, and evokes an attitude of trust and friendliness. He never expresses disapproval or disgust at any of the client's revelations, and never criticizes, lectures or advises. The counseling atmosphere is therefore a new social experience for the client. He finds after a few sessions that he does not have to be defensive and can talk freely about his fears, conflicts and aggressive tendencies without expecting censure.

As the client's social inhibitions are released by the counselor's attitude and method, he finds himself describing emotionally toned experiences about which he is ordinarily unable to talk, and remembering events whose recall had been repressed. In this phase of treatment, sometimes called *catharsis,* meaning purge, the client is responding to emotion-evoking stimuli in a nonreinforcing situation. Extinction of emotional responses takes place by unreinforced repetition, as in the conditioned reaction experiments (p. 142). The client now finds that he can face his conflicts with reduced anxiety.

The expression of previously inhibited emotional attitudes and the recall of repressed experiences permit the client to view his adjustive life more comprehensively than he could before the treatment. Thus he is led to gain *insight* about himself, his problem, his relationships to other people and the demands of his environment. Insight can sometimes be promoted by the counselor's interpretations, but it never can be forced. It has to be constructed by the client through his own problem-solving efforts. Insight is genuine and functional only when the client accepts it emotionally as well as intellectually. After insight has been achieved, the client usually makes his own self-initiated attempts toward readjustment. His new adjustments are superior to his old ones, because of his freedom from tension and his superior appreciation of reality. After all you can come to accept life—your own life—as it really is (1) *if* you can realize fully just what the reality of yourself in your world is like and (2) *if* you can get rid of the bitterness and emotion which go with not being able to have what you very much want. Psychotherapy helps you to learn how to want most what you can have.

MENTAL HYGIENE

The aim of mental hygiene is to aid people to achieve more satisfying and more productive lives, through the prevention of anxieties and maladjustments. It is unlikely that mental hygiene will ever be able to reach its goal completely, but much good can be done, comparable to the gains that medical hygiene has made in reducing the occurrence of disease.

Mental Hygiene in Childhood

The early years of life are most significant for mental hygiene because the initial habits of adjustment to human relationships are being formed during that period. A young child has limited resources for coping with his difficulties, as compared to an adult, and has a great need for understanding and assistance. Intense and unsolved conflicts in childhood can predispose an individual to adjustive difficulties throughout his life, just as the laboratory studies of experimental neurosis show that 'breakdown' leads to a continued impairment of the ability to resolve new conflicts. The relationships of the parents to a child are the basis of his principal early adjustments, because of the dependence of the child on his parents, the greater number of contacts he has with them and the emotional responses that the parent-child association evokes. Since parenthood is almost universal, progress in mental hygiene depends more on the understanding of children by parents than on any other factor.

Mental hygienists today agree that the most important characteristics of the parent-child relationship are *warmth* and *acceptance.* The child is inevitably dependent on his parents (or on parent substitutes) and experiences serious conflict if he feels that he is unwanted or unloved. This condition of rejection, leading to insecurity for the child, is probably the most important single cause of subsequent adjustive difficulties. Two causes of parental rejection of children can be distinguished. Some parents reject children because they are prevented from accepting and giving love by their own conflicts, or because the child represents to them a thwarting of their other motives. Such parents can be helped by working out their own problems with a counselor, but cannot be aided appreciably by books or advice. On the other hand, many parents reject children because they do not understand what a child needs, or because they have misconceptions concerning the value of 'discipline' and 'obedience' in character formation, or because they overvalue the child's need for independence. This kind of rejection is more easily remediable.

The acceptance of a child by his parents can be defined only in terms of the parents' real attitudes, not in terms of specific *do's* and *don't's* of child care. For example, there can be no rigid rule as to whether a child should be punished or not. It is true that continued and severe punishment almost always implies rejection and results in anxiety, aggressive antagonism or both. Occasional and appropriate punishment, however, may not be rejecting. It may actually relieve a child's anxiety when he feels guilty over his act, or it may show him that the parent cares about how he behaves. In fact a parent who never punishes may be rejecting, if his cold and excessive stress on independent responsibility shows that he does not care what happens to the child or what the child does. Warmth shows itself in a cumulative number of small expressions, not in accordance with any set of rules.

As in many other human problems, moderation is essential in the emotional development of children. Spinach may be healthful, but a whole diet of it is certainly not. Warmth and acceptance must be distinguished from a parental submission which fulfills a child's every whim, and is not hygienic. A mother who smothers a child with excessive affection is usually fulfilling some exaggerated need of her own and is not warmly accepting the child for his own worth. Acceptance implies not only the recognition of the child's need for dependence when he is very young, but also means the recognition of his need for independence as he grows older. An accepted child is, therefore, neither retarded nor pushed ahead in the development of his initiative but is permitted to grow to the adult state at his own pace. The child needs freedom as well as security and should not be prevented from growing up by the selfish needs of a dominating or possessive parent who wishes to maintain the child's dependence.

Another important aspect of the parent-child relationship is its *consistency*. The child's security depends on the dependability of his environment. He must know what he can count on. The most obvious inconsistencies are to be found in situations in which a child is praised for an act at one moment because it is 'cute' and punished at another time for substantially the same act because the parents are bored or annoyed. More subtle and frequent inconsistencies arise when a child is expected to be independent and capable in one respect, but is treated as immature and as requiring rigid supervision in another. Inconsistency prevents a child from learning his role in the family and from developing a clear conception of his own individuality. It may result in conflict, giving rise to either anxiety or aggression.

Another requirement for good mental hygiene is that a child must always be able to talk about his worries and problems with a parent, without fear of being ridiculed or rebuffed. A *confidential relationship* with a parent has the value of psychotherapy, in that the child can express his conflicts and get better insight into his own adjustments. Like a therapist, a good parent recognizes the child's problems calmly and also does not rob him of the opportunity to work them out on his own terms.

A handicap of many educated parents, especially of those who have studied psychology, is oversensitivity to a child's imperfections. If they recognize signs of anxiety in him, or defense mechanisms, they may be unduly disturbed about their own guilt and may rush in to make amends, often doing more harm than good with their emotional fervor. It must be remembered that a full acceptance of a child implies accepting him as the imperfect human being that every one of us is. A sense of proportion, and more than a touch of humor, will in these circumstances make a satisfactory therapist of the wayward parent.

Mental Hygiene for Adults

For adults who have anxieties, or who recognize evidences of poor adjustment in themselves, the most constructive step for mental hygiene is to secure professional help, from psychiatrists, consulting psychologists, college counselors or other qualified persons. Lacking such facilities, some aid can often be secured from friends who can be warm but objective listeners, from family physicians, teachers or clergymen. Recognizing the prevalence of the mechanism of projection, people who are having trouble with their parents, spouses, children or employers will also be wise to seek counseling for themselves. It is axiomatic at every child guidance clinic that the parents of a problem child need psychological aid as much as the child himself.

Most people do not need professional assistance, but can get some benefit from following some principles of mental hygiene, as indeed they do from knowing the common requirements of physical health. Just as acceptance is basic to the mental hygiene of childhood, so self-acceptance is a fundamental healthful factor in adult life. Self-acceptance does not mean smug complacency, but the recognition of faults and limitations that permits your living in peace with yourself. Most defenses and rationalizations are used for their individual adjustive value rather than for their social effect. Self-acceptance enables an individual to get along with a minimum of these hampering types of behavior and thought. For the more intellectually inclined, self-understanding, through a study of the psychology of personal adjustment, may contribute to acceptance. The study of your own behavior can become morbid if it leads you to feelings of inferiority. The person who sees himself reflected in a psychology book may be reassured, however, that he is reading of common human nature, and that untold numbers of other people, who are functioning effectively in life, show the same mechanisms.

Psychological principles and experience point to a number of other generalizations about adult mental hygiene. Social participation is invaluable for mental health, for a person who is a participant in a group forgets himself and directs his attention to reality and to the present. Everybody needs an experience of some success in self-expression. Many obtain it in their work, others in sports and hobbies. A rhythm of work, recreation and rest breaks up non-adjustive responses and gives you an opportunity to attack problems more effectively when the inhibitions arising from continued effort have been lessened.

A very general principle of mental hygiene is to apply the technique of scientific method, or of rational problem solving, to personal matters. Many people who are not markedly maladjusted rush into their interpersonal relationships with an unthinking abandon that they would condemn if it were applied to investing money, building a house or even to buying a new suit of clothes. The technique of defining the problem, gathering the data, making hypotheses and checking the results can profitably be applied by intelligent persons to the management of their own lives.

REFERENCES

1. Freud, S. Psychopathology of everyday life. *The basic writings of Sigmund Freud.* New York: Modern Library, 1938.

   Slips of the tongue, forgetting of names and similar events illustrate the common 'abnormalities' found in normal people.

2. Horney, K. *The neurotic personality of our time.* New York: Norton, 1937.

   A modified psychoanalytic theory, with emphasis on cultural conflicts as sources of maladjustment.

3. Hunt, J. McV. (Ed.). *Personality and the behavior disorders.* 2 vols. New York: Ronald Press, 1944.

These two volumes, the work of forty collaborators from psychology, medicine, anthropology and allied fields, give the most comprehensive survey of personality and its abnormalities.

4. Landis, C., and Bowles, M. M. *Textbook of abnormal psychology.* New York: Macmillan, 1946.

An excellent description of mental disorders, their explanation and treatment.

5. Lewin, K. Environmental forces. In C. Murchison (Ed.), *A handbook of child psychology.* (2nd ed.) Worcester, Mass.: Clark University Press, 1933. Chap. 14.

A clear introduction to the author's topological theory of personality.

6. Lewin, K. Behavior and development as a function of the total situation. In L. Carmichael (Ed.), *Manual of child psychology.* New York: Wiley, 1946. Chap. 16.

The 'field theory' or topological approach to personality and conflict, considered as an interaction between the individual and his environment.

7. Maslow, A. H., and Mittelmann, B. *Principles of abnormal psychology.* New York: Harper, 1941.

A good introduction to abnormal psychology which skillfully blends the experimental, psychoanalytic and cultural approaches.

8. Masserman, J. H. *Behavior and neurosis.* Chicago: University of Chicago Press, 1943.

Reports of ingenious experiments with cats clarify many problems of the production, effects and cure of conflicts.

9. McKinney, F. *Psychology of personal adjustment.* New York: Wiley, 1941.

Recommended to the college student who seeks help for his own academic, personal and social adjustments.

10. Rogers, C. R. *Counseling and psychotherapy.* Boston: Houghton Mifflin, 1942.

The book gives an excellent idea of the non-directive, client-centered method in interviewing by means of a full description of a series of eight interviews.

11. Rogers, C. R., and Wallen, J. L. *Counseling with returned servicemen.* New York: McGraw-Hill, 1946.

One of the clearest elementary descriptions of personal counseling, applicable to others as well as to servicemen.

12. Shaffer, L. F. *The psychology of adjustment.* Boston: Houghton Mifflin, 1936.

An account of the social and individual adjustment problems of normal people, from the point of view of objective psychology.

13. Shaffer, L. F. Abnormal psychology. In J. P. Guilford (Ed.), *Fields of psychology.* New York: Van Nostrand, 1940. Chaps. 9, 10 and 11.

The three chapters give a brief and clear survey of the significance, causes and varieties of abnormal behavior.

CHAPTER 23

Vocational Selection

THE individual's basic problem in life is his adjustment to the circumstances in which life places him, the personal adjustment which makes him—when it succeeds—what is called a 'well-adjusted person.' In the preceding chapter we have considered the psychological mechanisms by which that adjustment takes place.

Within the total area of his life, the individual usually—especially if he is a man—has to earn his living. He needs a job and, unless there is unemployment, he has a job. That, however, is not the same thing as having the right man in the right job. Some men are better fitted for one kind of work than another; different men have different aptitudes. And, if the men are properly fitted into their jobs, everyone benefits—the employee, the employer and society.

The employee benefits because either his work is easier or his production and pay are greater. Consequently his morale and job satisfaction are likely to be better. The employer benefits because he gets more work done. Either the worker produces more per hour or, because good morale reduces turnover, absenteeism and illness, the worker produces more per year. Society benefits because maximal efficiency and the maximal contentment are got by the best adjustment of men to their jobs.

Both the recent World Wars, with their shortages of manpower, have made it clear that aptitudes and skills are part of a nation's limited resources. They must, when short, be rationed and used with planned efficiency. This idea in itself is not new. As long ago as 1884 Francis Galton was sponsoring a plan to inventory the brains and abilities of all Englishmen so that his Government might know what resources it had for use in the promotion of British civilization. (He feared that the British were not so able as the ancient Greeks and hoped that, if the facts were known, selective parenthood might do something about the matter.) The Second World War with its manpower shortage forced attention to this basic problem of the use of human resources, and now vocational guidance and selection are used wherever practicable.

Since this development has grown out of psychological testing and is itself an important phase of modern applied psychology, the present chapter is devoted to an explanation of how in business and industry, and even in the professions, the right man can be got into the right job.

Contentment and satisfaction are not the proper criteria to use for this selection since employee and employer may easily not be satisfied with the same performance. For

This chapter was prepared by Carroll L. Shartle of Ohio State University.

example, a worker may consider that he is making a satisfactory vocational adjustment. He feels that he is earning a good living, he likes the kind of work and the work surroundings, and he considers he has reasonable security in his position. On the other hand, his employer may have quite a different view of the matter and reports that the worker, although steady and reliable, is a low producer compared with others. If the employee is then discharged, his union may present evidence that he is a success. In an arbitrated dispute it may be ruled that the employee was after all successful and must be retained by the employer. The employer, however, remains dissatisfied. It ought to be possible for all concerned to measure success more certainly.

Suppose we were making an occupational follow-up of graduates of a school. Should we consider the aforementioned worker successful in his chosen occupation? For such decisions criteria must be set up. Let us see what they may be.

CRITERIA

In studies of workers and their jobs a number of indices or criteria of success are usually explored. Sometimes a single criterion of success is chosen. In other cases two or more criteria are utilized, either singly or in combination. For example, success in selling a product may be judged by the number of new steady customers obtained during a given length of time, or the criterion may be put in terms of total sales or it may be a combination of both variables.

To a great extent the soundness of vocational selection depends upon how well the criteria of success have been developed and how they are interpreted in the applications of research findings to vocational guidance, vocational selection, training, promotion and other personnel procedures. For example, tests may be developed to measure the human characteristics required in a given occupation. The tests are administered to persons in the occupation. The scores of persons within the occupation who are most successful are then compared with those persons less successful. Is this a good method? It is, if we know how to assess success. The criteria of success are crucial. Let us see what some of them are.

Criteria of Vocational Success

Every person has his own set of values that he considers important in judging vocational success. Here are some of them.

Productivity. How much does the worker produce per hour, per day or per month? Wide differences are frequently found among workers in any given job. Figure 239 shows the distribution of sixty-two card-punch machine operators according to their criterion scores, the average number of cards punched per hour.

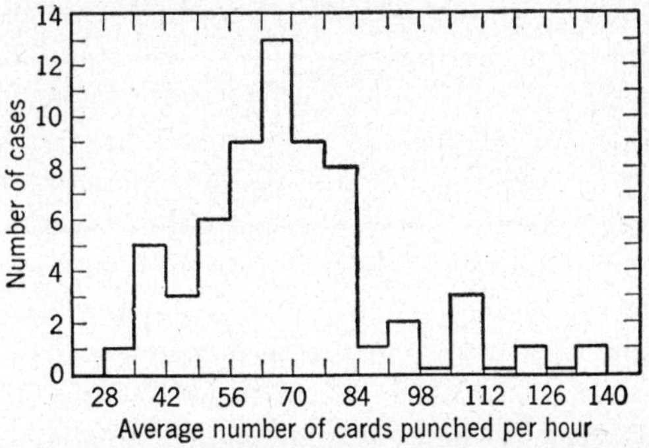

FIGURE 239. DISTRIBUTION OF CRITERION SCORES OF SIXTY-TWO CARD-PUNCH MACHINE OPERATORS

The criterion scores are average number of cards punched per hour.

Errors and accidents. Mistakes are often costly and, when adequate records of mistakes or errors are available, they may be used as one factor in judging success. Accidents are also sometimes used as a criterion. One worker may have several times as many accidents during a given period as another worker in the same job.

Tenure. Workers who are unsuccessful in a job may be discharged or may leave of their own accord. It is assumed in some occupational studies that, if a person remains in an occupation for several years, he is successful in it. For example, in standardizing an employment questionnaire, several hundred persons in each of several occupations filled in the items. It was decided to use five years of continuous experience in the occupation as the criterion for selecting the subjects.

Attendance. Workers who are frequently absent from a job or are tardy for work may be judged less successful than others. The employer wishes continuity and predictability. Moreover, frequent absence suggests discontent. Even illness can sometimes be had by wishing (p. 535).

Salary. Salary received has been used as a criterion of success, particularly in follow-up studies of college graduates. Persons, in occupations which have similar wage structures and where promotion is open to all, have been evaluated in terms of salary attained after a given length of time on the job. The individual worker often uses salary as a criterion in judging his own success. He may compare himself with others in his occupation or with associates in other occupations. His wife is likely to make similar comparisons.

Social values. A worker may evaluate his vocational success personally in terms of certain values outside of salary. The social position associated with various occupations is part of the psychological pay. What he lacks in dollars he gains in status. A worker also likes to feel that he is contributing something that society wants. Such values frequently come up in vocational counseling and may constitute a good reason for a worker's desire to change his occupation to one in which he believes his status will be better or where he believes he can make a greater social contribution.

Supervision. A man may be highly skilled in performing most of the tasks in his occupation, yet fail to work satisfactorily under supervision. He may have conflicts with his supervisor. Or the job may include the supervision of others, and the worker may fail in this respect. In a study made of jobs held by psychologists, proficiency in supervision was indicated as an important criterion of success in many of the jobs.

Cooperation with associates. Closely related to supervision is proficiency in working effectively with others. A man may be highly successful in all phases of his occupation but fail to work congenially as one of a group. Although his individual productivity is high, he may reduce cooperative activity and, for that reason, be judged relatively unsuccessful as an overall worker. These social factors often receive greater weight as a criterion of success than productiveness and tenure. Many employers believe that deficiencies in skill can be remedied by on-the-job training, but that it is difficult or impossible to train an uncooperative employee to work congenially with his associates.

Choice of Criterion

In problems of occupational adjustment the choice of a criterion or criteria of success depends upon many things. We may obtain an idea of some of the factors that must be considered from the following discussion of self-evaluation, employer-evaluation and kind of tasks.

Self-evaluation. One of the most frequent evaluations is made by the worker himself. He wants to know how successful or how unsuccessful he is in his job. He attempts to appraise his own progress not only in his present job but also in regard to his overall occupational plans. Such appraisals are usually highly subjective for they are likely to be based upon limited factual information. The worker hesitates to ask his supervisor for a frank appraisal of his performance or to seek advice from a competent vocational counselor. Supervisors are usually negligent in telling their subordinates exactly what is expected of them and how well they are progressing in the various phases of their jobs. It also may happen that events cause a worker to change his vocational plans and to apply a different set of values in attempting to judge his own progress. For example, the knowledge that a close friend has just received a substantial raise in salary may cause a worker to believe that he is quite unsuccessful and should change to some other kind of work. It is indeed seldom that any worker lists and attempts objectively to consider all the factors which are important in judging his own occupational achievement. He needs the help of a counselor.

A vocational counselor should be well informed concerning the various criteria frequently considered by workers as well as the criteria used by employers. The counselor can thus aid the counselee in evaluating his adjustment more objectively or in foreseeing the criteria which might be applied in the future if he entered a given occupation.

Employer evaluation. The employer frequently sets up criteria for evaluating job performance. Sometimes he uses rating scales, which are filled in by the supervisor at periodic intervals (p. 414). The results may be used as evidence in determining who shall be promoted, laid off, given additional training, transferred or demoted. Table XXX (p. 550) reproduces a rating form used by one employer for this purpose.

Employers also use rating scales in standardizing tests to discover the relationship of test scores to job performance. Production records, accident records and the appraisals of samples of work are likewise employed for the standardization of tests and are generally considered more objective and, therefore, better measures than ratings.

Kinds of tasks. The nature of the tasks in the job necessarily affects the kind of criteria which are available. In some occupations accidents occur so rarely that they are not a factor. In others the workers perform their tasks in groups, so that individual production records are not available. Sometimes a work-sample performance test is set up to allow the workers to perform for appraisal a sample of tasks that occur in the job. Each worker, of course, performs the same set of tasks under controlled conditions. This method has been used for establishing criteria for sewing machine operators, typists and package wrappers.

For standardizing tests an objective criterion is desirable. When that is not possible, ratings by supervisors must be used. If two or more criteria are available, the single best index of success is used or the several criteria are combined. Occasionally two criteria may be used independently. For example, in a study of bus operators, both the supervisors' ratings of

TABLE XXX

RATING FORM FOR VOCATIONAL COUNSELOR

Name____ Date employed________________

(Check the one item in each case which best describes the worker.)

1. How well informed is this counselor concerning occupational information, test score interpretation and other technical subject matter necessary for satisfactory performance?

____Fairly well informed but needs more background.
____About as well informed as one would expect for the work.
____Quite deficient, needs considerable training.
____Excellent knowledge, none could be better.

Comments____

2. In face to face situations how well does this counselor handle clients and their problems?

____Needs considerably more training and experience.
____One of the best in this phase of the work.
____Does an ordinary job.
____Can be counted upon to do better than average.

Comments____

3. In maintaining case records how successful is this counselor in understanding and following good practices?

____Records are complete and accurate at all times.
____Needs considerably more training.
____Does better than the average.
____Records are fairly well kept.

Comments____

4. How do you size up this counselor in following through and maintaining continued and effective counseling relationships with clients until the cases are closed?

____Does reasonably well.
____One of the best.
____Needs more supervision on this part than most other counselors.
____Seldom can be trusted.

Comments____

5. What is your overall appraisal of this counselor's work performance and prospects in the organization?

____Promising but needs more experience.
____Is ready for promotion now.
____Not very satisfactory, should be encouraged to try some other job.
____About an average worker.

Comments____

________________ Date

________________ Supervisor

performance and the accident records were available. In standardizing selection tests the overall rating of performance showed a satisfactory correlation with one set of tests and the accident records were positively related to another test. In the selection process applicants were required to pass *both* sets of measures. The personnel office hoped in this way to get men who would have both high performance ratings and good accident records.

JOB ANALYSIS

Two terms are frequently used in vocational psychology; they are *worker analysis* and *job analysis*. *Worker analysis* refers to a study of workers in jobs either individually or in groups. The workers may be given tests and interviews, and their backgrounds studied in order to discover their characteristics both on and off the job.

In *job analysis* the job is studied by observing what the workers do, by questioning supervisors and workers and by observing how the job fits into the organization and structure of the particular office or plant. The characteristics of the workers themselves are not studied, although the analyst may estimate what worker's characteristics appear important for the job. A job analysis is made to get the picture of the duties, the tools needed and machines used, the hiring requirements, the working conditions, the kind of supervision received and the apparent worker characteristics that are important for success in the job. The job analysis should precede a study of the workers, for it gives the essential background which the analyst must have to know what tests or other measures can be applied in a worker analysis.

In analyzing a job the investigator may actually learn the duties himself, becoming one of the workers, or he may act as an assistant to the worker whose position is being analyzed, or he may be only an observer. The first two methods are employed when detailed analysis is wanted, as in the development of testing procedures to measure the aptitudes required in an occupation. In other instances, job analysis may be very brief, being only such as is necessary to develop definitions or short descriptions of jobs. Sometimes a job specification is developed. That is a descrip-

TABLE XXXI

Job Specification for Personnel Assistant

Summary of Duties: After arrangements have been made by supervisor, analyzes jobs by observation of worker, by obtaining information from foremen and workers and other plant personnel. According to prescribed procedure, writes up each analysis and presents to supervisor for approval. Administers group tests to employed workers, scores tests and performs statistical analysis including computation of means, standard deviations and product-moment correlations.

Minimum Requirements

Educational: Graduate of an accredited college or university with at least 20 semester hours in psychology including one or more courses in tests and measurements and statistics.

Previous Experience: None. *Age:* 22–25. *Sex:* Male.

Special Characteristics: Must be able to write understandably and to work congenially with others in obtaining information.

Starting Salary: $175.00 per month. *Hours per week:* 40.

Promotional Possibilities: Top salary $225.00 after two years on the job. Ph.D. degree required for next higher position.

tion in which the hiring requirements are listed in some detail, although the description of the job is fairly brief. Table XXXI reproduces specification for the job of personnel assistant.

NATURE OF OCCUPATIONS

You begin to get some idea of the difficulty of vocational guidance when you discover how many different kinds of jobs there are.

A *job* is defined as a group of similar positions, and an *occupation* as a group of similar jobs. There are around 30,000 occupations in the United States. Of course, the number of jobs is many times that number, and there are as many positions as there are employed workers—58 million in 1947.

Dictionary of Occupations

Based upon job analyses, about 21,000 civilian occupations have been classified and defined. The classification structure and the definitions have been developed by the United States Employment Service and published in a document called the *Dictionary of Occupational Titles.*

The occupations defined in the Dictionary are grouped under seven major breakdowns. Table XXXII shows the major groups and the number of occupations defined in each.

Census Classification

Civilian occupations have been classified through the years by the Bureau of Census. This classification uses occupational and industrial titles only and does not include definitions, since in taking the federal census the respondents are not asked to list the duties of the job in which they are employed. Table XXXIII shows the major breakdown of the census classification and the total number of employed workers in each group.

The Army and Navy have also developed definitions of their various military specialties.

Characteristics of Occupations

In studying the characteristics of occupations it is found that occupations may be grouped in many types of classifications. Such special groupings are sometimes called *occupational families.* For example, occupations may be grouped according to the hiring specifications, types of machines used, special abilities required and other characteristics.

A study of the characteristics of occupa-

TABLE XXXII

Major Occupational Groupings and the Number of Occupations Defined under Each in Dictionary of Occupational Titles

Major Occupational Groups	*Number of Occupations Defined*
Professional and managerial occupations	1,837
Clerical and sales occupations	1,454
Service occupations	557
Agricultural, fishery, forestry and kindred occupations	297
Skilled occupations	3,820
Semiskilled occupations	7,819
Unskilled occupations	6,016
Total	21,800

TABLE XXXIII

Major Census Groupings and Number of Workers Employed in Each (1940)

	Total	Male	Female
Experienced Labor Force	*52,022,158*	*39,481,880*	*12,540,278*
Professional and semiprofessional workers	3,549,354	2,006,073	1,543,281
Proprietors, managers and officials, including farm	9,026,984	8,443,063	583,921
Clerical, sales and kindred workers	8,307,490	4,809,619	3,497,871
Craftsmen, foremen and kindred workers	5,877,094	5,751,857	125,237
Operatives and kindred workers	9,415,901	7,009,752	2,406,149
Protective service workers	740,876	733,420	7,456
Service workers, except protective	5,517,194	1,900,476	3,616,718
Laborers, including farm	8,605,256	8,139,309	465,947
Occupation not reported	982,009	688,311	293,698
Employed (except emergency work)	*45,166,083*	*34,027,905*	*11,138,178*

tions shows that the majority of them do not have any specific educational requirement although the ability to read and write is required for some of them. About half of occupations do not require previous work experience for entrance; more than half require an unusual amount of dexterity of hands, arms or fingers; and about a third are occupations requiring unusual strength. About 47 per cent of the occupations involve the use of machines, and about the same proportion involve the use of tools. Unusual keenness of vision is essential in about 20 per cent, and color discrimination is important in about 4 per cent of the occupations.

About 55 per cent of the working population are employed as machine operators, service workers and laborers, and about 7 per cent in the professional and semiprofessional occupations.

These figures outline the American scene. They do not show the resources of the United States in skills and aptitudes, but they show its needs. To maintain production requires plenty of manual dexterity and quite a little strength, but not so much education. It is with such qualities that the personnel expert concerns himself.

TRADE KNOWLEDGE AND PERFORMANCE

The measurement of trade knowledge and performance has been applied in industry, education and government to aid in the selection and assignment of persons to jobs which require previous experience or a specific skill. We have for use both *trade tests* and *performance tests.*

Oral Trade Tests

Oral trade tests were developed by the government for both World Wars to aid in evaluating the extent of knowledge in certain skilled trades, such as automobile mechanic or bartender. (The armed services do have uses for bartenders—with a change of name.) These tests measure knowledge only, and thus have definite limitations. Knowledge is not skill. A man may pick up a good deal of knowledge about an occupation from reading or conversation. It is also true that a highly skilled worker may be handicapped in his skill with language and do poorly on the test for that reason. Many a skilled craftsman does not quite know how he does what he does. He has his required skills but cannot verbalize them. Or he knows what he does without being able to state the general rule. He cannot tell you that the proper distance between the points on a timer is twenty thousandths of an inch, but he does know that a timer will work if you separate the points by the thickness of a tobacco tin.

Oral trade tests are composed of a series of trade questions which have been carefully worded and tried out on a group of subjects. The questions are put in simple language and in such a way that the correct answer can be given in a word or two. For example, it would be quite useless for a psychologist or interviewer to ask an applicant to describe how he would build a wooden structure. The answer would be long and detailed, and the interviewer, unless he was a skilled carpenter, could not judge its adequacy. On the other hand a specific question, such as, "What do you call the timbers that brace the studs?" could be evaluated at once by an interviewer if he had a key of correct answers. (The correct answer is, "Spacers," and in some localities "Bridgers" is just as good.)

Oral trade questions are standardized by administering them to skilled workers in a trade, to learners and helpers and to workers in closely related occupations who might in their work gain knowledge of the trade.

Table XXXIV shows how a set of fifteen oral trade questions differentiated expert machinists from apprentices and helpers, and apprentices and helpers from workers in related occupations. The median scores are shown by rows of x's. There is an overlapping of the scores between the experts and the apprentices and helpers, but the poorest of the experts scored higher than the best of the related group. In the standard-

TABLE XXXIV

Distribution of Scores on Oral Trade Test Questions

Score	Expert Machinists (Total: 101)	Apprentices and Helpers (Total: 50)	Related Group (Total: 50)
15	xxxxxxxxxxxxxxxxxx		
14	xxxxxxxxxxxxxxxxxxxxxxxxxxxxxxxxxx *		
13	xxxxxxxxxxxxxxxxxxxx	x	
12	xxxxxxxxxxx	xx	
11	xxxxxxxxx	x	
10	xxxxx	xx	
9	x	xxxx	
8	xxx	xx	
7		xxx	
6		x	
5		xxxxx	x
4		xxxxx *	xx
3		xxx	xx
2		xxxxxx	xxxxx
1		xxxxx	xxxxxxxx
0		xxxxxxxxxx	xxxxxxxxxxxxxxxxxxxxxxxxxxxxxxxx *

* Median score.

ization, each question was evaluated, and only those questions were retained which significantly differentiated both apprentices and helpers and the related group from the experts.

A satisfactory oral trade question is usually answered correctly by at least 80 per cent of the experts, by not more than 50 per cent of the apprentices and helpers and by less than 10 per cent of the related group.

Written tests have also been developed to measure occupational proficiency. Like the trade tests they are primarily tests of knowledge about the occupation. Civil service examinations are frequently of this type.

Performance Tests

Performance trade tests are a sample of the job performance. Stenographic and typing tests and performance tests for welders, automobile drivers and aircraft pilots are examples of performance tests which are frequently used.

Performance trade tests are used in vocational selection, in evaluating progress in learning an occupation and in appraising proficiency for granting permits or licenses.

Occupational proficiency can also be evaluated indirectly by appraising a person's experience or training in a personal interview or by a study of his work history and school record. Applicants for positions are more frequently examined by these less formal methods. In many instances, however, such records are not accurate or comparable, and it is difficult accurately to appraise job proficiency from them.

Actual tryout in the job itself is the best measure of proficiency. It is, however, usually an expensive procedure. Many employers have the practice, however, of hiring all new employees on a provisional basis. During this trial period the employee may be dismissed at once if he does not show the required proficiency.

VOCATIONAL POTENTIALITY

Everyone who works has at some time learned how to perform the tasks in a job. The preparation for professional occupations involves several years. In the simpler occupations where academic background is unimportant, often a worker would like to know how he would 'make out' if he entered a given job. Employers are reluctant to hire inexperienced workers unless there is evidence that the worker is capable of learning the job satisfactorily.

How well a vocationally untrained individual can learn and succeed in an occupation depends upon a number of factors and conditions. Psychologists have developed measures of potentiality that are useful as aids in attempting to estimate probable achievement.

Aptitude tests, for example, have been constructed to measure specific reactions which are analogous to those which occur in occupations. In the selection of streetcar motormen, applicants may be required to respond rapidly to signals with hand and foot levers in a laboratory. Such a test is not a measure of skill in street-car operation, but it does show in some degree how quickly and how well applicants could learn the job once they were employed.

Intelligence tests, interest tests, personality tests and *personal interview data* are also used as indicators of occupational potentiality to aid an individual in making vocational plans and to aid professional schools and employers in selecting individuals who will most likely succeed in training and in subsequent performance on the job. Measures of potentiality are not always sharply defined from tests of vocational knowledge and proficiency. For example, in one study a vocabulary test was found useful as an aid in predicting success in an engineering occupation. The test contained engineering and related terms. Although the test was used as one of potentiality, it contained some items of knowledge required directly in the occupation.

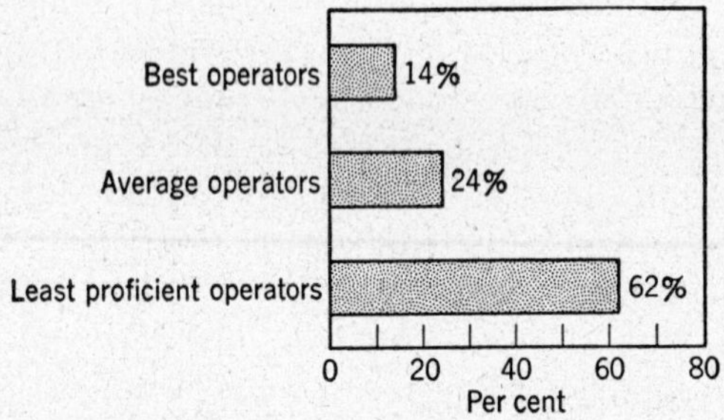

FIGURE 240. PERCENTAGE OF POWER SEWING-MACHINE OPERATORS WITH LOW TEST SCORES FOR EACH OF THREE GROUPS RATED DIFFERENTLY IN PROFICIENCY

Based on seventy-seven operators in two different plants.

Measures of potentiality must be standardized for any particular occupation. The usual method is to try out the measures on workers already in the occupation to discover the potentialities and what measures are related to them.

Figure 240 shows the results of administering a battery of aptitude tests to two groups of sewing-machine operators. It is noted that only 14 per cent of the best operators had low aptitude test scores, whereas 62 per cent of the least proficient operators had low scores. The supervisor of the workers in each sample compared each worker with every other worker, indicating which worker in each successive pair was the more proficient. The worker with the greatest number of 'firsts' received the highest rating.

The names given to tests do not always indicate what it is that the tests test. The tests given the sewing-machine operators included two subtests that are supposed to measure clerical aptitude and others that are meant for mechanical aptitude. A tester never knows what a test will do until after he has tried it out and determined its validity.

Intelligence

Intelligence tests have been related to occupational status more frequently by showing the differences in average test scores between occupational groups than by finding that they will differentiate the better from the poorer workers.

In both World Wars millions of men in uniform were given 'intelligence' tests. The scores made by soldiers who came from specific occupations were compared.

Table XXXV shows by civilian occupations the mean, standard deviation and range of Army General Classification Test scores for a sample of white enlisted men in the Army Air Forces. The differences between the mean scores of accountant and lawyer are not significant, but the means for these two occupations are significantly higher than those of any of the other occupations listed. In general, differences of five points or more between mean scores are significant in this sample. As in other such studies the overlapping of scores is considerable, but the overlapping up from the lower occupations is greater than down from the higher occupations. The upward overlapping may be due in part to the youth of so many of the subjects. Youth, lacking experience, seldom is

TABLE XXXV

MEAN GENERAL CLASSIFICATION TEST STANDARD SCORES, STANDARD DEVIATIONS AND RANGE OF SCORES FOR ARMY AIR FORCE WHITE ENLISTED MEN BY CIVILIAN OCCUPATION

[Data from T. W. Harrell and M. S. Harrell, *Educ. and psychol. Meas.*, 1945, **5**, 231–232.]

Civilian Occupation	*Number of Cases*	*Mean Score*	*Standard Deviation*	*Range of Scores*
Accountant	172	128.1	11.7	94–157
Lawyer	94	127.6	10.9	96–157
Teacher	256	122.8	12.8	76–155
Draftsman	153	122.0	12.8	74–155
Stenographer	147	121.0	12.5	66–151
Tabulating machine operator	140	120.1	13.3	80–151
Bookkeeper	272	120.0	13.1	70–157
Clerk, general	496	117.5	13.0	68–155
Clerk-typist	468	116.8	12.0	80–147
Radio repairman	267	115.3	14.5	56–151
Salesman	494	115.1	15.7	60–153
Manager, retail store	420	114.0	15.7	52–151
Machinist	456	110.1	16.1	38–153
Airplane mechanic	235	109.3	14.9	66–147
Receiving and shipping checker	281	107.6	15.8	52–151
Sheet metal worker	498	107.5	15.3	62–153
Auto serviceman	539	104.2	16.7	30–141
Butcher	259	102.9	17.1	42–147
Carpenter, construction	451	102.1	19.5	42–147
Auto mechanic	466	101.3	17.0	48–151
Truck driver	817	96.2	19.7	16–149
Laborer	856	95.8	20.1	26–145
Farmer	700	92.7	21.8	24–147
Farmhand	817	91.4	20.7	24–141
Miner	156	90.6	20.1	42–139

placed where all its intelligence can be used. Given time more men would rise in the occupational levels which the table shows than would fall, and eventually the spread about the average for each occupation would be just as much down as up.

In industry, intelligence tests are often administered to workers in order to determine hiring standards. Then lower limits and sometimes higher limits are set for employment. Sometimes a relationship has been found between intelligence test scores and job proficiency, but usually there are other better indicators of potentiality. (For a description of the Army General Classification Tests, see p. 405.)

Interests

Tests of vocational interest have been obtained by administering questionnaires to persons employed in various occupations. Items in the scales are then weighted so that in the scored test the client can see how his pattern of interests compares with the patterns for various occupations and fields of work.

In one interest test (Kuder Preference Record) scores are obtained for nine general areas: (1) mechanical, (2) computational, (3) scientific, (4) persuasive, (5) artistic, (6) literary, (7) musical, (8) social service, (9) clerical. Chemists have been found to be high in the scientific area, clergymen in the literary and social service areas and insurance agents in the persuasive area.

Occasionally items from interest questionnaires are used to differentiate poorer from better workers. For instance, in developing tests for the selection of salesmen, such items have been found useful. Each item is weighted by comparing the responses of the less proficient with the more proficient salesmen. In one study interest in music was found—surprisingly enough!—to differentiate salesmen significantly with respect to their proficiency.

Other Measures

Personality tests and personal data items (pp. 491–497) have been utilized as measures of occupational potentiality. Such items have been found useful, for example, in differentiating better from poorer salesmen. In one study of department store salespersons, the more proficient workers showed responses on personality test items which suggested that they were more 'extraverted' than the poorer salespersons.

In another study, place of birth, age at time of hiring, previous occupation, grade completed in school and other personal data were found, when weighted by statistical procedures, to differentiate better from poorer wholesale salesmen. That is a good example of how necessary it is to find out what the tests actually do. It is evident that you could not know which of these items would make up a suitable test until you had tested the test.

BASIC FACTORS IN OCCUPATIONAL SKILLS

When the scores on various measures of occupational potentiality are correlated with one another and given further statistical treatment, it is found that a relatively few factors seem to account for the numerous characteristics measured in the tests. Some of the factors found thus far in studies of aptitudes are indicated by the terms *dexterity, spatial, numerical, verbal, aiming, mechanical* and *speed*. Further research may result in the development some day of a basic test battery for occupational potentiality which will cover the essential factors now found in the various aptitude, intelligence, interest and personality tests. The amounts of these basic factors required for success in families of occupations can then be determined. It would become possible for a person, after taking the basic battery, to know how his potentialities measure up to the requirements in occupational families which cover thousands of separate occupations. And it would be just as possible for the employer, knowing the requirements of the job from his job analysis, to select the proper men for the job. The job and the worker can be brought together with the greatest efficiency and the greatest satisfaction to all concerned, when worker analysis and job analysis have shown clearly which belongs to which.

REFERENCES

1. Bingham, W. V. D. *Aptitudes and aptitude testing.* New York: Harper, 1937.

   An authoritative description of aptitudes and their measurement. A book widely used by vocational counselors.

2. Burtt, H. E. *Principles of employment psychology.* New York: Harper, 1942.

   Devoted to the descriptions of psychological techniques as applied to the selection of persons for jobs.

3. Shartle, C. L. *Occupational information.* New York: Prentice-Hall, 1946.

Describes how information about jobs is developed and applied, giving many examples.

4. Stead, W. H., Shartle, C. L., and Associates. *Occupational counseling techniques.* New York: American Book, 1940.

Describes the development of trade and aptitude tests for use in vocational counseling.

5. Tiffin, J. *Industrial psychology.* (2nd ed.) New York: Prentice-Hall, 1947.

Covers the use of tests in their application to industry, giving many examples.

6. Viteles, M. S. *Industrial psychology.* New York: Norton, 1932.

An older book, which nevertheless covers the field well.

CHAPTER 24

Attitudes and Opinions

EACH individual starts life in a particular culture composed of institutions, laws, fashions, language and objects of all kinds that are characteristic of it. To keep this seemingly obvious fact ever in mind is essential from the outset. If we propose to study our own culture, we must understand with as much objectivity and perspective as possible the basic assumptions and the predominant modes of thought and behavior that provide the framework for our observation. We must, somehow, jump out of our own skins in order to look at ourselves and our own kind as we would at laboratory subjects.

For example, suppose an American, interested in determining the attitudes of adolescents toward different occupations, finds that the banker and the business executive are most highly esteemed, the lawyer and the doctor next, the engineer and the carpenter and the mason last. Can he conclude that there is something about banking or the practice of law that makes its devotees more respectable than would carpentry or brick laying? He should not come to such a conclusion, although he often does. There is a fallacy here. The American is observing within a particular social framework—the United States—and it is only within this framework that his conclusions are valid. Were he to go to Soviet Russia, he might find his conclusions completely reversed. Or even were he to carry on his study in a small rural community where the local doctor was the outstanding citizen, his findings might likewise be upset.

If he decides to compare the vocational ambitions of children in different cultures, instead of inquiring what the attitudes of children are toward different occupations, the question which he must really ask turns out to be: How does the social framework within which an individual is born determine his attitude toward different vocations? In other words, unless an American has this perspective, he will fail to recognize some of the major problems in his field.

SOCIAL NORMS

Every culture surrounding every individual is, then, more or less specific. In some cases its limits are natural boundaries, such as mountains or oceans. In other cases it is limited by the imaginary lines separating one 'nation' from another. In still other situations, the boundaries are merely class, custom, language, income, education, sex or age. Two people living in the same city may, from the point of view of psychology, be living in quite different

This chapter was prepared by Hadley Cantril of Princeton University.

cultures, subjected to quite different social stimulus situations. To one man may come wealth, prestige, security, while no more than a block away there may live an unskilled laborer, poor, unknown and unsure of his job. The social frames of reference within which these two men think, feel and act will turn out to be almost as different as those of an Eskimo and an Australian Bushman—possibly, indeed, even more different. If both the Eskimo and the Bushman happen to be leaders or slaves, their social frames of reference may have a good deal more in common than those of the two neighbors in the city.

There are many assumptions, habits and customs that most people living in the United States at the present time take for granted but that would seem queer enough to many an outside observer unacquainted with our culture. A few examples are the following: that a man should have only one wife, a woman only one husband; that we should eat three times a day, using knives and forks; that we should regard roast beef and roast pork as delicacies but eschew whales' fins or dried mice; that most business and professional work should be done by men, and most housework by women; that we should elect people to govern us; that we should have a stock exchange.

Such basic assumptions, customs, institutional patterns of behavior—as well as forms of art, of buildings, and the characteristic shapes, sizes and uses of the products of our particular technological society in which we happen to live—may all be described by the term *social norms*. In our own culture these norms may be represented by such widely different examples as a football game, a skyscraper, democracy, a diatonic musical scale or an automobile, all of which may be regarded as social norms, since each has been created and accepted and passed on to the next generation by groups of individuals. Other cultures, however, have other norms: cricket, igloos, dictatorship, the five-interval musical scale or jinrikishas.

Particularly important for those who would study people's attitudes and opinions is the fact that, among these norms, there are standardized and accepted value judgments which are transmitted to the newborn individual. When, for example, we learn about democracy, we also learn that democracy is a 'good' thing; when we hear about football games, we infer that people 'approve' of them; when we learn about thieves, we are warned that they are 'bad' men. As we shall see, the fact that we learn how we should judge or evaluate a custom, an institution, a shape or a symbol at the same time that we learn *about* that custom, institution or shape is of the utmost importance if we are to understand social behavior.

It is these social norms that form a large share of the social stimulus situation to which a person responds. The person does not, to be sure, react to the abstract value or norm itself; he reacts to its concrete representation. We do not stop at a corner because of a vague norm called 'the law,' but because the policeman bars the way, because there is a traffic signal and because we ourselves fear what might happen to us if we did not stop. We are taught to salute the flag, to sing The Star-Spangled Banner, to buy Liberty Bonds, and in all these ways we learn the abstract value of patriotism. Yet each of these specific objects or modes of behavior must in the end be regarded merely as socially accepted representations of those more generalized ways of thinking or acting approved by our particular society.

These norms have emerged in the long process of human interaction. In spite of the fact that norms generally tend slowly to change, it is not true that there is anything absolute or fixed about them. If this were true, obviously, we should not experience the social change which is so characteristic of man's society.

We have seen that these norms make up the social stimulus situation for an individual. The importance of this fact must be underlined if we are to avoid the pitfalls of those writers who have tried to explain the behavior of different peoples by mystical racial theories or by typologies of one sort or another (pp. 431–433). For since norms are first external to the individual, the conclusion is inevitable that no person—and that means the members of no group nor of any particular nation or culture—is endowed at birth with any particular set of attitudes or opinions. They are all acquired (learned) in the process of socialization. Therefore, if we really want to understand what is meant by the phrase *human nature,* about which many laymen and political leaders make hasty generalizations, we must understand what this process of socialization involves. We shall trace this process briefly in the present chapter and leave for the next a more detailed account of some of the mechanisms involved and some of the consequences in terms of individual group relations and social adjustment.

THE PROCESS OF SOCIALIZATION

Social norms may be regarded as forming the *superstructure* of the society into which the individual is born. If he is to live satisfactorily in his society, avoiding jails and mental hospitals where the persons who deviate from the norms are isolated, he must as he grows up somehow make these values or norms a part of himself. Most of us have unwittingly incorporated in our conduct the behavior and thought patterns of our particular culture. What this means, essentially, is that somehow the norms of the culture, which, to repeat, are first external to us, have become an intimate part of us, have become *our* attitudes, attitudes that direct or determine our behavior and thoughts. We may define an attitude as *a mental set which directs an individual's response.* (On the relation of *attitude* to *need* and *set,* see p. 126.)

There are, of course, many ways in which we derive or learn our attitudes. If we really want to know how a particular person has acquired a particular attitude, we must probe deeply into his life history and personality make-up. The chances are that we would find his attitude was determined in one of the following three ways: (1) by the uncritical acceptance of social norms, usually through suggestion, (2) by the generalization of personal experience or (3) by some strong emotional experience.

Acceptance of Social Norms

The first and by far the most important and most common method is for the individual to accept an attitude whole from a culture before he has necessarily had any contact with the specific objects toward which the attitude is later directed. We learn, that is, how we *should* regard things before we see the things themselves. A demonstration of this fact is found in a study of the development of attitudes toward the Negro. An investigator was interested in determining the differences between the attitudes of northern and southern children toward the Negro. He obtained for his study different groups of children: groups in rural and in urban Georgia and Tennessee, children in an all-white school in New York City, children in a mixed school in New York City and children of Communist parents. His results indicated that there are no great differences in the attitudes of rural and urban children in the south, that children in both the north and the south have about the same prejudices at about the same age, that children in an all-white school develop the same prejudice as children in a mixed school, but that children of Communist parents do not develop an unfavorable attitude toward the Negro. On the basis of these results it was concluded that "attitudes toward Negroes are chiefly determined not by contact with Negroes, but by contact with the prevalent attitude toward Negroes." In other words, children accept in toto and uncritically the frame of reference provided in their immediate culture, and that without necessarily having had any experience whatsoever upon which to base the standards they accept. (See also p. 604.)

Another study illustrating the same point was made by investigators who had students place in rank order their preferences for various national and racial groups. A comparable set of students was asked to pick out from a long list of adjectives those terms they thought most characteristic of the same national and racial groups. Those groups that had been rated high by the first set of students were assigned the most favorable adjectives by the second set. Similarly the racial groups at the bottom of the list were characterized unfavorably. The important point of the experiment is that all the students who participated in this experiment made their judgments glibly and easily or selected their adjectives without any real knowledge of the racial or national groups or any previous experience with them. In other words, they blindly applied the traditional stereotypes of their culture to these groups. A *stereotype* is a conventional concept of the appearance, character or habitual behavior of a person or thing. It is derived—usually unwittingly—from the culture more than from experience and it is changed only with difficulty. (See p. 599.)

Suggestion

One of the most important basic concepts in the field of social relations is *suggestion,* for it is largely by its means that a person acquires the stereotyped norms of his community, his religion, his politics, his racial prejudices, his ethical and esthetic standards. If the majority of people in this country are Democrats or Republicans, it is not because they have made careful analyses of Anarchism, Socialism, Fascism or the other political points of view found in our modern world, not because they have decided on the facts of their study that the particular principles for which the Democrats or Republicans may stand are superior to those of other doctrines. On the contrary, they are Democrats or Republicans because they have acquired the particular norms of their culture.

The norms have the advantage of providing us with relatively fixed and limited standards of judgment by means of which we interpret or give meaning to specific events. Without such standards of judgment, which we may call *frames of reference,* we should be at a loss how to conduct ourselves in a complex world. Since the limits of time and energy forbid our reasoning out an opinion on every issue where we need to have some such opinion, we uncritically accept, instead, the prevailing norms and then try to rationalize them to ourselves.

We may define *suggestion* as the *acceptance by an individual of a frame of reference without the intervention of critical thought processes.* When a person has no standard of judgment but has a desire for some standard, he may accept a judgment uncritically. For example, a person, who, knowing nothing about music, nevertheless feels that he should know something about it, will accept the critic's judgment of an artist's performance or of a new symphony. Or an individual may accept a suggestion because it is consistent with some frame of reference (attitude, opinion, belief) which he already possesses. In this latter case, the suggestion merely reinforces his established opinion.

It is largely because of suggestion that advertising is so successful. Generally the advertiser tries to show how his product will help us attain some desired goal, how vital it is in achieving that end. If we use his soap, we shall all, he tells us, be social successes; if we smoke his cigarette, we shall be athletic; if we serve his whiskey, we shall impress business associates.

Frequently the advertiser makes use of what we know as *prestige suggestion* by telling us of the famous people who use his product. A recent automobile advertisement informs us, "During the past year, for instance, —— was chosen by 2 members of the English Royal Family, 33 diplomatic representatives of 21 countries, 8 government officials of Ecuador, a judge of the Supreme Court of China, etc." Such an advertisement not only calls attention to the product, it also provides a highly valued frame of reference (the prestige of the diplomat) by means of which the product may be judged.

The influence of prestige in the acceptance of dogmatic statements has frequently been demonstrated. In one study the experimenter first determined from his subjects what well-known persons they liked best and what ones least. Then he presented the subjects with a questionnaire containing thirty statements, such as the following, with instructions to mark on a five-point scale the degree to which they agreed or disagreed with the statement: "There is nothing sacred about the American Constitution. If it doesn't serve its purpose, it should be changed as often as necessary."

A third of the subjects were given the impression that the statement had been made by one of their best-liked people (like Mark Twain or Woodrow Wilson). Another third were given to understand that it had been made by one of their most disliked people (like Big Bill Thompson or Aimee Semple McPherson). For the third group the statement was attributed to no one. In this manner the investigators found that statements were in general more likely to be accepted when attributed to well-liked people than when attributed to disliked persons.

Suggestibility to majority opinion is also common in everyday life. In another experiment a test of attitudes was given to nine hundred people, who were subsequently divided into three groups, A, B and C. One month later the persons in Group A were told that the majority of people had answered a certain way in the previous test; Group B was told that certain experts had given unanimous opinions in a certain direction; and Group C, used as a control group, was told nothing. When the three groups were retested, it was found that those in Group A had changed their opinion in the direction of the majority about four times as much as the control group, whereas the people in Group B had changed almost twice as much as those in Group C.

Studies on the conditions of suggestibility have indicated that children are more suggestible than adults, that women are more suggestible than men, that certain primitive peoples are more suggestible than more civilized groups. It would be easy to draw false conclusions from these experiments. There is almost certainly nothing inherent in the child, the female or the primitive to make them more suggestible. These groups have merely had comparatively little experience in certain fields of activity and consequently possess less knowledge concerning the propositions on which tests are usually made. As their training and experience increase, so will their dependence and suggestibility diminish. Factors such as fatigue, depression, excitement and fear also increase suggestibility, inhibiting or interfering as they do with maximum critical thought. (For more on suggestion, see pp. 55 f. and 593.)

Formation of Attitudes

A second way in which we get our attitudes is the reverse of the uncritical acceptance of social norms. We generalize on the basis of our own present or past experience rather than accept a conventionality for the interpretation of later experience.

Experiments indicate that the pattern of behavior which we call *honesty* is, in our own culture, acquired by a person only after he has learned to react in specific ways in specific situations. A child can learn not to steal apples, not to copy from his neighbor's arithmetic, not to tell lies. He has, at first, no idea that these specific behaviors are called by society "dishonest." But, as he matures, he gradually learns the meaning of the concept honesty so that, by the time he is an adult, he is able to interpret a new possible behavior as honest or dishonest. A difficulty which an individual encounters in forming consistent attitudes derives from the fact that the norms of different reference or membership groups—groups with which the individual identifies himself—conflict with one another, so that what may be regarded as honest behavior by a child's classmate at school may be something quite different from what is regarded as honest behavior by the same child's neighborhood alley gang. An adult also may be subjected to a conflict of the norms of different membership groups to which he feels he belongs. A businessman who, as a church member, accepts the golden rule may, as a businessman in a sharply competitive system, find that he cannot survive unless he outwits his competitors.

Emotional Origin of Attitudes

A third way in which the individual may evolve an attitude is by means of some intense, traumatic experience. Though this particular method is comparatively rare, it may be of the utmost importance in determining certain attitudes of certain people. For example, a young American soldier who had believed strongly in God and had in civilian life attended church regularly was severely wounded in action during the Second World War. While lying on the battleground he prayed that the medics would reach him in time to bind his wounds and carry him to safety; but before they came a shell exploded near by, blinded the young man and tore off one of his arms. As he reports the case, at that point he became a confirmed atheist. Some persons may develop an attitude toward a certain race because they were once frightened (or imagined they were frightened) by a member of that race. Others may change their attitudes toward money because they have suddenly lost or suddenly acquired a fortune.

EFFECTS OF ATTITUDES

Once attitudes have been learned they determine to a large extent what an individual perceives and how he behaves. For example, two observers watching the same event take place may, if they differ in their attitudes toward the stimulating situation, perceive quite different things. An observer's set or readiness to perceive a certain thing, usually the thing he *wants* to perceive, may modify greatly his interpretation of the situation.

Two college students from two different schools watched representatives of their respective institutions engage in a boxing match in a college tournament. The fight was the last and deciding bout in a tournament to determine the Intercollegiate Championship. Although, as a matter of fact, the two boxers were very closely matched, they did not seem so to these two observers. Observer A thought that the boxer from his school gave his opponent a sound thrashing. His every punch landed with a thud, whereas the blows he himself received were but glancing blows that did not appear to bother him. Observer B thought that his school's representative was making such effective use of his right hand that the other fighter was groggy during the third round. When the judges decreed that A's boxer had won, B went home complaining about the poorly qualified judges. The attitude of each student toward anything identified with his college had determined in part what he would perceive.

An experimental study involving suggestion by prestige was made of the effect of attitude on perception with the use of the *autokinetic phenomenon* (p. 239). It will be recalled that this is the phenomenon in which an observer in a strange dark room watches a tiny stationary point of light, which, though actually immobile, is perceived to move. It has been found that induced attitudes will affect an observer's illusory perceptions of the movements of such a light. When a naive subject is asked to make judgments as to the amount and direction of the movement after hearing like judgments made by an advanced student in psychology, he tends to follow the sophisticated student in his judgment. That is prestige suggestion. An attitude, built up during the time the observer heard judgments being made, determines his perception of the ambiguous stimulus.

The literature of social psychology abounds in studies which show that our everyday behavior is directed by acquired attitudes and follows the same psychological principles that can be studied in strict experimental situations.

Experiments have demonstrated the effect of the attitudes of college students toward artists on their judgments of the esthetic value of pictures. To one large group of college students an experimenter showed eight pictures, to some of which were attached the names of artists known to be great (Raphael, Rubens, Rembrandt, da Vinci), whereas the others revealed names of little-known artists. The students rated each picture on a five-point scale (1 for 'best,' 2 for 'next-best,' etc.). A second comparable group of students rated the same pictures, with the famous names substituted for the unknown names, and conversely. The students tended to rate the pictures higher when the name of a person who was known to be a great artist was attached. Here the attitude of the observer toward certain artists consisted in part of a readiness to see beauty in a picture—a predisposition which resulted in his seeing what he expected to see. Suggestion by prestige depends on the fact that individuals acquire toward well-known people attitudes which influence favorably the interpretation of their statements.

Studies made on the voting behavior of American citizens show that, by and large, the overwhelming majority of people vote for the party they have learned to identify themselves with, the one for which they have acquired a favorable attitude. Only a very small percentage of American voters seem in any way to cast their ballots according to any logical analysis they make of the major issues of the day. They tend, on the other hand, to rationalize the particular point of view of their party or the particular candidate their party has proposed for a given office as the 'right' stand to take on the issue or as the 'best' candidate available. Over two-thirds of the people who actually vote a straight party ticket say, at the same time, that they always vote for the 'man' rather than the 'party.' Yet analysis of their past voting behavior shows that the 'man' they have voted for has always been a member of their party.

Other studies concerned with people's judgments of different occupations in terms of their social usefulness, their prestige and the like clearly indicate that these judgments are the result of acquired attitudes and have practically no relationship whatever to any experience a person has had with that occupation or any real knowledge of its requirements or social usefulness. Comparative studies of the values children in the United States and children in the Soviet Union place on different occupations show quite clearly how their preferences derive from social values uncritically accepted. American children, for example, tend to rate bankers and lawyers higher than skilled workers, whereas the reverse is true for children brought up under the Soviet system.

Studies of rumor show that the rumors we tend to believe are those that fit in with our preexisting attitudes and that rumors become changed, twisted or distorted as they are passed on according to the particular cultural traditions or group interests of the individuals who accept them and adjust them before passing them on.

DEVELOPMENT OF THE EGO

The attitudes a person acquires—whether they are widely accepted social attitudes or whether they are attitudes almost unique to a single individual and acquired from his own experience—do not exist in a vacuum, unrelated to one another. You can see from your own introspection that your attitudes have a peculiarly personal quality, that they are *your* attitudes, that they are in large part what you regard as *yourself.* If someone insults the parents whom you dearly love, *you* are insulted. If someone praises your college, *you* are pleased. If someone you regard highly receives a great public honor, *you* are happy. Most of our attitudes, then, can properly be described as ego attitudes, as attitudes that involve *us,* that form the constellation of our egos.

The development of the *ego* from the newborn child to the adult, although a long and complicated story, is nevertheless a clear story from the point of view of the psychological principles it reveals, for it shows that the formation of the ego in the individual is concomitant with the development of the perceptual processes and the formation of attitudes. The infant, for example, has to learn fairly early in life to differentiate his own body from the objects that surround him. And gradually he does learn that *he* is something somehow different from the things around him and something to which things happen and something which can cause things to happen. The child learns that *he* has a name; he learns that certain things are *his;* he learns that there is such a thing as *his* family, as *his* playmates, and *his* home, *his* school, *his* country, *his* race, *his* religion, *his* political party and the thousand and one other identifications which go to form the particular pattern of attitudes that become his ego—for that is what the ego is, a pattern of attitudes. (See also pp. 593 f.)

The ego we are considering here is, therefore, nothing innate or biologically determined as a person's sex, his abilities or the color of his hair is determined. The ego is acquired, and the particular ego an individual forms, the attitudes that constitute a large and important part of his *me,* depend to a very large extent on the particular cultural and group influences to which he has been exposed. And since the social stimuli that surround us are constantly changing, constantly varying as we grow up and are subjected to new influences or new social conditions, our egos can never be regarded as static. For example, in the important period of adolescence, when the individual is developing sexually and becoming conscious of a whole host of social conditions and groupings his culture has created to take account of sex distinctions, mating and the care of children, we can very properly say of the adolescent at this time that his ego is being re-formed.

Just as the ego develops in the child and becomes re-formed in the adolescent, so also it can break down, disintegrate or change radically under catastrophic or otherwise exceptional conditions. For example, there is ample evidence that the egos of many people who had been put in Nazi concentration camps became completely altered by the horrible experiences to which they were subjected. In time a number of people in these camps lost many of their old allegiances and identifications and, in order to survive in the camp at all, came gradually to accept new allegiances and identifications more in conformity to Gestapo standards and practices. In critical times—during severe depressions or periods when old social standards have so broken down that they no longer provide a person with the status his former ego identifications had given him—people are likely to seek new allegiances, identify themselves with new leaders, be attracted by new slogans or in other ways acquire new ego attitudes which give new direction to their behavior.

It is impossible to understand the motivation of a person in his social life unless we take into account these ego attitudes. these identifications which provide status and the goals which an individual thinks are worth striving for.

Effects of Ego Involvement

A few illustrations taken from the experimental laboratory and from everyday life will show the functional role played by ego involvement in determining perception and behavior.

In one experiment the degree of confidence which subjects felt with respect to various tasks they were asked to perform was clearly shown to be a function of ego involvement. The subjects in this experiment were asked in their first experimental session to perform various operations in volving mental addition, definition and the like. All were asked to indicate on a seven-point scale how much confidence they had in their answers. In this first session the subjects participated in a free and easy manner without any emotional strain. Then a few days later they were asked to participate in a second session, and this time they were told that the tests they were about to take were part of a general intelligence test and that the results of it were to be put on record in the personnel bureau of the college. All the subjects in this second sesson felt under strain and all exerted themselves considerably more than they did in the first session. The results of the whole experiment showed that in the first or 'neutral' session there were very low correlations between the scores on various tests and the confidence rating on those tests; whereas in the second or ego-involved session, although the correlations between the scores on the various tests remained low, the correlations of the subjects' confidence ratings were high. In other words, the introduction of ego involvement aroused a general level of confidence not aroused under a situation which was similar in all respects except the important one of motivation.

The effect of ego-involved attitudes on the learning and forgetting of material has been demonstrated in a number of different studies. We have already seen how, in one study, investigators measured their subjects with an attitude scale toward Communism, and then later asked the subjects to learn materials, some of which contained matter favorable to the Soviets and some matter unfavorable (p. 193). The subjects learned more and remembered more of the material that agreed with their beliefs. Usually it is harder to learn and harder to remember what you disbelieve.

The ego involvement in everyday life is apparent whenever we turn to look for it. For example, people who pay some attention to the clothes they wear (and that includes most of us) find that clothes offer one of the easiest and most concrete expressions of their status. Frequently those who are members of the 'upper class' or who are eager to distinguish themselves in some way from other people indulge in some kind of exclusive attire. Professors will display Phi Beta Kappa keys but not wear zoot suits. The enormous success of advertising in the United States cannot be accounted for unless we have regard to the ego attitudes, for a great deal of advertising is meant to show how your status—by your bodily appearance, your lack of bodily odor, the kind of radio you have or the kind of car you drive—can be maintained or enhanced if you will but buy the product the advertiser has to sell. Studies made on job satisfaction repeatedly show that a worker's satisfaction with hours and wages is not enough to give him real psychological satisfaction in his job. Although fair wages and hours are, of course, essential to job satisfaction, a major component of such satisfaction is the worker's own feeling of his importance, his role or his status and involvement in carrying out his job. He wants to feel that he is an active participant in the particular process of production or distribution with which he is associated, and he does not get complete satisfaction until he is able to identify himself with this process. (See pp. 482 f.)

The Ego and Group Loyalty

We have already noted how one of the important sources from which an individual acquires or learns his attitudes is the nexus of group relationships in which he participates. In understanding some of the group relationships discussed more in detail in the next chapter, it may be helpful here to make a distinction between what we may call an individual's *reference* groups and his *membership* groups. *Reference group* refers to a broad grouping, like a nation, a class, an occupation, an age group. *Membership group* refers to a smaller, more specific group, like the family, the school, the club, the union or the church. We all develop certain loyalties and allegiances to certain reference and membership groups. These loyalties and allegiances are ego-involved attitudes that, by and large, determine our general social status. Generally speaking, we achieve status by identifying ourselves with reference to membership groups that are socially acceptable. Some people at some times, however, find it difficult to satisfy their needs or achieve certain goals by accepting as *their* attitudes the norms of society or the norms of different groups that are socially acceptable.

Members of delinquent gangs, for example, are by and large members of such gangs not because of inborn personality traits or characteristics but because, for some reason or other, the socially approved ways of achieving status have been denied them or are inaccessible. So these boys and girls drift into already established groups or create groups of their own which have standards or norms that do not conform to those of the larger society that surrounds them. Within the microcosm of the gang they find they are able to achieve status by allowing the norms of the gang to determine the definition of what is right and wrong, what is honest and dishonest. They accept these standards as their own, identify themselves with them and become delinquents.

Many of the conflicts which the 'normal' individual experiences in our society are due to the fact that individuals identify themselves with membership or reference groups that have themselves contradictory or conflicting standards. Identification with a group in conflict means assimilation of the conflict. For example, one of the underlying psychological reasons for the difficulties encountered in forming an international organization, like the United Nations or some other form of world government, is that, although the majority of people want some form of international regulation, they have so identified themselves with their own countries that they are unwilling to give up what they regard as *their own* national sovereignty in favor of the larger grouping. In the same way, a man who is called out on strike often suffers from the conflicting allegiances he has to his union and to his family. The union uses these strikes as a weapon for eventual higher standards of living, but his family will suffer an immediate and perhaps prolonged lowered standard of living if the breadwinner goes on strike. The American college student may experience conflicts because of contending standards of different membership or reference groups with which he has identified himself. What is expected of him as a fraternity man may not completely conform to what is expected of him as a scholar. His desire to achieve a prominent place on an athletic team may interfere with his loyalty to his parents who expect of him an outstanding academic record. He may feel that some of the subjects he has to take in college in order to achieve the status of a college graduate conflict with his ideas of what he should be learning in order to achieve success in his chosen vocation.

ATTITUDES AND SOCIAL CHANGE

Broadly speaking, social change depends on the relationships that hold in any society or group between the superstructure of norms of that society or group and the needs of its individuals. These needs of the individual include not only the biological needs like the needs for food, sex, shelter, but also the learned needs, which are based on such attitudes as our desires for a certain kind of food, a certain kind of mate, a certain kind of house, as well as our ego strivings, which include our desires for status, for certain social rewards and a place within a group which we respect and with which we have learned to identify ourselves.

Most of these learned needs derive from social norms, and frequently the individual is frustrated in his attempt to satisfy the demands which his culture makes. It is our purpose here to enter into the many reasons for the discrepancies that exist in most societies between the needs of the individuals and their satisfaction. We should have to explain why it is that some people do not get all the food they want in countries potentially able to produce enough food for all, why more people cannot have as much education as they want and many other matters that depend on the structure of society and its functioning. The point that needs emphasizing here is that the frustration of needs, whether these needs are biologically rooted or whether they are socially derived like ego strivings, produce constant undercurrents tending to force changes in the established norms.

There are, however, two aspects of social change that are of special concern to psychologists. The first is the general effect of *technological inventions* upon our thinking and behavior. Changes of this sort are, by and large, unplanned alterations in our thought and behavior by the many products of man's inventive genius. A second force affecting change in our thought and behavior is what we have come to know as *propaganda*. Unlike the changes brought about by technological developments, propaganda is a planned and deliberate attempt on the part of some interested group to mold the attitudes of others in a specific direction.

The Effects of Technology on Thought and Behavior

Few of us realize the extent to which the ways we think and the ways we act are patterned by the man-made products of our physical environment. For example, we know that, by and large, people in the United States place more emphasis on cleanliness and personal hygiene than people in many other parts of the world. And some of us may flatter ourselves by thinking that we have these habits of cleanliness simply because we are 'as a people' somehow different in nature from people who live in certain other countries in conditions of comparative filth and squalor. We tend to forget that our modern habits of cleanliness in the United States are possible and came only as a consequence of technological developments connected with plumbing, sewage disposal and the invention of mass production which made possible the enormous supply of piping, hot water, soap and all the other things necessary for millions of people to keep themselves clean. The sociologist, W. F. Ogburn, has pointed out that "The Eskimos are dirty; but when one considers that they have to hang a bag of snow down their backs to melt it in order to get water, it is seen that it is not so easy to be clean as when one has only to turn on a faucet of hot or cold water and reach for the soap. In comparing peoples, therefore, cleanliness is seen to be a matter not of heredity but of the type of culture." *

Ogburn also points out how "Inventions such as the watch and the clock encourage the habit of punctuality. The American Indians who have no clocks or watches in their culture have little notion of keeping appointments with any exactness, whereas commuters working in any large city have a very acute sense of time. Appointments are regulated with precision and daily schedules are laid off in units of time. . . . Why primitive peoples have little use for punctuality and why it is so important in modern civilization depend on many other factors than the watch, of course, but promptness is in general a reaction to objective products of cultural life. Modern culture is loaded with tools like the radio, the railroad and the timeclock, all demanding punctuality of those who use them." †

Field studies made in this country and in Turkey show conclusively that people who live nearest large urban centers, where punctuality is necessary to carry on the business of life as determined by industrial activity, have much more precise conceptions of time than persons living in remote areas who may think of time, not in terms of days, hours or minutes, but in terms of the cycle of the moon, whether it is before or after dinner, the length of time it takes to walk a certain distance, or the length of time it takes to smoke a cigarette.

We need not consider in detail here the countless ways in which the thoughts and behavior of men have been affected during the past few decades by inventions that have revolutionized many of our ways of life. The student himself will be able to think of numerous examples. The advent of the railroad rapidly encouraged the growth of cities with all the social and psychological consequences. The automobile has brought us much greater flexibility of movement and, among hundreds of other effects, has tended further to emancipate women by making it easier for them to get away from their homes, to see their friends and to work in factories or offices. The radio has increased our musical knowledge and taste and made us aware of what is going on in other parts of the world.

The unleashing of atomic power appears to be the greatest technological advance made since the invention of the steam engine, and its enormous consequences are now the subject of much speculation. For just as the invention of the catapult tended to make obsolete the castles of feudal times with their high surrounding walls and their moats and played its role in breaking down the pattern of life and the norms of thought and behavior associated with feudalism, so the invention of the atomic bomb seems likely to have profound effects on international relationships, on the value of some sort of world organization and thus eventually on our conceptions of national sovereignty and national rights.

The effects of technology on thought and behavior are all of necessity subsequent to the technological improvements themselves. The point is obvious, yet it is important to bear it in mind. It means, as we have already noted, that the consequences of the technological developments of the past and of those yet to come are not deliberate, are not thoroughly planned out ahead of time. Instead they emerge slowly, after their causes have become fully established. Thus

* W. F. Ogburn and M. F. Nimkoff, *Sociology*, Houghton Mifflin, 1940, 194.

† W. F. Ogburn and M. F. Nimkoff, *op. cit.*, 193 f.

they appear to have about them a certain inevitability. We cannot reverse an invention or decide to do without its consequences.

Propaganda

No discussion of the processes of socialization and of social change would be complete without mention of propaganda. The widespread use of propaganda today is itself one of the by-products of our technological age and of the enormous developments that have taken place in the media of communication. Newspapers, the radio and the movies are all vehicles of propaganda. And propagandists of all sorts are competing for the attention of the bewildered layman, who is influenced by them much more than he is likely to suspect.

We may define propaganda as a deliberate attempt by interested individuals or groups to influence opinions or actions of other individuals or groups with reference to predetermined ends. As we have noted above, propaganda is a consciously planned attempt to affect opinion. It is also selfish, and it is one-sided, making use of suggestion and not reason. On this account it does not include formal education. It may be good or bad depending upon the point of view of the individual judging it.

Techniques of Propaganda

When you observe the work of the propagandist, you see essentially two psychological techniques employed in ingenious ways to influence the actions of people. The first of them is the very simple device of linking the object or idea to be propagandized with some attitude, symbol or value already known to an individual and already likely to effect emotional reaction. If the propagandist is to use this principle, he must, of course, first of all be thoroughly acquainted with the social values and symbols of the culture in which he works.

The clever propagandist generally tries to join his idea to vague values or symbols which people tend to be for or against, and about which they feel strongly without knowing precisely what the symbols mean. Take, for example, the often-repeated symbols of justice, beauty, liberty, economy, patriotism, security, happiness. To these and other such attitudes we find the propagandist connecting soaps, cigarettes, political campaigns, appeals to join the Army or to engage in some crusade. Vague emotionally toned words, such as *Fascist, Communist, Red, atheist, slacker,* are used to arouse us against government officials, labor leaders or any other individuals whom the propagandist thus freely labels.

Most people will agree that they either like or dislike what is implied by these vague words; and that is precisely why the propagandist is careful not to define them. If different individuals or groups should ask themselves what they mean by these terms, they might discover themselves in disagreement. The propagandist, if forced to define his words, would lose part of his group. For example, suppose he is appealing to *liberty* in a campaign. What is meant by that word? Liberty for whom? For workers or for business? For radicals or for conservatives? For Negroes or for whites? For you or for me? Most Americans claim they believe in *freedom of speech.* Yet almost every week there are instances of these same Americans' protesting to a broadcasting company because a Communist or a Catholic is allowed access to the studios or criticizing a newspaper because it has printed the speech of a CIO organizer, a pacifist or a capitalist. This first method of propaganda—the use of emotionally toned symbols—is illustrated in

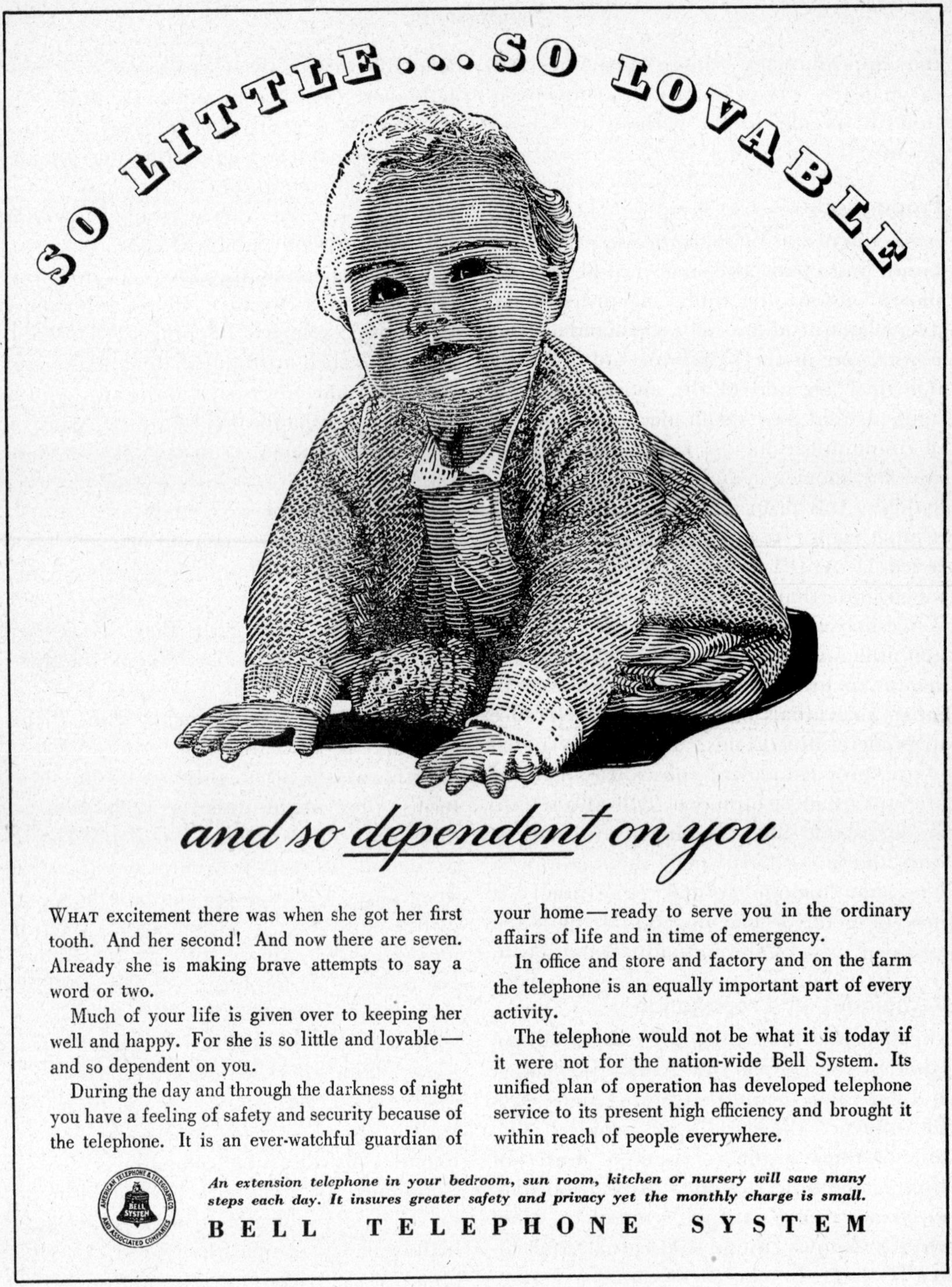

FIGURE 241. PROPAGANDA WHICH USES AN ESTABLISHED SYMBOL

[Reprinted by permission of the American Telephone and Telegraph Company.]

Fig. 241, where we see a symbol of something nearly everyone loves—a baby—used to catch the eye and to be associated with the services of a commercial organization.

The simple device of propaganda just described is so commonly employed that most people are by now aware of the trick. Thus, if the propagandist has some purpose to conceal because it is not socially acceptable, or if he believes he must use more subtle methods, he employs a second principle. He builds up an attitude or value around a product or an idea by means of indirect suggestion. The specific use of this principle is so varied and so changing that even the most expert analyst is often fooled unless he knows the selfish interests of the groups conducting the propaganda and carefully scrutinizes all that he reads and hears. In using this technique, for instance, the propagandist frequently gets his propaganda into newspapers as news or as editorial opinion. Another method used to build up an attitude or value for some idea is to disguise propaganda as explanation—explanation which is, however, distorted and incomplete. Since the use of this second principle is so dependent upon the situation in question and upon the tenor of the time, a great company, organization or government will hire an expert in propaganda who calls himself a public relations counsel, and whose business it is to feel the public's pulse in all classes and vocations and to find out where people are most suggestible. The public relations counsel, once hired, will work for his client through the newspapers, the radio, the medical journal, the textbook, the cut-out for the kiddies. This use of such indirect suggestion is illustrated in Fig. 242.

If we really want to understand this important force in modern life, however, a knowledge of the techniques of the propagandist is only half the story. As psychologists we must ask ourselves what it is in *us* that makes propaganda possible and effective. Why do the techniques work?

Quite a Handicap

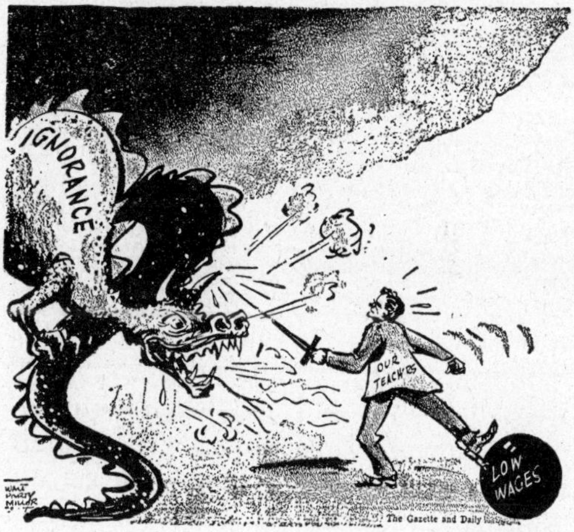

FIG. 242. PROPAGANDA DESIGNED TO BUILD UP AN ATTITUDE

Cartoon printed on the editorial page of a daily paper in a Pennsylvania town of about 100,000 population. [From the *Gazette and Daily,* York, Pa., April 21, 1947.]

Receptivity to Propaganda

There are several good psychological reasons for the success of propaganda. First, as we have already seen, the great majority of the words in our language or any other language are freighted with emotion. Most of the time we do not react to the dictionary meaning of the word, but to a whole complex of feeling that surrounds it. The word *love* can hardly be mentioned without arousing a host of sentiments in every individual. The word *Turk* will arouse in some Americans an unfavorable attitude even though most of these same Americans have never known a

Turk. We learn and accept these attitudes toward words, our society's value of words, at the same time that we learn their meaning. Our attitudes are determined for us by others.

A second reason why the propagandist is so successful is that most of us are unsure of ourselves. We seek a meaning for those things we do not understand. Since we usually have neither the time nor the facilities for studying problems ourselves and since we do not want to appear ignorant on many questions, we accept the judgment of some authority, of some official, of some newspaper editor, of some columnist or radio commentator. We feel that he must know more about the issue than we do, but we forget that the opinions of such experts are frequently only elaborated rationalizations of their own points of view, rationalizations which are given to us as objective, critical analyses. With life becoming more and more specialized, we have to depend more and more upon other people for our judgments. The propagandist snatches at this opportunity. He gives us *his* meaning. He satisfies our desire for a solution to such questions as what shall I buy, how shall I vote, what shall I believe—satisfies us so as to satisfy himself.

A third reason for his success is that nearly everyone is anxious to preserve his own position in life, to maintain or to enhance his status. A person has, therefore, a tendency to accept the type of propaganda which makes him feel superior to other persons or makes him feel that his own status is better than the other fellow's. One race likes to be reassured that it is superior to another race. Some rich people like to think of the poor as happy-go-lucky or as irresponsible. We accept the political philosophy best suited to our interests. That is one reason why most people read a newspaper whose editorials or news slants fit their prejudices, why many people turn off the radio if a speaker begins to tell them what they hope is not true.

In brief, the propagandist by appeals to a man's already existing frame of reference leads him to extend that frame to include the object or the idea in which the propagandist is interested. Or the propagandist may try to impose on the individual a frame of reference which he will accept because it gives meaning to his environment or because it enables him the better to rationalize his own position in life.

Social Bias of Propaganda

We must remember that the tools and facilities which provide the means for propaganda are mainly in the hands of those who own and control the mass media of communication or of those whose business interests or political power directly or indirectly control these mass media. In our own country, for example, the newspapers and radio are supported by advertisers who pay for space or time. Most of us have become so accustomed to this fact that we take it for granted, although in many countries of the world the radio is either a government monopoly or a public corporation, and in some the newspapers are government controlled.

Even our popular magazines tend to perpetuate, presumably unconsciously, our current majority biases. Figure 243, for example, based on an analysis of a sample of popular magazines which appeared between 1937 and 1943, shows how these magazines tend to misrepresent in their selection of characters the true complexion of our population. "The Americans" indicated in this figure are those people who are portrayed as "white Protestants with no distinguishable ancestry of foreign origin."

In this sense of an 'American' only sixty per cent of the people in the United States but ninety per cent of the people in the stories are 'Americans.'

Thus it comes about that public opinion is truly biased by propaganda. Insofar as propaganda is effective, public opinion has a dependence on wealth, for control of the sources of propaganda costs money, and the social norms of those who have control inevitably affect the way they use the control. No agency or government is likely to support views that lessen its own power. Thus in the United States the means of propaganda favor those attitudes which go along with belief in private enterprise, whereas the government-controlled propaganda of the Soviet Union favors a wholly different set of norms. As the inevitable biases come to be recognized there may be, as there is in the United States, an attempt to offset them by counterpropaganda, but the bias for self-defense of the controlling interests is as unavoidable as are the ego involvements that make propaganda effective.

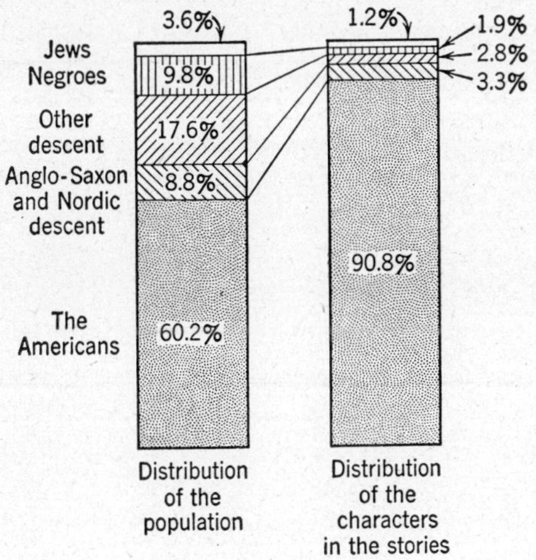

FIGURE 243. HOW MAGAZINE STORIES DISTORT THE POPULATION OF THE UNITED STATES

Shows the true distribution of the United States population about 1940 and the counts of fictional characters in magazine stories. Foreigners in the stories are omitted. An 'American' is anyone who does not fall in one of the other categories. In this sense only 60 per cent of the people in the United States, but 90 per cent of the people in the stories, are 'American.' [From B. Berelson and P. J. Salter, *Public Opinion Quarterly,* 1946, **10**, 175.]

The goals of propaganda are not necessarily evil. Propaganda may be directed toward the selfish ends of some small group or toward the enlightenment and the improvement of living conditions for a whole people. In either case the psychological role of propaganda is the same.

MEASUREMENT OF ATTITUDES AND OPINIONS

We have seen what attitudes do and where they come from. Our next topic is their measurement.

The word *opinion* is generally used to refer to attitudes which have been expressed. The measurement of attitudes is now generally termed *measurement of opinions,* and the most significant methods of measuring opinions today are those we associate with public opinion surveys.

Since the results of public opinion polls are becoming of increasing interest to the layman as he reads them in his newspapers or in a magazine and since the technique of appraising public opinion is now being widely used by psychologists and others in the social sciences, we can confine our discussion of attitude measurement to a discussion of the measurement of public opinion by the survey technique. It should be borne in mind, however, that the public opinion survey described here is, as a method, only one of many different methods available to the social scientist for gathering information. He also relies on case studies, on analyses of group situations, on developmental studies, on the comparative field studies of the ethnologist, as well as on experiments.

Sampling

There is nothing mysterious about a public opinion poll. It operates on the very simple principle that if an accurate miniature sample of the total population is made, the opinions of the people in that sample will faithfully reflect the opinions of the population as a whole. The basic problem of the public opinion poll is to select an accurate miniature sample—one that contains people of every variety, one that contains people who have all the different characteristics, occupational groupings, geographic distribution, religious affiliation or any other affiliations or identifications that might be expected to affect their opinions in a significant way. So every miniature sample of the population will have its fair share of old people and young people, of Protestants and Catholics, of Democrats and Republicans, of men and women, of people who live in cities, of farmers, of businessmen and skilled workers, etc.

Incredible as it seems, if 3000 properly representative voters in the United States are questioned, the statistical chances are 99 out of 100 that their answers to a question will not vary more than 4 or 5 per cent from the opinions of the whole voting population of 50,000,000. And the chances are 95 out of 100 that these opinions of a sample of 3000 will not vary more than 3 per cent in another sample of 3000. As the size of the sample is reduced, the size of the error increases but not, perhaps, as much as we might expect. For example, the chances are 95 out of 100 that, if 1500 people are included in a carefully selected sample, the maximum error due only to sampling would not be more than 5 per cent; with 500 people the maximum error would not be expected to be over 8 per cent; but with only 100 people the error expected from sampling alone would rise to 20 per cent.

How do we go about getting this miniature sample of the population? So far two major methods of sampling for opinion have been developed. One is known as *areal sampling,* the other as *quota sampling.* Areal sampling involves the careful selection ahead of time of specified people who live in specified dwelling units. This selection is made on the basis of maps from which specific counties may be chosen, on the basis of further information obtained about that county, on the basis of city directories and many other sources of data which tell the investigator how people are distributed in different dwelling units. The purpose of this specification is to increase the randomness of the sample and leave as little selection as possible to the individual interviewer. We can describe the method of quota sampling more in detail since it is less complicated and is mainly used by those organizations whose survey results are publicly known, such as the Gallup Poll, the *Fortune* survey, the National Opinion Research Center and many other investigators sampling on a statewide or local basis.

Suppose the poll administrator decides that he will have 3500 persons in his quota sample. First of all, the poll administrator determines on the basis of census figures what percentage of these persons should come from each of the major sections of the country—in other words, what quota to assign each sectional unit. Then, within each section, he decides on the basis of census figures what proportion of the interviews should be with farmers, what proportion should come from small towns, what proportion from large cities. Then, still on the basis of known information, he decides how many of these people should be in the upper income group, how many in the middle income group, how many in the lower income group, how many on relief. He also decides how many should be white and how many colored people. Most polling organizations have representatives scattered throughout the country who do their interviewing for them. Nearly all polls rely on personal contact rather than on mail ballots, for mail ballots are unreliable. They are generally returned in greater proportion by the better-educated, upper income group.

An interviewer in a certain town is then instructed from his central office to interview, let us say, 20 people. Of these, 4 are to be farmers, the rest are to be people living in the interviewer's own town. The interviewer is told to get so many people in the upper income group, so many in the middle and so many in the lower income group. He is also told to get about half men and half women, to divide his sample more or less evenly between people who are over 40 years of age and those who are under 40. We have, then, six 'controls' in determining this quota sample: section of the country, rural-urban distribution within each section, income distribution, race (white or Negro), sex and age. Such factors as education, religion or occupation are not used because, obviously, one cannot easily, if at all, judge these things by a person's appearance or by where he happens to live. But by and large it is found that, if the controls we have noted are used, the miniature sample thus obtained will faithfully reflect the educational, religious and occupational distribution of the total population.

Accuracy

One reason for the increasing use of public opinion surveys in commercial, government and scientific work is the accuracy they have demonstrated in predicting behavior. Their validity has been shown with respect to elections. So far the polls have made forecasts of 365 national or state elections, and their average error has been around 4 per cent. Improvement has gone on with the years. For example, the American Institute of Public Opinion (Gallup Poll), which has made 197 of these 365 forecasts, had, in 1936, an average error of 6 per cent. Between the years 1936 and 1940 its error was reduced to an average of 4½ per cent. From 1940 to the present writing, the Institute's average error has been only 2½ per cent.

Aside from occasional referenda, elections provide the only easy means for testing poll accuracy. In many ways this fact is unfortunate and unfair to the polls themselves, since there are so many variables that determine an election that cannot possibly be forecast by a poll. For example, elections are often determined by the weather, with bad weather tending to keep the farmers at home and thus reducing the Republican vote, since farmers, by and large, vote Republican. Furthermore, although an interview can determine with high accuracy how a person will vote, no sure-fire method has yet been discovered to determine whether or not a person will vote even though he says he will. Hence only about 2 per cent of an error made by a public opinion poll in forecasting an election can be charged to sampling; the rest is caused by such other factors as turnout, last-minute shifts and the effect of political party machines.

To illustrate how much more important is the selection of a sample than the size of a sample, two predictions based on extremely small samples may be cited. In one instance, with only 200 cases carefully distributed, the New York gubernatorial election in 1942 was forecast with an accuracy of 3 per cent. In the same year a referendum taken in Canada was correctly forecast within 4½ per cent with only 200 cases. Such small samples are, of course, not adequate substitutes for larger surveys. For one thing the investigator is likely to be accurate with so small a sample only when opinion is fairly uniform within the various population groups.

Setting the Problems and Questions

Certainly the most important, the most difficult and the most delicate operations connected with any survey of public opinion are slicing issues meaningfully and significantly and preparing questions that are clear and understandable and are so unbiased that they will not affect the answer itself. The investigator must be very certain in his own mind just what he is trying to find out, what relationships of opinion might exist, what possible determinants of opinion he can look for and the like. His questions must be neither vague nor obscure. They should not encourage stereotyped answers unless rigid stereotypes are part of the problem to be studied. Questions should avoid technical or unfamiliar words. They should not force answers into only a few categories unless and until the investigator knows by asking free and open questions what is the respondent's point of view before any alternatives for choice have been presented to him. Furthermore, before asking a person's opinion on some subject, it is of the utmost importance to find out if the person questioned has ever thought about that subject or has ever heard about it. And in addition to the problem of determining the direction of opinion, it is often important to discover another dimension of opinion, *its intensity,* if the investigator is interested in finding out how tenaciously that opinion is likely to be held and how much it means to the individual.

We can illustrate some of the problems encountered in constructing a survey by reference to an actual questionnaire prepared by the American Institute of Public Opinion in March, 1947. The purpose of this study was to find out what the reaction of the American people was to what has become known as the "Truman Doctrine" as enunciated by President Truman in his speech to Congress asking for loans to Greece and Turkey. The complete Gallup ballot follows. We may consider these questions in order.

THE GALLUP POLL

THE AMERICAN INSTITUTE OF PUBLIC OPINION

—WANTS YOUR OPINION—

---

1. If the question of national prohibition should come up again, would you vote wet or dry?

( ) WET ( ) DRY ( ) NO OPINION

---

2. Have you heard or read about Truman's speech to Congress asking for $400 million to help Greece and Turkey?

( ) YES ( ) NO

IF YES, ASK ALL OF THE FOLLOWING QUESTIONS; IF NO, SKIP TO QUESTION 16:

---

3. What do you think are the chief reasons FOR helping Greece and Turkey?

4. Can you tell me what are the chief reasons AGAINST helping Greece and Turkey?

5. What is your own feeling as to what we should do about this?

6. Why do you feel this way?

7*a*. Would you like to see your Congressman vote for or against the bill asking for $250 million to aid Greece?

( ) FOR ( ) AGAINST ( ) NO OPINION

b. How strongly do you feel about this—very strongly, fairly strongly, or not at all strongly?

( ) VERY ( ) FAIRLY ( ) NOT STRONGLY ( ) NO OPINION

c. And would you like to see your Congressman vote for or against the bill asking for $150 million to aid Turkey?

( ) FOR ( ) AGAINST ( ) NO OPINION

d. How strongly do you feel about this—very strongly, fairly strongly, or not at all strongly?

( ) VERY ( ) FAIRLY ( ) NOT STRONGLY ( ) NO OPINION

8*a*. Would you favor sending American civilian experts over to Greece to help supervise the uses to which this money will be put?

( ) YES ( ) NO ( ) NO OPINION

b. Would you favor sending American civilian experts over to Turkey to help supervise the uses to which this money will be put?

( ) YES ( ) NO ( ) NO OPINION

9*a*. Would you favor sending American military advisers to train the Greek army?

( ) YES ( ) NO ( ) NO OPINION

b. Would you favor sending them to train the Turkish army?

( ) YES ( ) NO ( ) NO OPINION

---

10. Why do you think this problem was not turned over to the United Nations Organization to handle?

11. Do you think it should have been turned over to the United Nations Organization?

( ) YES ( ) NO ( ) NO OPINION

---

12. If we aid Greece and Turkey, what do you think Russia will do?__________

13*a*. Do you think that lending money to aid Greece and Turkey is or is not likely to get us into war?

( ) IS ( ) IS NOT ( ) NO OPINION

b. Why do you feel this way?__________

14*a*. Do you think the present Greek government has the backing of the majority—that is, more than half—of the Greek people?

( ) YES ( ) NO ( ) NO OPINION

b. Do you think the present Turkish government has the backing of the majority—that is, more than half—of the Turkish people?

( ) YES ( ) NO ( ) NO OPINION

---

15. Suppose other nations find themselves in the same fix as Greece. Do you think the United States will have to do something about it?

( ) YES ( ) NO ( ) NO OPINION

---

16. Generally speaking, should the United States take a strong stand in European affairs, or should we try to get out of European affairs?

( ) TAKE STAND ( ) GET OUT ( ) NO OPINION

17*a*. Do you remember, FOR CERTAIN, whether or not you voted in the 1944 presidential election, or did something keep you from voting?

1( ) YES, VOTED
4( ) KEPT FROM VOTING
2( ) NO, DIDN'T VOTE
5( ) DON'T REMEMBER
3( ) NO, TOO YOUNG TO VOTE

IF YES, VOTED, ask:

b. Did you vote for Dewey, Roosevelt, or Thomas?

6( ) DEWEY 7( ) ROOSEVELT 8( ) THOMAS 9( ) OTHER

---

18. If a presidential election were being held TODAY, which party would you vote for—the Democratic or Republican?

( ) DEMOCRATIC ( ) REPUBLICAN

( ) SOCIALIST ( ) OTHER ( ) UNDECIDED

And now, just a question or two to help me keep track of the cross-section I'm getting:

19. What is the last grade or class you completed in school?

1( ) NO SCHOOLING

2( ) GRAMMAR SCHOOL (GRADES 1 THROUGH 8)

3( ) HIGH SCHOOL, INCOMPLETE (9th, 10th or 11th GRADE)
4( ) HIGH SCHOOL, GRADUATED (12th GRADE)
5( ) COLLEGE, INCOMPLETE }
6( ) COLLEGE, GRADUATED } ________ What type of college?

---

20. What is your occupation? (Record SPECIFIC occupation, not just industry or name of organization worked for.)________

(If housewife, widow or student, record occupation of head of family. If retired or unemployed give former occupation.)

21*a*. Is there a telephone in your home? ( ) YES ( ) NO
IF YES, ask:
b. Is the telephone listed either under your name or the name of a member of your immediate family?
( ) YES ( ) NO

PLEASE COMPLETE ALL VITAL INFORMATION BEFORE LEAVING RESPONDENT

Classify respondent as:			Check whether:		
( ) Wealthy	( ) Average	( ) Old Age Assistance	( ) Car	( ) Man	( ) White
( ) Average plus	( ) Poor	( ) On Relief	( ) No Car	( ) Woman	( ) Colored

---

Respondent's Age________ Address________
(Street and number)
City________ State________
Date of interview________, 1947 Interviewer________

We see that the first question has nothing whatever to do with the topic under consideration. Why, then, was it asked? The reason is that this particular question, dealing with national prohibition, has been found from experience to be one that people enjoy answering. In other words, it makes a good *opener*. People begin to think the interview is going to be fun. So this question is included only in order to enlist the cooperation of the respondent. In question 2, the respondents are asked if they have ever heard or read of President Truman's speech to Congress asking for the loans to Greece and Turkey. This is known as a *filter question*. Obviously, if people have never heard of the speech, there is no use asking them a lot of questions about it, for any opinions they might give would only be useless falsifications.

Questions 3, 4 and 5 are examples of what are known as *open-ended* or *free answer questions*. Here the investigator tries to find out before he asks any specific questions involving alternative courses of action, what the respondent himself thinks about President Truman's statement. What are the arguments for and against the Truman Doctrine and how does the respondent himself feel about it? Question 6 is a *probing question* in which the investigator tries to find out what some of the underlying reasons are for the person's opinion.

In questions 7*a* and 7*c*, the respondent is confronted with the same proposition that his Congressman must face, whether or not to vote for or against the bill asking for the loans. Although the respondent may have expressed one point of view or another with definite qualifications in question 5, and although similar qualifications may exist in the mind of his Congressman, both the citizen and the Congressman in the end have to choose one or the other course of action. Questions 7*b* and 7*d* are *intensity questions,* designed to find out how strongly a person feels the way he does. Questions 8*a* and 8*b* and 9*a* and 9*b* are designed to tap opinion on some of the more important qualifications which the pretesting (preliminary interviewing before the final ballot was prepared) had shown were important. Questions 10 through 15 are designed to find out what people see as some of the implications of the policy enunciated by President Truman and how the policy will affect the United Nations, the Soviet Union, and the likelihood of war. Question 16 is a question that has been asked many, many times by the Gallup Poll as one of its *trend questions.* These trend questions are particularly valuable in determining to what extent opinion changes with events. An illustration of the use of trend questions in public opinion studies is found in Fig. 244. All the rest of the Institute's ballot is made up of questions which give the 'background' data on the respondent.

Analysis of Results

With this information the sample population can be 'broken down' in a number of ways. The opinions of different groups of people may be compared; that is to say, we can compare the opinions of Republicans and Democrats, people of different occupations, people of different income groups, and, if we want a more elaborate analysis, we can make what are known as 'two-way' or 'three-way' breakdowns by further subdividing the population. For example, we could make a two-way breakdown and find out what differences, if any, appeared between Democrats and Republicans who were further classified according to their economic status. How the differences between rich and poor Democrats compared with the differences between rich and poor Republicans. Or we could make a three-way breakdown and find out how the opinions of the Democrats and Republicans, that we had divided into different income groups, compared when the population was further subdivided into educational levels. That would give us rich Democrats who had been to college, poor Democrats from college, rich Democrats who stopped at the eighth grade, and all the other combinations for Democrats and the corresponding combinations for Republicans. In making these elaborate breakdowns, the investigator must always watch the number of respondents who finally fall into one of the small subcategories obtained. For unless his sample has a large enough number of cases, he may end up with so few people in various categories that his results will be statistically insignificant. An example of a two-way break down by political party affiliation (as determined by how a person voted in 1944) and economic status on one of the questions asked is shown in Table XXXVI. It can be seen there that the people who did not vote in 1944 were more ignorant of Truman's speech to Congress proposing aid to Greece and Turkey than those who did vote, and that those who voted for Roosevelt were less aware of the speech than those who voted for Dewey. However, to infer from this that political affiliation as such is a 'cause' of ignorance of Truman's

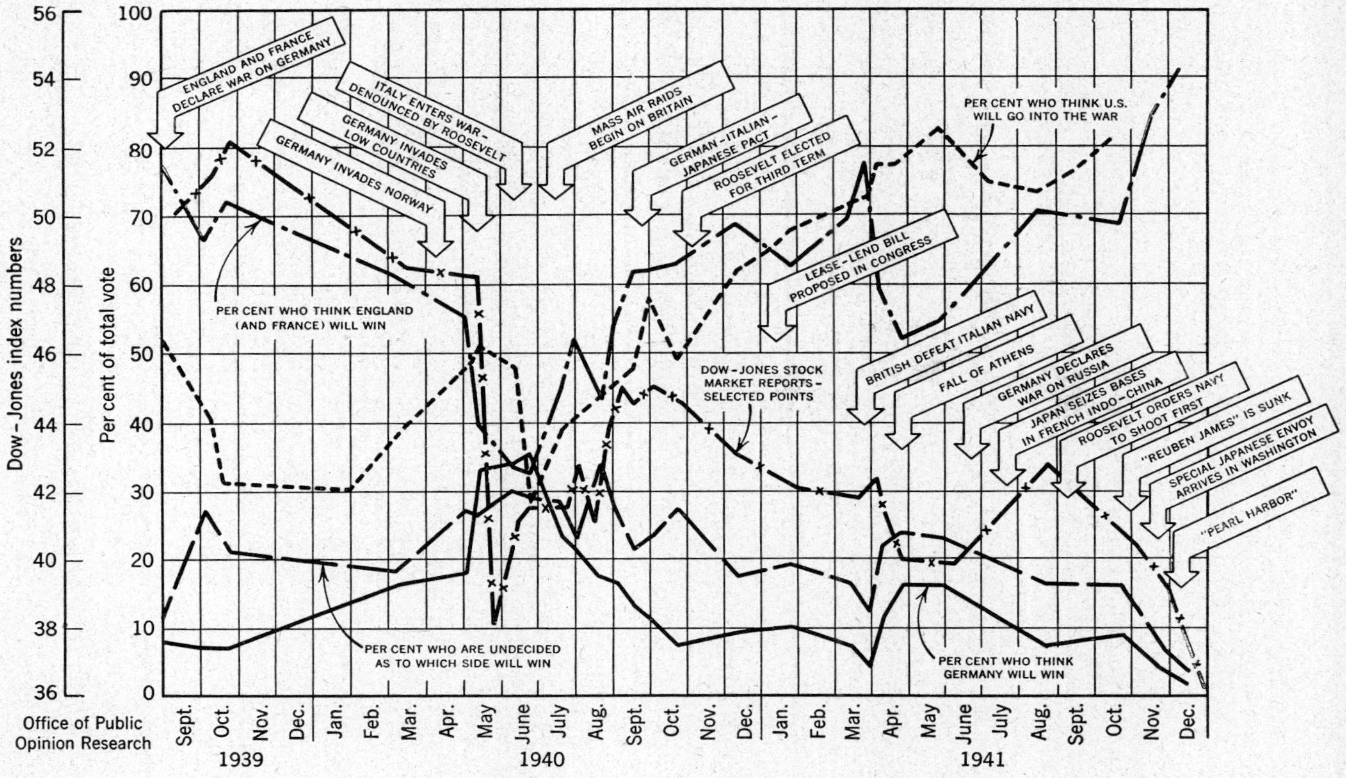

FIGURE 244. SOME TRENDS OF AMERICAN PUBLIC OPINION FROM THE OUTBREAK OF THE SECOND WORLD WAR TO THE DISASTER AT PEARL HARBOR

The data were obtained from the results of polls by the Office of Public Opinion Research. [From H. Cantril (Ed.), *Gauging public opinion,* Princeton University Press, 1944, p. 221.]

TABLE XXXVI

BREAKDOWN OF OPINION BY VOTE AND ECONOMIC STATUS

"Have you heard or read about Truman's speech to Congress asking for $400 million to help Greece and Turkey?"

	Number of Cases	*Yes*	*No*
Dewey: Total	806	92%	8%
Upper Income	186	100	0
Middle Income	309	93	7
Lower Income	311	86	14
Roosevelt: Total	1217	83	17
Upper Income	121	99	1
Middle Income	374	92	8
Lower Income	722	76	24
Didn't vote: Total	821	80	20
Upper Income	69	91	9
Middle Income	221	89	11
Lower Income	531	76	24

speech would be quite unjustified. For we find that people in the lower income groups, irrespective of whether or not they voted or how they voted, show significant and consistent variations. We can see in this table that Dewey voters represent a higher income group than Roosevelt voters, and we know from previous studies that economic status is correlated positively with education. So this two-way breakdown begins to show us what other factors to look for in order that our understanding of the figures obtained in the original question should be more complete.

Another useful method of analyzing the data obtained is to make a comparison of people's opinions on different questions. This gives the investigator some idea of how opinions hang together, which ones are related to which other ones, what some of the more basic attitudes of people are. In Table XXXVII we find from this cross-tabulation that those people who believe the problem of aiding Greece and Turkey

TABLE XXXVII

CROSS-TABULATION COMPARING OPINION ON LIKELIHOOD OF WAR AS CONSEQUENCE OF LOANS TO GREECE AND TURKEY AND ADVISABILITY OF TURNING PROBLEM OVER TO UNITED NATIONS

[Based only on those who had heard of Truman proposal.]

	Should problem of aiding Greece and Turkey be turned over to United Nations?		
	Yes	*No*	*No opinion*
Is loan likely to get us into war?			
Is	41%	30%	28%
Is not	47	61	28
No opinion	12	9	44

should be turned over to the United Nations are more inclined than others to believe the loans are likely to get us into war.

How to Poll

Suppose you wanted to carry out a public opinion survey. What steps would you have to follow? First of all, of course, you would have to find the money necessary to conduct your survey. In actual practice in this country, surveys are supported either by newspapers, magazines, government departments or agencies, foundations, business or labor organizations, or some group interested in obtaining information on a specific problem. You would then go about designing your sample according to the problem at hand on the basis of the quota or areal method or, possibly, some combination of the two. After your sample had been designed, you would know at what points you would need to have interviews made. Then, unless you had full-time interviewers to travel around from place to place, you would recruit an interviewing staff distributed among the localities you had selected as sample points.

These people would not be employed full time but would merely take on your interviewing assignment as an extra part-time job.

How would you go about finding interviewers? The most efficient method seems to be to write to reliable people in the different towns who are in a position to understand your problem and to recommend someone for the job of interviewing. Newspaper editors, school superintendents, principals have proved to be good 'recommenders.' Then you yourself or a highly trained representative in whom you have confidence would talk to each potential interviewer and try to judge him on the basis of his stability, his honesty, the ease and ability with which he meets people, the interest he is likely to have in his work, etc. It is known that housewives, school teachers, social service workers and students have proved to be conscientious interviewers, interested in the work, with extra time to spend and a desire to earn some extra money. When you have decided that a person is a good bet, he must be trained by you or your field representative. He must be told something of the whole method of public opinion polling, he must know how ballots are made up, he should watch you conduct several interviews and then conduct some himself while you watch him and until you are satisfied with his work. After the interviewers have been hired and trained, you must, from your central office, do all you can to keep up their interest and morale in such ways as providing them with results of surveys they have worked on, sending them newsletters in which their names are mentioned occasionally and some interesting experiences of interviewers are recited. You must keep a careful check on the quality of their work and on their integrity by reviewing the interviews they return, checking them against other interviewers in the same or comparable locality or, occasionally, using in your surveys questions known as 'trap' questions which will enable you to tell whether or not an interviewer has actually gone out and made interviews or whether he has sat at home filling out his ballots.

After your sample has been designed and your interviewers employed, you will be in a position to go ahead. But no matter how smart you are or how much experience you have had in the construction of actual questionnaires, you cannot merely sit in your office, write out questions and then send them to your interviewers. All the questions must be carefully *pretested* in your local area by you and others who are trained to detect flaws in the questions. You must be sure that the questions you are asking are completely unambiguous, that they are unbiased. Even the most experienced poll administrators will find in actual practice that new questions they ask have to be revised many times before they are properly stated for inclusion on the questionnaire.

When your questionnaire has been constructed, pretested and accepted, you have it printed or mimeographed. You send to each of your interviewers the number of copies he needs to complete his assignment, together with an instruction sheet which gives him his particular quota, that is to say, which tells him how many people and what types of people you want him to interview and explains to him some of the background of the particular questions contained on the survey. The interviewer is usually given three or four days in which to complete his assignment. He then returns the questionnaires to your office, where they go through the processes of coding (getting punch card numbers on them) and of actual transference of information to the punch cards. Then the cards are put through the sorting and tabulating machines. Your final job is analyzing and interpreting the data you have thus collected. It may be that you will find out that, after all, you have not asked the right questions or enough questions and that you will have to undertake more probing before you get what you think is a reliable answer to your original general query. Such is the modern method of opinion measurement.

REFERENCES

1. Allport, G. W. Attitudes. In C. Murchison (Ed.), *A handbook of social psychology*. Worcester, Mass.: Clark University Press, 1935. Chap. 17.

   A comprehensive review and evaluation of studies dealing with the nature of attitudes.

2. Cantril, H. (Ed.), *Gauging public opinion*. Princeton: Princeton University Press, 1944.

   A compilation of studies dealing with some of the major problems of measuring public opinion and interpreting data.

3. Coffin, T. E. Some conditions of suggestion and suggestibility: a study of some attitudinal and situational factors influencing the process of suggestion. *Psychol. Monogr.*, 1941, No. 241.

   An excellent study reporting experiments and studies based on questionnaires. The author brings all his data together in a systematic formulation.

4. Gallup, G. *A guide to public opinion polls*. Princeton: Princeton University Press, 1944.

   The best introduction yet written to the problems encountered in measuring public opinion. Prepared in question and answer form.

5. Horowitz, E. L. The development of attitude toward the Negro. *Arch. Psychol.*, 1936, No. 194.

   An excellent study of the way in which attitudes are formed. The study takes full account of the social context and reports data from different parts of the country.

6. Murphy, G., Murphy, L. B., and Newcomb, T. M. *Experimental social psychology*. New York: Harper, 1931.

   A monumental volume reviewing with some interpretation and evaluation much of the work in the field of social psychology up to 1937.

7. Sherif, M., and Cantril, H. *The psychology of ego-involvements*. New York: Wiley, 1947.

   A systematic discussion of the process of socialization, with the subtitle *Social attitudes and identifications*.

CHAPTER 25

Social Relations of the Individual

IT is a commonplace that society is delicately interrelated. What is not so widely understood is the consequence that the old philosophy (or absence of one) of letting problems of social relations resolve themselves through conflict and 'muddling through' no longer serves. Nowadays we all know how a small conflict between labor and management can tie up an entire economy. It takes no crystal ball to see that presently a small national conflict would 'atomize' civilization. The fact must be faced; civilization today must work efficiently to work at all. And it cannot work efficiently except through a knowledge of human relations.

The acquisition of the elements of that knowledge is the aim of this chapter. For the purposes of discussion it is convenient to treat social relations under three broad headings: (1) *primary social relations,* (2) *relations of the individual to the group,* both the assembled group and the dispersed group, and (3) *relations between groups,* the social interaction of groups upon each other. The special example of the relation of the individual to the group is found in *leadership* and of social interaction in *group prejudice.* The latter we shall consider in detail.

PRIMARY SOCIAL RELATIONS

Direct person-to-person relationships constitute the primary interactions of social life. They are primary in respect of time, directness and importance. They are primary in respect of time because person-to-person relations constitute the earliest social experiences of the organism in the history of both the individual and his group. They are primary in directness because as face-to-face relations they are the most influential point of contact between the individual and his culture. They are primary in importance because it is the early parent-child relationship which determines, in large part, the adult personality.

General Functions of the Family

The origin, as well as the most significant setting, of the primary social relations lies within the family. Largely through the medium of intimate face-to-face contacts the family serves three general functions in social life.

First, the family is the major agency for *socialization of the child.* The new recruit to life initially wants what he wants when he wants it. This biological egoism must be reduced to mutual give-and-take if society is to function efficiently. So the child is compelled to learn that to have his cake

This chapter was prepared by Leo P. Crespi of Princeton University.

he must drink his milk first, to enjoy his own toys he must respect the property of others. Through primary experience with frowns and smiles, cuffs and caresses, the child is ultimately domesticated to the requirements of social living.

Second, the family functions importantly in *transmitting the cultural heritage.* Through its intimate contacts, the specific ways of thinking, doing and feeling, which are the traditions of a society, are channeled into the individual. The child acquires *folkways*—the routine habits of life in his culture, like wearing shoes, addressing people as *Mr.* or *Mrs.* and eating with a knife and fork. He acquires *mores* —the customs buttressed with moral sanctions as codes of decency and respect for property. And, especially in primitive societies, he acquires *taboos*—prohibitions which arouse feelings of fear or horror at the thought of their violation, like the general incest taboo or the reaction in our society to cannibalism. Finally, among the most important of the child's acquisitions are *stereotypes* (p. 563) and *prejudices.* Prejudice is treated in the last half of the present chapter, which contains also numerous examples of stereotypes.

The processes of socialization and cultural transmission produce the overall similarity of social habits in a culture. It must not be forgotten, however, that they also produce the differences. The family is the main agency for perpetuating the social hierarchies of a society. In particular it inculcates class differences, the differences in social habits associated with differences in the income and occupational levels of parents. Although both of them wear shoes and eat with a knife and fork, there is a vast difference between the attitudes and actions of the boy brought up on the lower East side of New York City and those of his compatriot brought up on a Long Island estate. Upper class families perpetuate elaborate codes of etiquette which display their superior status, whereas lower classes lack the means to participate in such customs.

The third function of the family derives most directly from primary social relations. It is the provision of an *outlet for the expression of personality.* Group relationships dominate our modern life, and in them there is scant opportunity to express the whole personality. As a member of a business organization or a church or a political party, you generally participate only as a part of yourself. You reveal in the setting of each group only that facet of your personality which is advantageous. It is in the intimate family group that you can cease functioning as a cog in a machine. There you can be yourself. You can know and be known for what you really are as a whole personality. That there is a real need for such intimate groupings is shown by the substitutes for the family circle which a person quickly finds once he has departed from the home.

The Family in Relation to Social Control

The family, like the church, the school and the state, is an *institution.* That is to say, it is a grouping of individuals whose attitudes and actions are organized toward the cooperative pursuit of mutual ends. Yet, over and above being itself an institution, the family is also the matrix of all the other institutions in a society. This fact is obvious in many ways, especially in the manner in which *social control,* without which institutions could not exist, is itself rooted in the institution of the family.

Social control embraces the processes by means of which groups of people are manipulated, led and sometimes regimented into conformity with traditional social norms. It is a significant fact that people obey their institutional leaders in part because they have learned to obey their parents. It is no accident that the empire builder wishes to preserve the family.

Social control draws upon the family in four ways.

First, it feeds upon the *emotional attachments* which have developed in the family. Much of the hold of religion upon the individual, for example, stems from the fact that children generally absorb their religious attitudes at their mother's knee and hence unconsciously weave into them their affection for their parents. For a man later to reject religion may prove to be emotionally equivalent to his rejecting his mother.

Second, social control draws upon *fear and dependency* in family relationships. The child learns both to fear and to be dependent upon the authority of his parents. These reactions are later transferred to other sources of authority. In this connection it may be said that not a little of the German acceptance of an authoritarian regime can be traced to the habits of rigid obedience inculcated in German family life.

Third, the family makes social control possible through the *constancy and the personal quality of its relationships.* Where relations are shifting, retribution often fails to catch up with asocial acts. Where relations are impersonal, the individual tends to be indifferent to what others think of his actions. It is only through the constancy and intimacy of the primary social relations of the family that the conscience can develop which makes men responsive to social demands.

Finally, the family directly makes for social control in the adult life of the individual through the *responsibilities* that marriage and parenthood impose upon him. The necessities of bread winning curb irresponsibility and make more difficult the challenging of traditional values.

With the content of socialization and cultural transmission sketched in, we may now turn our attention to the mechanisms. The four of them which stand out in significance are *imitation, suggestion, identification* and *language.*

Imitation

Observers have long noted the similarities of behavior in a society, how its newly born members tend to mirror the patterns of behavior exhibited by those about them. To account for this mirroring some have supposed that there is an instinct of imitation, an innate tendency for individuals to behave in the manner in which others are behaving. The notion that imitativeness is innate and instinctive has, however, now been disproved. Imitation does not occur automatically whenever the opportunity arises, but only under particular conditions. For instance, the adolescent boy imitates the ball playing of his older brother, but he definitely does not imitate the doll playing of his younger sister.

Imitativeness is simply a learned mechanism of satisfying motives. People learn to imitate whenever it helps them to achieve satisfaction. They learn equally well not to imitate when imitation leads to no rewards or to punishment. Three types of imitation are distinguishable in terms of how it is learned. There are *simple imitation, matched-dependent behavior* and *copying.* Not all similarities in group behavior, however, need be cases of imitation. People may respond similarly to the same stimulus quite independently of one another. Good examples are the so-called *coenotropes.* All the members of a group may turn up their collars in the face of a blizzard not because of imitation, but because such a response is to each of them his obvious and compelling means of adjustment to the storm.

Simple imitation is a kind of conditioning. It is used in the acquisition of language by the child, a process which is described farther on.

Matched-dependent behavior develops from chance learning. An illustration of it might run as follows. Jim and Bobby are playing in a room when Jim hears his father's footfall on the stairs. He has learned that it means candy, so he runs to greet his father. His younger brother, Bobby, has not learned to use this clue, but by chance on this occasion he happened to be running in the same direction as his brother when his father arrived—so he too receives candy. The law of effect operates. Thereafter Bobby tends to run more frequently at the mere sight of his brother running, in this situation and eventually in others as well. In a word, Bobby has learned to imitate Jim because, more often than not, he has got candy for doing it.

The combination of learning and motivational conditions involved in matched-dependent behavior has been conveniently diagrammed in Table XXXVIII. Jim's response to his father's footfall is to run to him. Jim's running becomes the stimulus for a similar response by Bobby, who thus, being rewarded, has his response reinforced. Since Bobby can also hear the footfall, he will soon become conditioned to it, and then can get candy without having Jim for a stimulus.

Copying is an elaboration of matched-dependent behavior in which a critic functions as well as a model. For example, the model may sound a certain note which the imitator wishes to copy without being able to know when his attempted matchings are correct. Hence he needs a critic to point out similarities and differences. In copying, the critic is also a guide in the specification of such environmental clues as will ultimately enable the copier to become independent of the model. A matcher knows, for example, that at certain points in the ceremony he ought to stand or kneel in church but does not know the precise occasions. So he continues to match those who do. The copier, on the other hand, will have eventually learned not only to perform the proper responses but also to interpret the environmental signals for himself. He acquires the conditioned responses of those who know.

TABLE XXXVIII

MATCHED-DEPENDENT IMITATION

The model is already conditioned for running to the stimulus of the father's footfall, and the model's response becomes the stimulus to the same (imitative) response in the imitator. [Adapted from N. E. Miller and J. Dollard, *Social learning and imitation*, Yale University Press, 1941.]

	Model		*Imitator*
Motivating drive	appetite for candy		appetite for candy
Stimulus to response	father's football	↗dependent⟶	running of model
Conditioned response	running (of model)	—matched⟶	running (of imitator)
Reinforcing reward	eating candy		eating candy

Suggestion

Suggestion, as we have already learned (p. 564), can be looked upon most simply as the unreasoned acceptance of propositions. To the degree that an individual accepts ideas or courses of action without exercising his powers of reasoning or logical analysis, he is said to be influenced by suggestion.

Proneness to suggestion or suggestibility is promoted by conditions which produce either *inhibition* or *dissociation* of critical thought processes. The simplest kind of inhibition is caused by fatigue or emotional excitement. When a person is either too tired or too excited to think, he is ready prey to suggestion. That the Nazis knew this fact well is indicated by their care in scheduling party rallies in the evening when the people were weary, and by their calculated efforts to stir up excitement.

The most important inhibitory condition of suggestibility is not physiological or emotional in origin, like those above, but motivational. Reasoning gets inhibited by wishful thinking. In such cases individuals are suggestible because either (1) they badly need an interpretation for a bewildering situation or (2) they already have a fixed interpretation for a situation, and hence a 'will to believe.' It is for the first reason that perplexed citizens accept the oversimplified schemes of crackpot utopians. It is for the second that staunch party members accept without qualification the line laid down by party leaders.

Suggestibility through dissociation arises when the individual is thinking about something else. To secure his effects the magician often makes use of deliberate dissociation or misdirection. In the performance of a card trick, he may patter on about mathematical formulas to get his audience thinking in this vein so that he may plant other ideas about the pack of cards, ideas which they, otherwise occupied, fail to scrutinize critically.

Suggestion plays a very important part in *propaganda*. Since propaganda is essentially an attempt to secure acceptance of propositions through any and all means, propagandists find suggestion of great advantage, especially when the attitudes or actions they are seeking to promulgate are not likely to be accepted in the light of critical scrutiny. Education, unlike propaganda, minimizes suggestion as much as possible and aims, though not always with success, to have all propositions accepted only when they have passed critical examination.

Identification

In the preceding chapter we noted that, at the beginning of life, the individual cannot distinguish at all between himself and his environment. He never completely succeeds. Initially the infant is not able to distinguish what is his self from what is not. He does not know the boundaries of his body. He draws his thumb from his mouth and then cries because the thumb has got away. He pulls his toes so hard that they hurt and cries the while because something is hurting him. Since he can in some measure predict and control his parents, he feels that their qualities and actions are part of him.

Later through a process of learning the bodily self becomes differentiated. It is probably significant that when the child strikes his body, he receives two stimulations—one from the part struck and one from the offending member; but that, when he strikes an object, there is only one stimulation. He perceives also that he can both feel and see his own movements, whereas external movements can only be seen. Through these and further processes the bodily self becomes a stable individuated perception. But what is true in perception need not hold for emotion. From childhood on through adulthood to death, the things and actions that the individual likes and can control he still *feels* are a part of his ego, even though he *perceives* them as beyond the boundaries of his body. The workman regards his tools as part of himself, as extensions of his arms and fingers. The horseman feels his horse a part of himself as it responds to his slightest signal.

Language

One of the most significant factors in human socialization is language. It is itself a cultural acquisition, but once acquired it becomes the master key to vast stretches of culture beyond the individual in time and place. The development of language in the race is too uncertain a speculation to be considered here; but of its development in the individual we know a great deal. The four important stages in the development of language are as follows.

(1) *Random vocalization.* From the birth cry on, an infant's wiggling of toes and waving of arms are accompanied by the constituents of words—distinguishable vowels and consonants, 'clicks,' 'grunts' and 'gurgles.' This wide repertory of random vocalizations that the infant early exhibits is the raw material for his communication, all ready to be fashioned through learning into language.

(2) *Circular conditioned responses.* Between five and twelve months of age, the infant becomes repetitious in his vocalizations, uttering the same syllable repeatedly. This 'babbling' reflects, according to one accepted theory, an intricate process of learning, the circular conditioned response.

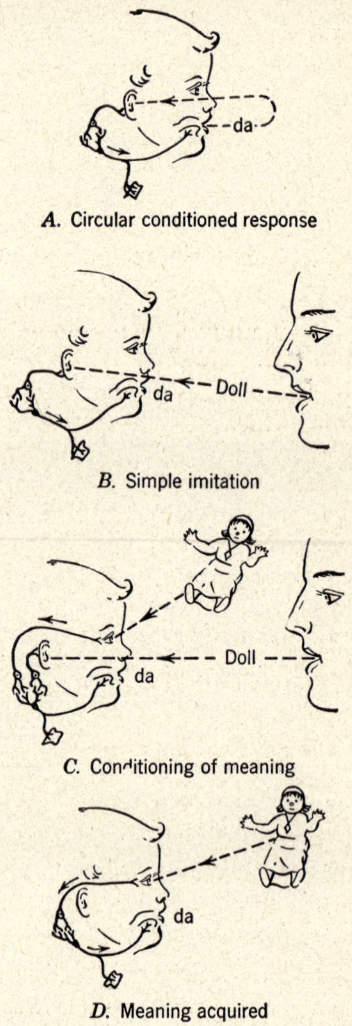

FIGURE 245. PROCESSES IN LANGUAGE DEVELOPMENT

[Adapted from J. F. Dashiell, *Fundamentals of general psychology,* Houghton Mifflin, 1937, p. 527.]

As shown in Fig. 245*A,* when the child articulates *da,* for example, he hears his own sound while he makes the response. Thus the sound *da* becomes a conditioned stimulus for saying *da.* So the infant keeps on hearing *da,* saying *da,* hearing *da,* saying *da,* a circular conditioning which continues indefinitely. Presumably the initial utterance was a matter of chance, and the cessation of babbling is a matter of fatigue.

(3) *Social selection of particular vocalizations.* The child will in this way establish through his own vocal play a wide variety of circular conditioned responses. Once they are established the adults around him begin to have a voice in which of them will be emphasized. If they utter the right conditioned stimuli, their sounds will activate in the child particular babbling chains. Suppose, as in Fig. 245*B*, the adult says *doll,* which may sound somewhat like *da* to the child. He starts babbling *da.* This event marks a case of *simple imitation,* the illustration of which was delayed until now. It rests simply upon activation of circular conditioned responses by some other person.

By virtue of this conditioning-born imitation, the sounds the child practices and thus makes his own are those which he hears about him. So it is that he acquires the linguistic stamp of his specific culture, be that anything from German with its gutturals to Hottentot with its clicks. The selection of the proper babblings is hastened by parental interest in the child's new 'words.' Let the child approximate any word of his mother's tongue and she will echo it back with enthusiasm, thus rewarding the child with attention and reinforcing the response.

(4) *Acquisition of meaning.* In prompting the child's babblings the mother will employ words in reference to specific objects. As shown in Fig. 245*C,* in saying *doll* she is likely to wave a doll in the child's face. Gradually through conditioning the sight of the doll comes to reinstate the verbal response to it (Fig. 245*D*). This is the birth of meaning. Through this process the child comes to name objects and situations. At first the naming is characteristically too general. The word *milk,* for example, may stand for the entire feeding situation. Soon, however, this vague meaning gives place to greater specificity as the child hears the word spoken in different contexts, yet always with reference to the same object.

With meaning initiated, vocabulary begins to form. Once the child catches on to the fact that everything has a name—an event which occasionally happens with great suddenness—vocabulary may grow by leaps and bounds. It is at this stage that the child begins to combine words into sentences. At first vocabulary is limited to nouns (the names of conditioned stimuli); later the child acquires verbs, and last the qualifying words and those denoting relationships.

Primarily we have been considering the acquisition of substantive meanings, but words can also have affective or emotional significance. Suppose little Bobby of fourteen months is being taken for a walk when a large dog trots up and tries to lick his face. Should Bobby be terrified by his nurse's screaming in fright, it is quite possible that a conditioned fear response will thereafter be associated with the word dog, one that may persist for years. Nor need all affective values be acquired so dramatically. Many of them are simply taken over from parental evaluations as embodied in pronouncements that this is *good* and that is *bad.*

Semantics

For centuries language has been largely taken for granted, but in recent years there has been a movement to overhaul language habits with the aim of improving social relations. This movement is called *semantics.*

One of the major contentions of the semanticists is that people fail to appreciate that the connection between symbols and their referents is purely arbitrary and conventional. To illustrate this confusion between words and things, they point to statements like "The pig is rightly named for it is such a dirty animal." Or better, the story of the Englishman who, in undertaking to prove that English is the best language, said: "Take the word *knife;* the French call it *couteau,* the Germans *Messer,* the Danes *kniv,* while the English say *knife,* and that's what it really is."

In advertising particularly, semanticists believe that people are being misdirected by word magic when they act as if naming things agreeably somehow makes them better. Three times as many men buy a felt hat when it is named *Tyrolia* as when it is unnamed. If sofas sell well, "snuggle sofas" of the same shape, appearance and quality sell better. Ten times more women buy hosiery when the shade of it is called *Gala* than when it is offered as just plain *beige.* Euphemisms, semanticists hold, also illustrate the confusion of words with things in that they rest upon the assumption that agreeable names for disagreeable things better the things.

Undoubtedly there is truth in the semanticists' indictment. To most of us a rose by another name does not smell so sweet. The Nazis in the Second World War made heavy use of the converse principle—that a stinkweed by another name does not smell so bad—when they called their retreats "planned withdrawals," "defensive successes," "successful disengagements" and "unencircling maneuvers." The semanticists' means for avoiding this 'primitive and infantile' use of words seems to be to get rid of all our euphemisms and other similar graceful distortions of language. It is doubtful, however, if people could be taught to face reality and truth simply by forbidding them all the ameliorating charm of figures of speech and pinning them down to harsh unimaginative description. If man were denied language as a medium for his repressions, suppressions and wishful distortions, he would find another way to be himself and to escape the unpleasant. Mankind, which made words for its purposes, is not likely to truckle to semanticists wishing to change human nature.

THE INDIVIDUAL IN RELATION TO THE ASSEMBLED GROUP

Persons have relations with—affect and are affected by—*assembled groups* and *dispersed groups.* An assembled group is all together physically, like a congregation in a church, or an audience in an auditorium; but it is not the 'audience' for whom a book is written, which is a dispersed group. A town meeting is an assembled group. A political party is a dispersed group, for most of its members never see one another. As the means of communication (air travel, radio, movies, etc.) get better and the world 'gets smaller,' as the phrase is, dispersed groups can be more closely integrated and so become more important than assembled groups. A dispersed group may consist of millions of persons, an assembled group is limited to a few thousands. In this section we are considering the individual in the assembled group.

Social Facilitation and Social Inhibition

Improvement of any aspect of a person's performance by virtue of the sight and sound of other persons simultaneously engaged in similar activities has been termed *social facilitation* (p. 124). When impairment results, *social inhibition* is said to have occurred. In everyday life social facilitation is illustrated in such obvious occurrences as people's eating more and drinking more in company than when alone. Experiments show the same relationship; workers turn out more work in a room with others busy at the same kind of task than they do working in isolation.

Social inhibition has been demonstrated in the same experiments which revealed social facilitation. For while the speed and amount of performance increases in a co-acting group, the quality of performance often goes down. These opposing trends are not illogical if it is remembered that the effect of a co-acting group upon the individual derives, in theory, from an increase in motivation. Gross motor responses profit from the whip, but accurate discrimination and thought are disrupted. It is for this reason that in tasks calling for thought the solitary performance of an individual is often better than his performance in a group.

Social inhibition may occur even in activities where facilitation is the rule if the individual happens to be particularly susceptible to emotional excitement or the competition is particularly intense. In one experiment fourteen out of fifteen normal subjects wrote more in the presence of co-workers than alone. But in another experiment eight out of ten stammerers—stammering is known to be caused in part by emotionality in social situations—produced more written material in isolation.

Crowds and Mobs

The most striking instances of the influences of assembled groups upon the individual are to be observed in crowd and mob behavior. Indeed, so different is the action of persons in mobs from their ordinary behavior that some early writers felt impelled to invoke a 'group mind' which presumably took over in an active crowd to bend the individual to its wishes. Such a notion is quite unacceptable as an explanation since minds pertain to individuals. It is also quite unnecessary.

A *crowd* may be said to come into being whenever an assembled group of people is attracted to a common focus of attention and shares similar emotions. They may be a group of curious and fearful spectators of a fire, or sympathetic onlookers at an accident or excited fans at a sports contest. If the common emotion is intense, especially if it is anger, and if concerted action eventuates, the crowd has turned into a *mob*.

We may now turn our attention to a consideration of some of the factors which seem to be instrumental in the development of mob action, drawing illustrations, when they are needed, from the formation of a lynching mob in the South.

(1) *Background factors.* Mob outbreaks are most likely to occur in areas where there exist long-standing frustrations, which create *general susceptibility* to mob action in pent-up hostility and *specific susceptibility* in antagonisms toward particular groups. Laying the background for lynching mobs, the depressed socio-economic conditions of the South have produced many potential white mob members, all with the generalized hostility of frustrated men and common antagonisms toward employers and possible Negro competitors.

(2) *Precipitating factors.* In such a situation some incident occurs. Let us say a Negro is presumed to have attacked a white woman. This incident generates a crowd by focalizing attention and initiating common emotions. People, stirred by the rumor, gather where talk of the matter is go-

ing on. Immediately, there is intensification of emotion, which is the most significant factor in changing a crowd into a mob. Crowd excitement increases in the milling or muttering stage, primarily through the process of social facilitation. The sights and sounds of others expressing similar emotions serve to heighten the feelings and demonstrativeness of the individual. His increased expressiveness intensifies the feelings of others. Thus there is a circular working up of anger from indignation to fury.

Strong emotion, as we have seen, inhibits critical thought and makes the individual highly suggestible. This suggestibility underlies the next stage of mob development, which is *directed action.* The infuriated group, probably with the most suggestible acting first, plunges into concerted action, if the course is obvious, or if a leader arises to voice the sentiment of the crowd by shouting "Break into the jail!" or "Get a rail and batter in the door!"

(3) *Reinforcing factors.* Primarily because it short-circuits critical thought, mob action usually produces psychological effects which reinforce the participants. Suppose you get caught, psychologically as well as physically, in a mob. What happens to you? First, you feel a *sense of universality.* Coursing along with the group, you are elated because you 'know' that everyone is with you in what you are doing. Second, you have the *sense of righteousness.* High-sounding rationalizations you hear and repeat with satisfaction. "Southern womanhood must be protected." "The Negro must learn to keep his place." With so many people sure, how could you be wrong? Third, you have a *sense of power* or righteous might. You know what to do, why you should do it, how it should be done and that you can do it. There is nothing left to stop you. Yet, if more reinforcement were needed, there is in addition your *sense of anonymity* and your consequent invulnerability to reprisals. "How could so many be punished?" you might ask yourself, thus becoming confident of immunity.

There is no need to invoke a mysterious group mind to understand why people will commit acts of violence in a mob which they would not dream of doing singly. The violence, the suggestibility and the inflexibility of mobs all derive from the extraordinary intensity of emotion which energizes action and inhibits both reason and conscience.

THE INDIVIDUAL IN RELATION TO THE DISPERSED GROUP

We come now to the individual's relation to the dispersed group—the questions of how and why he identifies himself with so invisible a being and just what he thinks this invisible group is like. A dispersed group may not seem the same to two men both of whom are loyal to it or antagonistic to it.

Group Attachment

The cement which binds spatially separate individuals into group membership flows from motivational and emotional conditions. Appreciation of common interests yields an intellectual sense of membership. Then the emotional process of identification can supervene to develop feelings of solidarity and loyalty. Particularly when the group members occasionally come together physically and there is some degree of formal organization, interested persons tend to identify themselves with the group leaders, the group symbols and the group values. Thus they become loyal Americans, Democrats, Rotarians or Presbyterians. Assembly of a part of a dispersed group is not essential for group identification, but it is an aid. A Presbyterian in Tibet may be less faithful than in Scotland. The faith of a Rotarian may weaken in Antarctica. Yet any of these persons can maintain a sense of group membership without a congregation. The Roman in conquered provinces never lost his sense of identity with Rome, nor did the British public servant of the Victorian empire ever forget he was British. He—the story has it—dressed for dinner in the remote provinces of India or in the wastes of the Sudan.

Perhaps the most significant expression of group identification today is *nationalism* —the identification of the individual with the national group or state. This kind of identification has the advantage of allowing the individual to share the prestige and power of the largest group of which he can claim to be a member. Especially do frustrated persons need the vicarious sense of greatness and achievement that can come from nationalistic identification. It has been remarked that the fiercest nationalism is found in the countries where the peoples' lives have been most hopeless and thwarted.

Nationalistic identification is also gratifying because it provides an opportunity for venting frustration-born hostility on the outgroups. The *ingroup* is the group with which you identify yourself. The other groups outside the boundaries or barriers of the ingroups are *outgroups*. The structuring of society into groups creates this social cleavage. The more closely its members identify themselves with their ingroup, the more they separate themselves from the outgroups which the formation of the ingroup has created. That is why an intense nationalism can be fierce. It directs hatred at those who are not of your kind, those who are not identified with your group. Hatred is satisfying, and frustrated people need it. The prerequisite for forming "one world" is not the abolition of hatred but its redirection against the true enemies of all mankind—want, fear, ignorance and disease.

Group Conception

The individual's conception of a dispersed group may be fairly well specified and it is generally much simpler than the reality which it represents. The individual never sees his total ingroup, and his outgroups may be so remote from him that he has no direct acquaintance with their members. Here is the situation in which ignorance and ego involvement favor the formation of rigid stereotypes, especially concerning outgroups. So it is that the white American picks up oversimplified, undiscriminating conceptions like "the shiftless Negro," "the sly Oriental," "the terrible Turk," and lets them serve him as outgroup representatives.

Ingroup stereotypes are more favorable to the insiders. No man identifies himself with what he disparages nor disparages what he has identified himself with. The Nazis accepted for themselves the Aryan stereotype of the blond Viking, thus affording an opportunity to those in their outgroups to retaliate by phrasing the lampoon, "as blond as Hitler, as tall as Goebbels and as slim as Goering."

LEADERSHIP

Leadership can arise in an individual's relation to either an assembled group or a dispersed group, but the requirements are different in the two cases. The leader of an infantry squad, as well as the chairman of a board of directors, are in a face-to-face relation with their groups. They can use simple emotional appeals, discussion and argument, peremptory demand or any of the subtler devices whereby the egos of the group members are moved toward identification with the leader. The president of a great institution, on the other hand, has a dispersed group to lead. He, too, through tactful propaganda, may appeal to the emotions of his group, but in general his procedure is more intellectualized. He attempts to get his group members to identify themselves with the institution, not with him. The boss of a political machine is intermediate between the squad leader and the president. His group is somewhat dispersed, but he deals face-to-face with many individuals and trusts them to spread the word about him to the others.

Leadership is a relation of an individual to a group, established in the interests of achieving some end. There are so many kinds of groups, and of ends, and of ways of achieving the same end and of securing the loyalty of the same group that the problem has turned out to be a sheaf of problems.

This much, however, can we say. The physical and personality characteristics of leaders may vary greatly from successful leader to successful leader, yet their successes seem to hinge upon two necessary conditions.

The first is that they possess *membership character* in the group they are undertaking to lead, that is to say, they must share the values, attitudes and interests of the group. This psychological similarity is necessary for the identification of the followers with the leader. Politicians know this fact well. When they run a candidate for office in a particular district, they make every effort to get a man with whom the district can readily identify itself. It is no accident that the late Governor Talmadge of Georgia appeared in red 'galluses' and shirtsleeves when he addressed his backwoods constituents. And no small part of Hitler's success as a leader was due to his reflection of the aspirations and experiences of so many of his countrymen.

The second condition of leadership is that the leader should be *somewhat superior* to the members of the group in the qualities esteemed by them. People are not satisfied to identify themselves with someone who is not greater than they. On the other hand, the superiority must be temperate and not so great or obvious that it destroys the leader's membership character in the group.

RELATIONS BETWEEN GROUPS

With the modern development of society it has become increasingly true that to be effective the individual must often act as a member of a group. Many of the most significant social interactions of today operate in and through group relations—national groups, political groups, social groups, racial or ethnic groups, etc. Two of the important groupings, which have been subjected to recent analysis are *socio-economic interest* groups and *social participation* groups.

Socio-economic Interest Groups

When a national sample of the population was polled as to whether they belonged to the upper, lower, middle or working class, only one per cent answered, "I don't believe in classes," and only one per cent said, "I don't know." So the existence of 'class consciousness' among the American people cannot be denied. The chief division lay between the *working class* with fifty-one per cent of the sample polled and the *middle class* with forty-three per cent. That these two classes exist as more than mere labels is shown by the occupations, and also attitudes and interests, of the respondents. In Fig. 246 it may be observed that members of the middle class come predominantly from business, professional and other white collar occupations, whereas members of the working class come from skilled and unskilled manual occupations.

Consistent with their differences in occupation, the middle class and working class divide in their attitudes. If opinions upon social, political and economic issues are classified as *radical* when desire for change is expressed, and *conservative* when adherence to the status quo is preferred, those who put themselves in the working class are, on the average, more radical than those who put themselves in the middle class. This result is graphed in Fig. 247 for a battery of six issues presented to a national sample.

The existence of class opposition in socio-economic interests makes plain the necessity of adjusting and compromising such differences before the classes pull widely apart. If the opposition increases, violent class struggle and revolutionary upheavals may be the result.

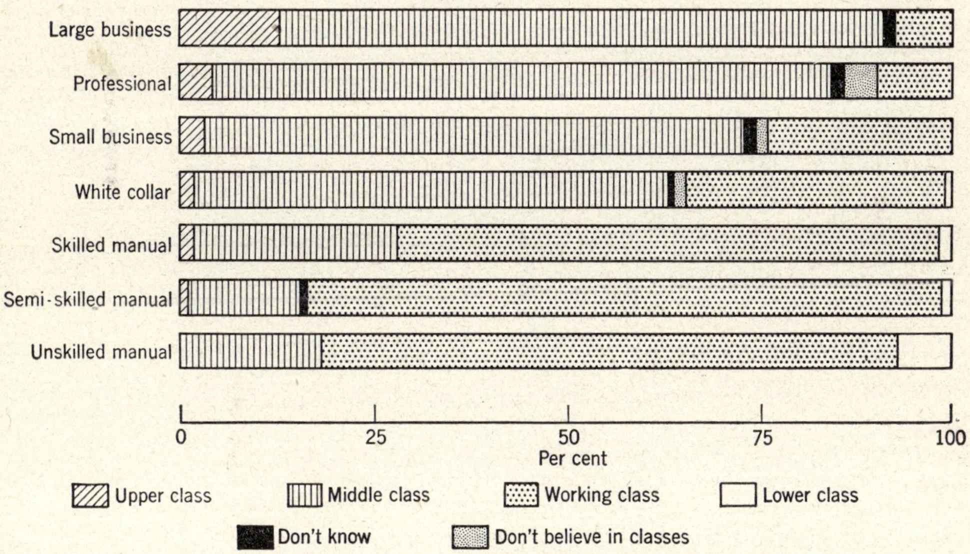

FIGURE 246. CLASS IDENTIFICATIONS OF OCCUPATIONAL STRATA

For simplicity rural groups have been eliminated from the above results. Otherwise they are based upon a national sample. [Adapted from R. T. Centers, *Psychological aspects of socio-economic stratification: an inquiry into the nature of class,* Princeton University Press, 1948; by permission.]

Social Participation Groups

A social participation group, in the sense of the present paragraph, is a class of people who associate together even to the extent of intermarriage and regard themselves, and are regarded by others, as similar in social status. Investigation has shown that there are three such main groups: the *upper class,* the *middle class* and the *lower class.* It is useful to subdivide each of these classes, as for example upper and lower middle class, to form a total of six groups. Some *social mobility* is possible among these classes, for individuals can, by their actions and achievements, raise or lower their class status.

In the study of participation classes in the South, the additional concept of *caste* has arisen. The Negro is of lower caste than the white in the sense that he cannot marry into the white group.

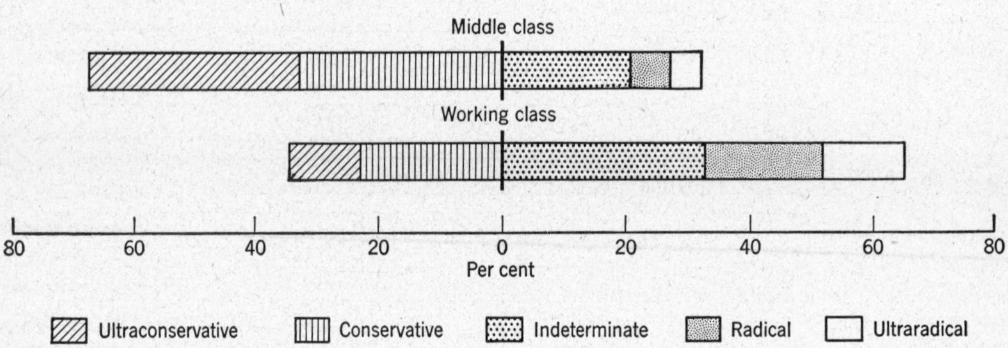

FIGURE 247. CLASS DIFFERENCES IN CONSERVATISM-RADICALISM

These results are based upon the responses of a national sample to six socio-economic issues. [Adapted from R. T. Centers, *Psychological aspects of socio-economic stratification: an inquiry into the nature of class,* Princeton University Press, 1948; by permission.]

A revealing chart of the relationship between caste and class in the South is reproduced in Fig. 248. The caste line separates the white and Negro groups; the dotted lines show the three general classes in each caste. The double-headed arrows represent the mobility which is socially acceptable between classes, but not between castes.

The most interesting feature of the diagram lies in the tilt of the caste line. At an earlier period this division was horizontal—the white man's floor was the Negro's ceiling. But the development of class strata in the Negro group since the days of slavery has gradually pushed the top Negro class above the lowest white class in wealth and the other desiderata of class status. The upper Negro class in the South is now in the anomalous and conflict-ridden position of being superior to many whites in class, but inferior in caste. When such Negroes engage in a social interaction with a low-class white, they can never be certain whether they will receive deferential treatment based upon class lines or arrogant treatment based on caste. The hypothesis has been advanced that the disproportionate amount of emotional instability in the upper-class Negro group is due to this objective instability in the social situation in which they live.

The conception of two parallel civilizations as the solution of the Negro problem envisions a time when the caste line shall have rotated to the vertical position *d–e.* The "two civilizations" would then be "separate but equal."

We turn next to the basic problem of relations between groups, the problem of social conflict which is rooted in social prejudice.

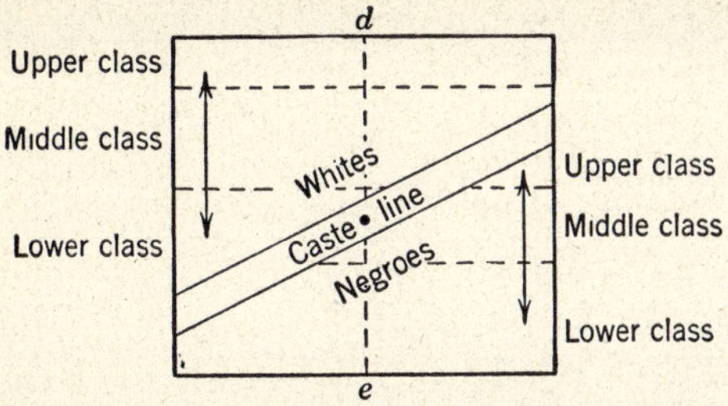

FIGURE 248. THE RELATION BETWEEN CASTE AND CLASS IN THE DEEP SOUTH

Relative class levels shown for each caste. The arrows represent the range of socially acceptable mobility between classes in each caste. Area roughly indicates numbers of persons. The caste line, once horizontal, is now tilted. If the castes were to form two parallel civilizations, the caste line would become vertical at *d–e*. This diagram does not portray quantitative relations. [Adapted from W. L. Warner, in A. Davis, B. B. Gardner and M. R. Gardner, *Deep South, a social anthropological study of caste and class,* Chicago University Press, 1941.]

SOCIAL PREJUDICE

With some understanding of the social relations between individuals and groups we can now push ahead into the difficult area of social conflict. Disputes today involve a much larger area and a greater population than formerly. Once they were nearly individual and settled with clubs or spears. Now that the individuals are identified with groups, the groups fight with total war and atomic techniques. The ultimate cost to civilization is incalculable. Some wise men and women think that the continuity of civilization itself is threatened by its own achievements. Fortunately this book does not have to provide an answer to that question.

Nevertheless it behooves not only the psychologist, but also all men who would be wise, to gain understanding of the nature of social conflict and of the never-ending war between the ingroup and the outgroup, for that is the pattern of every war. Why do men fight? Why do they contend? They contend with each other in order to defend and enlarge their egos. They fight because that is nature's rude technique for remedying frustration. Presumably they may stop fighting when education and emotional maturity of the two or three billion people who will probably then be occupying the five continents is sufficient to make it clear to all that mutual destruction does not pay in the long run. We advance in that direction when we seek to understand the nature of conflict.

Conflict is fundamentally psychological. Its tools are physical, but its origin and sustaining force lie in human hostility, in the opposition between ingroup and outgroup. The power to change such discord to concord among groups lies largely in whatever understanding and control can be won over the working of *prejudice,* for it is from the fires of prejudice that most human conflicts derive. It will serve us well, therefore, to scrutinize exhaustively prejudice as a primary threat to peace.

Nature of Prejudice

Fundamentally prejudices have their basis in preferences, the simple judgments of pleasantness and unpleasantness that everyone makes so easily. Such judgments are not rational. They depend upon the basic needs of the organism and upon learned needs. A person does not know why he dislikes yellow and prefers red, yet he may find that he cannot change his likes by any simple act of 'will' and that his preferences remain constant until he has some very unpleasant experience with red or some very great pleasure from yellow. Then, by conditioning, his preferences may be altered.

Literally *prejudice* means *prejudgment.* All individual action and choice is prejudged. It is prejudged in the constitution of the genes, insofar as heredity contributes to choice. It is prejudged in past experience insofar as conditioning affects preference. Prejudice is *need* and *set,* and basically it is irrational. Only a small part of human behavior has rational processes as its immediate antecedents, and these antecedents themselves have antecedents, being at the end of a chain of events that begins with the needs. In this sense all human action is prejudiced by what the organism is—by what every human organism is and also by what each particular organism has become.

There is, however, a *practical* problem of prejudice, which leads to a limiting definition of the word. Some of your learned needs and sets, some of your habits of thought and action are good, forming part of the behavior repertoire of the well-adjusted man and the good citizen. But you may have other sets and habits which need altering for your own good. They are 'irrational' in the sense that adhering to them works to your own disadvantage in the long run. Perhaps indulging them at the moment is pleasant, but in the long run they may make you lose friends and gain enemies or create trouble for you in some other way. You 'ought' to change them, that is to say, it would be best for you if you did change them. We shall not go far wrong if we limit the use of the word *prejudice* to those sets and preferences which 'ought' to be changed, which, if changed, would be of advantage to the individual or his ingroup or presumably both.

The assumption of the remainder of this chapter is that the extreme dislike of outgroups is a mark of immaturity in the ingroup and not to the advantage of the ingroup's members. It seems quite clear that tolerant understanding is the best mutual relation between groups, that social conflict, because it arouses emotion, tends to shut off the wise insight which might lead to the solution of the problem that caused the conflict. Nor shall we go far wrong if we lay down the rule that, whenever we hear that what the outgroup wants is bad and what the ingroup wants is good, we are facing an instance of prejudice, a set which could with advantage be changed.

Origin of Prejudice

In the early days of social psychology, when it was customary to invent 'instincts' to explain social behavior, many psychologists believed that prejudices were instinctive. They thought of race prejudice as a consequence of innate "consciousness of kind" associated with an instinctive "dislike of the unlike." Only a few of the considerations need be cited to show why this historically important but short-sighted theory could not persist.

(1) There is no evidence of race prejudice in very young children. On the contrary, as a classic study in a Tennessee community revealed, white and Negro children play together until forbidden to do so, and some continue to do so even after repeated punishment. A recent investigation found that not until the school years do prejudices begin to develop in any number. The average of remembered onset for cases of Negro prejudice in whites was 12.6 years, of Jewish prejudice in gentiles, 13.7 years.

(2) The visibility of differences between groups seems to be more an *effect* of prejudice than a cause. Anti-Semitism occurs even where, in large numbers of cases, Jews cannot be distinguished from non-

Jews. In such instances prejudice has had to create visibility through such means as requiring the Jews to wear distinctive garments or yellow badges.

Even where natural differences do exist between two groups, preexisting prejudice seems necessary to insure attention to them. Visibility depends upon learning. When racial differences mean little, they go unremarked. There is a story of six-year-old Tommy who asked his mother if he might bring his friend Sammy home to lunch. His mother, knowing that Tommy attended a 'mixed' school, asked if Sammy were white or colored. "I don't know," said Tommy, "but I'll look next time I see him and tell you."

A recent experiment supports the view that visibility depends on prejudice. Subjects were asked to judge which photographs of twenty presented were Jewish and which non-Jewish. It was found that the subjects who disliked Jews were both more 'suspicious' (judged more faces to be Jewish) and more accurate (better able to distinguish Jewish from non-Jewish faces). The unprejudiced were less sensitive to the ethnic affiliation of those whom they judged. That is natural. In perception you see what you use. Perception exists because it is useful to the organism.

(3) If anti-Negro prejudice were universal among whites, it might be regarded as associated with the white gene, and then it surely would be called 'instinctive.' But the prejudice is not universal. There is little, for example, in Brazil.

(4) Dislike-of-the-unlike cannot be an 'instinct.' Too many people desire new experiences. In some groups the foreign and the bizarre are welcomed. Strange people and things are liked when they enlarge the ego, disliked when their novelty threatens security.

(5) Finally, we may note that two professional musicians of different races have more 'consciousness of kind' than you could expect to find between either of them and, say, a peddler of the same race.

Since prejudice is not innate, the question arises as to what kind of experiences produce prejudices. Are the key experiences generally direct personal contacts with the members of minority groups? Certainly they may be. An intensely unpleasant episode with a Negro can leave a lasting antagonism to all Negroes. In general, however, the conclusion has been that the attitudes of whites toward Negroes are chiefly determined "not by contact with Negroes, but by contact with the prevalent attitude toward Negroes."

It is the culture that provides us with these many ready-made prejudices. It is true that some of them have sprung from experiences, but most of them are derived from second-hand experiences which have been passed on by the many who have used them. This fact has been brought into focus through the studies of what is called *social distance*. In these studies persons were asked to check the degree of intimacy with which they would be willing to admit members of various groups to association with themselves. In an early inquiry it was found that students showed the greatest prejudice toward the Turks, though most of them had never even seen a Turk. It developed, upon analysis, that the prejudices stemmed from the second-hand acceptance of traditions and current opinions.

The results of a study of racial preferences in 1939 are shown in Table XXXIX. The steps in the scale are listed at the top of the table. The general pattern of liking Canadians and English best (after Americans) and preferring Turks and Hindus

TABLE XXXIX

AVERAGE TOLERANCE OF PRINCETON STUDENTS TOWARD ETHNIC GROUPS AS MEASURED BY A SCALE OF SOCIAL DISTANCE

The Japanese are lower here than in earlier studies of social distance. The drop is due to the antagonism that was developing toward their foreign policy. These data are for 1939.

The scale runs as follows:

1. Would exclude from my country.
2. As visitors only to my country.
3. To citizenship in my country.
4. To employment in any occupation in any country.
5. To my school as classmates.
6. To my street as neighbors.
7. To my club as personal chums.
8. To close kinship by marriage.

[After E. L. Hartley, *Problems in prejudice*, Kings Crown Press, 1946.]

Nationality	Median tolerance	Nationality	Median tolerance
American	8.0	Russian	3.3
Canadian	8.0	Latvian	3.3
English	8.0	Polish	3.2
Irish	7.5	Portuguese	3.2
Swedish	7.3	Negro	3.1
Swiss	7.3	Lithuanian	3.0
German	6.8	Greek	2.9
French	6.6	Filipino	2.8
Danish	6.5	Arab	2.8
Austrian	6.4	Wallonian	2.8
Finn	5.9	Mexican	2.7
French Canadian	5.9	Chinese	2.7
American Indian	5.3	Turk	2.7
Argentine	5.1	Hindu	2.6
Czechoslovak	4.5	Danirean	2.6
Hungarian	4.0	Pirenean	2.4
Italian	3.6	Japanese	2.3
Rumanian	3.5		

least is almost an American custom. In 1928 a definitive survey of the country revealed this hierarchy, which has been verified ever since. A study of seven colleges from Florida to Washington produced coefficients of correlations among these rankings varying from +0.84 to +0.99. School children in St. Louis gave similar results. Among them the preferences were similar for Jews, Catholics and Protestants, for rural and urban children, for Negro and white children and for children of different economic levels.

The one limitation to the overall constancy in such a series is that members of minority groups who rank low in the hierarchy accept the pattern with the single modification that they place their own group at the top.

Such a national uniformity of ethnic preference, covering as it does a great diversity of individuals, makes the conclusion inescapable that personal experience plays at most a minor role in initiating race prejudice. Such prejudices come as part of the social heritage which the new recruits to society absorb from early childhood. Children, eager to be adults, emulate the prejudiced attitudes and discriminatory behaviors of their parents. Like conscience, these prejudices follow the parent pattern and are not easily changed.

Now what about the Pireneans, Danireans and Wallonians who are ranked low in Table XXXIX, along with the Turks and Hindus? These are entirely fictitious groups. Most of the subjects, however, evaluated them with the other groups, putting them at the bottom of their preference rankings. This apparent trick is in reality a significant finding. First, it shows that racial evaluations are prejudicial and not judicial, except insofar as complete ignorance about a man is a reason for disliking him. Second, it shows how uncritical is the absorption and how undiscriminating the application of these stereotyped racial attitudes. Third, it indicates how prejudice goes hand in hand with ignorance. There is a large measure of truth in the homely dictum, "Prejudice is being down on what you are not up on." On the other hand, it may be said that it is no great achievement on the part of the culture to make people feel a distaste for what is strange. Safety first and action second is the rule of survival. Conservatism is the first way of playing safe. Cultivating the novel comes under the rule of 'nothing ventured, nothing won.' If perceptions were not stereotypes—for that is what the principle of object constancy means (p. 231) —the organism would fail. The point here is that, although the fear of what is strange may be sound basic policy for the organism, social progress, nevertheless, lies along the path of liking what is novel.

One further point needs to be made. Though the reality is otherwise, most people *believe* that their prejudices flow from personal experiences. The explanation of this widespread discrepancy between belief and reality lies principally in the fact that adults do not remember how they learned their attitudes from their parents and the further fact that prejudice, since it is an ego defense, is itself preserved by a largely unconscious process of rationalization.

Motivations for Prejudice

A prejudice like race prejudice is likely to be ever so much more strongly held than a simple like or dislike as, for instance, the prejudice for tea instead of coffee. It is plain that such a strong prejudice is reinforced. All motives work because they promise gain to the organism—now or in the past when the habit was formed. Even conscience has this history. What then, we may ask, are the more important kinds of reinforcement which make a person dislike or hate the members of outgroups in these cases of 'race' prejudice?

There are three large advantages which 'race' prejudices seem to offer to some of those who have them. They are (1) *economic gain,* (2) *gain in status* and (3) *outlet for hostility*. All three are related, but we may consider them in order.

(1) *Economic gain.* It is a commonplace that ours is a competitive acquisitive society where often one man's success is predicated upon another man's failure. Playing the economic game by such rules puts a premium, of course, upon anything which gives an advantage in the struggle. And race prejudice definitely offers economic advantage to some members of the superior

group and may seem to offer advantages to all.

The economic motive for the dispossession of Jews in Nazi Germany was never far beneath the surface. Long before the Nazis took over the government they had promised their followers the jobs held by the Jews. By widening the term *Jew* to apply to anyone who could not prove pure 'Aryan' ancestry as far back as January 1, 1800, they greatly increased their gains. Later, as the necessity for subtlety disappeared, the Nazis began to expropriate all Jewish belongings.

The close dependence of group prejudice upon economic factors is also well illustrated by the manner in which group antagonisms fluctuate with changes in economic conditions. When the Chinese, as one study revealed, first came to the Pacific Coast, there was great need for their labor. During this era they were described as orderly, industrious, thrifty, adaptable, inoffensive and law abiding. Then came white competition for the jobs which the Chinese had. Soon they were being said to be clannish, servile, deceitful, vicious and generally undesirable. Prejudice appeared when there was work for it to do.

The same kind of revealing about-face occurred during the Second World War in connection with the Japanese evacuees at Poston, Arizona. When the ranchers of a near-by valley found that they needed evacuee help to harvest their cotton, there was in the space of a few weeks a remarkable shift of opinion. Whereas previously all evacuees had been regarded as treacherous enemies, now they were hailed as hard-working and cooperative Americans of Japanese ancestry. And, as the reporter dryly remarked, when the cotton picking was halted by military order, the drift back to former prejudices was equally noticeable.

(2) *Gain in social status.* Along with the economic competition in American society goes a struggle for social status. The two are related, for each helps the other. Still they can be distinguished. All of us have a desire for superiority and social recognition. All of us are pleased to look down upon those who seem to be beneath us in social status or who act as if they were.

For persons at the upper levels of the socio-economic hierarchy there are many people to whom they can feel superior. On the other hand, those at the bottom are hard put to gratify their desire for recognition and superiority. Their need for ego enhancement is, moreover, whipped up by the fact that there are so many others to whom they must defer. For the poor southern whites, who need inferiors, it is no trick at all to discover that the Negro exactly fits the role. So prejudice is reinforced by an undeniable gain in status.

There is the story about a little southern white girl who was found weeping bitterly over the news that the Negroes in that area were all departing for the North. Asked why she was crying over the Negroes' departure, she answered, "When all of them leave, we won't have nobody to be better than."

(3) *Outlet for hostility.* Frustration begets aggression—not always but usually (p. 513). When you see the sequence working it is almost as if they were parts of the same mechanism, as if frustration were a need and aggression were its satisfaction. At any rate, aggressive action does relieve frustration, and from that fact spring many social phenomena. There are two further facts about aggression that become important here.

In the first place, we must note that aggression may be *latent*. The need for it persists when it has no opportunity to exercise itself. The frustration may come and go, but the need for aggression persists and is reinforced if the same frustration recurs soon enough. Any man whom you see on the street has in him a great deal of bottled-up aggression which he would vent quickly were the object of his aggression to appear and were all restraint to be removed.

The other fact is that aggression may be *displaced*. Your needs do not require you to work off your aggression on the person or persons for whom it was intended. You can let go at someone else and very often you do (see Compensation, p. 517).

When the little boy who cannot go out fishing because of the downpour pulls his sister's hair and gives his hound a rough time, he is storing up and displacing aggression. The worker who, tongue-lashed by his boss, comes home and beats his wife is illustrating the same principle. Elaborate experimental evidence is not lacking.

Displacement is a failure of specification, a case of generalization in learning. Two rats were trained in aggression, trained to strike at each other on receiving a mild shock. A doll placed in the enclosure was ignored as long as two rats could strike each other; but, when one was removed and the shock administered, the other rat would strike the doll.

It is through displacement that *scapegoating* comes about. Vulnerable outgroups are scapegoated for the thwarting difficulties of the ingroup. When the price of cotton falls in the South, the number of Negro lynchings goes up. The process is bereft of logic—the Negro could hardly be even remotely the cause of the price of cotton—but it is psychologic. The scapegoater is seeking tension reduction, not justice. Unfortunately he does not know it.

Rationalizations about Prejudice

Persons are rationalizing when, instead of stating the actual motives for their attitudes or actions, they offer 'good' reasons. Rationalization is a reversal of the logical process of generating belief from evidence. Instead the belief generates evidence. It is a process not of verification, but of justification. Ordinarily people who are rationalizing do not know it (pp. 518 f.).

Rationalizations abound in the area of prejudice. The reason is not difficult to find. The more rigid prejudices, we have seen, involve the absorption of social traditions. Unfavorable stereotypes are uncritically taken over, particularly in childhood when critical abilities are meager and dependence upon parental instruction is great. Parental injunctions, regardless of supporting evidence, are accepted as beliefs. But, as children grow to be adults, developing their critical abilities, discomfort arises. We have learned that our judgments should follow from evidence for that is the method of reason and science, and these traditions are valued highly in our culture. This difficulty can, however, be resolved through rationalization. People find what they call 'good' reasons for their antagonisms.

Not only ideas but experiences can be found to fortify preconceived beliefs. Any anti-Semite can recount the time that he was tricked by a Jewish merchant. What he fails to remember are the times that he was treated fairly or with generosity. He may call the generosity "unctuous insincerity." If you project the prejudice into the issue, you will not see it in yourself.

That preconceived likes and dislikes can go far in influencing observations has been demonstrated in an experiment. The experimenter first ascertained in a classroom which children were almost universally liked, and which generally disliked. She then had subjects from each of these two groups perform calisthenics under her direction in front of the class. She had previously instructed the 'liked' children to make mistakes, the 'disliked' children to follow her signals precisely. After the performance she asked the class to indicate which group had done the exercises correctly. The striking outcome was that the majority of the votes went to the popular group. On the basis of subsequent interviews the experimenter decided that the children actually 'saw' the results they reported, were letting their own perceptions deceive them, in the way that perceptions, working in the interests of their owners, always do.

Since scientific investigation fails in general to support race prejudice, the process of distortion has gone to great lengths in this area in erecting defenses. Let us examine a series of alleged Negro-white racial differences to see how facts and logic can be twisted to provide the 'good' reasons for a prejudice.

(1) *Negroes naturally give off a characteristically unpleasant body odor.* This belief is as dubious as it is widespread. Results of experiments show that there was neither consistent preference for samples of perspiration from the whites nor for samples from Negroes.

(2) *Negro blood is different from the blood of whites.* Biologists have failed to find racial differences in blood.

(3) *Negro legs are different from the legs of whites so that the whites are penalized in athletic competition.* The legs of Negro athletes are longer than the legs of the average white man, but so are the legs of white athletes. The longer heel of the Negro, which is alleged to give him greater leverage in running and jumping, is the result of nothing more than a thick layer of subcutaneous fat.

(4) *The Negro is more apelike than the white.* Both the Negro and the ape have flat noses, but the lips of the ape are like those of the white man. In general body hairiness and in the size of the brow ridge, the white man is much more like the ape than the black man.

(5) *The Negroes are naturally inferior in intelligence to whites.* White children have, on the average, done better upon intelligence tests than Negro children, but the consensus of scientific opinion favors the view that the inferior performance of the Negro is due primarily to inferior environmental opportunities.

There is a certain circularity in the effects of prejudice. Prejudice can feed on what it creates. Hostility toward Jews has driven them into ghettos for self-protection. Then it is claimed that the Jews are seclusive and live by themselves, and prejudice is increased. Hostility toward Negroes has deprived them of educational advantages that are provided for white persons. Then it is claimed that Negroes are stupid, and prejudice against them is increased. It is hostility toward a bright and competent Jew that makes of him an insecure person, who shifts quickly from the self-assertion of competence to the submission of appeasement. Then it is said of him that he is inconsistent and insincere. This is the process that electronic engineers call positive feedback, the process that facilitates itself.

There are many situations in psychology where positive feedback builds up a situation and renders it stable. There are instances of perception and instances of motivation. Prejudice gets stabilized in the same way. There is nothing wrong about stability itself. The organism needs it. The only reason why we wish to get rid of prejudice, why we regret its stability, is that we defined prejudice at the outset as those sets or attitudes which 'ought' to be changed. An *ought* does not, however, mean a psychological difference, and there really are both good prejudices and bad, as those who are prejudiced against prejudice presumably know.

Individual Differences in Prejudice

Common experience shows that people differ in prejudice. Habitually we distinguish between tolerant and intolerant persons. There is not much experimental evidence on this point, but we already know enough about the mechanisms of motivation and personality to understand why these differences should exist.

There are really two reasons for the growth of tolerance, one negative and one positive. Tolerance may be caused by lack of frustration in the personal life or by specific motivation which sets up tolerance as a goal.

(1) Persons who experience many frustrations accumulate a supply of latent aggression. The frustration may be constantly recurring in the same situation, as it often is with the very poor man or can be with the richer ambitious man who is much poorer than his level of aspiration would have him be. Or the frustrations may occur in many different areas. Some people seem to be *frustration-prone,* just as others are accident-prone. It is hard to say why they are, yet it is clear that persons who have set their ambitions high above their abilities would be perpetually refrustrated by having 'bitten off more than they can chew.'

The recurrence of frustration, whether for the same cause or for different ones, builds up a stock of latent aggression. Here again there are individual differences, for some persons are known to have more *frustration tolerance* than others, that is to say, they can accept more frustration without gaining commensurately in latent aggression. Given enough of it, latent aggression comes out when there is an opportunity. Aggression called *latent* is readily displaced; it is 'looking for' a victim. Mobs are formed by frustrated persons with aggression waiting for use. Scapegoating is a common relief for latent aggression. So is that mild form of half-conscious scapegoating called *gossip.* Why is gossip usually more unfavorable to its subject—to its 'victim'? Because it is a means of relieving latent aggression.

Not all prejudice operates in this general way. It may occur within a specific area or between two people only. Divorce cases show how one spouse—perhaps with misdirected hopes and aspirations—can come to be perpetually frustrated by the other until his love has changed to hatred. No professional counselor expects to get an objective account of the unloved spouse from the unloving one. In such a case prejudice is normal, and insight is offered as a partial remedy.

It is obvious that one way to get rid of prejudice is to remove or diminish the frustrations. Sometimes that method works. A man changes to a job at which he is more likely to succeed. People take vacations to dodge the daily round of frustration. It is hoped that the diminution of the frustrations of the working classes by raising the standard of their living will reduce social conflict.

(2) The other way in which tolerance is substituted for prejudice is by *motivation.*

Many people have the insight into the nature of prejudice. They see how wasteful prejudice is and seek to substitute understanding for it. They form groups and associations to promote understanding and get support from their members and from foundations. Nowadays the old-fashioned pacifists have become the international understanders. Such persons accept tolerance as a goal and succeed in avoiding many common prejudices. They usually side with the under-dog in a social conflict because they feel that the top-dog, being on top, must accept responsibility for it. If at times they overcompensate in furthering the equality of status which must precede mutual understanding, they are being human and illustrating a common mechanism of motivation.

In the individual, tolerance accompanies emotional maturity. Not all physiologically mature persons are, however, emotionally mature. Many old people are embittered by frustration. The Second World War showed us how much latent aggression can issue suddenly from men in their thirties, forties and fifties who have come suddenly to power. Yet, for all this, there is a psychological and emotional maturity which makes for tolerance and understanding; and some young men are further along in this development than others of their age. These people believe in tolerance and are against prejudice. They believe in insight into themselves, and by constant self-criticism and psychological learning they achieve a fair amount of self-understanding. They are shamed by their own prejudices, when they find them, and try to eliminate them. Being unprejudiced is not always simple for them, for often they lack the wisdom or the evidence which is necessary for a decision between conflicting prejudices. The point is, however, that there are these individual differences in motivation and that motivation is not impotent in the operation of rooting out personal intolerance.

Elimination of Prejudice

Have we hope of getting rid of those social prejudices which are known to hinder social progress by producing social conflict? A positive answer to that question would consist of a practicable program of social engineering. Many men could formulate a program, but each would have his own. Most of the factors to be considered and changed would not be psychological. Getting frustration reduced involves sociology, economics and government—all the social sciences. It involves engineering and agriculture too—getting cheap houses and plenty of food—and is plainly not a topic for consideration in this book, even if it could be reduced to a statement of facts.

The chief psychological factors that can be used for the elimination of conflict-producing prejudice have been stated in the preceding section. *Reduce frustration. Promote the understanding of outgroups.* To these rules the psychologist has no other magic to add.

Social science can supplement psychology if it can find ways to reduce the economic gain and the gain in personal status, which are supported by the maintenance of group prejudice. Education can be aimed directly at the increase of social tolerance and also at the acceptance of that social engineering which bids fair to reduce group conflict. The present situation in the United States is by no means hopeless, and it is fortunate that the social entrepreneurs are angry about the status quo and are trying vehemently to change it. Their prejudice against prejudice shows us that not all prejudice is to be condemned, even though it may seem better to find another word than *prejudice* for the personal drive which makes some men devote their lives to striving for the greatest good to the greatest number.

REFERENCES

1. Benedict, R. *Race: science and politics.* New York: Viking Press, 1945.

   A compact treatment of the problems of defining and classifying races, and of the nature and history of race prejudice.

2. Cantril, H. *The psychology of social movements.* New York: Wiley, 1938.

   A very readable psychological analysis of some of the more significant contemporary social movements.

3. Centers, R. T. *Psychological aspects of socio-economic stratification: an inquiry into the nature of class.* Princeton, N. J.: Princeton University Press, 1948.

   A detailed public opinion study directed toward the analysis of status and class relationships in American life.

4. Davis, A., Gardner, B. B., and Gardner, M. R. *Deep South. A social anthropological study of caste and class.* Chicago: Chicago University Press, 1941.

   A revealing application of the methods of anthropology to the study of a segment of our own American culture.

5. Freeman, E. *Social psychology.* New York: Holt, 1936.

   A critical exposition of social psychology with special emphasis upon the analysis of conventional social values.

6. Graeber, I., and Britt, S. H. (Eds.). *Jews in a gentile world.* New York: Macmillan, 1942.

   A series of searching essays by outstanding authorities upon the biological, sociological, psychological and economic aspects of anti-Semitism.

7. Hartley, E. L. *Problems in prejudice.* New York: Kings Crown Press, 1946.

   An informative presentation and discussion of a series of large-scale studies in prejudice.

8. Katz, D., and Schanck, R. L. *Social psychology.* New York: Wiley, 1938.

   A systematic and thoroughly documented textbook of social psychology with careful and precise handling of basic concepts.

9. Klineberg, O. *Social psychology.* New York: Holt, 1940.

   An illuminating comparative treatment of social psychology from the perspective of social anthropology.

10. Miller, N. E., and Dollard, J. *Social learning and imitation.* New Haven: Yale University Press, 1941.

    A fresh and closely reasoned analysis of learning in social situations and the problem of imitation.

11. Montague, M. F. A. *Man's most dangerous myth: the fallacy of race.* (2nd ed.) New York: Columbia University Press, 1945.

    A critical analysis of the concept of race and its dangerous implications in group life.

12. Warner, W. L., Havighurst, R. J., and Loeb, M. B. *Who shall be educated?* New York: Harper, 1944.

    A brief discussion of the status system in American culture and its implications for educational policy.

INDEX

Names. The full names with dates of birth and death are given for a few of the very important psychologists whose names are cited. After any names, abbreviated terms have these meanings: "auth." = contribution to this book as collaborator; "bk." = a book or contribution to a book, cited in the book lists at the ends of the chapters; "ref." = a reference to the literature occurring usually in a legend to a figure or table; "inc." = the mention is incidental and of minor importance.